Ambulatory Anesthesia and Perioperative Analgesia

Notice

Medicine is an ever-changing science. As new research and clinical experience broaden our knowledge, changes in treatment and drug therapy are required. The authors and the publisher of this work have checked with sources believed to be reliable in their efforts to provide information that is complete and generally in accord with the standards accepted at the time of publication. However, in view of the possibility of human error or changes in medical sciences, neither the authors nor the publisher nor any other party who has been involved in the preparation or publication of this work warrants that the information contained herein is in every respect accurate or complete, and they disclaim all responsibility for any errors or omissions or for the results obtained from use of the information contained in this work. Readers are encouraged to confirm the information contained herein with other sources. For example and in particular, readers are advised to check the product information sheet included in the package of each drug they plan to administer to be certain that the information contained in this work is accurate and that changes have not been made in the recommended dose or in the contraindications for administration. This recommendation is of particular importance in connection with new or infrequently used drugs.

Ambulatory Anesthesia and Perioperative Analgesia

Susan M. Steele, MD

Associate Professor
Department of Anesthesiology
Chief, Division of Ambulatory Anesthesiology
Medical Director, Ambulatory Surgery Center
Duke University Medical Center
Durham, North Carolina

Karen C. Nielsen, MD

Assistant Professor
Department of Anesthesiology
Division of Ambulatory Anesthesiology
Duke University Medical Center
Durham, North Carolina

Stephen M. Klein, MD

Assistant Professor
Department of Anesthesiology
Division of Ambulatory Anesthesiology
Duke University Medical Center
Durham, North Carolina

McGraw-Hill

Medical Publishing Division

New York   Chicago   San Francisco   Lisbon   London   Madrid
Mexico City   Milan   New Delhi   San Juan   Seoul   Singapore   Sydney   Toronto

Ambulatory Anesthesia and Perioperative Analgesia

Copyright © 2005 by The McGraw-Hill Companies, Inc. All rights reserved. Printed in the United States of America. Except as permitted under the United States Copyright Act of 1976, no part of this publication may be reproduced or distributed in any form or by any means, or stored in a data base or retrieval system, without the prior written permission of the publisher.

1 2 3 4 5 6 7 8 9 0   KPT/KPT   0 9 8 7 6 5 4

ISBN: 0-07-141240-9

This book was set in Berkeley by Westchester Book Group.
The editors were James Shanahan and Michelle Watt.
The production supervisor was Rick Ruzycka.
Project management was provided by Westchester Book Group.
The cover designer was Pehrsson Design.
The indexer was Sandi Schroeder.
Quebecor Kingsport was printer and binder.

This book is printed on acid-free paper.

Library of Congress Cataloging-in-Publication Data

Ambulatory anesthesia & perioperative analgesia / edited by Susan M. Steele,
   Karen C. Nielsen, Stephen M. Klein.
      p. ; cm.
   Includes bibliographical references and index.
   ISBN 0-07-141240-9
   1. Anesthesia—Handbooks, manuals, etc.   2. Ambulatory surgery—Handbooks, manuals,
etc.   3. Postoperative care—Handbooks, manuals, etc.   I. Title: Ambulatory anesthesia and
perioperative analgesia.   II. Steele, Susan M.   III. Nielsen, Karen, M.D.   IV. Klein,
Stephen, M.D.
      [DNLM: 1. Anesthesia—methods.   2. Ambulatory Care—methods.   3. Perioperative
Care—methods.   WO 200 A4978 2005]
   RD82.A654   2005
   617.9'6—dc22   2004045913

About the cover: A sculpture from Auguste Rodin, *Walking Man* (*L'homme qui marche*), c. 1900.

To our teachers and mentors,
thank you for your endless support and guidance. For the gift of your wisdom
and devotion to patient care we will be forever grateful.

To our colleagues and students,
thank you for your inspiration. Continue the legacy with innovation and compassion.

We wish all of you happiness, peace, and health.

Susan M. Steele, Karen C. Nielsen, and Stephen M. Klein

To Mark, Eric, and Ryan, my love always.
Susan

To Ricardo, who brought me alive and showed me a world without limits.
With all my heart, Karen

To my family, friends, and teachers, thank you for your limitless love and support,
upon which all great projects are built.
Stephen

The hands of time and perchance of life turn in a circle. After several decades of advances in anesthesiology, with new techniques and amazing strides in pain management, we would like to reflect on the pioneers who led the way in regional anesthesia and pain management. The concepts of anesthesia and pain control may seem new, but the brilliant minds and intellects of our predecessors redefined perioperative patient care and gave us the foundations for success. They focused on the total well-being of the patient. Through their insight, new avenues of pain relief and management were brought to fruition. Using their depth of knowledge in physiology and anatomy, these great minds gave birth to the artistry of regional anesthesia and pain management. Yes, they are truly artists.

At Duke University Medical Center in our Department of Anesthesiology, there are several individuals who stand out and have broadly influenced how we practice regional anesthesia and apply it to surgery. We are grateful to pioneers Sir Robert Macintosh, Dr. Merel Harmel, Dr. LeRoy D. Vandam, Dr. Philip R. Bromage, Dr. Alon P. Winnie, Dr. P. Prithvi Raj, Dr. Benjamin G. Covino, and Dr. Mercedes Concepcion. This esteemed group formed the concepts that have enriched our practice in perioperative care and pain control. These heroes of anesthesia revealed to us the importance of attending to the total well-being of the patient in a compassionate manner. They are the lineage from which we evolved. What a treasured inheritance.

One individual embodies the spirit of what we all seek to achieve. He is a person called on to exhibit boundless strength, courage, and tenacity just to face his situation in life. A lesser man may have been bitter, but Dr. Alon P. Winnie chose to be magnificent. We make a special dedication of this work to him.

Dr. Winnie had a happy childhood. He had a warm family relationship, loved sports, and possessed a brilliant intellect. His interest in medicine was encouraged by his father, who wanted a son to go into medicine. To be close to home he attended Northwestern University. During his junior year in medical school the Salk polio vaccine was offered, and Dr. Winnie received all three installments of the Salk vaccine. He had a childhood memory of the seriousness of polio. The Sabin vaccine was not yet available.

Upon graduation from Northwestern, Dr. Winnie went to Cook County Hospital, an event he recounts as one of the smartest things that he ever did. It was an opportunity to see patients with every disease he had studied. He was fascinated. It was hard for him to choose a specialty because he liked them all. His last rotation was Ear, Nose, and Throat, and as a young intern he spent an October morning examining a long line of pediatric sore throats. One of those children must have had the poliovirus, and coughed it into the future of Dr. Winnie. Within twenty-four hours after sore throat exams he awoke with a terrible backache. He developed dysesthesia and felt horrible—even his clothes caused discomfort. Twelve hours later he had leg paralysis, and twelve hours after that he was paralyzed up to his chin. Dr. Winnie remarks that it was a terrific experience. "It's like the war, if you survive it, it's a great experience. If you don't, you're dead."

His positive pressure ventilator had no alarms; however, Dr. Winnie had a team of human alarms, his colleagues, who surrounded his bed around the clock. He attributes his life being saved five times to the compassionate care of his colleagues. Dr. Morch, the head of anesthesia and the chief surgical resident, performed a life-saving tracheostomy on Dr.Winnie. Ironically, the local anesthetic Novacaine, repeatedly re-autoclaved, had lost its activity. During the tracheostomy the chief resident stated in horror, "There is no anesthesia." Dr. Morch literally slit Dr. Winnie's throat, quickly placing the tube. Dr. Winnie recalls, "It really hurt, but they did a great job." Dr. Winnie recounted, "One day I awoke and felt I knew I was going to die." The ventilator had malfunctioned, preventing exhalation. Luckily an intern and good friend of Dr. Winnie's took the initiative; he disconnected the ventilator, hooked up a bag and mask, and ventilated him slowly to allow him to exhale. Anesthesia was called, and the trach tube was replaced with the discovery that a round clot hanging on the tip of the tube was acting as a perfect ball valve. Again,

Dr. Winnie's life was saved. Dr. Winnie states that he "is indebted for life itself to his fellow interns and residents of Cook County Hospital, who exhausted from their own demanding call schedules, took an additional call to protect me from the possible malfunction of the ventilator upon which my life depended."

Now paralyzed, Dr. Winnie was advised to enter a sedentary field of medicine, perhaps radiology. Dr. Winnie felt that those fields "just weren't people-oriented enough." Dr. Morch asked Dr. Winnie about a career in anesthesia. The rest is history—despite rejections and discouragements, Dr. Winnie met with Dr. Vincent Collins and became the first anesthesia resident at Cook County Hospital in Chicago. Dr. Winnie overcame his physical disabilities with great ingenuity, hoisting IV bags on poles like flags. He resourcefully and imaginatively used periscopes to see the surgical field. As the first and sole resident he recalls just having fun, but the greatest fun was regional anesthesia. He would study Danny Moore's book in the hallway outside of the operating room. He would read about femoral, lateral femoral cutaneous, and obturator nerve blocks. He would select an appropriate case, go in with the book, and do the block the way Danny Moore instructed. And the blocks worked! At this point he realized how much simpler regional anesthesia was than general anesthesia, and how much safer. He had the opportunity to develop the teaching program at Cook County Hospital. Dr. Winnie remarks that "To teach people you have to know it better than they do, and you have to have answers to their questions." What an extraordinary teacher of regional anesthesia he became.

While dissecting cadavers in the laboratory Dr. Winnie stumbled onto a fantastic concept—the plexus coming down between the scalene muscles in a common fascial plane. He realized that "Peripheral regional anesthesia for an arm could be accomplished by placing the needle in the space between the scalenes, like putting the needle into the epidural space; injecting once and have a volume relationship the way we do with epidural anesthesia." It worked, and the beginning of *plexus anesthesia* was born. Dr. Winnie's first published technique was presented at the Midwest Residents' Conference and was entitled "The Subclavian Perivascular Technique of Brachial Plexus Block," which was really a descriptive term for a *single-injection supraclavicular* block. Later Dr. Winnie developed the interscalene block and the cervical plexus block. Dissections in the anatomy lab continued to intrigue Dr. Winnie. He continued with this passion and soon developed analogous concepts for the lower-extremity and the "3-in-1" block. Dr. Robert Macintosh states, "For the twenty years I have known Alon Winnie, the disposition of the fascia surrounding muscle, nerves, and vessels has been one of his main interests in his professional life." Dr. Winnie describes the concept in the dedication of his book—"Plexus anesthesia to me represents the epitome of the science of anesthesiology, the application of fundamental anatomic principles to form a clinical concept, which carried out with sufficient technical skill and clinical judgment, results in enhanced safety for the surgical patient."

After joining the faculty at Cook County Hospital, Dr. Winnie worked with Dr. Collins and founded the first pain clinic in the Midwest. With Dr. Bonica's clinic the only other well-recognized pain clinic of the day, the two forged modern pain medicine. He states, "Loving regional anesthesia as I did, and I think you would agree, the roots of anesthesiologists in pain management go back to their roots in regional anesthesia at the beginning." He felt that pain management is doing something outside of the operating room that causes a change in the attitude of other specialists toward you. You really become involved in the welfare of the patient.

As Dr. Winnie's career burgeoned, he continued to be an innovator in regional anesthesia. With deft skill he learned new blocks, developed new concepts, and taught countless students worldwide. Dr. Winnie realized that his polio was a blessing in a tragic way. "If it weren't for polio, I would not be doing what I love to do." Although he could not stand at the bedside of a patient, he was standing tall in the fields of pain management and regional anesthesia.

Dr. Winnie values his work with epidural steroids as some of the most rewarding work he has done in medicine. Dr. Winnie, a recipient of epidural steroids himself, realized that when used properly and for the right indications it is a very effective modality.

Dr. Winnie, still doing major impact science, reported in 1997 the compassionate transplantation of allogeneic adrenal medullary chromaffin cells into the cerebrospinal fluid of patients with intractable pain and terminal cancer. These chromaffin cells act as a constant source of endogenous opiod peptides and catecholamines that drastically reduced the pain scores and exogenous morphine requirements in these patients. This extraordinary contribution to patient care has remarkably improved the quality of life for terminal patients, allowing them to live their last days with greater dignity.

Dr. Winnie has been instrumental in the formation of several societies. Most notably he was a founder of the American Society of Regional Anesthesia (ASRA). Dr. Winnie states that at the time of the society's formation only 10% of anesthesiologists had training in regional anesthesia and pain management. ASRA helped many anesthesiologists add regional anesthesia to their practices. ASRA has effectively encouraged institutions into teaching regional anesthesia as a part of every residency program. ASRA has also been successful in promoting research in regional anesthesia.

Dr. Winnie regards the education and training of young anesthesiologists as his greatest professional accomplishment. Three children and five grandchildren are his most precious accomplishments. His ultimate accomplishment is his victorious triumph over his physical limitations, although it is hard to imagine Dr. Winnie as one with limitations.

It is hard to determine if Dr. Winnie's dedication to relieving pain is a result of his personal painful experiences or his indomitable spirit. Perhaps it is a marvelous blending of both. His true grit, brilliant mind, gentle poetic spirit, resourcefulness, and compassion for his fellow man have made his overwhelming contributions to the field of regional anesthesia and pain management even more esteemed. Dr. Winnie continues to face the hard times in life with his usual strong determination. He has recently battled colon cancer, undergoing surgery and chemotherapy treatments with the strength and grace with which he has lived his life. He continues to write and is currently working on a second edition of *Plexus Anesthesia*. Dr. Winnie is a living testimony to the saying that "What doesn't kill us makes us stronger."

Dr. Winnie, you are our hero. Dr. Macintosh refers to *Plexus Anesthesia* as a "splendid masterpiece." We think that is a fit description for your life both personally and professionally. Thank you for providing such a stalwart example for us to encompass in our personal lives as well as in our anesthesia practices.

With admiration and appreciation, Susan M. Steele, MD, Karen C. Nielsen, MD, Stephen M. Klein, MD, and LuAnne Latta.

Love on Wheels

Triumph over the agony of pain and sadness; admission of the ways of the Creator and "happy to be alive"; optimism with brilliant accomplishments from a wheelchair; "breathing happiness" and "cultivating love" are but few of the myriad of faculties endowed upon my dearest friend, Alon P. Winnie.

Anis Baraka, MD
Professor and Chairman
American University of Beirut
Beirut, Lebanon

CONTENTS

PART II
GENERAL ADMINISTRATIVE PRINCIPLES

PART III
GENERAL SEDATION AND ANALGESIA PRINCIPLES

PART IV

SPECIFIC AMBULATORY PROCEDURES

PART V

PATIENT SAFETY, SPECIAL SITUATIONS, AND CRISIS MANAGEMENT

PART VI

EMERGING TECHNIQUES

COLOR PLATES APPEAR BETWEEN PAGES 552 AND 553

Tom Archer, MD, MBA

Staff Physician
Stanford University Medical Center
Stanford, California

Angela M. Bader, MD

Associate Professor of Anaesthesia
Harvard Medical School
Director, Pre Admitting Test Center
Brigham and Women's Hospital
Boston, Massachusetts

Terrance W. Breen, MD

Assistant Professor
Department of Anesthesiology
Division of Women's Anesthesia
Duke University Medical Center
Durham, North Carolina

Chester C. Buckenmaier III, MD

Chief, Regional Anesthesia Section
Anesthesia and Operative Service
Walter Reed Army Medical Center
Washington, DC

Pamela Campbell, MD

Senior Resident in Anesthesiology
Department of Anesthesiology and Perioperative Medicine
Oregon Health and Science University
Portland, Oregon

Xavier Capdevila, MD, PhD

Professor and Chairman
Department of Anesthesia and Critical Care Medicine
Lapeyronie University Hospital
Montpellier, France

Vincent W.S. Chan, MD, FRCPC

Associate Professor
Department of Anesthesia
Toronto Western Hospital
University Health Network
University of Toronto
Toronto, Ontario, Canada

Jacques E. Chelly, MD, PhD, MBA

Professor
Departments of Anesthesiology and Orthopaedic Surgery
University of Pittsburgh
Director, Orthopedic Anesthesia and Acute Pain Services
University of Pittsburgh Medical Center–Shadyside
Pittsburgh, Pennsylvania

Frances Chung, MD, FRCPC

Professor
Department of Anesthesia
Toronto Western Hospital
University Health Network
University of Toronto
Toronto, Ontario, Canada

Claudia Coimbra, MD

Assistant Professor
Department of Anesthesia and Critical Care Medicine
Lapeyronie University Hospital
Montpellier, France

Lydia A. Conlay, MD, PhD, MBA

Professor and Chairman
Department of Anesthesiology
Baylor College of Medicine
Houston, Texas

James C. Crews, MD

Associate Professor
Director, Acute Pain Management
Division of Regional Anesthesia and Acute Pain Management
Department of Anesthesiology
Wake Forest University School of Medicine
Winston-Salem, North Carolina

Scott M. Croll, MD

Clinical Fellow
Division of Ambulatory Anesthesiology
Department of Anesthesiology
Duke University Medical Center
Durham, North Carolina

Oscar A. de Leon-Casasola, MD

Professor and Vice-Chair of Clinical Affairs
Department of Anesthesiology
State University of New York at Buffalo, School of Medicine
Chief of Pain Medicine
Roswell Park Cancer Institute
Buffalo, New York

Étienne de Médicis, MSc, MD, FRCP(C)

Associate Professor of Anesthesiology
Université de Sherbrooke
Chief of Acute Pain Service
Centre Hospitalier Universitaire de Sherbrooke
Sherbrooke, Québec, Canada

Mark Dershwitz, MD, PhD

Professor and Vice Chair of Anesthesiology
Professor of Biochemistry and Molecular Pharmacology
University of Massachusetts School of Medicine
Worcester, Massachusetts

Meena S. Desai, MD

Managing Partner
Nova Anesthesia Professionals
Villanova, Pennsylvania

Brett Dickinson, RN, OCN

Duke Ambulatory Surgery Center
Duke University Medical Center
Durham, North Carolina

D. John Doyle, MD, PhD, FRCPC

Staff Anesthesiologist
Department of General Anesthesiology
The Cleveland Clinic Foundation
Cleveland, Ohio

John B. Eck, MD

Associate Clinical Professor
Department of Anesthesiology
Division of Pediatric Anesthesia and Critical Care Medicine
Duke University Medical Center
Durham, North Carolina

Lee A. Fleisher, MD

Professor and Chairman
Department of Anesthesiology and Critical Care Medicine
Johns Hopkins Medical Institutions
Baltimore, Maryland

Tong J. Gan, MB, FRCA, FFARCS

Associate Professor
Department of Anesthesiology
Duke University Medical Center
Durham, North Carolina

Sugantha Ganapathy, FRCA, FRCPC

Professor
Department of Anesthesiology and Perioperative Medicine
Director, Regional Anesthesia
Director, Regional Anesthesia and Pain Research
University of Western Ontario
St. Joseph's Health Care
London, Ontario, Canada

Ralf E. Gebhard, MD

Associate Professor
Department of Anesthesiology
The University of Texas Medical School at Houston
Medical Director, Day Surgery Unit
Memorial Herman Hospital
Houston, Texas

Ralph Gertler, MD

Resident in Anesthesiology
Department of Anesthesiology and Pain Management
University of Texas Southwestern Medical Center
Dallas, Texas

Peter S.A. Glass, MB, ChB

Professor and Chairman
Department of Anesthesiology
Stony Brook University
Health Sciences Center
Stony Brook, New York

Roy A. Greengrass, MD, FRCP
Associate Professor
Department of Anesthesiology
Mayo Clinic
Jacksonville, Florida

Jason Gregory, DO
Resident in Anesthesiology
Department of Anesthesiology
New York Medical College/Westchester Medical Center
Valhalla, New York

Anil Gupta, MD, FRCA, PhD
Associate Professor
Department of Anesthesiology and Intensive Care
University Hospital
Örebro, Sweden

Ashraf S. Habib, MBBCh, MSc, FRCA
Assistant Professor
Department of Anesthesiology
Duke University Medical Center
Durham, North Carolina

Admir Hadzic, MD, PhD
Associate Professor
Department of Anesthesiology
St. Luke's–Roosevelt Hospital Center
New York, New York

Steven C. Hall, MD
Professor of Anesthesia
Feinberg School of Medicine, Northwestern University
Associate Chair
Department of Anesthesiology and Critical Care
Feinberg School of Medicine, Northestern University
Chicago, Illinois

Scott E. Helsley, MD, PhD
Staff Anesthesiologist
Hamot Medical Center
Erie, Pennsylvania

Jean-Louis Horn, MD
Associate Professor
Department of Anesthesiology and Perioperative Medicine
Oregon Health and Science University
Portland, Oregon

Girish P. Joshi, MB, BS, MD, FFARCSI
Professor of Anesthesiology and Pain Management
Director of Perioperative Medicine and Ambulatory Anesthesia
University of Texas Southwestern Medical Center
Dallas, Texas

Michael L. Kentor, MD
Assistant Professor
Department of Anesthesiology
University of Pittsburgh
Chief of Anesthesiology
University of Pittsburgh Medical Center–South Side
Pittsburgh, Pennsylvania

Michael Kerner, DO
Instructor in Anesthesiology
Jefferson Medical College
Thomas Jefferson University
Philadelphia, Pennsylvania

Stephen M. Klein, MD
Assistant Professor
Department of Anesthesiology
Division of Ambulatory Anesthesiology
Duke University Medical Center
Durham, North Carolina

Spencer S. Liu, MD
Clinical Professor of Anesthesiology
Virginia Mason Medical Center
Seattle, Washington

Jody Locke, CPC
Vice President
Anesthesia Business Consultants, LLC
El Cajon, California

David A. Lubarsky, MD, MBA
Professor and Chairman
Department of Anesthesiology, Perioperative Medicine and
Pain Management
University of Miami School of Medicine
Miami, Florida

Alex Macario, MD, MBA
Associate Professor
Department of Anesthesiology
Stanford University School of Medicine
Stanford, California

Steve Mannis, MD, MBA
Medical Director
Health South Surgery Centers
Sacramento, California

Donald M. Mathews, MD

Assistant Professor
Department of Anesthesiology
New York Medical College
Valhalla, New York
Chief of Ambulatory Anesthesia Services
St. Vincent Catholic Medical Center–St. Vincent's Manhattan
New York, New York

Kathryn E. McGoldrick, MD

Professor and Chairman
Department of Anesthesiology
New York Medical College
Director of Anesthesiology
Westchester Medical Center
Valhalla, New York

Daryn H. Moller, MD

Assistant Professor
Department of Anesthesiology
Stony Brook University
Health Sciences Center
Stony Brook, New York

Holly A. Muir, MD, FRCPC

Assistant Professor
Department of Anesthesiology
Chief, Division of Women's Anesthesia
Duke University Medical Center
Durham, North Carolina

Jeanellen Newkirk, RN, BSN, CCRN

Perioperative Clinical Information System Specialist
Duke Health Technology Solutions
Duke University Health System
Durham, North Carolina

Elaine Nichols, RN

Duke Ambulatory Surgery Center
Duke University Medical Center
Durham, North Carolina

Karen C. Nielsen, MD

Assistant Professor
Department of Anesthesiology
Division of Ambulatory Anesthesiology
Duke University Medical Center
Durham, North Carolina

Matthew Oldman, MBBS, FRCA

Department of Anaesthesia
Derriford Hospital
Plymouth, England

Adeyemi J. Olufolabi, MB.BS, DCH, FRCA

Assistant Professor
Department of Anesthesiology
Division of Women's Anesthesia
Duke University Medical Center
Durham, North Carolina

Moeen K. Panni, MD, PhD

Assistant Professor
Department of Anesthesiology
Division of Women's Anesthesia
Duke University Medical Center
Durham, North Carolina

D. Janet Pavlin, MD

Associate Professor
Department of Anesthesiology
University of Washington Medical Center
Seattle, Washington

Anahi Perlas, MD, FRCPC

Lecturer
Department of Anesthesia
Toronto Western Hospital
University Health Network
University of Toronto
Toronto, Ontario, Canada

Beverly K. Philip, MD

Professor of Anesthesia
Department of Anesthesiology, Perioperative and Pain Medicine
Harvard Medical School
Director, Day Surgery Unit
Brigham and Women's Hospital
Boston, Massachusetts

P. Prithvi Raj, MD, DABPM

Professor of Anesthesiology
Department of Anesthesiology
Co-Director of Pain Services, International Pain Institutes
Texas Tech University Health Sciences Center School of Medicine
Lubbock, Texas

Narinder Rawal, MD, PhD

Professor
Department of Anesthesiology and Intensive Care
University Hospital
Örebro, Sweden

Jeffrey M. Richman, MD

Assistant Professor
Department of Anesthesiology and Critical Care Medicine
Johns Hopkins University
Baltimore, Maryland

Michael Ronayne, MD, FFARCSI

Department of Anesthesia
Toronto Western Hospital
University Health Network
University of Toronto
Toronto, Ontario, Canada

Allison K. Ross, MD

Associate Professor
Department of Anesthesiology
Chief, Division of Pediatric Anesthesia and Critical Care
Medicine
Duke University Medical Center
Durham, North Carolina

Yair Rubin, MD, FRCPC

Assistant Clinical Professor
Department of Anesthesia
Rockyview General Hospital
University of Calgary
Calgary, Alberta, Canada

Iain S. Sanderson, MB, ChB, FRCA

Associate Professor
Department of Anesthesiology
Duke University Medical Center
Durham, North Carolina

Robert J. Schlosser, MD

Clinical Fellow
Division of Ambulatory Anesthesiology
Department of Anesthesiology
Duke University Medical Center
Durham, North Carolina

Dianne L. Scott, MD

Associate Professor
Department of Anesthesiology
Duke University Medical Center
Durham, North Carolina

Shruti Shah, MD, FCPS

Research Fellow, Regional Anesthesia
Department of Anesthesiology
College of Physicians and Surgeons of Columbia University
St. Luke's–Roosevelt Hospital Center
New York, New York

Michael Simon-Baker, MD

Resident in Anesthesiology
Department of Anesthesiology
Thomas Jefferson University Hospital
Philadelphia, Pennsylvania

Thomas F. Slaughter, MD

Professor of Anesthesiology
Department of Anesthesiology
Section on Cardiothoracic Anesthesiology
Wake Forest University School of Memdicine
Winston-Salem, North Carolina

Karen J. Souter, MB, BS, MSc, FRCA

Assistant Professor
Department of Anesthesiology
University of Washington Medical Center
Seattle, Washington

Susan M. Steele, MD

Associate Professor
Department of Anesthesiology
Chief, Division of Ambulatory Anesthesiology
Medical Director, Ambulatory Surgery Center
Duke University Medical Center
Durham, North Carolina

Lila Ann A. Sueda, MD

Staff Anesthesiologist
Virginia Mason Medical Center
Seattle, Washington

Christopher Swide, MD

Associate Professor
Department of Anesthesiology and Perioperative Medicine
Oregon Health and Science University
Portland, Oregon

John E. Tetzlaff, MD

Director, Center for Anesthesiology Education
The Cleveland Clinic Foundation
Cleveland, Ohio

Marcy S. Tucker, MD, PhD

Assistant Professor
Department of Anesthesiology
Division of Ambulatory Anesthesiology
Duke University Medical Center
Durham, North Carolina

Rebecca S. Twersky, MD

Professor of Clinical Anesthesiology
Vice-Chair for Research
Director, Division of Ambulatory Anesthesia
State University of New York–Downstate Medical Center
Medical Director, Ambulatory Surgery Unit
Long Island College Hospital
Brooklyn, New York

Hector Vila, Jr., MD

Assistant Professor of Anesthesiology and Oncology
University of South Florida College of Medicine
Service Chief, Anesthesiology
H. Lee Moffitt Cancer Center
Program Leader, Anesthesiology
Department of Interdisciplinary Oncology
University of South Florida College of Medicine
Tampa, Florida

Cynthia Vincent, RN, BSN

Clinical Manager, Surgical Services
Rex Surgery Center of Cary
Cary, North Carolina

Eugene R. Viscusi, MD

Director, Acute Pain Management Service
Jefferson Medical College
Thomas Jefferson University
Philadelphia, Pennsylvania

Jerry D. Vloka, MD, PhD

Associate Professor
Department of Anesthesiology
St. Luke's–Roosevelt Hospital Center
New York, New York

Brian A. Williams, MD, MBA

Associate Professor
Department of Anesthesiology
University of Pittsburgh
Director, Outpatient Regional Anesthesia Services
University of Pittsburgh Medical Center–South Side
Pittsburgh, Pennsylvania

Christopher L. Wu, MD

Associate Professor
Department of Anesthesiology
Johns Hopkins Hospital
Baltimore, Maryland

PREFACE

Over the last three decades, ambulatory surgery has grown exponentially and now accounts for the majority of surgery performed in the United States. At the moment, 70–75% of all surgical procedures in this country are performed on an outpatient basis. In fact, major surgical procedures are being performed on a routine basis in many ambulatory surgery centers. The rapid growth in ambulatory surgery has been an enormous success and has proved to be cost-effective without affecting patient safety or satisfaction. Improvements in perioperative anesthetic care have allowed surgeons to perform an increasing range of more extensive surgical procedures in the ambulatory setting. Much of this has been attributed to the introduction of short-acting, rapid-elimination sedatives, opioids, volatile anesthetics, and muscle relaxants. Nevertheless, these changes are not the only areas of expansion. The new ambulatory environment has demanded the rapid progression of all anesthetic techniques to serve the growing outpatient population, including remarkable advances in regional anesthesia and analgesia. Regional anesthesia techniques are site-specific; they provide superior analgesia with few side effects, which are very important components of successful ambulatory care. In fact, these techniques may be the ultimate solution for providing extended non-opioid analgesia after ambulatory surgery, a primary obstacle for performing extensive outpatient surgery in a compassionate manner.

This book is designed to fill the enormous need for an updated resource focusing on ambulatory anesthesia and analgesia techniques. Because postoperative pain is the leading cause of prolonged stay and unanticipated hospital admissions after ambulatory surgery, one of the main focuses of this book will be to define regional anesthesia and analgesia techniques specifically applied to the ambulatory setting.

This textbook, a compilation of 81 authors, has seven major divisions which total 51 chapters. These sections include the following: (1) history and development of ambulatory anesthesia; (2) general clinical principles of ambulatory anesthesia; (3) general administrative principles; (4) general sedation and analgesia principles; (5) specific ambulatory procedures; (6) patient safety, special situation, and crisis management; and (7) emerging techniques. These book sections will supply anesthesiologists with the knowledge to assist them in providing optimal perioperative ambulatory care by becoming actively involved in all aspects of ambulatory care including administrative, regulatory, economic, and especially clinical aspects.

This book intends to provide a balanced and innovative view, with a critical analysis of the literature, of the safe and effective use of ambulatory anesthesia and analgesia techniques to provide advanced patient care in the day-case setting. The result is a unique tool, a practical resource that can serve as an educational tool as well as a daily guide for novices and experts equally. Finally, the ultimate goal of this review is to provide advanced patient care and improve outcomes with every ambulatory anesthetic technique. The editors believe that this textbook will successfully achieve this essential goal.

This textbook would not be possible without the innovative talents of the contributors and their enthusiasm to participate. These experts not only share their vast practical clinical expertise as leaders in this field but also present a comprehensive review of the literature. The accomplishment of this exciting venture is theirs. In addition, we would like to acknowledge the exceptional administrative support of LuAnne Latta and Katheryn Clifton, without which this project could not have been possible.

Susan M. Steele, MD
Karen C. Nielsen, MD
Stephen M. Klein, MD

Ambulatory Anesthesia and Perioperative Analgesia

HISTORY AND DEVELOPMENT OF AMBULATORY ANESTHESIA

Ambulatory Anesthesia: Then and Now

LYDIA A. CONLAY

In the early 1970s, one of the earliest ambulatory facilities was founded at George Washington University Hospital, where Dr. Marie-Louise Levy was asked to anesthetize difficult dental patients. Dr. Levy stated that she was put in charge of the effort because "It was going to be a small, well contained project."[1] That statement certainly proved to be less than prophetic. In fact, it is estimated that between 60 and 70% of all surgical procedures are performed in the outpatient setting today.[2] Even the Anesthesiology Residency Review Committee has recently dropped its requirement for residents to care for a certain number of ambulatory patients during their training—not because such experience is unimportant, but rather because it is ever-present. This chapter will review some of the major questions facing ambulatory anesthesiologists today, and present challenges as the specialty matures and seeks newer venues.

IN THE BEGINNING

The concept of ambulatory anesthesia and surgery has come a long way since its inception at the Phoenix Surgicenter some 35 years ago. Our beginnings were not very noble, or particularly auspicious. In fact, an early sketch of the first "Freestanding" Surgicenter in Phoenix was drawn on the back of a napkin from the Smuggler's Inn by Drs. Wallace Reed and John Ford in 1969 (Fig. 1-1). Dr. Reed considered himself to be a medical and political strategist, and thought that by serving on hospital committees, he could show that an anesthesiologist was "more than just an etherizer, he was also a real doctor." Ground was broken on the Phoenix Ambulatory Surgery Center on Lincoln's birthday in 1970, and shortly thereafter its index cases were performed.

Some seven years later, in 1977, the Methodist Ambulatory Surgery Center opened for business in Peoria, Illinois. It was headed by a young anesthesiologist named Bernie Wetchler, and 10 nurse anesthetists.[3] According to Dr. Wetchler, "It proved easier to convince surgeons and patients that ambulatory care was the wave of the present and the future, than it was to get the third party payors on board." In fact, it took two years of negotiations with Caterpillar Inc., the world's largest manufacturer of bulldozers and earth-moving equipment and the major employer in Peoria, to allow their unionized employees to undergo surgery on an ambulatory basis. It seems that to have done so would have potentially caused a strike, since the union's contract had specified hospitalization in the event of surgery. In 1979, this provision was changed, Caterpillar employees were finally able to become outpatients, and the field of ambulatory anesthesia moved forward.

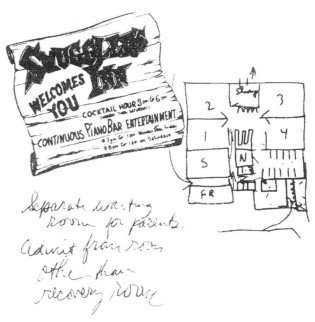

Figure 1-1 Early sketch of the Phoenix Ambulatory Surgery Center. (Reprinted with permission from Dr. Wallace Reed.)

FACTORS AFFECTING THE PRACTICE OF AMBULATORY ANESTHESIA TODAY

Practices Precede Data

Ambulatory practice patterns have quickly shifted over the past decade, sometimes driven by changes in reimbursement, which in some instances has changed just as rapidly. Thus, practices may well have changed before any clear advantages had been demonstrated for patient care, and indeed, perhaps even before there was any evidence that the change was actually safe. Once data had been gathered, practices are typically re-evaluated in light of the new information. This scenario is possible because all too often we as humans tend to place too much value on an anecdotal experience, perhaps because it is such personal knowledge for each of us. We are particularly prone to errors in judgment when evaluating probabilities, and tend to value information that is novel, unusual, or all too often, anecdotal, and we do so even at the expense of the familiar or the status quo.[4]

Evidence-based medicine accounts for these innate characteristics in our decision making. Whether it is providing postoperative care in a physician's office by leaving behind a postanesthesia care unit (PACU) nurse, or testing the limits of a 23-hr stay, evidence-based medicine has become an increasingly important tool to aid practitioners in attempting to understand the limits within which we can safely operate. For example, in some states minor procedures are not typically approved for surgicenter venues by third-party payors even in patients with significant comorbidities who may require extensive sedation. Thus patients who, even a short time ago, would have received care in a hospital by virtue of their comorbidities have found themselves receiving care in a doctor's office.

A stellar example of a decision that was not related to evidence-based thinking involved the Food and Drug Administration's (FDA) recent "black box" warning for droperidol.[4] Even after large, randomized, and well-controlled studies had shown that droperidol was as safe as ondansetron and/or placebo in low doses, the "black box" warning was still issued for the drug. It was based on 10 anecdotal reports from patients simultaneously receiving a number of other drugs including general anesthetics, many of which could also have precipitated the catastrophic event.[5] Unfortunately, the "black box" warning for droperidol has changed practice of administering an efficacious and cost-effective drug in many venues.

Public interest regarding the safety of surgical procedures, particularly those performed in a physician's office, has recently increased following publicity from a few high-profile adverse events.[6,7] Office surgery is not a new concept: for many years, almost half of the cosmetic surgery in the United States was performed in this venue.[8] Yet the majority of states do not regulate procedures performed in the surgeon's office. Vila et al. recently observed a 10-fold higher likelihood of death in the State of Florida if a patient's surgery was performed in an office when compared to an ambulatory surgery center.[9] This finding, coupled with another similar study and their own investigation, led the state to require the presence of an anesthesiologist for patients with an American Society of Anesthesiologists (ASA) physical status of III or above. The duration of office procedures was also limited to 8 hr, and the simultaneous performance of liposuction and abdominoplasty in the same patient was prohibited.

From Hospital to Surgicenter, From Surgicenter to Office

Just as two decades ago hospitals witnessed flight of simple (and often profitable) cases into ambulatory surgery centers, the past half decade has witnessed the transfer of many of these cases from the ambulatory surgery center environment to the physician's office. Indeed, one of the most common challenges for ambulatory anesthesiologists today is the match of patient to surgical venue, whether it be hospital-based ambulatory surgery center, a freestanding ambulatory surgery center, or a physician's office.

Fleisher et al. asked these very questions in a landmark study examining risk factors for ambulatory surgery in a Medicare database.[10] The good news was that outpatient anesthesia was found to be very safe. In a cohort of over 1.2 million patients, the major predictor of inpatient admission was the history of a previous inpatient hospitalization. Similarly, an age of over 85 years also predicted hospital admission and death within seven days of a surgical procedure. Thus, a history of prior hospitalization, or advanced age—even if looks are deceptive—suggests that a patient might be less suitable for surgery in a freestanding facility. The risks of death were also associated with the duration of the surgical time, the presence of cardiovascular disease, presence of malignancy, or an HIV-positive status. The exception to this rule remains cataract surgery, which has a very low morbidity and mortality even in patients with significant disease.[11] The relative safety of cataract surgery has led many centers to limit the preoperative testing for this procedure, even despite significant preexisting comorbidities.

As attention is paid to cases moving from the ambulatory environment to the doctor's office, it is perhaps less noted that cases traditionally performed as inpatients are being transferred to ambulatory surgery centers. Thus, patients undergo lumbar discectomy, transurethral resection of the prostate, and laparoscopic cholecystectomy, and are successfully discharged within 24 hr.[12,13] Of course, such an early discharge following these types of surgery necessitates special attention to detail, especially the careful control of pain and emesis.

In Ambulatory Patients, "Little Things" Matter

Inpatients undergoing major surgical procedures may worry about the malignancy of a biopsy, the loss of life or limb, or other potential major medical sequelae. In contrast, ambulatory patients notice comparably "small" things as parts of their overall experience. Perhaps it is because the risks of their procedures are less. Or perhaps the ambulatory procedure is the patient's first experience with surgery. Nevertheless, outpatients are exquisitely sensitive

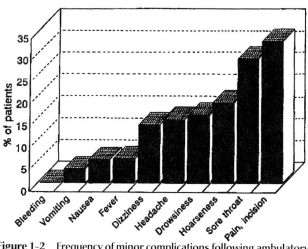

Figure 1-2 Frequency of minor complications following ambulatory surgery. (From Chung F. Recovery pattern and home-readiness after ambulatory surgery. Anesth Analg 1995;80:896–902. Reprinted with permission from Williams & Wilkins.[15])

Table 1-1   Predictors for Postoperative Nausea and Vomiting (PONV)

Female gender

Young age

History of previous PONV

General anesthesia

Anesthesia > 30 min

Surgical procedure
    Breast augmentation
    Gynecologic surgery
    Eye surgery
    Ear, nose, and/or throat surgery

SOURCE: Sinclair DR, Chung F, Mezei G. Can postoperative nausea and vomiting be predicted? Anesthesiology 1999;91:109–18.

to their surroundings—whether it be the demeanor of the receptionist at the front desk, the fragments of conversations from physicians that are overheard, or the patience of a recovery room nurse as he/she explains the discharge instructions. Indeed, Phillip observed that almost 90% of patients report at least one minor complication following their discharge.[14] Such complaints typically include pain, sore throat, hoarseness, drowsiness, headache, dizziness, fever, and nausea and vomiting[15] (Fig. 1-2).

Postoperative Nausea and Vomiting Is *Not* a "Little Thing"

Few complications are as dreaded by patients as postoperative nausea and vomiting (PONV). Indeed, many patients would be willing to trade other complications such as pain, dysphoria, and/or sedation if they could be guaranteed to experience less PONV instead.[16,17] This "minor" but all-too unpleasant complication is predicted by a number of factors, including gender, age, a previous history of PONV, and the surgical procedure (Table 1-1).[18]

The standard therapies for PONV are, by and large, combinations of antiemetic drugs. Thus, droperidol, in doses of 0.625 and 1.25 mg, and 8 mg of dexamethasone reduce the incidence of PONV similarly to 4 mg of ondansetron.[19,20] The optimal doses of droperidol and ondansetron have been carefully validated, but the optimal dose of dexamethasone has been less well defined in adults. Nevertheless, each of these drugs is generally effective in only 40–50% of patients, while placebo was effective in almost 30%. So although the antiemetics significantly reduce the incidence of PONV, when administered alone, their effects are evident in only 10–20% more patients than placebo.

A variety of studies has now confirmed the superiority of antiemetic agents used in combination.[4] Indeed, in patients at significant risk for PONV, such as those undergoing gynecologic laparoscopy, a combination of drugs is needed to reduce the incidence of PONV to within the 10–20% range.[21–23] Similarly, if a drug is not an effective

antiemetic, using it in combination with another drug is not likely to produce an optimal effect. For example, metoclopramide has never been shown to be as effective as droperidol or ondansetron, and is indistinguishable from placebo in some studies.[24] Thus, it is not surprising that the combination of metoclopramide and dexamethasone is not as effective as ondansetron and dexamethasone.[25]

Several studies have demonstrated an increase in patient satisfaction when patients at high risk for PONV received antiemetic prophylaxis with either ondansetron or droperidol.[19,26] Because the risk of prophylaxis is so very small and the benefit demonstrable, prophylaxis is recommended for patients at high risk for PONV.[27] Prophylaxis may be accomplished by using a single drug, or by combination therapy for patients with multiple risk factors. The question arises as to whether any benefit might accrue from treating patients symptomatic for PONV despite previous treatment with a drug from the same class. At least with respect to the 5-hydroxytriptamine 3 (5-HT$_3$) receptor antagonists and in specific granisetron, two rationales suggest an additional efficacy despite previous treatment with another 5-HT$_3$ antagonist.[28] First, differences in molecular structure, particularly of the side chains, confers an additional specificity and an enhanced affinity for the 5-HT$_3$ receptor. Differences in metabolism may also distinguish between drug actions within that class. So, at least within the class of 5-HT$_3$ antagonists, rescue may well be possible by using a related antiemetic agent.[28]

"Alternative therapies" to treat PONV include (but are certainly not limited to) acupuncture, supplemental oxygen, fluid administration, and aromatherapy. Acupuncture has been shown to reduce the incidence of PONV by 30% after major gynecologic surgery.[29] However, when studied in a randomized, controlled, and blinded trial, no significant difference was noted with acupuncture in patients undergoing gynecologic or breast surgery. Acupuncture at the P6 point did offer a small advantage of about 10% of patients when compared to placebo in the gynecologic group[30] and after laparoscopic cholecystectomy,[31] but no advantage during breast surgery was observed. The Relief-

Band was observed to significantly increase the efficacy of ondansetron.[32]

Supplemental oxygen has been reported to reduce the incidence of nausea and vomiting in patients who have undergone colectomy,[33] during transport of elderly victims of minor trauma to the hospital,[34] and in patients undergoing gynecologic laparoscopy in one study,[35] but not another.[36] It is thought to work by preventing possible ischemia of the intestine. In support of this hypothesis, supplemental oxygen did not reduce the incidence of PONV in patients undergoing thyroid surgery.[37] Aromatherapy with peppermint and isopropyl alcohol were also found to be effective at relieving PONV. However, placebo was similarly effective at relieving these symptoms, suggesting that the controlled breathing patterns and/or the placebo effect may be responsible for aromatherapy's action.[38] Supplemental preoperative fluids, 15 ml/kg, have also been shown to reduce PONV in patients undergoing laparoscopic cholecystectomy.[39,40]

Pain

Pain is a major factor affecting the outcome of ambulatory patients and accounts for nearly one third of nonelective returns to the hospital.[41] Pain also seems to continue as a challenge, despite a significant interest in pain control for ambulatory patients over the past 15 years. In 1989, Gold and colleagues reported in the *Journal of the American Medical Association (JAMA)* that almost 20% of patients undergoing ambulatory procedures were admitted to the hospital unexpectedly from pain.[42] Although significant advances have been made in pain management since that time, improvements in analgesia have not necessarily kept pace with the increasing complexity of the surgical procedures performed in the ambulatory setting. Not surprisingly, certain procedures seem to be associated with more pain than others, and it is not surprising that this may be true for the most complicated procedure recently deemed suitable for ambulatory care. For example, patients undergoing lumbar microdiscectomy have an unusually high readmission rate to the hospital (5.7%). Fully 61% of these patients complain of postoperative nausea, and 75% complain of pain in the PACU.[43]

In a recent article by Pavlin and co-workers, the surgical procedure was indeed the major predictor of postoperative pain. Pain was, in turn, the major predictor of recovery time.[44] Gebhard and colleagues demonstrated that almost 40% of ambulatory patients had significant pain during the first 24 hr postoperatively, but the pain was attenuated in some orthopedic patients receiving peripheral nerve blocks.[45] Atiyeh and Philip reported a high percentage of both pain and PONV following central neuraxial blockade, thus demonstrating the importance of remembering to provide for the management of pain following discharge after receiving a central neuraxial block.[46]

No doubt one of the most exciting entries into the anesthesiologist's armamentarium is the cyclooxygenase-2 (COX-2) selective inhibitors. Clearly superior to acetaminophen or placebo, COX-2 inhibitors reduce pain, are associated with less PONV, improve the ability to eat and drink following surgery, and speed the return to normal activity. These compounds may also reduce the resources necessary to manage postoperative pain, as well as other indices of outcomes such as length of stay and patient satisfaction.[47,48] To date, COX-2 inhibitors are suitable exclusively for oral administration. It is anticipated that a parenteral version shall be available soon. For celecoxib, 400 mg was superior to a 200-mg dose.[49]

Perineural infusion is also a novel method of controlling pain in ambulatory patients. This technique is well accepted: with one physician phone call each night, 97% of patients reported that they felt "safe." Only 4% said that they would have preferred to return for catheter removal, and 43% would have been comfortable with written instructions for removal at home.[50] Similarly, the intraperitoneal administration of ropivacaine prior to laparoscopic tubal ligation reduced not only postoperative pain, but PONV as well.[51] Such approaches to the management of pain may indeed represent the way of the future. Ketamine (in small doses) is also a novel analgesic in the ambulatory setting. For example, 0.15 mg/kg administered intravenously just following induction improved analgesia and functional outcome after arthroscopy of the knee.[52]

With respect to relieving the symptoms of pain, no one agent is as effective as combination therapy. Thus "multimodal therapy," particularly if administered prior to a surgical procedure, seems to be the most advantageous approach.[53] For example, outpatients undergoing inguinal hernia repair under general anesthesia typically report a moderate to severe intensity of postoperative pain. Multimodal therapy with a COX-2 inhibitor, a N-methyl-D-aspartate (NMDA) antagonist, and a local anesthetic field block reduced postoperative pain in the perioperative period and in the first 24 hr after surgery.[54]

HAS THE CONCEPT OF AMBULATORY SURGERY GONE TOO FAR?

Over the past half decade, care has shifted from more tertiary venues to more primary or less complex, and away from hospitals to the physician's office. Indeed, it has been said that "any patient can be an outpatient." Yet although perhaps possible, is it really best to perform transurethral sections of the prostate, lumbar laminectomies, and even total joint replacements as ambulatory or 23-hr procedures? Has the concept of ambulatory care finally gone too far?

We, as physicians, often validate the shift toward ambulatory surgery by the fact that patients prefer to recover from their procedures in the privacy of their own homes, and thus they prefer outpatient surgery as well. Perhaps a more cynical view would attribute the change in clinical venues to the cost shifting from payors to individuals, presumably to keep insurance premiums low, or at least as low as possible given the spiral of increasing costs of medical care.

Patient factors also influence the suitability of individuals for ambulatory surgery, but germane social factors may well go unnoticed. Outpatient surgery works best in middle- or upper-class patients, with a home environment and support to care for the patient as he or she recovers. It works less well in young, single people living alone, in the elderly, or in patients receiving care outside their native language. For example, a college student or young professional undergoing a procedure away from family may have difficulties with self-care and other basic needs such as shopping and transportation. For college students, this need can be met by the school infirmary, but the young professional may have a more difficult time. Similarly, an elderly patient with impaired vision may be almost unable to cope after cataract surgery in his or her "better" eye. He or she may also need to be cared for, or themselves be the caregiver for a spouse with significant illnesses and who may be even less self-sufficient. Patients receiving care outside their native language may have difficulties understanding printed material or explanations given to them even with an interpreter. They may also have difficulty communicating with their caregivers by phone. Society is attempting to address these issues at some levels. Indeed, almost all home care for Medicare recipients is now covered as a service. But as ambulatory surgery continues to mature as a concept, perhaps the next level in its evolution will be to increase the inclusion of social factors in outcome studies as well.

So can any patient be an outpatient? The answer to this question is increasingly "yes." But should any patient be an outpatient? The answer to this question is increasingly less clear.

REFERENCES

1. Levy ML. The beginning of modern day ambulatory surgery. SAMBA Newsletter 1994;9(3):5.
2. Owings MF, Kozak LJ. Ambulatory and inpatient procedures in the United States, 1996. Vital Health Stat Series 1998;13(139):1–119.
3. Wetchler BV, Jacoby J, Moore DC. Careers in Anesthesiology: Autobiographical Memoirs, vol VII. Park Ridge, IL: Wood Library–Museum of Anesthesiology, 2002.
4. Conlay LA, Gurnaney H. Vomiting or happiness: have we taken surrogate endpoints too far? Semin Anesth Perioper Med Pain 2001;20(4):283–87.
5. Habib AS, Gan TJ. Food and drug administration black box warning on the perioperative use of droperidol: a review of these cases. Anesth Analg 2003;96(5):1377–79.
6. Orecklin M. At what cost beauty? Plastic surgery may have lost some of its stigma, but that doesn't mean the risks have vanished too. Time, March 1, 2004.
7. Fields H. Patient safety. Health hazards of office-based surgery. US News & World Rpt 2003;135(11):54.
8. Courtiss EH, Goldwyn RM, Joffe JM, et al. Anesthetic practices in ambulatory aesthetic surgery. Plast Reconstr Surg 1994;93:792–801.
9. Vila H, Soto R, Cantor AB, et al. Comparative outcomes analysis of procedures performed in physician offices and ambulatory surgery centers. Arch Surg 2003;138(9):991–95.
10. Fleisher LA, Pasternak LR, Herbert R, et al. Inpatient hospital admission and death after outpatient surgery in elderly patients: importance of patient and system characteristics and location of care. Arch Surg 2004;139(1):67–72.
11. Schein OD, Katz J, Bass EB, et al. The value of routine preoperative

12. medical testing before cataract surgery. N Engl J Med 2000;342(3):168–75.
13. Chander J, Vanitha V, Lal P, et al. Transurethral resection of the prostate as catheter-free day-care surgery. BJU Internat 2003;92(4):422–25.
14. Shaikh S, Chung F, Imarengiaye C, et al. Pain, nausea, vomiting and ocular complications delay discharge following ambulatory microdiscectomy. Can J Anaesth 2003;50(5):514–18.
15. Philip BK. Patients' assessment of ambulatory anesthesia and surgery. J Clin Anesth 1992;4(5):355–58.
16. Chung F. Recovery pattern and home-readiness after ambulatory surgery. Anesth Analg 1995;80:896–902.
17. Macario A, Weinger M, Carney S, et al. Which clinical anesthesia outcomes are important to avoid? The perspective of patients. Anesth Analg 1999;89(3):652–58.
18. Orkin FK. What do patients want? Preferences for immediate postoperative recovery. Anesth Analg 1992;74:S225 (suppl 1) (abstr).
19. Sinclair DR, Chung F, Mezei G. Can postoperative nausea and vomiting be predicted? Anesthesiology 1999;91:109–18.
20. Fortney JT, Gan TJ, Graczyk S, et al. A comparison of the efficacy, safety, and patient satisfaction of ondansetron versus droperidol as antiemetics for elective outpatient surgical procedures. Anesth Analg 1998;86(4):731–38.
21. Elhakim M, Nafie M, Mahmoud K, et al. Dexamethasone 8 mg in combination with ondansetron 4 mg appears to be the optimal dose for the prevention of nausea and vomiting after laparoscopic cholecystectomy. Can J Anaesth 2002;49(9):922–26.
22. Wu O, Belo SE, Koutsoukos G. Additive anti-emetic efficacy of prophylactic ondansetron with droperidol in out-patient gynecological laparoscopy. Can J Anaesth 2000;47(6):529–36.
23. McKenzie R, Riley TJ, Tantisira B, et al. Effect of propofol for induction and ondansetron with or without dexamethasone for the prevention of nausea and vomiting after major gynecologic surgery. J Clin Anesth 1997;9(1):15–20.
24. Pueyo FJ, Carrascosa F, Lopez L, et al. Combination of ondansetron and droperidol in the prophylaxis of postoperative nausea and vomiting. Anesth Analg 1996;83(1):117–22.
25. Domino KB, Anderson EA, Polissar NL, et al. Comparative efficacy and safety of ondansetron, droperidol, and metoclopramide for preventing postoperative nausea and vomiting: a meta-analysis. Anesth Analg 1999;88(6):1370–79.
26. Maddali MM, Mathew J, Fahr J, et al. Postoperative nausea and vomiting in diagnostic gynaecological laparoscopic procedures: comparison of the efficacy of the combination of dexamethasone and metoclopramide with that of dexamethasone and ondansetron. J Postgrad Med 2003;49(4):302–6.
27. Scuderi PE, James RL, Harris L, et al. Antiemetic prophylaxis does not improve outcomes after outpatient surgery when compared to symptomatic treatment. Anesthesiology 1999;90(2):360–71.
28. White PF, Watcha MF. Postoperative nausea and vomiting: prophylaxis versus treatment. Anesth Analg 1999;89(6):1337–39.
29. Kovac AL. Is there rationale to use an antiemetic in the same class for the treatment of patients who experience postoperative nausea and vomiting despite prophylaxis? Anesth Analg 2003;97(6):1857.
30. Kim Y, Kim CW, Kim KS. Clinical observations on postoperative vomiting treated by auricular acupuncture. Am J Chinese Med 2003;31(3):475–80.
31. Streitberger K, Diefenbacher M, Bauer A, et al. Acupuncture compared to placebo-acupuncture for postoperative nausea and vomiting prophylaxis: a randomised placebo-controlled patient and observer blind trial. Anaesthesia 2004;59(2):142–49.
32. Agarwal A, Bose N, Gaur A, et al. Acupressure and ondansetron for postoperative nausea and vomiting after laparoscopic cholecystectomy. Can J Anaesth 2002;49(6):554–60.
33. White PF, Issioui T, Hu J, et al. Comparative efficacy of acustimulation (ReliefBand) versus ondansetron (Zofran) in combination

with droperidol for preventing nausea and vomiting. Anesthesiology 2002;97(5):1075–81.

33. Greif R, Laciny S, Rapf B, et al. Supplemental oxygen reduces the incidence of postoperative nausea and vomiting. Anesthesiology 1999;91(5):1246–52.

34. Kober A, Fleischackl R, Scheck T, et al. A randomized controlled trial of oxygen for reducing nausea and vomiting during emergency transport of patients older than 60 years with minor trauma. Mayo Clin Proc 2002;77(1):35–38.

35. Goll V, Akca O, Greif R, et al. Ondansetron is no more effective than supplemental intraoperative oxygen for prevention of postoperative nausea and vomiting. Anesth Analg 2001;92(1):112–17.

36. Purhonen S, Turunen M, Ruohoaho UM, et al. Supplemental oxygen does not reduce the incidence of postoperative nausea and vomiting after ambulatory gynecologic laparoscopy. Anesth Analg 2003;96(1):91–96.

37. Joris JL, Poth NJ, Djamadar AM, et al. Supplemental oxygen does not reduce postoperative nausea and vomiting after thyroidectomy. Br J Anaesth 2003;91(6):857–61.

38. Anderson LA, Gross JB. Aromatherapy with peppermint, isopropyl alcohol, or placebo is equally effective in relieving postoperative nausea. J Perianesth Nurs 2004;19(1):29–35.

39. Ali SZ, Taguchi A, Holtmann B, et al. Effect of supplemental pre-operative fluid on postoperative nausea and vomiting. Anaesthesia 2003;58(8):780–84.

40. McCaul C, Moran C, O'Cronin D, et al. Intravenous fluid loading with or without supplementary dextrose does not prevent nausea, vomiting and pain after laparoscopy. Can J Anaesth 2003;50(5):440–44.

41. Coley KC, Williams BA, DaPos SV, et al. Retrospective evaluation of unanticipated admissions and readmissions after same day surgery and associated costs. J Clin Anesth 2002;14(5):349–53.

42. Gold BS, Kitz DS, Lecky JH, et al. Unanticipated admission to the hospital following ambulatory surgery. JAMA 1989;262(21):3008–10.

43. Shaikh S, Chung F, Imarengiaye C, et al. Pain, nausea, vomiting and ocular complications delay discharge following ambulatory microdiscectomy. Can J Anaesth 2003;50(5):514–18.

44. Pavlin DJ, Chen C, Penaloza DA, et al. Pain as a factor complicating recovery and discharge after ambulatory surgery. Anesth Analg 2002;95(3):627–34.

45. Gebhard RE; Pivalizza EG; Warters RD, et al. Pain after discharge from ambulatory surgery—orthopedic patients benefit from peripheral nerve blocks. Anesthesiology 2002 Oct; A-25.

46. Atiyeh L, Philip BK. Adverse outcomes after ambulatory anesthesia: surprising results. Anesthesiology 2002 Oct; A-30.

47. Joshi GP, Viscusi ER, Gan TJ, et al. Effective treatment of laparoscopic cholecystectomy pain with intravenous followed by oral COX-2 specific inhibitor. Anesth Analg 2004;98(2):336–42.

48. Klein KW, Issioui T, White PF, et al. Role of Cox-2 inhibitors in preventing pain after outpatient ENT surgery. Anesthesiology 2002 Oct; A-36.

49. Recart A, Issioui T, White PF. The efficacy of celecoxib premedication on postoperative pain and recovery times after ambulatory surgery: a dose-ranging study. Anesth Analg 2003;96(6):1631–35.

50. Ilfeld BM, Morey TE, Enneking FK. Infraclavicular perineural local anesthetic infusion: a comparison of three dosing regimens for postoperative analgesia. Anesthesiology 2004;100(2):395–402.

51. Dreher JK, Nemeth D, Limb R. Pain relief following day case laparoscopic tubal ligation with intra-peritoneal ropivacaine: a randomised double blind control study. Aust NZJ Obstet Gynecol 2000;40(4):434–37.

52. Menigaux C, Guignard B, Fletcher D, et al. Intraoperative small-dose ketamine enhances analgesia after outpatient knee arthroscopy. Anesth Analg 2001;93(3):606–12.

53. Crews JC. Multimodal pain management strategies for office-based and ambulatory procedures. JAMA 2002;288(5):629–32.

54. Pavlin DJ, Horvath KD, Pavlin EG, et al. Preincisional treatment to prevent pain after ambulatory hernia surgery. Anesth Analg 2003;97(6):1627–32.

Historical Aspects of Regional Anesthesia, Ambulatory Anesthesia, and Continuous Outpatient Infusions

P. PRITHVI RAJ

HISTORY OF DEVELOPMENT OF REGIONAL ANESTHESIA

Regional nerve blocks are based on the concept that pain is conveyed by nerve fibers, which are amenable to interruption anywhere in their pathway. The idea that pain is conducted in the nervous system originated with the specific theory of Johannes P. Müller, described in 1826.[1] This was followed by alternate intensity theory of Erb in 1874[2] and later culminated in gate theory of pain by Wall and Melzack in 1965.[3]

Regional anesthesia was not available when general anesthesia was first successfully administered in 1846. It had to wait until 1855 when Rynd described the idea of introducing a solution of morphine hypodermically around a peripheral nerve.[4] Since he did not have needle or a syringe, he improvised by introducing a trocar and canula into the region and then allowing the solution to reach the nerves by gravity. Wood in 1855 was the first to perform a subcutaneous injection with a graduated glass syringe and a hollow needle, developed initially by Pravaz for injection of ferric chloride into an aneurysm to produce a coagulation[5,6] (Fig. 2-1).

Development of Regional Anesthesia

The idea that drugs might diminish local pain not only by their action on the central nervous system but also by their direct effect on the nerve endings or on the nerves themselves was put to trial after syringes for injection were made available in the middle of the nineteenth century. Thus ethyl alcohol was used in neuritis when injected in relatively high concentrations (over 50%), and when applied to the nerve it was killed, resulting in the alleviation of pain. The method is still recommended today in certain cases.[7] Injections of opium suspensions and later of solutions of morphium chloride in the vicinity of the nerves were also tried, but with poor results. As has been demonstrated by Macht and his collaborators,[8,9] the peripheral action of the opium alkaloids is—in contrast to the central effect—not prominent, and it was also shown that morphine had a smaller effect in this respect than papaverine and narcotine.

Cocaine

From the leaves of the coca bush known by the Incas before the conquest of Peru by Francesco Pizarro in 1532 and used to stimulate the general feeling of well-being and prevent hunger, a small quantity of an amorphous mixture was prepared by Gaedcke,[10] which on somewhat uncertain grounds was believed to be an alkaloid that he called erythroxyline. He thought that it might be related to caffeine without, however, being able to prove this. A few years later Niemann[11] obtained from coca leaves a crystalline alkaloid to which he gave the name cocaine. He found that the substance, upon degradation, gave rise to a weak base, ecgonine, and also to benzoic acid. After Niemann's death, the work was continued by Lossen,[12] who also split off methyl alcohol.

It has often been suggested that the anesthetic properties of the coca leaves had been used by the Incas to diminish local pain during certain surgical procedures. Thus Singer and Underwood state that "from early times the natives of Peru knew about the anesthetic qualities of the

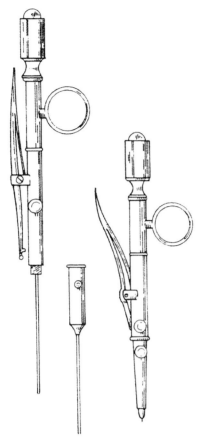

Figure 2-1   Syringe and needle as used in 1855. (From Raj PP [ed.], *Textbook of Regional Anesthesia*. New York: Churchill Livingstone, 2002, p. 4. Reproduced with permission.)

coca plant, and they used to chew leaves and allow the saliva to run over the part of the body, which had to be cut."[13] Killian[14] goes further and says that "it seems that the juice of the leaves of the Coca plant was dropped into painful wounds in order to decrease pain when trephining the skull." Some time earlier, Leake[15] in an historical review made the following statement:

> Local anesthesia was established upon a firm basis with the demonstration of the local anesthetic properties of cocaine. The aboriginal inhabitants of the highland of South America were acquainted with these properties. Roy L. Moodie has reconstructed an early surgical operation among the Incas, showing a blanket-clad shaman using a cautery to make a cruciform incision in the scalp of a woman suffering from melancholia. The operator chewed a cud of coca leaves, the juice from which he could drop upon the wound if the pain became severe.

To this might be added that another picture of trephining in ancient Peru, as imagined by R.A. Thom,[16] depicts the corresponding situation without the use of the coca leaves, nor is it mentioned in the accompanying text (written by Bender and checked by the historian E.H. Ackerknecht). No reference to early observations on the actual use of the coca leaves for the purpose mentioned has been given by any of the authors quoted. Nor had Dr. S.H.

Wassén of the Ethnographical Museum of Gothenburg, who has kindly consulted the ethnographic literature to ascertain if any mention is made on this point, been able to find any indication that such was the case. It seems that the whole story is only the result of imagination, not of definite knowledge.

But even if the aborigines of Peru should have applied coca leaves in any form to wounds to allay pain, it has undoubtedly been completely forgotten shortly after the conquest of Peru by the Spaniards. It is, of course, possible that this could have been a consequence of the intense efforts from the representatives of the church to eradicate what they considered as superstitious.[17] As is well known, this led for some time to the prohibition of the chewing of coca leaves as a stimulating agent. Later experience showed definitely the considerable stimulating effect of chewing coca on the working capacity of the Indian laborers, and the situation changed, but then there may not have been any understanding of the value of the juice in lessening sensibility.

Niemann described that cocaine on the tongue caused a kind of anesthesia, so that it became temporarily insensible to touch. He tried it on his own eye and observed no effects from it. Eight years later Moréno y Maiz, later to become the physician-in-chief of the Peruvian army, wrote a fairly extensive paper on cocaine.[18] Using frogs and guinea pigs he not only confirmed the increase in irritability of the brain with convulsions, but he also observed in experiments its effects on the general feeling of well-being, leading him to conclude: "these were the most blessed moments of my life." He also observed a peripheral effect leading to insensibility after local injection of the alkaloid in the calf muscle. Though he did not follow this finding closely, he understood its possibilities, since he remarked in a footnote, "Could we use it as a local anesthetic? It is not possible to give an answer after such a small number of experiments; the future will have to decide this." Bennett[19] carried out a comparative study of caffeine (and the identical theine), guaranine, theobromine, and cocaine and found that they were to all appearances identical in pharmacologic action. In small doses they produced cerebral excitement and partial loss of sensibility; in large doses, complete paralysis. Nothing is mentioned about local effects. With this background, it is perhaps not so remarkable that a British medical commission in 1881 reported on cocaine as merely being a poor substitute for caffeine.[20] In 1880, a detailed report by von Anrep[21] was published in which he described a number of experiments with the new substance on mammals, birds, and even on himself. He confirmed earlier findings on the general stimulating effects on animals. About the studies on himself he said:

> Local Action.
> (a) On cutaneous nerves, I have injected a weak solution (0.003–0.5) under the skin of my arm and at first experienced a feeling of heat; then insensibility to rather strong pin-pricks at the place of injection; after about 15 minutes the skin became quite red, and after about 25 to 30 minutes all these manifestations disappeared again.
> (b) On the nerves of the tongue: painting the tongue with a somewhat stronger solution (0.005–0.5) acts anesthetizing

on the taste nerves; after 15 minutes I was unable to differentiate between sugar, salt and acids. Pinpricks gave not rise to pain, whereas the other not painted side of the tongue reacted normally. . . .

(c) On the pupil: with local use on the pupil in mammals there always sets in mydriasis. In frogs not constantly. . . .

von Anrep concluded his report on the experiments in the following terms:

I have had the intention after the study of the physiological effects of cocaine on animals also to make experiments on man. Other engagements until now have prevented me from doing so, and the animal experiments do not permit practical conclusions. In spite of this I would like to recommend cocaine as a local anesthetic and in melancholiacs.

Thus von Anrep has pointed very definitely to the possibility of using cocaine for local anesthesia as well as for its psychic effects. When one remembers that the disappearance of hunger after coca chewing was considered the result of a local anesthetic effect on the mucous membrane of the stomach, it seems remarkable that von Anrep's advice did not lead to anything for several years, especially since some valuable results of treatment of pain had been obtained with cocaine already before von Anrep's work. Thus Collin[22] reported on experiments by Ch. Fauvel on the anesthetic action of coca on the mucous membrane of the mouth and also by him and others on the useful application of preparations containing cocaine, especially in cases of granulatous pharyngitis and angina tonsillaris. The preparations used were made by A. Mariani, who had erected a plantation of coca bushes close to Paris and made Mariani wine, as well as paste and lozenges. The wine was Bordeaux and it was thought to be especially valuable. Einhorn[23] mentioned—without any reference to Mariani— that Bordeaux wine often causes a local anesthesia of short duration on the tongue and supposed this to be due to esters of aromatic acids, though he did not think their presence had been proved. One is tempted to question the remark by Clark when he discussed the history of general anesthesia: "Indeed, an enemy of our profession might claim that it showed extreme slowness and conservatism in accepting the gift offered by science."[24]

The Birth of Regional Anesthesia

As is well known, the decisive step in this direction was taken by C. Koller (1858–1944), a young physician in Vienna who had been working for some time in S. Stricker's laboratory for experimental pathology, and who also devoted himself to ophthalmology. Both these circumstances were of importance, since he became familiar with experimental methods and also acquired personal experience in the need for local anesthesia when operating on the eyes, having seen

the unsuitability of general narcosis for eye operations; for not only is the cooperation of the patient greatly desirable in these operations, but the sequelae of general narcosis—vomiting, retching and general restlessness—are frequently such as to

constitute a grave danger to the operated eye; and this was especially the case at the time when narcosis was not so skillfully administered as it is now, by trained experts. Eye operations were formerly being done without any anesthesia whatsoever.

The quotation is from Koller's retrospective survey written many years later.[25] He therefore started experiments using chloral hydrate, bromide, morphine, and other substances but without success, so he gave up the experiments for the time being. In the summer of 1884 Sigmund Freud, later so famous as a psychiatrist, who was also attached to the general hospital in Vienna as a "Sekundararzt" and had been treating a colleague who was a morphine addict by the substitution of cocaine, asked Koller to cooperate in some studies on the effect of cocaine on muscular strength and the degree of fatigue, measured with the dynamometer. Koller thus became familiar with cocaine and decided to try it on the eye. Some interesting details have recently been told by Koller's daughter,[26] who quotes an untitled paper from 1919 by her father, showing how the numbing effect of cocaine on the tongue suddenly evoked in him the idea that he was carrying in his pocket the local anesthetic he had searched for years earlier, and how he immediately went to S. Stricker's laboratory with the well-known result. This story is supported by the only witness to the discovery, the assistant of the laboratory, J. Gaertner.[27]

Freud took a vacation, and before he left, he asked his friend L. Königstein, assistant professor of ophthalmology, to try cocaine in diseases of the eye. When Freud came back, the preliminary communication by Koller had already been given. Thus in 1884 Koller's famous communication about cocaine as a local anesthetic took place. He was naturally very anxious to report on his findings as soon as possible, and not being able to go in person to the German Ophthalmological Society's meeting in Heidelberg on September 15–16, he invited Dr. Brettauer from Triest to read the communication at the session. This brief classical report[28] will be quoted in full from the translation published in *Archives of Ophthalmology*:

It is a well-known fact that the alkaloid cocaine, which is obtained from Coca leaves (*Erythroxylon coca*) makes the mucous membrane of the throat and mouth anesthetic when brought in contact with it, and this led me to investigate the action of this agent on the eye. I have reached the following conclusions:

After a few drops of cocaine hydrochloride (I used a 2% watery solution of cocaine in my experiments) are applied to the cornea of a rabbit or a dog, or after the solution is instilled into the conjunctival sac in the usual manner, a stage of irritation develops which generally lasts from one-half to one minute, as shown by the contraction of the eye-lids, and the cornea and the conjunctiva of the eyeball become insensitive to contact. All reflexes, which usually develop on touching the cornea, such as closure of the lid, eversion of the eyeball and drawing back of the head, are eliminated. Insensitiveness is complete and lasts ten minutes. During this time the cornea can be scratched with a needle, punctured or cauterized with silver nitrate until it becomes white, or deep incisions can be made without the animal reacting in any way. Not until the aqueous escapes or the iris is touched is there a sensation of pain. Whether additional drops of cocaine hydrochloride applied after a corneal section, or cocaine administered by some other procedure will also produce anesthesia of the iris has not been investigated on account of the difficulties of examining sensation in animals. In my experiments with animals I found that when anesthesia ceases there exists a moderate and not always well pronounced dilatation of the pupil.

As these experiments on animals succeeded, I tried the action of cocaine on myself and on a colleague, with the following results: The immediate effect of the instillation of 1 or 2 drops of a 2 percent solution of cocaine was a moderate burning, which lasted for one-half minute and was succeeded by a feeling of dryness. The palpebral fissure appeared wider than that of the untreated eye. If the cornea or the conjunctiva of the eyeball was touched with the head of a pin one or two minutes after beginning the experiment, this contact was appreciated only to the slightest degree. When the sensation and the reflexes were not completely exhausted, this effect could be obtained by the instillation of additional drops of cocaine hydrochloride. A depression could be produced in the cornea by pressure on the conjunctiva, or the eyeball could be grasped with the forceps without producing any sensation whatever.

The state of anesthesia lasted ten minutes. This was followed by a weakened sensitivity, which was lost after several hours. During the period of anesthesia, the function of the eye was in no way disturbed. After twenty or thirty minutes following the instillation, the pupil began to dilate. The dilatation increased during the course of an hour to a moderate grade; in the second hour it gradually disappeared, and after several more hours (up to twelve hours) was entirely overcome. During this entire period the pupil reacted promptly to light and to convergence. The weakness of accommodation disappeared earlier than the difference in the size of the pupil. I have not had any opportunity to perform experiments on diseased eyes, though I could convince myself that the anesthetic action of cocaine also took place in animals in which I had produced keratitis by the introduction of a foreign body.

Perhaps it is not too bold to hope that cocaine can be used with success as an anesthetic in the removal of foreign bodies from the cornea as well as in more extensive operations, or as a narcotic in diseases of the cornea and conjunctiva. As I performed these experiments only during the past two weeks, I shall have to take up in a later publication the work which has previously been done on this subject.[29]

A facsimile of the original German text was placed at the disposal of Dr. Brettauer by Mrs. Koller-Becker. This communication, a model of scientific accuracy, cautious conclusions, and hopeful optimism, was obviously very well received by the meeting, especially after demonstrations by Brettauer of the remarkable anesthetic effect of a 2% solution of cocaine hydrochloride on the cornea and conjunctiva of one of the patients of the Heidelberg Eye Clinic.

The detailed publication mentioned by Koller took the form of a lecture before the Viennese medical association on October 17, 1884. He could then report that his results had already been confirmed in various places in Germany, and he pointed out that "for us Viennese, cocaine has be-

come a favorite topic because of the thorough review and interesting therapeutic work of my colleague at the general hospital, Dr. Sigmund Freud."

He could also add several important observations, such as ischemia occurring in the normal conjunctiva after cocaine administration; he saw that the widening of the palpebral fissure preceded the actions on the muscles in the iris and the ciliary body and therefore should be attributed to removal of stimuli, which determine the width of the fissure by acting on the cornea and the conjunctiva. He also concluded from the late effects on the pupil and on accommodation that a slow absorption had taken place. He never saw any signs of stimulation after the administration of cocaine to the eye.[30]

In Vienna, Koller's findings were confirmed immediately after his lecture by Königstein, and Koller persuaded Jellinek to try cocaine in laryngology, with the result that he could publish a paper[31] on its useful application in the extirpation of polypous and papillomatous growth. Fränkel soon afterward found that cocaine was well suited for anesthetizing the genital mucosa, even if it was inflamed.[32] But this was only the beginning. Before the end of the year, numerous "letters from the readers" appeared about the subject in England in the *Lancet*, and also in other countries the interest was obviously very great. Perhaps this is best illustrated from the United States. Already on October 11, 1884 a report about the Heidelberg meeting written by H.D. Noyes, professor of ophthalmology in New York, was published in a well-known medical journal.[33] He expressed himself enthusiastically about Koller's discovery, and a stream of communications on the subject soon came forth. As shown in the careful retrospect by Matas,[34] the first use of cocaine in the United States as an anesthetic for the eye took place already on October 8, as a consequence of a letter from Noyes (the case was not published at the time). Knapp, also professor of ophthalmology in New York and editor of the *Archives of Ophthalmology*, at the end of the year published an article starting with the following words: "No modern remedy has been received with such general enthusiasm, none has been so rapidly popular, and scarcely any one has shown so extensive a field of useful application as cocaine, the local anesthetic introduced by Dr. C. Koller of Vienna."[35] Knapp then gave the translation mentioned above "not only as an acknowledgment of a debt of gratitude we all owe to him but also as an appropriate introduction." In conclusion, he said that cocaine had been found useful in ophthalmology, otology, rhinolaryngology, pharyngology, urology, gynecology, and also in general surgery. It was, of course, to be expected, especially after von Anrep's experiments, that the subcutaneous application of cocaine would also be of value. This was definitely shown by Halsted, who also in the year 1884 successfully established regional anesthesia by blocking the corresponding nerve, as evident from a letter to the *New York Medical Journal* by his collaborator.[36] In the autumn of 1885 Halsted, during a visit to Vienna, demonstrated how to use cocaine with the result that A. Wölffler, assistant at Billroth's clinic, who had at first declared cocaine to be without value in surgery, now wrote an enthusiastic article about it in a daily paper. Also regional anesthesia with cocaine was demonstrated in Vienna by Halsted.[37] Later, because of his ignorance of the dangers associated with cocaine, he became an addict as the result of numerous experiments on himself. In 1885 he published the first part of an article on the use and abuse of cocaine,[38] but the last part of it never appeared. He had become a victim of his scientific enthusiasm, and only after great difficulties did he succeed in recovering from the addiction.[39] In 1885 Corning called attention to the considerable prolongation of the effect of cocaine injections in the arm brought about by the application of a tourniquet shortly after the injection.[40]

It is of interest to discuss the criticism of Koller by Jones in his chapter on "The Cocaine Episode." He starts with this remark: "When publishing the paper he had read in Vienna in October 1884, he quoted Freud's monograph as dating from August instead of July, giving thus the impression that his work was simultaneous with Freud's and not after it." To this one must remark that Koller in his article mentions Freud's review, pointing out that it and the therapeutic papers had brought cocaine to the notice of Viennese physicians. Every careful reader must understand that he therefore had no intention of giving the impression that Jones insinuated. Such a slip as Koller made may easily happen; a good example is given by Königstein, who in his article of October 19, 1884 make the same mistake. Furthermore, Koller stated in the Heidelberg report that he had performed his experiments "during the past two weeks," thus mainly in September. Jones continues his criticism in the following words: "As time went on, Koller presented the discrepancy in still grosser terms, even asserting that Freud's monograph appeared a whole year *after* his own discovery, which was therefore made quite independently of anything that Freud had ever done." This is completely wrong. The paper referred to by Jones is presumably the letter written in 1941 to M.D. Seelig where Koller says: "The facts are that Freud did not have anything whatever to do with cocaine anesthesia, nor did he write a single word about cocaine in 1885 (whereas my work dates from 1884) that had not been done better and more scientifically by von Anrep in 1878."[25] Obviously Koller here is not concerned with Freud's "monograph" at all—the word has simply been added here by Jones—the indirect influence of which he had already mentioned on various earlier occasions,[25,28,29] but with the reports of 1885 on Freud's own somewhat ill-fated experimental work.[41] Jones has erroneously assumed that Koller must have meant the literary review of 1884. For a psychoanalyst, the several mistakes made by Jones might be interesting to analyze.

Though there can be no doubt about the priority of Koller, one often sees even in modern literature[15,66] that Koller started his work at the suggestion of Freud. This is quite erroneous as is evident already from the well-established fact that Freud had turned to Königstein, the elder of the two ophthalmologists and the one with the better opportunities for working on patients, and it would have been remarkable if Freud had asked both to do the same job. Moreover, we have Freud's own words that Koller made his discovery on his own initiative and without any suggestion from Freud. On the other hand, Koller, as we have seen, emphasized that Freud's work on cocaine and

his reveiw[41] had influenced the interest in Vienna on cocaine.

It is not astonishing that Freud personally regretted that he had missed the opportunity of himself making the great discovery that fell on Koller, though it is probably true, as pointed out by Jones, that "it is not altogether likely that Freud, even with more time at his disposal, would have thought of the surgical application, one foreign to his interests."

The similarity between the two great discoveries considered here was also reflected in the unusually rapid acceptance of the new possibilities and in the early-observed dangers, which led to new progress on the foundation that had been laid. But it also happened that the men who had fought for the new methods were fated personally to suffer rather disagreeable hardships. As is well known of the pioneers for general anesthesia, Morton died in poverty, and exhausted from his efforts to get the appreciation he had hoped for, Wells committed suicide, and Jackson's life ended in an asylum. Only Long lived in peace, but he never had fought for the new insight, which he kept for himself. The fate of Koller was certainly influenced by the work he had performed, and the difficulties he met with in Vienna, which he speaks about as "distress and continuous humiliating enmities,"[42] were added to the fact that he did not even get the position of an assistant at the eye clinic as he—with good reason one might say—had hoped. He therefore immigrated to the United States where he at last found a refuge.

Development of Cocaine Anesthesia

Cocaine came into general use in 1884, not only in application to mucous membranes, but also for subcutaneous injections, and by blocking of nerves it found use in regional anesthesia. New methods for its administration were soon added to those mentioned. Thus in 1885 Corning published a paper where he described experiments on dogs on which he had injected 1.18 mL of a 2% solution of cocaine hydrochloride into the space "situated between the spinous processes of two inferior dorsal vertebrae" with the result that the animals did not react for several hours afterward if a stimulus was applied from a powerful faradic battery or through pinching or pricking the hind limbs.[40] One human experiment gave a similar local effect, and the author concluded: "Whether the method will ever find an application as a substitute for etherization in genito-urinary or other branches of surgery further experiments alone can show." Corning came back to the problem three years later.[43] His main interest was, however, the alleviation of pain in certain nervous diseases, and from the last of the papers mentioned, it is obvious that he succeeded with this in four cases. The reservations that were entertained about his first publication—it seemed uncertain whether he had really been in the subarachnoid space—were removed, and there can be little doubt that Corning was the first to apply cocaine (and some other substances) to the nerves at their origin in the spinal cord. But the pioneer in introducing the method for surgical purposes was Bier,[44] who was of the opinion that this kind of "spinal anesthesia" is due to an action on the unmediated fibers and perhaps also on the ganglion cells. He carefully described six patients he had operated on for osteomyelitis, resections, and so forth, with success under spinal anesthesia, obtained with 0.005–0.015 g cocaine injections. Since, however, several of the patients suffered from considerable postoperative effects (headache, vomiting), he decided to make some experiments on himself. Since much of the cerebrospinal fluid had escaped from Bier during administration of the solution, and since part of this had also been lost, the experiment was continued on his assistant, Dr. Hildebrandt. The two subjects would confirm that injection of as little as 5 mg of cocaine into the lumbar theca reduced the sensibility in approximately two-thirds of the body to such an extent that major operations without the patient feeling any pain must have been feasible. It was also found, however, that some very unpleasant aftereffects occurred.

The work of Bier stimulated the interest of many surgeons, and fairly soon spinal anesthesia was tried by others as well. The aftereffects, however, sometimes mild or absent, sometimes heavy and even fatal, caused certain hesitation. Presumably, the effects were due to attack on the medulla oblongata by the cocaine that had diffused into the liquor and also the slow normal circulation of the liquor, which after being "secreted" in the choroid plexus slowly passes via the ventricles into the epidural space and back through the subarachnoid space, ending in the Pacchionian bodies where it is partly transferred into the blood. This circulation takes several hours and is greatly influenced by the body position. When sitting or standing, the pressure of the cerebrospinal fluid increases considerably, and the circulation time consequently increases. This may partly explain the fact that in the cases of Bier and Hildebrandt it took a longer time for the aftereffects to appear and disappear than in the patients who were lying in bed. To counteract such effects Pitkin[45] added to the solution of the anesthetic—he used procaine—a mucilaginous substance and ethyl alcohol in such proportions that the specific gravity and viscosity of the "spinocaine" could be held above that of the cerebrospinal fluid. Solutions of high specific gravity were used when the upper part of the body was elevated, and the light one when the operation took place with the pelvis high. Special measures were also taken to prevent the blood pressure from decreasing too much.

A different method was indicated for certain cases. Sicard,[46] having used the method of Bier, tried a less dangerous technique. After trials on dogs he found it possible to reach the nerve trunks at their exit from the medulla by injections into the extradural space (i.e., between the dura and the bone). He then injected cocaine in this way in nine patients suffering from pain of various kinds (lumbar, sciatica, and even tabetic pain) and obtained a certain relief of varying duration. He pointed out that it belonged to the surgeon's domain to ascertain whether the method ("sacral anesthesia") could be improved sufficiently to evoke analgesia of the lower limbs. Shortly afterward Cathelin[47] reported similar animal experiments. He also claimed that he had tried the method in four patients with inguinal hernia, but the resulting reduction in sensibility was not sufficient for grave operations. This, he pointed out, was

probably due to the fact that the nerves passing through the extradural space are still surrounded by a cover of dura. Since, however, complete analgesia had occurred in the dog, the same result would be expected in humans by increasing the dose or by diluting the solution.

Several workers tried sacral anesthesia in humans without any evident success, until in 1910 Läwen[48] solved the problem. He used a 2% solution of procaine-bicarbonate, varying the amount of the injected fluid after the desired degree of anesthesia. Gros had demonstrated that the effect of some local anesthetics, like cocaine, procaine, and so forth, is highly dependent on the pH, so that the effect became smaller if the acidity rose[49]—a fact already observed by Königstein in 1884. Owing to its greater lipid solubility, the free base probably penetrates much more easily into the nerve than salts such as the hydrochloride. By injecting in this way he obtained better penetration into the nerve. Together with von Gaza he proved that procaine applied intramurally in rabbits was considerably more toxic than when introduced extramurally; thus the prospects for a useful application of the sacral block were greatly improved.[50] That variations in the amount of fluid infected determine the area affected is illustrated by the fact that 10 mL gave a saddle block, whereas 50 mL caused the anesthesia to reach the nipple.[7]

Other new and modified methods of application of the anesthetics have been announced, such as paravertebral, parasacral, venous, and arterial injections, but they need not be discussed here.

The heavy toll that cocainization for surgical purposes took in the form of grave intoxications and even several deaths during the early years of its general use caused a great distrust in the new methods when the substance was injected or applied to certain mucous membranes whence it was easily absorbed. But it also led to important investigations aiming to reduce the amount of cocaine applied without unduly decreasing the anesthetizing effect. Careful studies in this direction were made by Reclus,[51] who was able to show that the concentration of the solutions used could be considerably lowered. Whereas in the early days cocaine solutions of 2–5% were used in general surgery and on certain mucous membranes even as high as 20%, Reclus found 1–2% to be enough, and he communicated that he had performed about 3200 operations in this way without a single death, and even without disturbing the physical equilibrium of his patients. Some technical changes were necessary with the lower concentrations, such as anesthetizing layer after layer, as the operation proceeded, and waiting longer before the effect became strong enough. Even concentrations as low as 0.5% were sometimes sufficient.

The idea of using still more dilute solutions was further developed by Schleich[52] with the introduction of "infiltration anesthesia." He used three solutions, one (solution 2) for general purposes and two for special occasions (Table 2-1).

Schleich had observed (the well-known phenomenon) that the injection of water first caused heavy pain followed by local anesthesia, and since physiologic saline (0.9%) has no pain-inducing action, he tried to find an intermediate concentration at which no pain would appear, but which

Table 2-1   Schleich's Solutions

	Sol. 1	Sol. 2	Sol. 3
Cocaine hydrochloride	0.2	0.1	0.01
Morphine hydrochloride	0.02	0.02	0.005
Sodium chloride	0.2	0.2	0.2
Distilled water to 100.0	100.0	100.0	

would still cause some swelling in the surrounding cells with consequent disturbance in the functional activity of the nerve endings, and thus decrease sensibility. The effect was thus intended to be a summation of the actions of the hypotonicity and of cocaine; morphine has so small peripheral effect that it seems rather improbable that it has any effect in this connection. Schleich tried the method of infiltrating the tissues with these solutions and found a good anesthesia permitting numerous operations without pain. His work was at first met with the greatest distrust, but especially Braun (1897) showed convincingly that the method had a great prospect of useful action, even in fairly large operations. He denied, however, the results obtained with 0.2% saline, and he preferred eukaine B to cocaine, but there was no doubt that the principle of infiltrations with low concentrations was correct.

Development of Other Local Anesthetics

It was only natural that the progress made in organic chemistry, both analytic and synthetic, should have led to efforts to find preparations with good anesthetic properties but without the drawbacks of cocaine. In addition to its high acute toxicity and the risk of addiction, which had come to play a greater role as time went on, cocaine is easily decomposed when the solution is sterilized. It is also fairly expensive.

As emphasized by Willstätter, the vegetable bases, like cocaine, are often so complicated that the imagination of the chemist is not equal to shape them without the natural model, "at least in our time."[53] The constitutional formula of cocaine and its synthesis were not completed before 1934, i.e., 60 years after the isolation of the alkaloid by Niemann. For a long time the ideas about the structure of the base ecgonine were quite erroneous, but this did not prevent great progress from being made in the field of new local anesthetics. The points of departure were the observations of the split products from cocaine, namely benzoic acid and methyl alcohol. As early as 1887 Filehne[54] called attention to a certain analogy between cocaine and atropine—an ester between tropic acid and the complex organic base tropine or tropanol. According to Filehne, a weak local anesthetizing effect is exercised by atropine, and this was increased if mandelic acid was substituted for tropic acid (homatropine). If the still simpler benzoic acid was introduced into the molecule instead of tropic acid, the compound obtained (benzoyltropine) became a strong lo-

cal anesthetic. With ecgonine—obtained from Lossen himself—no anesthetic action at all was observed. Benzoyl derivatives of several alkaloids, such as quinine and morphine, on other hand, were highly active. Benzoic acid must therefore play a fundamental role in the anesthetic effect of cocaine. Soon afterward Poulsson[55] found that the local anesthetic effect of cocaine disappeared if the esterifying alcohol group was removed; the general effects then changed, and the toxicity decreased considerably, especially for mammals. If an ethyl or propyl group was introduced instead of the methyl group, the usual cocaine activity remained on the whole unchanged; hence esterification of the acidic group was of great importance for the anesthetic action. A second methyl group, attached to a nitrogen atom, can be removed without any loss of activity; indeed its removal rather increased cocaine's activity.

Ehrlich[56] could confirm that mice fed on cakes containing varying amounts of cocaine developed pathologic changes in the liver (great enlargement and vacuolization) and that this effect was much influenced by changing special groups in the molecule. The intermediate compounds leading from ecgonine to cocaine were only about 1/20 as toxic as cocaine itself. Soon afterward Ehrlich and Einhorn[57] observed that not only the sterifying methyl group in cocaine could be substituted by other alcoholic radicals, but that the benzoyl group could also be replaced by other acidic groups, belonging to the aliphatic or to the aromatic series, without the anesthetizing action being lost. These observations, combined with the imperfect knowledge of the structure of ecgonine, led to the development of hundreds of new synthetic anesthetics since then, many of them being less toxic than cocaine relative to their anesthetic action. It is of course impossible to go into details here, and the reader is referred to the works of Poulsson,[55] Laubender,[58] Braun and Läwen,[59] and Killian[14] for more specific information. Only a few typical examples illustrating the trend of the evolution will be given here. Einhorn and Heinz[60] found that even relatively simple derivatives of amino esters were anesthetic, but whereas their salts could not be used owing to their acidity and consequent irritating effects, the free amino esters were excellent local anesthetics on wounds. Since the preparations were only with difficulty soluble in water, the effect lasted for a long time, which was most desirable in the treatment mentioned. Many of the new substances, in contrast to cocaine, caused no contraction of the blood vessels, which led to fairly rapid absorption. Thanks to the important discovery by Braun[61] that the addition of small amounts of adrenaline to the solutions could often act as a "chemical tourniquet," an increase in the anesthetic action could be obtained.

As a further example it might be mentioned that Einhorn and Uhlfelder[62] described a new product, *p*-aminobenzoic acid diethylaminoethylester or Novocaine (procaine), which was carefully tried on humans by Braun,[63] who procured wheals on the skin of the forearm by an injection and could state that the new compound exhibited potent local anesthetic action with almost no irritation. The general toxicity was relatively lower than that of cocaine, its solution could be boiled without decomposition, and the effect was potentiated with adrenaline. Numerous modifications of procaine have since been developed, but it is still a valuable anesthetic in many cases.

When the final steps in the synthesis of cocaine had been taken by Willstätter and his collaborators, the former also succeeded in synthesizing a number of its numerous optical isomers.[53] These were studied pharmacologically by Gottlieb,[64,65] who found the dextrorotatory cocaine (with *cis*-transisomery) to be somewhat less toxic than the natural product, probably because the "unnatural" isomers are often metabolized more rapidly than those occurring in nature. At the same time it was about twice as active as cocaine on the sciatic nerve of the frog, which was explained by its greater lipid solubility; it also had the advantage that the solution could stand sterilization well. In contrast to cocaine, however, it caused no contraction of the blood vessels, but this could be changed by Brown's method. Psicaine, as the product was named, seemed to be suited at least in use on mucous membranes. On the whole, however, the intimate knowledge of the structure of cocaine did not yield the harvest one had hoped for with regard to new and better local anesthetics.

A valuable impetus in the search for new local anesthetics came from an unexpected quarter. In 1935 von Euler and Erdtman[66] in a study on the structure of the alkaloid gramine observed that whereas this substance had no such effect, its isomer, isogramine of 2-(dimethylaminomethyl)-indole at first tasted bittersweet and then caused anesthesia on the tongue. This time the observation was duly appreciated on a series of investigations started beginning with Erdtman and Löfgren.[67] Numerous compounds with local anesthetic action were synthesized, but often they also caused irritation or had other effects that precluded practical use. Löfgren and his collaborators (Löfgren, 1946, 1948) continued the work, with great energy, and after more than 100 compounds had been investigated, they found in 2-diethylamine-2',y'-acetoxylidide (xylocaine or lidocaine) a preparation that marked a considerable advance.[68,69] It had great stability, no irritating action, and had good anesthetic effects. This was confirmed by extensive pharmacologic studies, especially by Goldberg[70] and by Björn,[71] who evolved an elegant method for estimating the effect of local anesthetics in dentistry. In collaboration with Huldt,[72] he demonstrated the value of xylocaine in dentistry, while Gordh[73] and others made corresponding communications from surgical quarters. At present lidocaine is used extensively throughout the world.

Development of the Technique in Regional Anesthesia

In 1908, August Bier[74] devised a very effective method of bringing about complete anesthesia and motor paralysis of a limb. He injected a solution of procaine into one of the subcutaneous veins that were exposed between two constricting bands in a space that had previously been rendered bloodless by an elastic rubber bandage extending from fingers or toes. The injected solution permeated the entire section of the limb very quickly, producing what Bier called *direct vein anesthesia* in 5–15 min. The anesthesia lasted as long as the upper constricting band was kept in place. After it was removed, sensation returned in a few minutes.

Interestingly, the first spinal anesthesia occurred five years prior to the first lumbar puncture. The term *spinal anesthesia* was introduced by Corning in his famous second paper of 1885. Unfortunately, what he had in mind was neither spinal nor epidural anesthesia as now understood. Corning was under the mistaken impression that the interspinal blood vessels communicated with those of the spinal cord, and his intention was to inject cocaine into the minute interspinal vessels and have it carried by communicating vessels into the spinal cord. He made no mention of the cerebrospinal fluid, nor of how far he introduced the needle into the spinal space.

It fell to Heinrich Quincke to do the first lumbar puncture. He based his approach on the anatomic ground that the subarachnoid spaces of the brain and spinal cord were continuous and ended in the adult at the level of S2, whereas the spinal cord extended only to L2. Thus, a puncture effected in the third or fourth lumbar intervertebral space would not damage the spinal cord.

Lumbar puncture was invented as a treatment for hydrocephalus. Quincke acknowledged in his communication that he followed Essex Wynter, who six months earlier had described the use of a Southey's tube and trocar for a similar purpose.[75] This device was originally designed to drain edema fluid in cases of dropsy. Wynter introduced the tube between the lumbar vertebrae, after making a small incision in the skin, for the purpose of instituting drainage of the fluid in two cases of tuberculous meningitis. Quincke prescribed bed rest for the 24 hr following the puncture. It is interesting to note that he entered the skin 5–10 mm from the midline. Thus, the paramedian approach is and has always been the classic one, and not the median approach as is sometimes taught.

August Bier published his celebrated paper on spinal anesthesia in 1899, under the title "Versuche uber Cocainisirung des Ruckenmarkes" ("Research on Cocainization of the Spinal Cord"). Bier assumed that intrathecal injection of cocaine produced anesthesia by a direct action on the spinal cord. Bier wanted to apply cocaine anesthesia for major operations and saw spinal anesthesia as a way to safely produce a maximum area of anesthesia with a minimum amount of drug. It was his opinion that the anesthesia evoked by small amounts of cocaine injected into the dural sac resulted from its spread in the cerebrospinal fluid and that it acted not only on the surface of the spinal cord but especially on the unsheathed nerves that traverse the intramembranous space. The extent of the anesthesia produced was somewhat unpredictable, so Bier decided to experiment on himself. His assistant, Hildebrandt, performed the lumbar puncture on Bier, but when the time came to attach the syringe to the needle, a crisis developed: the needle did not fit. A considerable amount of cerebrospinal fluid and most of the cocaine dripped onto the floor. To salvage the experiment, Hildebrandt volunteered his own body. This time there was a good fit and complete success.

However, the incident did not end there. After both of them celebrated the success with wine and cigars, Bier suffered an oppressive headache the next day that lasted for nine days. Hildebrandt's "hangover" developed even before the night ended.

News of Bier's work spread quickly, and, although he abandoned it himself, his method of subarachnoid spinal anesthesia was soon brought into prominence by Tuffier.[76] In 1900, in a report on 63 operations, Tuffier enunciated the rule "never inject the cocaine solution until the cerebrospinal fluid is distinctly recognized."[77] The sensation caused by Tuffier's demonstrations is well conveyed by Hopkins, who wrote: "To be able to converse with a patient during the performance of a hysterectomy, the patient all the while evincing not the slightest indication of pain (and even being unable to tell where the knife was being applied) was certainly a marvel, and was well worth crossing the Atlantic to see."[78] Rudolph Matas,[34] in his description of spinal anesthesia, used cocaine hydrochloride, 10–20 mg, dissolved in distilled water. The solution instilled was therefore clearly hypotonic. Fowler[79] preferred to have his patients in the sitting position for the injection and not surprisingly was often astonished by the rapidity and completeness of the anesthesia. Gravity methods were not yet understood.

Aseptic precautions were strictly observed, and Lee mentions that the injection he used consisted of 12–20 minims of a 2% sterilized solution prepared in hermetically sealed tubes by Truax, Green, and Company of Chicago.[80] This appears to be the earliest published reference to this method of packaging, an important advance because previously it was necessary for the surgeon to prepare his own solution from tablets and sterilize it.

In 1912, Gray and Parsons of Birmingham, England undertook an extensive study of variations in blood pressure associated with the induction of spinal anesthesia.[81] They concluded that the bulk of the fall in arterial blood pressure during high spinal anesthesia is attributable to the diminished negative intrathoracic pressure during inspiration, which is dependent on abdominal and lower thoracic paralysis. They noted that when the negative pressure in the thorax is increased, the arterial blood pressure rises.

It was by then quite clear that one of the principal dangers of spinal anesthesia is the lowering of the blood pressure. Smith and Porter[82] found that the quantity of anesthetic solution was more important for diffusion than its concentration, dilute solutions usually spreading farther than concentrated ones. The introduction of procaine beneath the dura in the region in which the splanchnic nerves arise caused as profound a fall in blood pressure as was caused by complete resection of the cord in the upper thoracic region. This, they thought, proved that the fall in blood pressure was not due to toxicity of the drug or to paralysis of the bulbar vasomotor center but to paralysis of the vasomotor fibers that regulate the tonus of the blood vessels in the splanchnic area. Since these nerve roots originate between T2 and T7, Smith and Porter believed that the main clinical objective was to prevent cephalad diffusion of the drug from reaching this height and paralyzing these nerve roots.

The idea of marking the injected solution hyperbaric with glucose, to obtain control over the intrathecal spread of the solution, originated with Arthur E. Barker.[83] Barker employed stovaine.[83] It was less toxic than cocaine but was slightly irritating, and was eventually superseded by procaine.

Pitkin, in 1928, and Etherington-Wilson, in 1934, experimented with a glass model of the spinal canal to obtain control over the rate of ascent of the drug by making the injected solution hypobaric. Control was achieved by varying the time the model was kept sitting upright after the injection. Pitkin did this by mixing alcohol with the procaine solutions, a mixture he called *spinocaine*, but he categorically warned against having the patient in the sitting position during injection. He controlled level of blockade by tilting the table and illustrated this with a figure showing an "altimeter" attachment.[45]

Barker stressed such points of technique as raising the head on pillows: whenever he injected a heavy fluid intradurally, he kept the level of analgesia below the transverse nipple line.

Barker advocated puncture in the midline as being easier and allowing more even spread of the injected fluid than the paramedian approach. He, too, emphasized that in no case should the analgesic solution be injected unless the cerebrospinal fluid ran satisfactorily. Above all else, perfect asepsis throughout the entire procedure was absolutely necessary. Moreover, no trace of germicides should be left on the skin, because they could be conveyed by the needle into the spinal canal, where their irritating qualities were particularly undesirable.

Barker's rational approach to the use of a hyperbaric solution for spinal anesthesia was apparently forgotten when stovaine was replaced by improved drugs and had to be rediscovered after trials of quasi-isobaric solutions of several new drugs led to unsatisfactory control of level. The lessons of the past were ignored or forgotten by surgeons and not yet learned by anesthesiologists. Indeed, at that time there were few anesthesiologists to learn. In 1920, W.G. Hepburn[84] revived Barker's technique with stovaine, and Sise, an anesthesiologist at the Lahey Clinic, applied it to procaine in 1928 and to tetracaine in 1935.

Tetracaine's great advantage as a spinal anesthetic was its relatively prolonged duration of action without undue toxic effects, but this advantage was partly negated by the vagaries of its segmental spread, which resulted from its being used in approximately isobaric solution. Therefore, Sise mixed the solution with an equal or greater volume of 10% glucose and injected it while the patient lay on his/her side on a table tilted head down 10°. The patient was then turned on his/her back and a good-sized pillow inserted under his/her head and shoulders to flex the cervical spine forward as much as possible; the slope of the table was adjusted during the next few minutes as dictated by the level of analgesia needed.[85]

A refinement of this technique was the saddle block method described in detail by Adriani and Roman-Vega.[86] Anesthesia deliberately confined to the perineal area was obtained by performing the lumbar puncture and injection of hyperbaric solution with the patient sitting on the operating table and remaining so for 35–40 sec after the injection.

The technique of hypobaric spinal anesthesia was published by W.W. Babcock in 1912. He dissolved 80 mg of stovaine in 2 mL of 10% alcohol, thus obtaining a solution whose specific gravity was less than 1.000, well below that of the cerebrospinal fluid, which he took to be 1.0065. He believed that the anesthesia that resulted was chiefly a nerve root anesthesia and not the "true spinal cord anesthesia" obtained with the standard solutions.

A method for continuous spinal anesthesia was described by W.T. Lemmon in 1940.[87] It was performed with the aid of a special mattress, a malleable needle, and special tubing, and was proposed for long operations that required abdominal relaxation. In 1907, H.P. Dean wrote of having so arranged the exploring needle that it could be left in situ during the operation and another dose injected without moving the patient beyond a slight degree. He proposed that additional injections be made postoperatively to treat pain or abdominal distention.[88] Lemmon's technique was simplified by Tuohy. He performed continuous spinal anesthesia by means of a ureteral catheter introduced in the subarachnoid space through a needle with a Huber point.

Tuffier's favorable experience with spinal anesthesia for surgery on the lower limbs and urogenital organs led O. Kreis of Basel to try it in childbirth.[89] He injected 10 mg of cocaine at the L4–5 level, in five parturients, and claimed that this alleviated pain with little impairment of muscular power or uterine motility; however, he recommended the method particularly for forceps delivery. S. Marx[90] in the United States quickly followed with several reports praising the ability of lumbar cocainization. All of this occurred in the year 1900, but the enthusiasm soon waned.

Interest in obstetric regional anesthesia was revived when W. Stoeckel[91] developed sacral anesthesia with procaine. The feasibility of injecting a local anesthetic by the caudal route was demonstrated by Fernand Cathelin in 1901. He found that fluids injected into the extradural space through the sacral hiatus rose to a height proportional to the amount and speed of injection. His objective was to develop a method that would be less dangerous but just as effective as subarachnoid lumbar anesthesia. He was successful in reducing the danger, but his efforts to demonstrate the efficiency of the caudal injection for surgical operations were disappointing.

In 1909, Stoeckel described his experience with caudal anesthesia in the management of labor.[91] He wrote that various concentrations of procaine and epinephrine produced predictably varying degrees of success after a single injection. Pain relief averaged 1–1.5 hr in duration, but Stoeckel warned the greater the analgesic effect, the greater the hazard of impairing the forces of labor. These reservations, of course, would not apply to the use of caudal anesthesia for surgical operations, and Läwen, in 1910, described how he used Stoeckel's experience and Cathelin's ideas to perform a variety of surgical operations in the perineum.

Matas, the eminent American pioneer and historian of regional anesthesia, recorded that Sellheim, injecting close to the posterior roots of T8–T12, in addition to the ilioinguinal and iliohypogastric nerves, was able to perform abdominal operations successfully.[34] Sellheim was, therefore, credited by Matas as being the originator of the paravertebral method of anesthesia.

Kappis described posterior approaches to the lower seven cervical nerves for the purposes of cervical and brachial plexus block. The method of paravertebral block of the thoracic nerves and the first four lumbar nerves was also described by Kappis, and was used in a great many upper abdominal operations. He pointed out that these techniques could be used to treat acute and chronic pain with procaine, or even with alcohol if motor function could be disregarded. Kappis was also responsible for the posterior approach to the splanchnic plexus.[92]

In 1922, Läwen found unilateral paravertebral block of selected spinal nerves useful in the differential diagnosis of intra-abdominal disease.[93] In 1925 Mandl reported 16 cases of angina pectoris in which he injected procaine, 0.5%, paravertebrally with excellent results.[94] The next year Swetlow[95] attempted to destroy the afferent sensory fibers altogether by substituting 85% alcohol for the procaine and for the most part obtained satisfactory relief of pain for several months.

The pioneer of alcohol injection for the purpose of producing a long-lasting interruption of neural conduction was Schloesser. Schloesser presented the method as a means of managing convulsive facial tic; he obtained paralysis that lasted from days to months, according to the quantity of alcohol injected. He suggested that the method would also be useful for supraorbital neuralgia and tic douloureux.[96]

Segmental peridural anesthesia, under the name of metameric anesthesia, was used for the first time in 1921 by Fidel Pagés, a Spanish military surgeon.[97] Dogliotti, however, popularized segmental epidural spinal anesthesia.[98,99] He emphasized that if the anesthetic solution is injected in sufficient quantity (50–60 mL) and under adequate pressure, it will be quite easy to subject the spinal nerves to the action of the injected fluid throughout their length in the spinal canal and the intervertebral foramina, and even beyond. Dogliotti's method was easier and, without question, simpler than paravertebral regional block, since only one puncture was needed. He stressed the sudden loss of resistance when the point of the needle, having pierced the ligamentum flavum, entered the epidural space. The usefulness of this technique was extended further when Curbelo decided to apply the Tuohy armamentarium for continuous spinal anesthesia to continuous segmental peridural anesthesia.[100] In one case, he left the catheter in place for as long as four days and administered a total of 10 injections of 15 mL each of 2% procaine solution for the production of a continuous sympathetic lumbar block.

It was but a short step from diagnostic block to therapeutic block, and indeed the step was taken by von Gaza and by Brunn and Mandl in 1924 in the management of visceral pain. Long-term pain relief by neurolytic injection of alcohol was developed by Swetlow for the interruption of cardiac afferent inflow and subsequently applied to paravertebral sympathetic block in the treatment of severe intractable pain, particularly the pain of malignant disease.

Dogliotti, in 1930, took the bold step of injecting absolute alcohol into the subarachnoid space, hoping to produce by simple chemical means a posterior rhizotomy equivalent to that previously attainable only by surgery. At the opposite end of the local anesthetic concentration spectrum, Sarnoff and Arrowood exploited the continuous subarachnoid injection of dilute procaine (0.2%) to obtain a differential block limited to efferent sympathetic fibers and afferent fibers subserving pain.[101]

Summary

Local anesthesia by chemical means has come to play a great role in surgery. Today almost no part of the body is inaccessible to it. Whether general or local anesthesia is to be used in the special case depends on many factors and must be carefully considered by the surgeon. According to Braun and Läwen,[59] the proportion of operations performed under local anesthesia in Germany increased considerably during the first decades of this century, and in some clinics reached as high as 50%. The demands on anesthesiologists have risen a great deal: they must master several different methods and also the controls that are regularly performed on the patient's reactions during the operation. This has necessitated special training of anesthesiologists who are now appointed in modern surgical clinics.

Thus on the foundation once laid by Carl Koller, a new and important branch of medical science has developed. It is the old story about the young man who became fascinated by a great idea and was ready to grasp the opportunity when it presented itself. But it is also an illustration of the truth in the famous words of Pasteur that chance only favors those whose mind has been prepared.

HISTORY OF DEVELOPMENT OF AMBULATORY ANESTHESIA

Modern ambulatory (outpatient or day-case) anesthetic practices evolved from the early efforts of dental surgeons. Although dental anesthesia is recognized as a specialized form of ambulatory anesthesia, the true beginnings of ambulatory surgery can be traced to the early 1900s. A pioneering pediatric surgeon from Scotland, James Nicoll (Fig. 2-2) reported operating on a series of 8988 children as day cases at the Glasgow Royal Hospital for Sick Children over a 10-year period at the turn of the century.[102] In 1916, a legendary American anesthesiologist, Ralph Waters (Fig. 2-3), opened his Downtown Anesthesia Clinic in Sioux City, Iowa.[103] This facility, which provided care for dental and minor surgery cases, is generally regarded as the prototype for the modern freestanding ambulatory surgery center. Although other practitioners also reported favorable results with ambulatory surgery, little interest was directed toward ambulatory surgical care until the 1960s.

Hospital-based ambulatory surgery units were first described in the United States in 1962 with the development of a formal ambulatory surgery program at the University of California at Los Angeles, and the opening of similar facilities at George Washington University in 1966 and in Providence, Rhode Island, in 1968.[104] The first successful "freestanding" ambulatory facility was the Surgicenter in Phoenix, Arizona that was established by Wallace Reed and John Ford

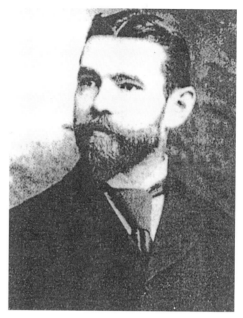

Figure 2-2   James Nicoll, Glasgow Royal Hospital for Sick Children, a pioneer in ambulatory surgery. (From White PF [ed.], *Ambulatory Anesthesia and Surgery*. Philadelphia: WB Saunders, 1997, p. 3. Reproduced with permission.)

in 1969. Over the past two decades, there has been a dramatic growth in our knowledge regarding ambulatory anesthesia and surgery practices.[105–109] Numerous articles describing newer drugs and anesthetic techniques for ambulatory anesthesia have appeared in the peer-reviewed medical literature.[110,111] The formal development of ambula-

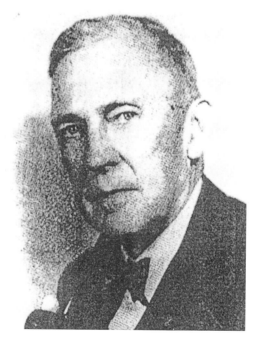

Figure 2-3   Ralph M. Waters, a pioneer in ambulatory anesthesia. (From White PF [ed.], *Ambulatory Anesthesia and Surgery*. Philadelphia: WB Saunders, 1997, p. 3. Reproduced with permission.)

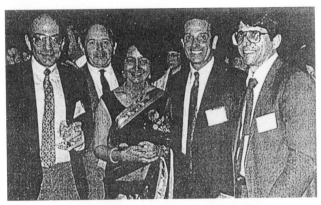

Figure 2-4   The first Annual Meeting of the Society for Ambulatory Anesthesia (SAMBA) in Williamsburg, Virginia. Members of the Board of Directors included Drs. R. Hannallah, H. Weintraub, S. Kallar, B. Wetchler, and P.F. White. (From White PF [ed.], *Ambulatory Anesthesia and Surgery*. Philadelphia: WB Saunders, 1997, p. 5. Reproduced with permission.)

tory anesthesia as a subspecialty occurred with the establishment of the Society for Ambulatory Anesthesia (SAMBA) in 1984 (Fig. 2-4). By 1985, 7.3 million operations in the United States (representing 34% of all elective surgical procedures) were performed on an ambulatory basis. In 1990, this figure had increased to over 11 million, with less than 10% of these cases performed in freestanding units. In 1994, over 16 million ambulatory operations (61.3% of all elective surgical procedures) were performed in the United States alone. By the end of the century, 70% of all elective operations were performed on an ambulatory basis.

In other parts of the world, the growth in ambulatory surgery has occurred at a much slower pace. The initial growth of ambulatory surgery in the United States was a result of the efforts of the private medical insurance companies to curtail rising health care costs. In Europe and Asia, tradition has favored the retention of an overnight stay even after "minor" surgical procedures. However, in recent years significant growth in ambulatory surgery has occurred in Europe.[112] In the United Kingdom, the growth in ambulatory surgery is likely to accelerate with the move toward a purchaser-provider system under the recent health care reforms. At present, ambulatory surgery accounts for less than 20% of all elective operations in Great Britain, but the Royal College of Surgeons has recommended that this should increase to 50–60% by the end of the decade.

In 1988, a multidisciplinary organization consisting of surgeons, radiologists, and anesthesiologists formed the Society for Minimally Invasive Therapy (SMIT) and held its first meeting in London. The growth of this international organization has been aided by the rapid development of endoscopic surgical techniques. In 1995, the International Association for Ambulatory Surgery (IAAS) held an organizational meeting in Brussels, Belgium. The purpose of this "organization of organizations" is to facilitate the worldwide development of ambulatory surgery practices. This multidisciplinary organization will hopefully provide practitioners with more accurate information regarding the types of procedures judged suitable for the ambulatory setting. The list of procedures that are considered appropriate day cases is changing rapidly and varies considerably between different countries, and even with different regions of a country. Although decisions regarding appropriate procedures will depend on political and social conditions, so-called Third World countries can benefit from the extensive experience with ambulatory surgery in the United States.

Choice of Anesthetic Technique

Ambulatory surgery can be performed under general, regional, or local anesthesia.[107,113–115] In addition, sedation may be used to supplement local anesthetic-based techniques as part of a so-called monitored anesthesia care (MAC) technique. The choice of the anesthetic technique depends on both surgical and patient factors. For many ambulatory procedures, general anesthesia remains the most popular technique with patients and staff. While central neuraxial blocks have traditionally been popular for many ambulatory procedures (e.g., herniorrhaphy, arthroscopy, and cystoscopy), their use in the ambulatory setting can delay discharge compared to the use of general anesthetic or MAC techniques as a result of the residual sympathetic blockade, which can contribute to postural hypotension, nausea, vomiting, and inability to void. On the other hand, use of peripheral nerve block procedures can clearly facilitate the recovery process after ambulatory surgery.[116–118] Not surprisingly, an increasing percentage of ambulatory cases are being performed using a combination of local anesthesia with intravenous sedation.[119,120] Although midazolam-ketamine has been widely used for sedation-analgesia during office-based plastic surgery procedures,[121] propofol alone,[122] or in combination with ketamine,[123] has become increasingly popular in the office setting. Infusions of short-acting intravenous anesthetics and analgesics can improve titration, enhance patient safety, and facilitate the recovery process.[124]

The increasing availability of intravenous, inhaled, analgesic, and muscle-relaxant drugs with a rapid onset of action, short and highly predictable duration of effect, lack of accumulation, and minimal side effects has made brief surgical procedures safer and more pleasant for patients, and permits longer and more complex operations to be performed on an ambulatory basis.[125,126] Intravenous agents are now used routinely for induction of anesthesia in both adults and older children (Table 2-2). Intravenous anesthetics are becoming increasingly popular for maintenance of anesthesia and sedation using continuous infusion techniques.[124,127,128] Thiopental has long been the gold standard for induction and maintenance of general anesthesia during brief ambulatory procedures. However, thiopental can impair fine motor skills for several hours and produce a "hangover" sensation even after short procedures.[129,130] Although methohexital has a shorter elimination half-life than thiopental, its use is associated with a variety of undesirable excitatory side effects (e.g., hiccoughing, myoclonic activity), as well as pain on injection. Etomidate has also been used for induction and maintenance of general anesthesia for short ambulatory procedures.[131] However, use of etomidate was associated with a high incidence of pain on injection, myoclonic movements, and postoperative nausea and vomiting (PONV).[12]

Table 2-2   Comparison of Currently Available Intravenous Anesthetics for Use during Ambulatory Anesthesia

Drug Name	Dose (mg/kg)	Onset of Action	Recovery Profile	Side Effects
Thiopental	3–6	Rapid	Immediate	Drowsiness ("hangover")
Methohexital	1.5–3	Rapid	Rapid	Pain; excitatory activity
Etomidate	0.15–0.3	Rapid	Immediate	Excitatory activity; emesis
Ketamine	0.75–1.5	Immediate	Immediate	Emergence reactions
Midazolam	0.1–0.2	Slow	Slow	Drowsiness; amnesia
Propofol	1.5–2.5	Rapid	Rapid	Pain; cardiovascular depression

Propofol has become the intravenous induction agent of choice for ambulatory anesthesia.[132] Its use is associated with a rapid emergence (as a result of its rapid redistribution and short elimination half-life) and low incidence of postoperative side effects.[133] After induction of propofol, emergence and recovery of psychomotor function are more rapid than with thiopental, methohexital, or etomidate.[134–136] Because of its favorable pharmacokinetic-dynamic profile, propofol can also be administered by a continuous, variable-rate infusion for maintenance of ambulatory anesthesia as an alternative to the volatile agents.[137,138] In addition, propofol is frequently associated with a degree of euphoria on emergence and a low incidence of PONV.[139,140] It has been suggested that propofol has direct antiemetic properties at subhypnotic levels.[141] The use of propofol for maintenance of anesthesia has been alleged to reduce blood loss during endoscopic sinus surgery.[142] Although propofol has been an extremely valuable drug for ambulatory anesthesia, it does produce pain on injection, cardiovascular and respiratory depression, and decreases the duration of electroconvulsive therapy–induced seizure activity.[143,144] In spite of the widespread acceptance of propofol, the search for an improved intravenous anesthetic is continuing (e.g., eltanolone [pregnanolone]).[145] However, preliminary studies suggest that emergence from eltanolone anesthesia may be slower than from propofol.[146]

In spite of the increased interest in intravenous anesthetic techniques, in particular total intravenous anesthesia (TIVA) for maintenance of general anesthesia,[147–149] volatile agents (Table 2-3) remain the most popular maintenance anesthetics because of their ease of administration and favorable recovery profile.[150,151] The use of inhaled anesthetics has compared favorably to TIVA for laparoscopic cholycystectomy.[152] The newer halogenated ether compounds (e.g., sevoflurane, desflurane) have lower blood:gas solubility characteristics, thereby permitting a more rapid onset and termination of their clinical effects.[153–155] In addition, the less-soluble volatile agents provide a greater degree of intraoperative hemodynamic stability secondary to their enhanced titrability. For short ambulatory procedures, most investigators have found only minor differences between halothane, enflurane, and isoflurane. However, the use of enflurane may be associated with the most rapid recovery and lowest incidence of postoperative side effects.[156,157] Desflurane has become an increasingly popular drug for maintenance of ambulatory anesthesia because of its superior recovery characteristics.[153,154,158,159] This agent has the lowest blood:gas solubility of all inhaled anesthetics and is associated with a more rapid awakening than isoflurane, enflurane, or propofol.[159,160] Sevoflurane is useful for both induction and maintenance of anesthesia in the ambulatory setting as an alternative to halothane,[161,162] isoflurane,[163] desflurane,[164] and even propofol.[165] Because it is nonirritating to the airway, sevoflurane is particularly useful for induction of anesthesia in children and outpatients without venous access.[161,162] Desflurane is particularly valuable in situations where a rapid emergence is required.[15]

Table 2-3   Comparison of Currently Available Inhaled Anesthetics for Use during Ambulatory Anesthesia

Drug Name	Concentration (%)	Onset of Action	Recovery Profile	Side Effects
Halothane	0.5–1.5	Slow	Slow	Sedation
Enflurane	0.75–1.5	Intermediate	Intermediate	Shivering
Isoflurane	0.5–1	Intermediate	Intermediate	Coughing
Desflurane	3–6	Very rapid	Very rapid	Coughing; tachycardia
Sevoflurane	1–2	Rapid	Rapid	± Metabolites
Nitrous oxide	50–70	Very rapid	Very rapid	± Nausea/emesis

Table 2-4   Comparison of Currently Available Opioid Analgesics for Use during Ambulatory Anesthesia

Drug Name	Dose (μg/kg)	Onset of Action	Recovery Profile	Side Effects
Morphine	50–100	Slow	Slow	Sedation; dizziness; nausea/emesis, ileus
Fentanyl	1–2	Intermediate	Intermediate	Sedation; nausea/emesis
Sufentanil	0.1–0.2	Rapid	Intermediate	Sedation; nausea/emesis
Alfentanil	7.5–15	Very rapid	Rapid	Nausea/emesis
Remifentanil	2–4	Very rapid	Very rapid	Transient ventilatory depression

Nitrous oxide (N_2O) 60–67% is commonly administered in combination with both intravenous and volatile drugs to reduce their anesthetic requirements and to facilitate the early recovery process.[159,166] Concerns regarding the potential adverse effects of N_2O on bowel distention during laparoscopic surgery were not validated.[167] Although early ambulatory studies suggested that N_2O increased the incidence of PONV,[168,169] more recent studies have failed to find a significant increase in PONV when N_2O was used to supplement halothane,[170] isoflurane,[167,171] desflurane,[159] or propofol.[166] Although low-dose propofol infusions (25–75 μg/kg/min) are being used during the maintenance period in combination with inhaled agents to improve the quality of recovery and to decrease PONV following inhalation anesthesia,[172] their concomitant use may contribute to a slower emergence from anesthesia compared to either drug alone. However, the antiemetic effect of subhypnotic doses of propofol[141] should facilitate the recovery process.[134] The use of the so-called propofol "sandwich" technique (i.e., administering propofol for induction and prior to emergence from anesthesia) may reduce the incidence of PONV following maintenance of anesthesia with the volatile anesthetics.[173]

Opioid analgesics are widely used adjuvants during ambulatory anesthesia to improve hemodynamic stability and their anesthetic-sparing effects can facilitate a more rapid emergence from anesthesia (Table 2-4). Although intravenous fentanyl 1–3 μg/kg remains the most popular opioid analgesic in the ambulatory setting, both intravenous sufentanil 0.15–0.3 μg/kg and alfentanil 10–20 μg/kg may have advantages over fentanyl with respect to their recovery characteristics in outpatients.[106,174] Alfentanil (15 μg/kg) can also be used to suppress coughing during emergence from inhalation anesthesia.[175] The newest fentanyl derivative, remifentanil, is metabolized by tissue esterases, resulting in an ultrashort duration of action.[176] This unique opioid analgesic can be used as an adjuvant during both general and regional anesthesia.[177] However, concerns regarding the emetogenic properties of the opioid analgesics have led to renewed interest in nonopioid analgesics (e.g., nonsteroidal anti-inflammatory drugs [NSAIDs]) and sympatholytic drugs (e.g., α_2-agonists, β-blockers, and calcium channel antagonists). Although the parenterally active NSAID ketorolac has no anesthetic-sparing affects, its use can facilitate the recovery process as a result of its ability to decrease the postoperative opioid analgesic requirement and reduce the incidence of PONV.[139,178,179] However, other studies have failed to report improved outcome when NSAIDs were administered during ambulatory surgery.[179,180] Furthermore, concerns regarding bleeding and renal dysfunction have discouraged the use of NSAIDs prior to ambulatory surgery.[181] The sympatholytic drugs can be used as alternatives to the opioids to improve hemodynamic stability, attenuate the stress hormone responses, and decrease PONV.[182,183] When cardiovascular drugs (e.g., β-blockers, α_2-agonists, β- and calcium channel blockers) are used to maintain intraoperative hemodynamic stability, concomitant use of NSAIDs and local anesthetics is essential to minimize pain upon emergence from anesthesia.

Muscle relaxants are used to facilitate tracheal intubation and optimize surgical conditions during intracavitary and laparoscopic procedures (Table 2-5). Although suc-

Table 2-5   Comparison of Currently Available Muscle Relaxants for Use during Ambulatory Anesthesia

Drug Name	Dose (mg/kg)	Onset of Block	Duration of Block	Side Effects
Succinylcholine	0.75–1.5	Very rapid	Very short	Phase II block, myalgias
Atracurium	0.3–0.6	Intermediate	Intermediate	Histamine release
Mivacurium	0.15–0.25	Intermediate	Short	Histamine release
Vecuronium	0.06–0.12	Intermediate	Intermediate	Variable recovery
Rocuronium	0.5–0.8	Rapid	Intermediate	None known
Cisatracurium	0.1–0.2	Intermediate	Intermediate	None known

cinylcholine is still widely used for intubation,[184] its well-known side-effect profile has led to increasing use of the nondepolarizing muscle relaxants atracurium and vecuronium. Yet, muscle pain occurs after ambulatory laparoscopy despite the substitution of vecuronium for succinylcholine.[184,185] Because of the slow onset and lack of spontaneous recovery with the intermediate-acting relaxants, the newer more rapid and shorter-acting nondepolarizing compounds rocuronium and mivacurium are rapidly becoming the muscle relaxants of choice for ambulatory anesthesia.[186,187] Rocuronium (0.6 mg/kg) can produce intubating conditions similar to succinylcholine (1 mg/kg).[188] However, the duration of effect produced by this dose of rocuronium necessitates the routine use of reversal drugs after short ambulatory procedures.[187] On the other hand, the use of mivacurium for maintenance of anesthesia can obviate the need for neuromuscular blockade reversal drugs. Avoiding reversal drugs (e.g., neostigmine/glycopyrrolate) may decrease the incidence of PONV after ambulatory laparoscopy.[189,190] The availability of more titratable muscle relaxants should reduce morbidity due to residual neuromuscular blockade when these compounds are used in the ambulatory setting.

Face masks and oral airways are frequently employed for brief ambulatory procedures. However, the use of tracheal intubation remains popular in the ambulatory surgery setting because it "frees up" the practitioner's hand for other tasks. Although virtually all types of ambulatory surgery can be managed with either a face mask or tracheal tube, both techniques have disadvantages. Therefore, the laryngeal mask airway (LMA) is now being employed in situations where either a face mask or tracheal tube would have been used in the past.[191,192] The advantages of the LMA include a clearer, "hands-free" airway compared to a face mask and oral airway,[193] and reduced requirement for anesthetic drugs, a lower incidence of postoperative sore throat, decreased acute hemodynamic changes during induction and emergence, reduced work of breathing, and avoidance of muscle relaxants and reversal agents compared to an endotracheal tube.[194,195] Although the laryngeal mask does not offer the same protection against aspiration as the tracheal tube (Fig. 2-5),[196] the incidence of passive regurgitation does not appear to be increased compared to patients undergoing similar procedures using a tracheal tube or face mask for airway management.[195,197] Although the acquisition cost of the LMA is high, it is alleged to be a cost-effective alternative to the tracheal tube if it can be reused at least 40 times.[195,198]

Regional Anesthetic Techniques

The flexibility of ambulatory surgery is greatly enhanced by the use of a wide variety of local and regional anesthetic techniques.[199] The alleged beneficial impact of epidural (vs. general) anesthesia on recovery after ambulatory arthroscopy includes a shorter postanesthetic care unit (PACU) stay, less postoperative pain, and decreased PONV.[200] With local anesthesia, the side effects associated with general anesthesia (e.g., nausea, vomiting, dizziness, lethargy) can be avoided, the risk of aspiration pneumoni-

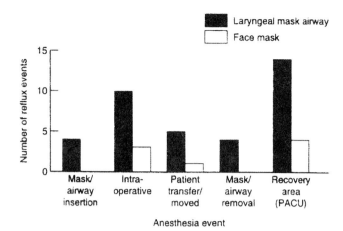

Figure 2-5   Number of gastroesophageal reflux events occurring during five different phases of anesthesia: (1) laryngeal mask insertion; (2) intraoperative period; (3) patient transfer; (4) laryngeal mask removal; and (5) postanesthesia care unit (PACU). Some patients experienced more than one reflux event. (From White PF [ed.], *Ambulatory Anesthesia and Surgery*. Philadelphia: WB Saunders, 1997, p. 15. Reproduced with permission.)

tis is minimized, postanesthesia nursing care may be decreased, and residual analgesia is provided in the early postoperative period. Superficial surgical procedures can be performed using wound infiltration (or instillation), whereas more extensive operations can be undertaken using field blocks, intravenous regional block (Bier block), and peripheral nerve block techniques. For lower-body procedures, spinal and epidural techniques are frequently utilized. In general, subarachnoid blockade is preferable to an epidural block because it is more readily performed and produces more rapid and consistent anesthetic effects.[201] Although the risk of postdural puncture headache (PDPH) has limited the popularity of this technique in younger outpatients, the availability of fine (e.g., 27 ga), pencil-pointed (e.g., Sprotte and Whitacre) needles, has significantly decreased the incidence of PDPH.[202] When spinal anesthesia is utilized in the ambulatory setting, 1.5% hyperbaric lidocaine is associated with significantly shorter recovery times than 5% hyperbaric lidocaine.[203] For ambulatory epidural anesthesia, use of chloroprocaine and lidocaine is associated with a decreased hospital stay and lower admission rate compared to the longer-acting local anesthetics.[204] Patient acceptance of regional anesthesia can be enhanced by the adjunctive use of sedative-hypnotic infusions.[132,205]

The use of peripheral nerve block techniques (Table 2-6) can provide both intra- and postoperative analgesia without the side effects associated with central neuroaxial blockade (e.g., postural hypotension and PONV upon ambulation, inability to void, residual leg weakness). For brief procedures involving the upper or lower extremity, intravenous regional anesthesia with 0.5% lidocaine is highly effective. The addition of ketorolac to the local anesthetic mixture has been alleged to reduce tourniquet pain and to decrease postoperative analgesic requirements.[206] For more extensive extremities procedures, axillary,[116] interscalene,[117,118] and "3 in 1" femoral[207] blocks have been shown to be cost-effective alternatives to general anesthesia. In outpatients undergoing inguinal herniorrhaphy, use of a

Table 2-6 Common Techniques for Administering Local Anesthesia during Monitored Anesthesia Care

Peripheral nerve blocks
  Ilioinguinal/hypogastric (e.g., herniorrhaphy)
  Paracervical (e.g., dilation and curettage, cone biopsy)
  Dorsal penis (e.g., circumcision)
  Peroneal/femoral/saphenous/tibial/sural (e.g., podiatric
    procedures)
  Axillary/ulnar/median/radial (e.g., hand procedures)
  Peribulbar/retrobulbar (e.g., ophthalmologic
    procedures)
  Mandibular/maxillary (e.g., oral surgery)
  Intravenous regional (Bier block) (e.g., arms, legs)

Tissue infiltration and wound instillation
  Cosmetic and ear, nose, and throat procedures (e.g.,
    blepharoplasty, nasal, septum, endosinus)
  Excision of masses and biopsies (e.g., breast, axilla,
    lipomas)
  Field blocks or "splash" technique (e.g.,
    herniorrhaphy, vasovasotomy)
  Laparoscopic procedures (e.g., cholecystectomy,
    laparoscopic tubal ligation)
  Arthroscopic procedures (e.g., knees, shoulders)

Topical analgesia
  Eutectic mixture of local anesthetics (EMLA) (e.g.,
    lithothripsy, skin grafts)
  Lidocaine spray (e.g., bronchoscopy, endoscopy,
    herniorrhaphy)
  Lidocaine gel or cream (e.g., circumcision, urological,
    oral surgery)
  Cocaine paste (e.g., nasal, endosinus surgery)

SOURCE: Adapted with permission from White PF, Smith I. Use of sedation techniques during local and regional anesthesia. Can J Anaesth 1995;42:R38–R46.

peripheral nerve block and wound infiltration with local anesthetics offers advantages over both general[208] and spinal[209] anesthesia. The residual analgesia can decrease the requirement for oral analgesics after discharge.[210]

Many outpatients find the use of local anesthetic techniques highly acceptable alternatives to both general and regional anesthesia when adjuvant drugs are administered to provide sedation and anxiolysis.[119,120,211,212] Infusions of methohexital, etomidate, midazolam, and propofol have been used for sedation during local and regional anesthesia.[205,209,213] When laparoscopic sterilization was performed under local (vs. general) anesthesia, the operating and recovery times were shorter, and the incidence of postoperative side effects was decreased.[214,215] A paracervical block supplemented with midazolam-alfentanil for sedation-analgesia was associated with improved intraoperative conditions and less postoperative pain compared to propofol anesthesia.[216] The availability of more rapid and shorter-acting intravenous sedative-anxiolytic and analgesic drugs

can further enhance patient comfort during a wide variety of ambulatory procedures.[132,217–220] Although the benzodiazepine antagonist flumazenil can rapidly and effectively reverse benzodiazepine-induced sedation and amnesia,[221] the duration of its clinical action is short because of its rapid elimination. Use of flumazenil after large doses of midazolam for sedation during local anesthesia facilitated the early recovery process and decreased the discharge times.[222] Although the early recovery following a midazolam-flumazenil combination is similar to propofol, outpatients receiving flumazenil may experience a higher incidence of resedation after discharge from the ambulatory surgery unit. Furthermore, flumazenil is less effective in reversing respiratory depression than residual sedation and amnesia.[223,224]

Midazolam, 25 mg intravenously, combined with propofol, 25–75 μg/kg/min, has been shown to provide a predictable level of sedation, amnesia, and anxiolysis during procedures performed under local anesthesia without delaying recovery.[225] Although intermittent bolus injections of propofol can be as effective as a continuous infusion, the infusion technique is more convenient and provides a stable level of sedation.[226] Even in elderly outpatients, use of low-dose infusions of propofol (0.5–2 mg/kg/hr) produces a stable level of sedation and permits a rapid recovery and early discharge.[132] Compared to traditional barbiturate-base sedation techniques, the use of a propofol infusion for sedation of children is reported to be cost-effective because of its more favorable recovery profile (Fig. 2-6).[227] A combination of propofol and alfentanil (or remifentanil) by infusion provides highly titratable sedation-analgesia during more painful procedures.[219,220] Pain directly impacts on recovery even after "minor" ambulatory procedures.[228,229] Although ketamine is less costly than propofol when used for sedation,[230] its use is associated with a higher incidence of perioperative side effects.[217] However, use of ketamine af-

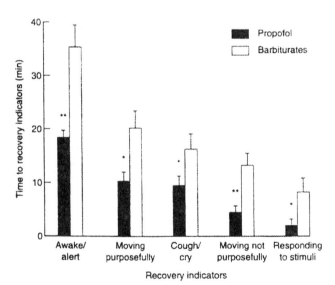

Figure 2-6 Time required to achieve recovery endpoints after sedation with either propofol or barbiturates in children undergoing magnetic resonance imaging (MRI) procedures. *$p < 0.05$ between two drug treatment groups. (From White PF [ed.], *Ambulatory Anesthesia and Surgery*. Philadelphia: WB Saunders, 1997, p. 17. Reproduced with permission.)

ter premedication with a benzodiazepine has become a popular adjuvant to local anesthesia for plastic surgery.[121,231,232] Furthermore, the S(+) isomer of ketamine appears to be associated with fewer side effects than the correctly used racemic mixture.[233] Combining midazolam and ketamine may provide a superior condition for a peribulbar block than methohexital.[234] For brief painful procedures (e.g., retrobulbar injections), use of a rapid short-acting opioid may offer advantages over a sedative-hypnotic.[235] The intraoperative use of patient-controlled analgesia with alfentanil during uncomfortable diagnostic and therapeutic procedures was comparable to physician-controlled drug administration.[236] More recently, patient-controlled administration of midazolam and propofol has also been described during ambulatory surgery procedures performed under local anesthesia.[237]

HISTORY OF CONTINUOUS INFUSIONS IN THE OUTPATIENT SETTING[238]

The ability to provide continuous peripheral nerve blocks to patients safely on an outpatient basis has been a major advance in ambulatory surgery over the past several years. The first reports of patients self-administering local anesthetic via wound and perineural catheters were published in 1998.[239] Such infusions have now become a necessary component for the success of various ambulatory procedures. The rapid development of these techniques has been based on advances in equipment manufacturing, drug development, and the need to provide a greater degree of analgesia for patients in the ambulatory setting. Many of the concepts used to provide safe ambulatory infusion have been drawn from studies of patients receiving these types of therapies in a hospital setting. Few studies have actually examined these techniques in an outpatient environment. However, the advantages of these analgesic techniques over traditional oral opioids for patients undergoing major surgery in the ambulatory environment have led to their rapid acceptance as a standard of care at many institutions.

Continuous regional analgesia has been extensively used over the last decade as physicians have come to appreciate the important role of pain control in postoperative rehabilitation and surgical outcome. For many years, continuous regional analgesia implied central neuraxial techniques. However, several key factors have shifted the focus from neuraxial to peripheral nerve block techniques. The factors leading to this change of focus include the continued expansion of procedures appropriate for an ambulatory environment. Pain control is often the primary reason for hospital admission following orthopedic procedures. Continuous peripheral nerve blocks have been successfully used to control pain after ambulatory orthopedic surgery for an ever-increasing variety of operations. Another element in the shift from neuraxial to peripheral nerve blocks was the U.S. Food and Drug Administration (FDA) black box warning, issued in 1997, regarding the risk of spinal hematoma in patients receiving low-molecular-weight heparin and epidural anesthesia. This change in the risk-benefit ratio for epidural analgesia has

led to a greater interest in the development and use of continuous peripheral nerve block techniques for inpatients, which has then "spilled over" into the ambulatory setting. Finally, the equipment to provide routine, successful continuous peripheral nerve blockade has only recently been developed and made available to practitioners. These factors—the need for profound nonopioid ambulatory analgesia, the change in acceptable risk for a well-established practice, and the development of new equipment—have brought us to the current level of interest in continuous peripheral nerve blocks today. Rawal et al. reported on the first use of continuous regional analgesia for patients in the home environment in 1998.[239] Since that time, several studies and case reports have been published demonstrating the efficacy of these techniques.

The Application of Continuous Regional Analgesia Techniques in the Ambulatory Environment

Several studies have compared the use of continuous epidural analgesia, continuous lumbar plexus blockade, and intravenous opioid analgesia in patients following major open-knee surgery, primarily total knee replacement.[240-242] In all of these studies the continuous lumbar plexus and epidural groups had equivalent analgesia, which was demonstrated to be superior to analgesia in the intravenous opioid groups. In addition, rehabilitation was achieved earlier for the patients in the regional analgesia groups.[240,241] However, when compared with the epidural groups, the lumbar plexus groups had fewer side effects and improved patient satisfaction.[240,241]

In ambulatory surgery, continuous lumbar plexus blocks, either as a femoral nerve block or psoas compartment block, have been used for extensive knee surgery, including arthroscopically assisted anterior cruciate ligament (ACL) reconstruction.[243-245] These studies also demonstrated a high degree of patient satisfaction and low supplemental opioid requirement using these techniques.

Shoulder surgery frequently results in a significant degree of pain in ambulatory patients.[246] Continuous interscalene brachial plexus blockade has proved to be a valuable asset for patients undergoing major shoulder surgery in an ambulatory environment, including rotator cuff repair, total shoulder arthroplasty, and frozen-shoulder release.[247-249] These procedures are frequently painful for several days postoperatively and often require intensive and immediate physical therapy. Cohen et al. reported on the success of this technique in 100 consecutive frozen-shoulder surgeries.[248] In this group of refractory patients, they reported improvement in movement for nearly 80%. This high success rate was directly attributed to the high degree of analgesia provided by the continuous interscalene perineural local-anesthetic infusion. Borgeat et al. have reported higher patient satisfaction, lower additional opioid usage, and improved rehabilitation following major open-shoulder surgery for patients who received postoperative patient-controlled interscalene brachial plexus blocks versus intravenous opioids.[250] One major difference between

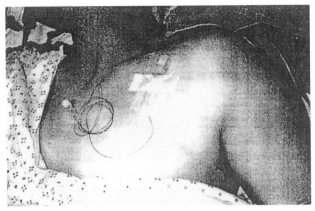

Figure 2-7   Infraclavicular catheter. (From Enneking FK, Ilfeld BM [eds.], *Major surgery in the ambulatory environment: continuous catheters and home infusions*. In: Van Aken H [ed.], *Clinical Anaesthesiology*. London: Ballière Tindall, 2002, p. 287. Reproduced with permission.)

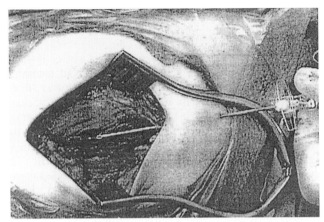

Figure 2-8   The catheter is placed at the base of the wound. (From Enneking FK, Ilfeld BM [eds.], *Major surgery in the ambulatory environment: continuous catheters and home infusions*. In: Van Aken H [ed.], *Clinical Anaesthesiology*. London: Ballière Tindall, 2002, p. 288. Reproduced with permission.)

the groups was the improved ability to participate in physical therapy.

Upper extremity analgesia below the shoulder can be effectively applied with the use of infraclavicular brachial plexus catheter placement (Fig. 2-7). Some clinicians use the coracoid technique initially described by Whiffler,[251] and later by Wilson et al.[252] This approach to the brachial plexus places a catheter at the level of the brachial plexus cords. The landmark for this block, the coracoid process, is readily identifiable even in obese patients. The technique is simple to perform[251,252] and has a high success rate.[251] Compared to catheters placed in the axillary region, infraclavicular catheters are more comfortable for patients and are resistant to dislodgment because the catheter transverses the mass of the pectoralis muscles.[253] The improvement in analgesia with infraclavicular catheter analgesia has recently been demonstrated following ambulatory hand surgery by Ilfeld et al.[254] These authors compared pain scores, opioid use, sleep disturbances, and satisfaction in patients receiving either ropivacaine or normal saline via infraclavicular catheters. In all categories, the patients in the ropivacaine group had improvement compared to the placebo group. This is the only double-blind, randomized, placebo-controlled trial of the efficacy of continuous peripheral nerve blocks.

Foot and ankle surgery can also be exquisitely painful and lends itself to continuous sciatic nerve block.[255,256] Singelyn et al. first described the use of continuous popliteal blockade for patients undergoing extensive foot and ankle surgery.[255] Consistent with other reports of continuous peripheral nerve blocks, these authors reported decreased supplemental opioid requirements and higher patient satisfaction compared to a control group receiving patient-controlled intravenous opioids. For patients in whom the territory of the saphenous nerve is not trespassed during surgery, this technique works extraordinarily well, with average visual analog scale (VAS) scores consistently less than 2 on a 10-point scale.[255,256]

There are data to suggest that direct local anesthetic perfusion of the wound bed via a surgically placed catheter improves analgesia following iliac bone crest harvesting and

subacromial decompression.[257,258] Brull et al. demonstrated a difference in pain at the iliac crest graft harvest site during long-term follow-up when a local anesthetic wound perfusion group was compared to a control group.[257] Compared to placement of perineural catheters, wound catheter insertion is technically much simpler. The catheter is placed under direct vision by the surgeon at the conclusion of the procedure (Fig. 2-8). This may make these techniques more widely applicable than perineural catheter techniques. However, they have not been studied as extensively as perineural techniques. From the limited data available, the degree of analgesia provided by wound catheters does not appear to be as profound as that provided by perineural catheters. A comparison of these two techniques is outlined in Table 2-7.

Table 2-7   Comparative Advantages and Disadvantages of Continuous Regional Analgesia Techniques

	Continuous Peripheral Nerve Block	Continuous Wound Perfusion
Visual analog scale	0–1	3–4
Sensory block	Yes	No
Motor block	Some degree	No
Patient-controlled bolus	Yes	Not studied
Difficulty of placement	Skilled anesthesiologist	Technically simple
Risk of infection	Yes, soft tissue	Yes, wound or bony

SOURCE: Modified and reprinted from Enneking FK, Ilfeld BM. Continuous wound infusions for analgesia. In: Chelly JE, Casati A, Fanelli G (eds.), *Continuous Peripheral Nerve Block Techniques*. Italy: Mosby, 2001, pp. 81–84. Reproduced with permission.

INFUSION DEVICES AND LOCAL ANESTHETIC SOLUTIONS

The choices of equipment and anesthetic are critical to the success of continuous regional analgesia in the ambulatory environment. There is a current boom in the infusion devices available to practitioners. For ambulatory infusions there are currently two categories of pump: battery-powered electronic and spring/vacuum/elastometric-powered nonelectronic pumps (Fig. 2-9). There are advantages and disadvantages for each type of infusion device. Balloon or vacuum pump technology is simple and easy to explain to the patient. The main disadvantages of these pumps are the inaccuracy of the infusion rates,[259] the inability to change or tailor the infusion rate, and, in most models, the inability to provide for patient-controlled boluses. Battery-powered electronic pumps that allow variable infusion rates and patient-controlled boluses are more complicated to explain to patients but allow for a lower basal infusion rate because of the patient-controlled bolus function. Continuous infusion of local anesthetic with a high basal infusion rate can lead to higher local anesthetic blood levels when compared to intermittent boluses using the same dosage of medication.[260]

The preferred mode of infusion is a low basal infusion rate with intermittent patient-controlled boluses. Singelyn and colleagues studied the mode of infusion delivery in patients following shoulder, hip, and knee surgery. They found higher patient satisfaction and lower local anesthetic consumption when the low basal infusion with patient-controlled bolus mode was compared to high basal infusion rate or patient-controlled intermittent boluses with no basal infusion modes.[249,261,262] The basal rate should be the lowest rate that provides patient comfort at rest. Clinical experience indicates that this rate varies according to the site of insertion, although it has not been extensively investigated (Table 2-8). The lower local anesthetic consumption is particularly important for outpatient therapy in which a set anesthetic reservoir frequently limits the infusion duration. The ideal drug for continuous regional analgesia in the ambulatory environment should have the following properties: it should be nontoxic if inadvertently overdosed, and it should produce a nociceptive block exclusively, preserve motor strength, and allow some degree of sensory perception. Currently, no ideal drug is available. Bupivacaine and ropivacaine are the most commonly used drugs for nerve blocks reported in the literature. Although ropivacaine is less cardiotoxic than bupivacaine when equal dosages are compared, there is intense debate over the relative potencies of the two drugs.[263,264] There are few studies comparing drugs using continuous peripheral nerve blocks. Borgeat et al. compared the use of 0.2% ropivacaine to 0.15% bupivacaine for infusion via indwelling interscalene catheters following major shoulder surgery.[265] They found that both drugs provided a similar degree of analgesia. However, those patients receiving ropivacaine had better preserved hand strength compared to those patients receiving bupivacaine. These results are similar to those from a study comparing epidural ropivacaine and bupivacaine in volunteers. In this investigation, motor strength of the lower extremity was preserved in the ropivacaine group as compared to the progressive motor block observed in all the bupivacaine groups.[266] This difference in motor strength may be an advantage of using ropivacaine over bupivacaine. However, further study regarding this issue is necessary.

Many different drugs have been added to single-injection regional blocks to improve onset time, density, and duration. For continuous peripheral nerve blockade, the α_2-agonist clonidine and multiple opioids have been used in an attempt to improve the quality of analgesia provided by the local anesthetic.[240,255,267] None of these drugs has been studied in a rigorous manner to validate their use. If a specific drug can be shown to reduce the hourly consumption of local anesthetic, this would be an important advantage for ambulatory patients. Theoretically, a reduc-

Table 2-8   Typical Infusion Settings for Various Catheter Sites

Catheter Location	Basal Rate (mL/hr)	Patient-Controlled Bolus (mL)
Axillary	8–12	4
Interscalene	5–8	2
Infraclavicular	5–10	2–4
Psoas compartment	8–12	4
Femoral	6–10	2–4
Sciatic	5–8	2–4
Popliteal	6–10	2–4
Wound	2–6	?

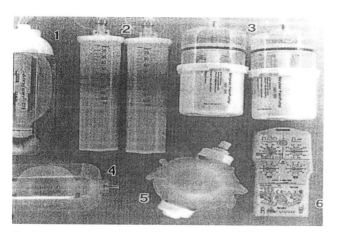

Figure 2-9   Ambulatory infusion devices. (1) McKinley Accufuser elastometric pump; (2) Sgarlato Labs spring-powered pump; (3) Stryker Instruments vacuum-powered pump; (4) MPS acacia Med-Flo II elastometric pump; (5) I-Flow C-Block elastometric pump; and (6) Sorenson Microject PCA electronic pump. (From Enneking FK, Ilfeld BM [eds.], Major surgery in the ambulatory environment: continuous catheters and home infusions. In: Van Aken H [ed.], *Clinical Anaesthesiology.* London: Ballière Tindall, 2002, p. 290. Reproduced with permission.)

tion in the hourly local anesthetic consumption would reduce the risk of toxicity from high local anesthetic levels and the duration of the infusion could be extended. With the current pump technology available, the amount of infusion solution is usually limited to 250–500 mL.

PATIENT EDUCATION

Perhaps the single most important factor for success of continuous perineural and wound infusion in the ambulatory environment is education of its consumers, both patients and physicians. Patient selection is of the utmost importance when considering the application of these techniques (Table 2-9). Instructions, including cautions and limitations of continuous regional analgesia, should be discussed with the patient and caregiver prior to discharge from an ambulatory facility. A written copy of these instructions should also be given to the patient and caregiver as a reference following discharge. Telephone communication must be available to the patient at all times. Typically, the instructions vary slightly depending on the site of catheter placement. Patients with upper-extremity catheters should be instructed to protect their arm in a sling, if possible. Patients with lower-extremity catheters must be instructed to always have an aid for ambulation and to avoid weight bearing on the surgical extremity. After foot and ankle surgery, patients must be specifically cautioned about the necessity of extremity elevation. These precautions, along with standard ambulatory instructions, including driving restrictions, must be emphasized to both the patient and candidate for outpatient perineural analgesia.

Surgeons must be aware of the limitations of continuous local anesthetic infusion therapy in the ambulatory environment. This technique for providing analgesia works best in concert with a multimodal regimen of analgesics. Traditional oral analgesics must be prescribed to treat pain in areas not covered by the site-specific catheter and breakthrough pain. Dressings must be carefully applied to allow for anticipated edema formation. Patients with continuous local anesthetic infusions may not notice the same degree

Table 2-9   Important Elements in Patient Selection for Continuous Ambulatory Local Anesthetic Infusions

- Surgery of such magnitude that pain is unlikely to be controlled by oral analgesics.
- Patient or caregiver must be able to understand instructions and warnings.
- Telecommunication device must be available at all times.
- Communication with administering physician must occur at least every 24 hr.
- Must be able to demonstrate ambulation with or without aids prior to discharge.
- Transportation must be readily available.

of compressive pressure. If drains are placed in the wound bed along with a wound catheter much of the local anesthetic may be recovered in the drain. This should be considered when examining wound drainage volumes.

CURRENT CONTROVERSIES

Should one allow patients to receive home local anesthetic infusion therapy? Although ambulatory application of continuous local anesthetic infusions is the basis of this discussion, these techniques are in their infancy in many regards. For practitioners with many years of experience using continuous regional analgesic techniques, the transition from in-hospital care of these patients to the ambulatory setting has been seen as a natural progression.[239,268] For the novice practitioner of these techniques, the lack of experience with the nuances of catheter placement, dressing, pump capabilities and limitations, and organized patient follow-up may require an initial period of in-hospital use. There are several caveats that must be observed for the safe practice of these techniques in an ambulatory environment:

1. Patients should be carefully selected for compliance.
2. The pump device must have a mechanical or electronic flow restrictor to ensure appropriate local anesthetic administration. Devices that rely on the patient to start and stop the infusion of local anesthetic are less desirable as the patient may inadvertently dispense more medication than desired.
3. Physicians or their representatives must be available at all times for consultation.

Will continuous local anesthetic infusions be supplanted by microsphere encapsulated local anesthetic preparations in the future? Encapsulated local anesthetic preparations certainly have the potential to provide analgesia comparable to that attainable with continuous peripheral nerve blockade.[269] The development of these preparations has progressed slowly and they are currently not available to patients. Research into ideal concentrations and delivery vehicles remains to be done. The biggest advantage these preparations may offer is the simplicity of a standard single-injection technique. However, they may not offer the flexibility of patient-controlled bolus or variable infusion rates that continuous catheter techniques offer. Experience with continuous perineural local anesthetic infusions will surely be applicable to the care of patients receiving encapsulated local anesthetics in the future.

SUMMARY

Continuous peripheral nerve blocks are an exciting area of analgesia that is in its infancy. There have been remarkably few complications attributed to these techniques.[270,271] The improvement in patient satisfaction, rehabilitation, and low complication rates should encourage the continued development of these techniques.

REFERENCES

1. Riese W, Arrington GE, Jr. The history of Johannes Müller's doctrine of the specific energies of the senses: original and later versions. Bull Hist Med 1963;37:179–83.

2. Dallenbach KM. Pain: History and present status. Am J Psychol 1939;52:331.

3. Melzack R, Wall PD. Pain mechanisms: A new theory. Science 1965;150:971–75.

4. Rynd F. Neuralgia—Introduction of fluid to the nerve. Dublin Med Press 1855;13:167.

5. Pravaz CG. Sur un nouveau moyen d'operer la coagulation du sang dans les arteres, applicable a la guerison des aneurismes. CR Acad Sci (Paris) 1853;36:88.

6. Wood A. New method of treating neuralgia by the direct application of opiates to the painful points. Edinb Med Surg J 1855;82:265.

7. Bonica JJ. *The Management of Pain*. Philadelphia: Lea & Febiger, 1953.

8. Macht DI, Herman NB, Levy CS. A quantitative study of the analgesia produced by opium alkaloids individually and in combination with each other. J Pharmacol 1916;8:1–37.

9. Macht DI, Johnson SL, Bollinger HG. On the peripheral action of the opium alkaloids. Effect on the sensory nerve terminals. J. Pharmacol 1916;8:451–63.

10. Gaedcke F. Uber das Erythroxylin, dargestellt aus den blattern des in Sudamerika cultiverten straucheserythroxylon coca lam. Arch Pharm 1885;132:141–50.

11. Niemann A. Ueber eine neue organische Base in den Cocablättern. *Inaug-diss*. Göttingen, 1860, p. 52. A preliminary report is given by F. Wöhler: Ueber eine organische Base in der Coca. Justus Liebigs Ann Chem 1860;114:213.

12. Lossen W. Ueber das Cocain. Ann Chem Pharm 1865;133:351–71.

13. Singer C, Underwood EA. *A Short History of Medicine*, 2nd ed. Oxford; Clarendon Press, 1962, quote p. 349.

14. Killian H. *Lokalanästhesie und Lokalanästhetika*. Stuttgart: G. Thieme, 1959.

15. Leake CD. The historical development of surgical anesthesia. Sci Month 1925;20:304–28.

16. Bender GA, Thom RA. *Great Moments in Medicine*. Detroit: Parke-Davis, 1961.

17. Mortimer WG. *Peru History of Coca*. New York: JH Bvail, 1901.

18. Moreno y Maiz T. Recherches chimiques et physiologiques sur l'Erythroxylum Coca du Pérou. Thèse de Paris, 1868, p. 91.

19. Bennett A. An experimental inquiry into the physiological actions of caffeine, theine, guaranine, cocaine, and theobromine. Edinb Med J 1873;19:323–41.

20. Sollmann T. *A Manual of Pharmacology*, 8th ed. Philadelphia: WB Saunders, 1957, quote from p. 323.

21. von Anrep B. Ueber die physiologische Wirking des Cocain. Pflügers Arch Physiol 1880;21:38–77.

22. Collin P. De la Coca et ses véeritables propriététes thérapeutiques. Méd Prat Franc 1877;24:239–40.

23. Einhorn A. Ueber neue Arzneimittel. Fünfte Abhandlung. Justus Liebigs Ann Chem 1909;371:125–31, quote from p. 127.

24. Clark AJ. Aspects of the history of anaesthetics. Br Med J 1938;II:1029–34.

25. Koller C. Historical notes on the beginning of local anesthesia. JAMA 1928;90:1742–43. The article was also published in German (1928) in Wien Med Wschr 78:601–2 and again in 1934 in the same journal 84:1179–80.

26. Koller-Becker H. Carl Koller and cocaine. Psychoanal Q 1963; 32–309–73.

27. Gaertner J. Die Entdeckung der Localanästesie. Der neue Tag, 1919. Also in Neue freie Presse under Unterhaltung. Quoted from Koller-Becker, 1963, p. 331.

28. Koller C. Verläufige Mitteilung über lokale Anästhesierung am Auge. Bericht über die 16. Versammlung der ophthalmologischen Gesellschaft. Heidelberg. Beilageheft zu Klin Mbl Augenh 1884; 60–63.

29. Koller C. Preliminary report on local anesthesia of the eye. Arch Ophthalmol 1934;12:473–74.

30. Koller C. Nachträgliche Bemerkungen über die ersten Anfänge der Lokalanästhesie. Wien Med Wschr 1935;85–708. Also: History of cocaine as a local anesthetic. JAMA 1941;117:1284–87.

31. Jellinek E. Das Cocain als Anaestheticum und Analgeticum für den Pharynx und Larynx. Wien Med Wschr 1884;34:1334–48, 1364–67.

32. Fränkel E. Über Cocain als Mittel zur Anästhesierung der Genitalschleimhaut. Wien Med Wschr 1884;34:1535.

33. Noyes HD. The Ophthalmologic Congress in Heidelberg. Med Rec 1884;26:417–18.

34. Matas R. Local and regional anesthesia: a retrospect and prospect. Am J Surg 1934;65:189–98, 362–79.

35. Knapp H. On cocaine and its use in ophthalmic and general surgery. Arch Ophthalmol 1884;13:402–48.

36. Hall RJ. Letter to the Editor. NY Med J 1884;41:643.

37. Fulton JF. *Harvey Cushing. A Biography*. Springfield, IL: CC Thomas, 1946, quote pp. 142–44 (Letter from Halsted to Cushing).

38. Halsted WS. Practical comments on the use and abuse of cocaine. Suggested by its invariably successful employment in more than a thousand minor surgical operations. NY Med J 1885;42:294–95.

39. MacCallum WG. *William Stewart Halsted Surgeon*. Baltimore: Johns Hopkins Press, 1930, quote pp. 54–57.

40. Corning JL. On the prolongation of the anaesthetic effects of the hydrochloride of cocaine when subcutaneously injected. NY Med J 1885;42:317–19.

41. Freud S. Ueber Coca. Cbl Ges Ther 2:289–314. Further (1885). Beitrag zur Kenntnis der Cocawirkung. Wien Med Wschr 1884;35:129–33, and (1885). Ueber die Allgemeinwirkung des Cocains. Med-chir Cbl 20:374–75. English translations in S Freud (1963). *The Cocaine Papers*: 1:26, 35–41 and 45–49. Vienna and Zürich: Dunquin Press.

42. Liljestrand G. Briefe von Carl Koller an Erik Nordenson. Arch Gesch Med 1965;49:280–306.

43. Corning JL. A further contribution on local medication of the spinal cord. Med Rec (NY) 1888;33:291–93.

44. Bier A. Versuche über Cocainisieurung des Rückenmarks. Dtsch Z Chir 1899;51.

45. Pitkin G. Controllable spinal anesthesia. Am J Surg 1928;5:537–53.

46. Sicard A. Les injections medicamenteuses extra-durales par Voie sacro-coccygienne. CR Soc Biol (Paris) 1901;53:396–98.

47. Cathelin F. Une nouvelle voie d'injection rachidienne. Méthodes des injections épidurales par le procédé du canal sacré. Applications à l'homme. CR Soc Biol (Paris) 1901;53:452–53.

48. Läwen A. Uber Extraduralanänsthesie für chirurgische Operationen. Dtsch Z Chir 1910;108:1–43.

49. Gros O. Ueber die Narkotika und Lokalanästhetika. Arch Exp Path Pharmak 1910;63:80–106.

50. Läwen A, Gaza W von. Experimentelle Untersuchungen über Extraduralanästhesie. Dtsch Z Chir 1911;111:289–307.

51. Reclus P. De l'anesthésie locale par la cocaine. Gax Hebd Méd Chir 1890;27:146–48.

52. Schleich CL. *Schmerzlose Operationen. Örtliche Betäubung mit indifferenten Flössigkeiten*. Berlin: Springer, 1894, (5th ed., 1906).

53. Willstätter R. Ueber die Synthese des Psikains. Münich Med Wschr 1924;71:849–50.

54. Filehne W. Die local-anästhesirende Wirkung von Benzoyl-derivaten. Berl Klin Wschr 1887;24:107–8.

55. Poulsson E. Beiträge zur Kenntniss der pharmakologischen Gruppe des Cocains. Arch Exp Path Pharmak 1890;27:301–13.

56. Ehrlich P. Studien in der Cocainreihe. Dtsch Med Wschr 1890;16:717–19.

57. Ehrlich P, Einhorn A. Ueber die physiologische Wirkung der Verbindungen der Cocainreihe. Ber Dtsch Chem Ges 1894;27:1870–73.

58. Laubender W. Lokalanaesthetica. Heffter's Handb Exp Pharmakol, Erg.-werk, 1939;8:1–78.

59. Braun H, Läwen A. Die örtliche Betäbung, 8th ed. Leipzig; JA Barth, 1933.

60. Einhorn A, Heinz R. Orthoform. Ein Lokalanaestheticum für Wundschmerz, Brandwunden, Geschwüre, etc. Münch Med Wschr 1897;44:931–34.

61. Braun H. Ueber die Bedeutung des Adrenalins für die Chirurgie. Münch Med Wschr 1903;50:352–53.

62. Einhorn A, Uhlfelder E. Ueber den p-Aminobenzoesäure-diäthyl-amino- and Piperidoäthylester. Justus Liebigs Ann Chem 1909;371:131–42.

63. Braun H. Die Lokalanästhesie, ihre wissenschaftlichen Grundlagen und praktische Anwendung. Leipzig; JA Barth, 1905.

64. Gottlieb R. Pharmakologische Untersuchungen über die Stereoiso-merie der Kokaine. Arch Exp Path Pharmak 1923;97:113–46.

65. Gottlieb R. Ueber die pharmakologische Bedeutung des Psikains als Lokalanästhetikum. Münch Med Wschr 1924;71:850–51.

66. Euler H von, Erdtman H. Ueber Gramin aus Schwedischen Ger-stensippen. Justis Liebigs Ann Chem 1935;520:1–10.

67. Erdtman H, Löfgren N. Ueber eine neue Gruppe von lokalanäs-thetisch wirksamen Verbindungen. a-N-Dialkylaminosäureanilide. Svensk Kem T 1937;49:163–74.

68. Löfgren N. Studies in Local Anesthetics. Xylocaine, a New Synthetic Drug. Thesis I. Haeggström, Stockholm, 1948. Reprinted. Worcester, MA, 1958.

69. Löfgren N. Studien über Lokalanästhetica. Ark Kemi Mineral Geol 1946;22:No. 18:1–30.

70. Goldberg L. Studies on local anesthetics: pharmacological proper-ties of homologues and isomers of xylocain (alkyl aminoacyl de-rivatives). Acta Physiol Scand 1949;18:1–18.

71. Björn H. Electrical excitation of teeth and its application to den-tistry. Diss. Stockholm. Also as Suppl 4 to Svensk Tandläk-T 1946;39:1–101.

72. Björn H, Huldt S. The efficiency of xylocaine as a dental terminal anesthetic, compared to that of procain. Svensk Tandläk-T 1947;40:831–52.

73. Gordh T. Xylocaine—a new local analgesic. Anaesthesia 1949;4:4–9, 21.

74. Bier A. Ueber einen neuen Weg Localanasthesie an den Glied-massen zu erzeugen. Arch Klin Chir 1908;86:1007.

75. Wynter WE. Four cases of tuberculosus meningitis in which para-centesis of the theca vertebralis was performed for the relief of fluid pressure. Lancet 1891;1:981.

76. Tuffier T. Analgesie chirurgicale par l'injection sous-arachnoidienne lombaire de cocaine. CR Soc Biol 11th Series, 1899;1:882.

77. Tuffier T. Anesthesie medullaire chirurgicale par injection sous-arachnoidienne lombaire de cocaine; technique et resultats. Sem med 1900;20:167.

78. Hopkins GS. Anesthesia by cocainization of the spinal cord. Philadelphia Med J 1900;6:864.

79. Fowler RG. Cocaine analgesia from subarachnoid injection, with a report of forty-four cases together with a report of a case in which antipyrin was used. Philadelphia Med J 1900;6:843.

80. Lee EW. Subarachnoidean injections of cocaine as a substitute for general anesthesia in operations below the diaphragm, with report of seven cases. Philadelphia Med J 1900;6:865.

81. Gray HT, Parsons L. Blood pressure variations associated with lum-bar puncture and the induction of spinal anesthesia. Q J Med 1912;5:339.

82. Smith GS, Porter WT. Spinal anesthesia in the cat. Am J Physiol 1915;38:108.

83. Barker AE. Clinical experiences with spinal analgesia in 100 cases and some reflections on the procedure. Br Med J 1907;1:665.

84. Hepburn WG. Stovain spinal analgesia. Am J Surg 1920;34:87.

85. Sise LF. Spinal anesthesia for upper and lower abdominal opera-tions. N Engl J Med 1928;199:61.

86. Adriani J, Roman-Vega D. Saddle block anesthesia. Am J Surg 1946;71:12.

87. Lemmon WT. A method for continuous spinal anesthesia. Ann Surg 1940;111:141.

88. Dean HP. Relative value of inhalation and injection methods of in-ducing anaesthesia. Br Med J 1907;2:869.

89. Kreis O. Ueber Medullarnarkose bei Gebarenden. Zentralbl Gy-nakol 1900;24:724.

90. Marx S. Analgesia in obstetrics produced by medullary injections of cocaine. Philadelphia Med J 1900;6:857.

91. Stoeckel W. Ueber sakrale Anasthesie. Zentralbl Gynaekol 1909;33:1.

92. Kappis M. Erfahrungen mit Lokalanasthesie bei Bauchoperatio-nen. Verh Dtsch Ges Chir 1914;43:87.

93. Läwen A. Ueber segmentare Schmerzaufhebung durch paraverte-brale Novokaininjektionen zur Differentialdiagnose intra-abdominaler Erkrankungen. Med Wochenschr 1922;69:1423.

94. Mandl F. Die Wirkung der paravertebralen Injektion bei "Angina pectoris." Arch Klin Chir 1925;136:495.

95. Swetlow GI. Paravertebral alcohol block in cardiac pain. Am Heart J 1926;1:393.

96. Schloesser. Heilung peripharer Reizzustande sensibler und mo-torischer Nerven. Klin Monatsbl Augenheilkd 1903;41:244.

97. Pagés F. Anestesia metamerica. Rev Sanid Milit Argent 1921;11:351–65.

98. Dogliotti AM. Eine neue Methode der regionaren Anasthesie: "Die peridurale segmentare Anasthesie." Zentralbl Chir 1931;58:3141.

99. Dogliotti AM. A new method of block anesthesia: segmental peridural spinal anesthesia. Am J Surg 1933;20:107.

100. Curbelo MM. Continuous peridural segmental anesthesia by means of a ureteral catheter. Anesth Analg 1949;28:13.

101. Sarnoff SJ, Arrowood JG. Differential spinal block. Surgery 1946;20:150.

102. Nicoll JH. The surgery of infancy. Br Med J 1909;2:753.

103. Waters RM. The down-town anesthesia clinic. Am J Surg (Anes-thesia Suppl) 1919;33:71–73.

104. Cohen D, Dillon JB. Anesthesia for outpatient surgery. JAMA 1966;196:98–100.

105. White PF. Anesthesia for ambulatory surgery. In: Stoelting RK (ed.), Advances in Anesthesia. Chicago: Year Book, 1985, pp. 1–29.

106. White PF. Outpatient anesthesia. In: Miller RD (ed.), Anesthesia. New York: Churchill Livingstone, 1985, pp. 1895–920.

107. White PF. Newer anesthetic drugs and techniques for outpatient anesthesia. Anesth Rev 1990;17:53–63.

108. White PF. Outpatient anesthesia—an overview. In: White PF (ed.). Outpatient Anesthesia. New York: Churchill Livingstone, 1990, pp. 1–56.

109. Östman PL, White PF. Outpatient anesthesia. In: Miller RD (ed.), Anesthesia. New York: Churchill Livingstone, 1994, pp. 2213–46.

110. Smith I, White PF. Anaesthesia for day-case surgery. Curr Anaesth Crit Care 1992;3:77–83.

111. Smith I, White PF. Impact of newer drugs and techniques on the quality of ambulatory anesthesia. J Clin Anesth 1993;5:3S–13S.

112. Saint-Maurice C, Kong-Ky BH, Hamza J, et al. Pediatric surgery and anesthesia in a day hospital. Cahiers d'Anesth 1993;41:407–11.

113. Chung F. Outpatient anesthesia: which is the best anaesthetic tech-nique? Can J Anaesth 1991;38(7):882–86.

114. White PF. Anesthetic techniques for the elderly outpatient. Anaes-thesiol Clin 1988;26:105–11.

115. Vessey JA, Bogetz MS, Caserza CL, et al. Parental upset associated with participation in induction of anaesthesia in children. Can J Anaesth 1994;41(4):276–80.

116. Allen HW, Mulroy MF, Fundis K, et al. Regional versus propofol

anesthesia for outpatient hand surgery. Anesthesiology 1993; 79:A1.

117. Brown AR, Weiss R, Greenberg CP, et al. Interscalene block for shoulder arthroscopy: a comparison with general anesthesia. J Arthro Relat Surg 1993;9:295–300.

118. D'Alessio JG, Rosenblum M, Shea KP, et al. A retrospective comparison of interscalene block and general anesthesia for ambulatory surgery shoulder arthroscopy. Reg Anesth 1995;20:62–68.

119. Smith I, White PF. Monitored anaesthesia care: use of adjuvant drugs. Mimimally Invasive Therapy 1994;3:5.

120. White PF, Smith I. Use of sedation techniques during local and regional anesthesia. Can J Anaesth 1995;42:R38–R46.

121. White PF. Use of ketamine for sedation and analgesia during the injection of local anesthetics. Am Plast Surg 1985;15:53–56.

122. Davies BW, Pennington GA, Guyuron B. Clinical office anesthesia: the use of propofol for the induction and maintenance of general anesthesia. Aesthetic Plast Surg 1993;17:125–28.

123. Friedberg BL. Propofol-ketamine technique. Aesthetic Plast Surg 1993;17:297–300.

124. White PF. Use of continuous infusion versus intermittent bolus administration of fentanyl or ketamine during outpatient anesthesia. Anesthesiology 1983;59:294–300.

125. Shafer A, White PF. New agents and techniques for outpatient anesthesia. Anesthesiol Rep 1990;3:82–96.

126. Smith I, Zelcer J, White PF. Anaesthesia for day-case surgery. Curr Opin Anaesth 1992;5:760–66.

127. White PF. Clinical uses of intravenous anesthetic and analgesic infusions. Anesth Rev 1989;68:161–71.

128. White PF, Shaler A, Boyle WA, et al. Benzodiazepine antagonism does not provoke a stress response. Anesthesiology 1989;70:636–39.

129. White PF. Continuous infusions of thiopental, methohexital, or etomidate as adjuvants to nitrous oxide for outpatient anesthesia. Anesth Analg 1984;63:282.

130. White PF. Outpatient anesthesia techniques—continuous infusions of intravenous anesthetics. West J Med 1984;140:437–38.

131. Wagner RL, White PF. Etomidate inhibits adrenocortical function in surgical patients. Anesthesiology 1984;61:647–51.

132. Smith I, Monk TG, White PF, et al. Propofol infusion during regional anesthesia: sedative, amnestic and anxiolytic properties. Anesth Analg 1994;79:313–19.

133. Watcha MF, Ramirez-Ruiz M, Jones MB, et al. Comparison of postoperative oxygen saturation following propofol-nitrous oxide halothane-nitrous oxide anesthesia in children. J Pediatr Anesth 1994;4:383–89.

134. Doze VA, Westphal LM, White PF. Comparison of propofol with methohexital for outpatient anesthesia. Anesth Analg 1986; 65:1189–95.

135. Fletcher JE, Sebel PS, Murphy MR, et al. Psychomotor performance after desflurane anesthesia: a comparison with isoflurane. Anesth Analg 1991;73:260–65.

136. Korttila K, Nuotto EJ, Lichtor JL, et al. Clinical recovery and psychomotor function after brief anesthesia with propofol or thiopental. Anesthesiology 1992;76:676–81.

137. Doze VA, Shafer A, White PF. Propofol-nitrous oxide versus thiopental-isoflurane-nitrous oxide for general anesthesia. Anesthesiology 1988;69:63–71.

138. Pace NA, Victory RA, White PF. Anesthetic infusion techniques—how to do it. J Clin Anesth 1992;4:45S–52S.

139. Watcha MF, Simeon RM, White PF, et al. Effect of propofol on the incidence of postoperative vomiting after strabismus surgery in pediatric outpatients. Anesthesiology 1991;75:204–9.

140. Weir PM, Munro HM, Reynolds PI, et al. Propofol infusion and the incidence of emesis in pediatric outpatient strabismus surgery. Anesth Analg 1993;76:760–64.

141. Borgeat A, Wilder-Smith OHG, Saiah M, et al. Subhypnotic doses of propofol possess direct antiemetic properties. Anesth Analg 1992;74:539–41.

142. Blackwell KE, Ross DA, Kapur P, et al. Propofol for maintenance of general anesthesia: a technique to limit blood loss during endoscopic sinus surgery. Am J Otolaryng 1993;14:262–66.

143. Fredman B, Nathanson MH, Wang J, et al. Use of sevoflurane vs. propofol for outpatient anesthesia: recovery profiles. Anesth Analg 1994;78:S121.

144. Avramov M, White PF. The comparative effects of methohexital, propofol and etomidate for electroconvulsive therapy. Anesth Analg 1995;81:596–602.

145. Van Hemelrijck J, Muller P, Van Aken H, et al. Relative potency of eltanolone, propofol, and thiopental for induction of anesthesia. Anesthesiology 1994;80:36–41.

146. Kallela H, Haasio J, Korttila K. Comparison of eltanolone and propofol in anesthesia for termination of pregnancy. Anesth Analg 1994;79:512–16.

147. Raeder J, Hole A, Arnulf V, et al. Total intravenous anaesthesia with midazolam and flumazenil in outpatient clinics: a comparison with isoflurane or thiopentone. Acta Anaesthesiol Scand 1987;31:634–41.

148. Van Hemelrijck J, White PF. Intravenous anesthesia for day-care surgery. In: Kay B (ed.), *Total Intravenous Anaesthesia*. Amsterdam: Elsevier, 1991, pp. 323–350.

149. Raftery S, Sherry E. Total intravenous anaesthesia with propofol and alfentanil protects against post operative nausea and vomiting. Can J Anaesth 1992;39(1):37–40.

150. Fredman B, Ding Y, White PF. Day-care surgery and anesthesia: recovery of mental and psychomotor function. Curr Opin Anaesth 6:659–64.

151. White PF. In defense of volatile anesthetics for outpatient surgery. Anesthesiology 1984;60:605–6.

152. Blobner M, Schneck HJ, Felber AR, et al. Comparative study of the recovery phase. Laparoscopic cholecystectomy following isoflurane, methohexital and propofol anesthesia. Anaesthesist 1994; 43:573–81.

153. White PF. Studies of desflurane in outpatient anesthesia. Anesth Analg 1992;75:S47–S54.

154. Smith I, Taylor E, White PF. Comparison of tracheal extubation in patients deeply anesthetized with desflurane and isoflurane. Anesth Analg 1994;79:642–45.

155. Smith I, Nathanson MH, White PF. The role of sevoflurane in outpatient anesthesia. Anesth Analg 1995;81:567–72.

156. Carter JA, Dye AM, Cooper GM. Recovery from day-case anaesthesia: the effect of different inhalational anaesthetic agents. Anaesthesia 1985;40:545–48.

157. Fisher DM, Robinson S, Brett CM, et al. Comparison of enflurane, halothane, and isoflurane for diagnostic and therapeutic procedures in children with malignancies. Anesthesiology 1985;63: 647–50.

158. Ghouri AF, Bodner M, White PF. Recovery profile following desflurane-nitrous oxide versus isoflurane-nitrous oxide in outpatients. Anesthesiology 1991;74:419–24.

159. Van Helmelrijck J, Smith I, White PF. Use of desflurane for outpatient anesthesia: a comparison with propofol and nitrous oxide. Anesthesiology 1991;75:197–203.

160. Rapp SE, Conahan TJ, Pavlin DJ, et al. Comparison of desflurane with propofol in outpatients undergoing peripheral orthopedic surgery. Anesth Analg 1992;75:572–79.

161. Piat V, Dubois MC, Johanet S, et al. Induction and recovery characteristics and hemodynamic responses to sevoflurane and halothane in children. Anesth Analg 1994;79:841–43.

162. Sarner JB, Levine M, Davis PJ, et al. Clinical characteristics of sevoflurane in children—a comparison with halothane. Anesthesiology 1995;83:38–46.

163. Smith I, Ding Y, White PF. Comparison of induction, maintenance and recovery characteristics of sevoflurane-N_2O and propofol sevoflurane-N_2O with propofol-isoflurane-N_2O anesthesia. Anesth Analg 1992;74:253–59.

164. Nathanson MH, Fredman B, Smith I, et al. Sevoflurane vs desflurane for outpatient anesthesia: a comparison of maintenance and recovery profiles. Anesth Analg 1995;81:1186–90.

165. Fredman B, Nathanson MH, Smith I, et al. Sevoflurane for outpatient anesthesia: a comparison with propofol. Anesth Analg 1995;81:823–28.

166. Sukhani R, Lurie J, Jabamoni R. Propofol for ambulatory gynecologic laparoscopy: does omission of nitrous oxide alter postoperative emetic sequelae and recovery? Anesth Analg 1994;78:831–35.

167. Taylor E, Feinstein R, White PF, et al. Anesthesia for laparoscopic cholecystectomy—is nitrous oxide contraindicated? Anesthesiology 1992;76:541–43.

168. Lonie DS, Harper NJN. Nitrous oxide anaesthesia and vomiting—the effect of nitrous oxide anaesthesia on the incidence of vomiting following gynaecological laparoscopy. Anaesthesia 1986;41:703–7.

169. Melnick BM, Johnson LS. Effects of eliminating nitrous oxide in outpatient anesthesia. Anesthesiology 1987;67:982–84.

170. Pandit UA, Malviya S, Lewis IH. Vomiting after outpatient tonsillectomy and adenoidectomy in children: the role of nitrous oxide. Anesth Analg 1995;80:230–33.

171. Hovorka J, Korttila K, Erkola O. Nitrous oxide does not increase nausea and vomiting following gynaecological laparoscopy. Can J Anaesth 1989;36:145–48.

172. White PF, Stanley TH, Apfelbaum JL, et al. Effects on recovery when isoflurane is used to supplement propofol-nitrous oxide anesthesia. Anesth Analg 1993;77:S15–20.

173. White PF. Practical issues in outpatient anaesthesia—management of postoperative pain and emesis. Can J Anaesth 1995;42:1053–55.

174. Chang T-L, Dworsky WA, White PF. Use of continuous electromyography for monitoring depth of anesthesia. Anesth Analg 1988;67:521–25.

175. Mendel HG, Guarnieri KM, Sundt LM, et al. The effects of ketorolac and fentanyl on postoperative vomiting and analgesic requirements in children undergoing strabismus surgery. Anesth Analg 1995;80:1129–33.

176. Rosow CE, DiBiase PM, Zaslavsky A, et al. Propofol vs. thiopental in in-patients: comparison of recovery after general anesthesia. Anesthesiology 1993;79:A336.

177. Avramov MN, White PF. Use of alfentanil and propofol for monitored anesthesia care—determining the optimal dosing regimen for ambulatory surgery. Anesthesiology 1995;83:A15.

178. Watcha MF, White PF. Increased cost of ketorolac versus morphine sulphate. Anesthesiology 1992;70:61.

179. Ding Y, Fredman B, White PF. Use of ketorolac and fentanyl during outpatient gynecologic surgery. Anesth Analg 1993;77:205–10.

180. Higgins MS, Givogre JL, Marco AP, et al. Recovery from outpatient laparoscopic tubal ligation is not improved by preoperative administration of ketorolac or ibuprofen. Anesth Analg 1994;79:274–80.

181. Souter A, Fredman B, White PF. Controversies in the perioperative use of non-steroidal antiinflammatory drugs. Anesth Analg 1994;79:1178–90.

182. Smith I, Van Hemelrijck J, White PF. Efficacy of esmolol versus alfentanil as a supplement to propofol-nitrous oxide anesthesia. Anesth Analg 1991;73:540–46.

183. Aho M, Scheinin M, Lehtinen AM, et al. Intramuscularly administered dexmedetomidine attenuates hemodynamic and stress hormone responses to gynecologic laparoscopy. Anesth Analg 1992;76(6):932–39.

184. Smith K, Halliwell RMT, Lawrence S, et al. Acute renal failure associated with intramuscular ketorolac. Anaesth Intens Care 1993;21:700–703.

185. Zahl K, Apfelbaum JL. Muscle pain occurs after outpatient laparoscopy despite the substitution of vecuronium for succinylcholine. Anesthesiology 1989;70:408–11.

186. Poler SM, Watcha MF, White PF. Use of mivacurium as an alternative to succinylcholine during outpatient laparoscopy. J Clin Anesth 1992;4:127–33.

187. Tang J, Joshi G, White PF. Comparison of rocuronium and mivacurium to succinylcholine during laparoscopic surgery. Anesthesiology 1995;83:A2.

188. Pühringer FK, Khuenl-Brady KS, Koler J, et al. Evaluation of the endotracheal intubating conditions of rocuronium and succinylcholine in outpatient surgery. Anesth Analg 1992;75:37–40.

189. Ding Y, Fredman B, White PF. Use of mivacurium during laparoscopic surgery: effect of reversal drugs on postoperative recovery. Anesth Analg 1994;78:450–54.

190. Watcha MB, White PF. Nausea and vomiting: pharmacology and clinical uses of antiemetic drugs. In: Brown BR, Prys-Roberts C (eds.), General Anaesthesia. London: Butterworth-Heinemann, 1995.

191. Pennant JH, White PF. The laryngeal mask airway: its uses in anesthesiology. Anesthesiology 1993;79:144–63.

192. Watcha MF, Garner FT, White PF, et al. Laryngeal mask airway vs face mask and guedel airway during pediatric myringotomy. Arch Otolaryngol Head Neck Surg 1994;120:877–80.

193. Smith I, White PF. Use of the laryngeal mask airway as an alternative to a face mask during outpatient arthroscopy. Anesthesiology 1992;77:850–55.

194. Cork RC, Depa RM, Standen JR. Prospective comparison of the use of the laryngeal mask and tracheal tube for ambulatory surgery. Anesth Analg 1994;79:719–27.

195. Joshi GP, Smith I, Watcha MF, et al. A model for studying the cost-effectiveness of airway devices: laryngeal mask airway vs tracheal tube. Anesth Analg 1995;80:S219.

196. Owens TM, Robertson P, Twomey C, et al. The incidence of gastroesophageal reflux with the laryngeal mask: a comparison with the face mask using esophageal lumen pH electrodes. Anesth Analg 1995;80:980–84.

197. Brimacombe JR, Berry A. The incidence of aspiration associated with the laryngeal mask airway: a meta-analysis of published literature. J Clin Anesth 1995;7:297–305.

198. Macario A, Chang PC, Stempel DB, et al. A cost analysis of the laryngeal mask airway for elective surgery in adult outpatients. Anesthesiology 1995;83:250–57.

199. Ryan JA, Adye BA, Jolly PC, et al. Outpatient inguinal herniorrhaphy with both regional and local anesthesia. Am J Surg 1984;148:313.

200. Parnass SM, McCarthy RJ, Bach BR Jr, et al. Beneficial impact of epidural anesthesia on recovery after outpatient arthroscopy. Arthroscopy 1993;9:91–95.

201. Seeberger MD, Lang MJ, Drewe J, et al. Comparison of spinal and epidural anesthesia in patients younger than 50 years of age. Anesth Analg 1994;78:667–73.

202. Kang SB, Goodnough DE, Lee YK, et al. Comparison of 26- and 27-G needles for spinal anesthesia for ambulatory surgery patients. Anesthesiology 1992;76:734–38.

203. Manica VS, Bader AM, Fragneto R, et al. Anesthesia for in vitro fertilization: a comparison of 1.5% and 5% spinal lidocaine for ultrasonically guided oocyte retrieval. Anesth Analg 1993;77:453–56.

204. Kopacz DJ, Mulroy MF. Chloroprocaine and lidocaine decrease hospital stay and admission rate after outpatient epidural anesthesia. Reg Anesth 1990;15:19–25.

205. Urquhart ML, White PF. Comparison of sedative infusions during regional anesthesia—methohexital, etomidate, and midazolam. Anesth Analg 1989;68:249–54.

206. Reuben SS, Steinberg RB, Kreitzer JM, et al. Intravenous regional anesthesia using lidocaine and ketorolac. Anesth Analg 1995;81:110–13.

207. Flanagan JFK, Edkin B, Spindler K. 3 in 1 femoral nerve block following ACL reconstruction allows predictably earlier discharge and significant cost savings. Anesthesiology 1994;81:A950.

208. Behnia R, Hashemi F, Stryker SJ, et al. A comparison of general versus local anesthesia during inguinal herniorrhaphy. Surg Gynecol Obstet 1992;174:277–80.

209. White PF, Negus JB. Sedative infusions during local and regional anesthesia: a comparison of midazolam and propofol. J Clin Anesth 1991;3:32–39.

210. Ding Y, White PF. Post-herniorrhaphy pain in outpatients after preincision ilioinguinal-hypogastric nerve block during monitored anaesthesia care. Can J Anaesth 1995;42:12–15.

211. Stevens MH, White PF. Monitored anesthesia care. In: Miller RD (ed.), *Anesthesia*, 3rd ed. New York: Churchill Livingstone, 1994, pp. 1465–90.

212. Ramirez-Ruiz M, Smith I, White PF. Use of analgesics during propofol sedation: a comparison of ketorolac, dezocine and fentanyl. J Clin Anesth 1995;7:481–85.

213. Smith I, White PF, Nathanson M, et al. Propofol: an update on its clinical uses. Anesthesiology 1994;81:1005–43.

214. Bordahl PE, Raeder JC, Nordentoft J, et al. Laparoscopic sterilization under local or general anesthesia? A randomized study. Obst Gynecol 1993;81:137–41.

215. Raeder JC, Bordahl PE, Nordentoft J, et al. Ambulatory laparoscopic sterilization—should local analgesia and intravenous sedation replace general anesthesia: a comparative clinical trial. Den Norske Laegeforening 1993;113:1559–62.

216. Raeder JC. Propofol anaesthesia versus paracervical blockade with alfentanil and midazolam sedation for outpatient abortion. Acta Anaesthesiol Scand 1992;36:31–37.

217. Monk TG, Bouré B, White PF, et al. Comparison of intravenous sedative-analgesic techniques for outpatient immersion lithotripsy. Anesth Analg 1991;72:616–21.

218. Monk TG, Rader JM, White PF. Comparison of alfentanil and ketamine infusions in combination with midazolam for outpatient lithotripsy. Anesthesiology 1991;74:1023–28.

219. Avramov M, Smith I, White PF. Influence of sedation level on side effects and recovery after outpatient monitored anesthesia care. Anesth Analg 1995;80:S23.

220. Avramov M, Smith I, White PF. Use of midazolam and remifentanil during monitored anesthesia care (MAC). Anesth Analg 1995;80:S24.

221. White PF, Shafer A, Boyle WA, et al. Benzodiazepine antagonism does not provoke a stress response. Anesthesiology 1989;70:636–39.

222. Ghouri AF, Ramirez-Ruiz MS, White PF. Effect of flumazenil on recovery after midazolam and propofol sedation. Anesthesiology 1994;81:333–39.

223. Mora CT, Torjman M, White PF. Effects of diazepam and flumazenil on sedation and hypoxic ventilatory response. Anesth Analg 1989;68:473–78.

224. Mora CT, Torjman M, White PF. Sedative and ventilatory effects of midazolam infusion: effect of flumazenil reversal. Can J Anaesth 1995;42:677–84.

225. Taylor E, Ghouri AF, White PF. Midazolam in combination with propofol for sedation during local anesthesia. J Clin Anesth 1992;4:213–16.

226. Newson C, Joshi GP, Victory R, et al. Comparison of propofol administration techniques for sedation during monitored anesthesia care. Anesth Analg 1995;81:486–91.

227. Kain ZN, Gaal W, Kain TS, et al. A first-pass cost analysis of propofol versus barbiturates for children undergoing magnetic resonance imaging. Anesth Analg 1994;79:1102–6.

228. Fraser RA, Hotz SB, Hurtig JB, et al. The prevalence and impact of pain after day-care tubal ligation surgery. Pain 1989;39:189–201.

229. Joshi G, Fredman B, White PF. Role of non-opioid analgesic techniques in outpatient anesthesia. In: Stanley TH, Ashburn MA (eds.), *Anesthesiology and Pain Management*. Amsterdam: Kluwer, 1994, pp. 151–169.

230. Watcha MS, White PF. Economics of anesthetic practice. Anesthesiology 1997;86(5):1170–96.

231. White PF, Way WL, Trevor AJ. Ketamine—its pharmacology and therapeutic uses. Anesthesiology 1982;56:119–36.

232. White PF, Vasconez LO, Mathes S, et al. Comparison of alfentanil with fentanyl as adjuvants during outpatient surgery. Anesthesiology 1988;81:703–10.

233. White PF, Ham J, Way WL, et al. Pharmacology of ketamine isomers in surgical patients. Anesthesiology 1981;52:731–68.

234. Rosenberg MK, Raymond C, Bridge PD. Comparison of midazolam/ketamine with methohexital for sedation during peribulbar block. Anesth Analg 1995;81:173–74.

235. Yee JB, Schafer PG, Crandall AS, et al. Comparison of methohexital and alfentanil on movement during placement of retrobulbar nerve block. Anesth Analg 1994;79:320–23.

236. Zelcer J, White PF, Paull JD, et al. Intraoperative PCA: A comparison with alfentanil bolus and infusion techniques during outpatient monitored anesthesia care. Anesth Analg 1992;75:41–44.

237. Ghouri AF, Taylor E, White PF. Patient-controlled sedation—a comparison of midazolam, propofol and alfentanil during local anesthesia. J Clin Anesth 1992;4:476–79.

238. Enneking FK, Ilfeld BM. Major surgery in the ambulatory environment: continuous catheters and home infusions. Best Pract Res Clin Anaesth 2002;16(2):285–94.

239. Rawal N, Axelsson K, Hylander J, et al. Postoperative patient-controlled local anesthetic administration at home. Anesth Analg 1998;86:86–89.

240. Singelyn FJ, Deyaert M, Joris D, et al. Effects of intravenous patient-controlled analgesia with morphine, continuous epidural analgesia, and continuous three-in-one block on postoperative pain and knee rehabilitation after unilateral total knee arthroplasty. Anesth Analg 1998;87:88–92.

241. Capdevila X, Barthelet P, Ryckwaert Y, et al. Effects of perioperative analgesic technique on the surgical outcome and duration of rehabilitation after major knee surgery. Anesthesiology 1999; 91:8–15.

242. Edwards ND, Wright EM. Continuous low-dose 3-in-1 nerve blockade for postoperative pain relief after total knee replacement. Anesth Analg 1992;75:265–67.

243. Klein SM, Greengrass RA, Grant SA, et al. Ambulatory surgery for multi-ligament knee reconstruction with continuous dual catheter peripheral nerve blockade. Can J Anaesth 2001;48:375–78.

244. Ilfeld BM, Morey TE, Enneking FK. Outpatient use of patient-controlled local anesthetic administration via a psoas compartment catheter to improve pain control and patient satisfaction after anterior cruciate ligament reconstruction. Anesthesiology 201;95: A38.

245. Tetzlaff JE, Andrish J, O'Hara J, et al. Effectiveness of bupivacaine administered via femoral nerve catheter for pain control after anterior cruciate ligament repair. J Clin Anesth 1997;9:542–45.

246. Chung F, Richie ED, Su J. Postoperative pain in ambulatory surgery. Anesth Analg 1997;85:808–16.

247. Klein SM, Grant SA, Greengrass R, et al. Interscalene brachial plexus block with a continuous catheter insertion system and a disposable infusion pump. Anesth Analg 2000;91:1473–78.

248. Cohen NP, Levine WN, Marra G, et al. Indwelling interscalene catheter anesthesia in the surgical management of stiff shoulder: a report of 100 consecutive cases. J Shoulder Elbow Surg 2000;9:268–74.

249. Singelyn FJ, Seguy S, Gouverneur JM. Interscalene brachial plexus analgesia after open shoulder surgery: continuous versus patient-controlled infusion. Anesth Analg 1999;89:1216–20.

250. Borgeat A, Schappi B. Biasca N, et al. Patient-controlled analgesia after major shoulder surgery. Anesthesiology 1997;87:1343–47.

251. Whiffler K. Coracoid block—a safe and easy technique. Br J Anaesth 1981;53:845–48.

252. Wilson JL, Brown DL, Wong GY, et al. Infraclavicular brachial plexus block: parasagittal anatomy important to the coracoid technique. Anesth Analg 1998;87:870–73.

253. Brown DK. Brachial plexus anesthesia: an analysis of options. Yale J Biol Med 1993;66:415–31.

254. Ilfeld BM, Morey TE, Enneking FK. Continuous infraclavicular brachial plexus block for postoperative pain control at home: a randomized, double blinded, placebo-controlled study. Anesthesiology 2002;96(6):1297–1384.

255. Singelyn FJ, Deyaert M, Joris D, et al. Continuous popliteal sciatic nerve block: an original technique to provide postoperative analgesia after foot surgery. Anesth Analg 1997;84:383–86.

256. Sutherland ID. Continuous sciatic nerve infusion: expanded case report describing a new approach. Reg Anesth Pain Med 1998;23: 496–501.

257. Brull SJ, Lieponis JV, Murphy MJ, et al. Acute and long-term benefits of iliac crest donor site perfusion with local anesthetics. Anesth Analg 1992;74:145–47.

258. Savoie FH, Field LD, Jenkins RN, et al. The pain control infusion pump for postoperative pain control in shoulder surgery. Arthroscopy 2000;16:339–42.

259. Valente MJ, Aldrete JA. Efficiency study of the rate of delivery of disposable non-mechanical pumps used for epidural infusions. Reg Anesth 1995;20:2S.

260. Mezzatesta JP, Scott DA, Schweitzer SA, et al. Continuous axillary brachial plexus block for postoperative pain relief: intermittent bolus versus continuous infusion. Reg Anesth 1997;22:357–62.

261. Singelyn FJ, Gouverneur JM. Extended "three-in-one" block after total knee arthroplasty: continuous versus patient-controlled techniques. Anesth Analg 2000;91:176–80.

262. Singelyn FJ, van der Elst P. Continuous "3-in-1" block after total hip replacement: continuous or patient-controlled infusion. Anesth Analg 1998;86S:315.

263. Casati A, Fanelli G, Magistris L, et al. Minimum local anesthetic volume blocking the femoral nerve in 50% of cases: a double blinded comparison between 0.5% ropivacaine and 0.5% bupivacaine. Anesth Analg 2001;92:205–8.

264. Capogna G, Celleno D, Fusco P, et al. Relative potencies of bupivacaine and ropivacaine for analgesia in labour. Br J Anaesth 1999;82:371–73.

265. Borgeat A, Kalberer F, Jacob H, et al. Patient-controlled interscalene analgesia with ropivacaine 0.2% versus bupivacaine 0.15% after major open shoulder surgery; the effects on hand motor function. Anesth Analg 2001;92:218–23.

266. Scott DA, Emanuelsson BM, Mooney PH, et al. Pharmacokinetics and efficacy of long-term epidural ropivacaine infusion for postoperative analgesia. Anesth Analg 1997;85:1322–30.

267. Fischer HB, Peters TM, Fleming IM, et al. Peripheral nerve catheterization in the management of terminal cancer pain. Reg Anesth 1996;21:482–85.

268. Corda DM, Enneking FK. A unique approach to postoperative analgesia following ambulatory surgery. J Clin Anesth 200;12:595–99.

269. Estebe JP, Le-Corre P, DuPlessis L, et al. The pharmacokinetics and pharmacodynamics of bupivacaine-loaded microspheres on a brachial plexus block model in sheep. Anesth Analg 2001;93:447–55.

270. Horlocker TT, O'Driscoll SW, Dinapoli RP. Recurring brachial plexus neuropathy in a diabetic patient after shoulder surgery and continuous interscalene block. Anesth Analg 2000;91:688–90.

271. Singelyn FJ, Contreras V, Gouverneur JM. Epidural anesthesia complicating continuous 3-in-1 lumbar plexus blockade. Anesthesiology 1995;83:217–20.

Philosophy of the Use of Regional Anesthesia and Continuous Peripheral Analgesia in Ambulatory Surgery

ROY A. GREENGRASS

INTRODUCTION

In order to advocate performance of regional anesthesia for ambulatory procedures, a discussion of both theoretical and evidence-based advantages compared with more traditional techniques must be presented. For completeness a discussion of possible disadvantages of regional anesthesia must also be included.

Exuberance following the initial demonstrations of the effectiveness of general (William Thomas Green Morton) and local (Karl Koller) methods of anesthesia has been tempered by a variety of complications associated with their use, e.g., hepatotoxicity associated with general anesthesia and arachnoiditis associated with spinal anesthesia. General anesthesia, by still debated mechanisms (a Nobel prize awaits the discoverer), creates a state of cortical unawareness that allows performance of surgical procedures. Unfortunately, volatile and most intravenous general anesthetics have no analgesic properties and, in fact, may lead to hyperalgesia early postoperatively.[1] This deficiency of general anesthesia mandates the use of ancillary agents, most commonly opioids, for treatment of postoperative pain. Currently most opioids utilized are mu receptor agonists that alter perception of pain. Unfortunately mu receptors are ubiquitous throughout the body and thus, besides the wanted analgesic effects, there is a variety of unwanted side effects the treatment of which is time-consuming and expensive.

Many of the attributes of regional anesthesia have been extensively studied. There is evidence-based medicine to support the following advantages of regional anesthesia: (1) a reduction in thromboembolic complications,[2] (2) better preservation of functional residual capacity (FRC)

and oxygenation,[3] (3) attenuation of the surgical stress response,[4] (4) enhancement of visceral blood flow after gastrointestinal surgery,[5] (5) earlier recovery of gastrointestinal function after postoperative ileus following surgery,[6] (6) as well as many examples of superior pain control.[7]

While all these attributes are important in an inpatient setting, the latter attribute, i.e., superior pain control, is most relevant to an ambulatory setting where any delay in discharge due to inadequate pain control assumes greater prominence.

Pain associated with ambulatory procedures is variable and thus often unpredictable for a given procedure. In an effort to better define procedures at high risk for significant postoperative pain, Rawal et al. conducted a survey of postoperative pain after ambulatory procedures. Their survey revealed that, in particular, orthopedic procedures and inguinal herniorrhaphy were associated with moderate to severe postoperative pain. Their survey also revealed that sleep disturbances were common with 30% of patients waking up due to pain.[8]

An early study comparing general versus regional anesthesia for shoulder surgery confirmed the difficulty of controlling pain in patients who received general anesthesia. Inadequate analgesia resulted in a significant incidence of unanticipated hospital admissions in the general anesthesia group.[9]

A complication of ambulatory surgery almost unique to general anesthesia and opioids is postoperative nausea and vomiting (PONV). Nausea and vomiting are, by far, the most important determinants of prolonged postanesthesia care unit (PACU) stay in ambulatory anesthesia.[10] This complication has been described by patients as more debilitating than pain.[11] Unfortunately, polypharmacy with antiemetics is often ineffective for many procedures and, even if initially effective, may not provide protection against symptoms occurring soon after discharge. In a large retrospective study of PONV related to specific surgical procedures, Larsson and Lundberg found a significant benefit to having a procedure performed under regional anesthesia.[12] Similarly, a large prospective study of 1000 ambulatory patients demonstrated significantly less pain and nausea and vomiting resulting in less PACU time and significant savings in patients receiving regional anesthesia for specific surgical procedures.[13] When properly utilized regional anesthesia can result in significant cost savings compared with similar procedures performed under general anesthesia. Significant cost savings were realized utilizing a local anesthetic technique for ambulatory knee arthroscopy versus the same procedure performed under general anesthesia.[14] D'Alessio et al. found for shoulder procedures that after performance of an interscalene brachial plexus block in the preoperative holding area, anesthetic time in the operating room, surgical times, and times till PACU discharge were all significantly shorter compared to similar procedures performed under general anesthesia. The time saved by interscalene brachial plexus anesthesia allowed the opportunity to schedule more surgical cases for shoulder surgery. Additionally, unanticipated admissions for pain and PONV were unique in the general anesthetic group.[15] Utilizing lumbar plexus block versus general anesthesia for outpatient knee arthroscopy resulted in significantly earlier discharge from the PACU due mainly to a significant reduction in need for postoperative analgesia.[16]

Gebhard et al. determined that, for outpatient carpal tunnel surgery, distal peripheral nerve blocks resulted in hospital discharge 1 hr earlier than the same procedure performed under general anesthesia, with potential savings of $260.00 per patient.[17]

Thus, with the caveat that regional anesthetic procedures be performed in a dedicated preoperative holding area, it appears that regional anesthesia accords significant advantages of enhancing efficiency and reducing costs compared with general anesthetic techniques.

What, then, are the risks associated with performance of peripheral regional anesthesia? In an analysis of closed claims, Cheney and colleagues reported that the highest risk of nerve injury was ulnar neuropathy associated with general anesthesia. Intermediate was central neuraxial injury. The least frequent injury was peripheral nerve injury most frequently associated with brachial plexus injury.[18]

In a large study evaluating 103,730 regional anesthetic techniques, Auroy et al. also determined that peripheral anesthesia techniques were associated with the least frequent incidence of neuropathy.[19] Of note, in both the closed claims and Auroy study, almost every case of neuropathy was associated with paresthesia or pain during injection of the local anesthetic.

The theoretical concern of ambulatory discharge of patients having an insensate limb has been addressed by Klein et al. in a large series of 2382 patients discharged after receiving a long-acting local anesthetic block. At 1 week follow-up they found that 0.25% had a persistent paresthesia that may have been related to the block. This incidence compares favorably to other series of patients receiving regional anesthesia who were hospital-based. It is important to note that in this study the patients had the insensate limb protected against injury. Furthermore, all patients were given an immediate contact number for medical attention if necessary.[20]

It is the author's opinion that nerve injury associated with performance of peripheral regional anesthesia would be very unusual if the following caveats were appreciated: (1) in adults regional anesthesia should not be performed under general anesthesia; (2) peripheral nerve stimulators should be utilized for performance of regional anesthesia; (3) after an appropriate motor stimulation end point, a 1-ml test dose of local anesthetic should be administered. If the patient complains of significant discomfort with this injection, the needle should not be "repositioned," as stated in many texts, but should be removed from the patient and the block either abandoned or repeated at an alternate site.

Continuous regional anesthesia has added a new dimension to the performance of ambulatory regional anesthetic techniques. Formerly, procedures associated with moderate to severe pain simply had their complication of inadequate pain control transferred into the later postoperative period after the single injection block had receded. Continuous regional anesthesia presents an exciting new modality for ambulatory pain control for many procedures.[21]

Although no large multicenter evaluation of possible complications of continuous regional analgesia has been published, the combined experience of Duke University and Mayo Clinic Jacksonville has not revealed a single case of a significant peripheral nerve injury related to the continuous technique.

SUMMARY

In summary, the philosophy of regional anesthesia for ambulatory surgery tends to support the premise, introduced by others, that multimodal analgesia utilizing a local anesthetic base confers great advantages over traditional anesthetic techniques. Further research is required to evaluate novel interventions introduced into the nociceptive pathway that will provide optimal analgesia while according minimal risks.

REFERENCES

1. Zhang Y, Eger E, Dutton RC, Sonner JM. Inhaled anesthetics have hyperalgesic effects at 0.1 minimum alveolar anesthetic concentration. Anesth Anal 2000;91:462–66.
2. Tuman KJ, McCarthy RJ, March PJ, et al. Effects of epidural anesthesia and analgesia on coagulation and outcome after major vascular surgery. Anesth Analg 1991;73:696–704.
3. Ballantyne JC, deFerranti S, Suarez T, et al. The comparative effects of postoperative analgesic therapies on pulmonary outcome: cumulative meta-analyses of randomized, controlled trials. Anesth Analg 1998;86:598–612.

4. Kehlet HK. Effect of pain relief on the surgical stress response. Reg Anesth 1996;21(6S):35–37.

5. Johansson K, Ahn H, Lindhagen J, et al. Effect of epidural anaesthesia on intestinal blood flow. Br J Surg 1988;75:73–76.

6. Liu SS, Carpenter RL, Mackey DC, et al. Effects of perioperative analgesic technique on rate of recovery after colon surgery. Anesthesiology 1995;83:757–65.

7. Singelyn FJ, Dyaert M, Joris D, et al. Effects of intravenous patient controlled analgesia with morphine, continuous epidural analgesia and continuous three-in-one block on postoperative pain and knee rehabilitation after unilateral total knee arthroplasty. Anesth Analg 1998;87:88–92.

8. Rawal N, Hylander J, Nydahl PA, et al. Survey of postoperative analgesia following ambulatory surgery. Acta Anaesthesiol Scand 1997; 41:1017–22.

9. Brown AR, Weiss R, Greenberg C, Flatow El, Bigliani LU. Interscalene block for shoulder arthroscopy: comparison with general anesthesia. Arthroscopy 1993;9:295–300.

10. Green G, Jonsson L. Nausea: the most important factor determining length of stay after ambulatory anaesthesia: a comparative study of isoflurane and/or propofol techniques. Acta Anaesthesiol Scand 1993; 37:742–46.

11. Hirsch J. Impact of postoperative nausea and vomiting. Anesthesiology 1994;49:30–33.

12. Larsson S, Lundberg D. A prospective survey of post-operative nausea and vomiting with special regard to incidence and relations to patient characteristics, anesthetic routines and surgical procedures. Acta Anaesthesiol Scand 1995;39:539–45.

13. Pavlin DJ, Rapp SE, Polissar NL, et al. Factors affecting discharge time in adult outpatients. Anesth Analg 1998;87:816–26.

14. Lintner S, Shawen S, Lohnes J, et al. Local anesthesia in outpatient knee arthroscopy: a comparison of efficacy and cost. Arthroscopy 1996;12:482–88.

15. D'Alessio JG, Rosenblum M, Shea KP, et al. A retrospective comparison of interscalene block and general anesthesia for ambulatory surgery shoulder arthroscopy. Reg Anesth 1995;20:62–68.

16. Patel NJ, Flashburg MH, Paskin S, Grossman R. A regional anesthetic technique compared to general anesthesia for outpatient knee arthroscopy. Anesth Analg 1986;65:185–87.

17. Gebhard RE, Al-Samsam T, Greg J, Khan A, Chelly, JE. Distal nerve blocks at the wrist for outpatient carpal tunnel surgery offer intraoperative cardiovascular stability and reduce discharge time. Anesth Analg 2002;95:351–55.

18. Cheney FW, Domino KB, Caplan RA, et al. Nerve injury associated with anesthesia; a closed claims analysis. Anesthesiology 1999; 90(4):1062–68.

19. Auroy Y, Benhamou D, Bargues L, Ecoffey C, Falissard B, Mercier FJ, Bouaziz H, Samii K, Mercier F. Major complications of regional anesthesia in France: the SOS Regional Anesthesia Hotline Service. Anesthesiology 2002;97:1274–80.

20. Klein SM, Nielsen KC, Greengrass RA, Warner DS, Martin A, Steele S. Ambulatory discharge after long-acting peripheral nerve blockade: 2382 blocks with ropivacaine. Anesth Analg 2002;94:65–70.

21. Grant SA, Nielsen KC, Greengrass RA, Steele SM, Klein SM. Continuous peripheral nerve block for ambulatory surgery. Reg Anesth Pain Med 2001;26(3):209–14.

GENERAL CLINICAL PRINCIPLES OF AMBULATORY ANESTHESIA

Ideal Ambulatory Surgery Center Structure and Function

ROBERT J. SCHLOSSER • SUSAN M. STEELE

A BRIEF HISTORY OF THE AMBULATORY SURGERY CENTER

Ambulatory surgery as we know it has occurred for centuries, though one could argue that it has gone on for thousands of years. Documented only by evidentiary skeletal remains, the healed skulls of trepanation patients suggest successful Stone Age neurosurgeries.[1] Occurring long before the development of hospitals, outpatient surgery is, by definition, the oldest known surgery.[2]

The dawn of anesthesia broke in the United States on March 30, 1842 with the first delivery of ether by Crawford W. Long for the extraction of neck tumors. While the lack of notoriety surrounding this event thwarted Long's shot at fame, it did not prevent the establishment of this date as Doctors' Day 91 years later.

The observation by Gardner Q. Colton at one of his infamous "nitrous parties" of analgesia in the intoxicated prompted Horace Wells to publicly demonstrate general anesthesia in Boston. This clearly helped to make ambulatory surgery more plentiful and much more popular with the masses. Colton himself also administered nitrous oxide to 121,709 outpatients from 1863 to 1881 without a single death.[3] Ensuing reports of successful outpatient surgeries arrived from twentieth century Scotland, where James Nicoll, over a 10-year period, documented a series of 8988 successful outpatient pediatric surgeries at the Glasgow Royal Hospital for Sick Children.[4]

Subsequent American pioneers, such as Ralph M. Waters of Sioux City, Iowa, frequently engendered contempt and scorn for their attempts.

Nonetheless, even in 1916, Waters had stumbled upon the basic needs for a successful endeavor: "An office was equipped with a waiting room and a small operating room with an adjoining room containing a cot on which a patient could lie down after his anesthetic."[5] He gauged the success of this center on many fronts, stating that "the men who are familiar with the place are well pleased. The place has been running in its present location now for eight months and is paying my total expenses. . . . Our fees are considerabl[y] less than for similar work in the hospital because less time and trouble is involved."[5]

Eventually hospital based outpatient surgery began to emerge. In 1961, Butterworth Hospital in Grand Rapids, Michigan first established an outpatient surgical program.[6] David Cohen and John Dillon quickly followed suit, founding a similar program at University of California Los Angeles in 1962,[7] as did Marie-Louise Levy at George Washington University in 1966.[8]

The year 1970 saw outpatient surgery's return from academic circles to the environment of private practice, with Drs. Wallace Reed and John Ford earning credit for establishing the classic model for freestanding surgery centers. By opening the doors to the first successful American freestanding center, the Surgicenter of Phoenix, Arizona, they ushered in a revolution in American medicine. This revolution answered the call from government, insurance companies, and patients to find a safe and more affordable way to perform surgical procedures without sacrificing patient care. Although the Surgicenter of Phoenix has certainly been remodeled and rebuilt since its inception, it remains a flourishing and productive organization to this day.[9,10]

Following on the heels of this work was an explosion in the utilization of ambulatory surgery. By 1980, 16.3% of all surgeries were performed on an outpatient basis. By 1984 this number rose to 30%, and the Society for Ambulatory Anesthesia (SAMBA) was born. The total outpatient rate approached 50% by 1990 and achieved 60% in 1997.[11,12] It is believed that a 70% rate was attained in the year 2003.[13]

WHY AN AMBULATORY SURGERY CENTER?

"With a population expanding faster than the number of hospital beds, a bed shortage of indefinite duration [confronted] the medical profession."[7] This realization led the pioneers of ambulatory anesthesia and surgery to create ambulatory surgery centers (ASCs) in order to perform

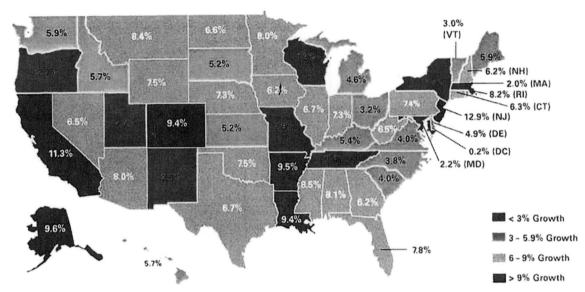

Figure 4-1   Annual growth in inpatient expenditures per health plan member, 1998–2001, based on the experience of a large, nationally representative private group health plan. (http://bcbshealthissues.com/cost/pdf/hospital.pdf.)

needed surgeries in a bottlenecked system of medicine. This new surgical venue was devoted to "the principle that high-quality outpatient surgery can be provided in a caring, personal environment . . . at a lower cost than other alternatives."[10]

Today, ASCs continue to provide advantages. Health care cost containment is one of these. If anything, the outlook for cost of inpatient care is bleaker than ever before. As an analysis of data collected from major medical insurance providers shows, the disturbing growth in inpatient expenditures is of national concern (Fig. 4-1).

Expanding the purview of collected data to include that of the last decade reveals this worrisome trend of rising inpatient costs to be accelerating on an annual basis (Fig. 4-2). This is in spite of the medical community's best efforts at containing cost by decreasing the length of inpatient stay (Fig. 4-3).

The national trend toward increased inpatient costs is likely to continue given the increasing dependence on costly technology, enforcement of the 80-hr resident work week, and most important, a devastating shortage of nursing staff (Fig. 4-4).

While job security has never been a real problem for physicians, the national shift to increased outpatient care has the fringe benefit of assuring ASC physicians bountiful work opportunity. Technologic improvements in medicine, as in anesthesia and surgery, have allowed for a safe, money-saving shift in the burden of care away from the inpatient setting and to patients and their families. The trend toward an increased use of outpatient facilities is demonstrated in Figure 4-5.

This trend applies to outpatient surgery as well, as can be seen in Figure 4-6.

Apart from the market-driven economic advantages of performing surgeries in ASCs, a host of other factors spur ASC development. These include advantages to the physician, nursing staff, and patient who work or receive health care in an ASC.

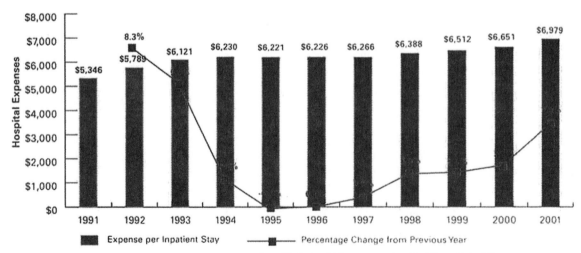

Figure 4-2   Hospital expenses per inpatient stay, 1991–2001. (http://bcbshealthissues.com/cost/pdf/hospital.pdf.)

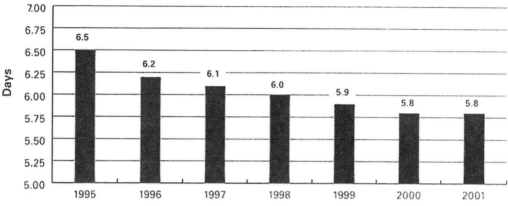

Figure 4-3   Average length of stay in days, 1995–2001. (http://bcbshealthissues.com/cost/pdf/hospital.pdf.)

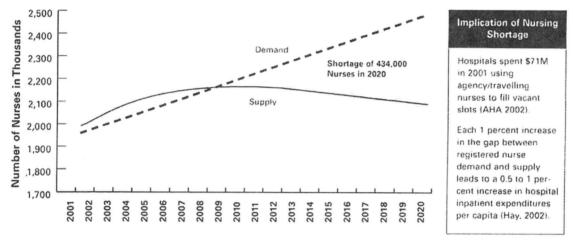

Figure 4-4   Forecast of total RN full-time equivalents vs. hospital requirements, 2001–2020. (http://bcbshealthissues.com/cost/pdf/hospital.pdf.)

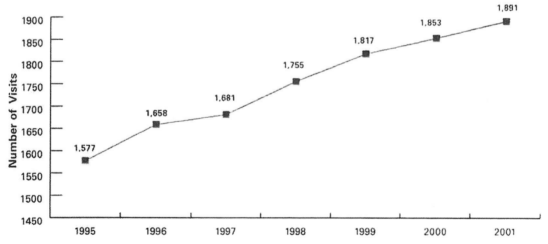

Figure 4-5   Number of outpatient visits per 1000 population. (http://bcbshealthissues.com/cost/pdf/hospital.pdf.)

For example, many physicians justifiably feel a loss of control over decision making in patient care, which results in a lack of ownership for the delivery of quality health care. Also, weighty bureaucratic regulations and the inefficiencies built into a hospital's inpatient surgical program can make work frustrating and burdensome. With increased autonomy and a renewed sense of personal re-

sponsibility for process as well as outcome, physicians at an ASC can regain a sense of practicing the art as well as the science of medicine. In addition, newer construction of ASCs, compared to inpatient hospital centers, allows for the incorporation of current technologies into the surgical suites that can be tailor-made for their intended use. By being built in areas close to clinician office space, the con-

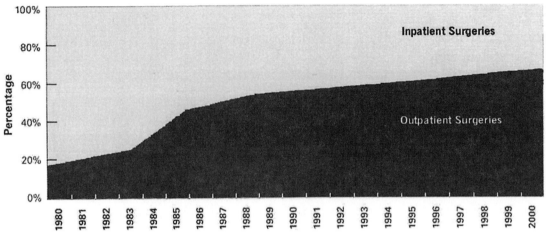

Figure 4-6 Distribution of hospital outpatient and inpatient surgeries, 1980–2001. (http://bcbshealthissues.com/cost/pdf/hospital.pdf.)

venience of an ASC can also be very attractive to surgeons. Finally, with its more limited hours of operation, the ASC provides a venue for medical professionals to balance their desires for professional satisfaction with family lifestyle issues.

Schedule flexibility, shorter nursing shifts, the lack of night or weekend calls, and a positive work environment also make ASCs attractive to nursing staff.

Patients have several reasons to be excited about ASCs as well. Today's population has increasingly become accustomed to paying for convenience and efficiency. Patients generally expect medical or even surgical problems to be solved without disruption to their schedules, preferably in locales convenient to their homes, which have clean and friendly atmospheres. Patients also increasingly expect surgery with minimal postoperative discomfort. It is difficult to accomplish these desires in a hospital setting today; however, an ASC is able to fulfill many of these aspirations.

Regardless of the reasoning behind the decision to build, entrepreneurs will need to undertake four steps. First among these is to determine the regional need for (and hence the viability of) an ASC. The second is to select a model or philosophy for the future center. This model will largely be guided by ASC ownership. Third, a team must be selected to achieve the fourth and final step of carefully designing the new ASC as a structure that ideally fits its function.

DETERMINING VIABILITY

The first step in determining the potential viability of an ASC is to estimate how much surgery will be performed in a given service area. Historically, successful statistical methodologies estimate that 84 total surgeries would be performed for every 1000 people annually and assume a population growth of 2.5%. Some planners suggest that 80% of surgical cases stem from a 4-mile radius,[14] while others suggest a 30-min driving radius as an estimate of the outer limits of one's service area. Competition from other medical centers, however, needs to be taken into ac-

count for both methodologies. In addition, no more than two hospitals within 6 miles and zero ASCs within 8 miles should exist from the center of the defined region.

Conservative planners have historically estimated that 20–40% of all surgeries in their region could be done in a same-day-surgery setting.[15] Setting up an ASC as a single rather than multispecialty center applies another incidence- and demographically related variable to the equation.

As aforementioned, this sort of surgical volume determination has worked well in the past. The numbers and calculations in today's market, however, show some of these variables to be far too conservative. *Outpatient surgical rates alone* have swelled to a national average of 58 per 1000 people in 1999, ranging from 35 per 1000 in California to 108 per 1000 in West Virginia.[16] This is much more consistent with the fact that 60% of all surgeries nationally were performed on an outpatient basis in 2000,[12] and with projections that by 2006 the national inpatient surgery rate will average roughly 37 per 1000 people.[17] Other factors that ensure ASC viability over time include: ample surgeons willing to utilize an ASC, an average combined household income exceeding $40,000 a year (1986 prices), a large regional population of children, a population growth of at least 2% per year, a strong local economy, and demographics not too skewed toward the elderly. While the elderly certainly require more surgeries than their children, their comorbidities, decreased support network, and habitual use of inpatient facilities may sway them to preferentially utilize inpatient surgery. When analyzing several different potential locations for an ASC, all of the above factors should be assigned a weight and applied schematically to determine the site most favorable to development.[14]

A final geographic consideration that will ultimately impact upon ASC revenue and viability is the regional rate for reimbursement of surgeries. A hallmark of ASC performance is providing surgery at a decreased cost to its patients. While most ASCs determine set charges for procedures based on cost plus a markup for profit, others set prices based on what other ASCs charge.[18] Regardless of method, this fee for service should allow for both ASC profit and for marketability in the region where it is established.

SELECTING A MODEL

Examination of the particulars of one's situation will aid in the matching of desired goals to outcomes and the marrying of the type of ambulatory surgery center to its philosophy. Apart from a doctor's office there are four basic models for the performance of ambulatory surgery: hospital integrated, hospital adjacent, hospital satellite, and freestanding autonomous. The determination of which model is most suitable for a given setting can be ascertained by ranking the importance of several factors. These include facility ownership, construction costs, and time frame for development, physician/patient satisfaction, and physician autonomy. The pros and cons of each of the four models are summarized below.[2,18–20]

1. Hospital Integrated
   Advantages
   - Low-cost, quick construction since operating and recovery rooms are preexistent.
   - Minimal financial risk to the hospital. Flexibility to abandon outpatient surgery if unsuccessful.
   - Less stringent requirements for selecting the ambulatory patient may spur utilization. Even if surgery becomes more extensive than anticipated, hospital admission is an easy option.
   - Certificate of Need unnecessary.
   Disadvantages
   - A decrease in patient dignity and quality of care as a result of staff directing their attention to the more critical needs of inpatients.
   - Delays in the commencement of surgery ranging from causes as diverse as parking difficulties, admission overloads, major inpatient surgeries exceeding expected duration, and the prioritization of emergency surgeries over elective cases.
   - Increased cost to the patient from subsidizing the cost of unused ancillary staff, inpatient overhead, and equipment.
   - Patient stress increased from receiving care in an institution "of the sick."
   - Increased risk of nosocomial infection.
2. Hospital Adjacent
   Advantages
   - Streamlined admissions process and separate pre- and postoperative areas decrease delays and increase patient satisfaction.
   - Less actual and patient-perceived cost of care than in the above situation.
   - Increased efficiency improves physician and patient satisfaction.
   - High morale.
   - Marketable to nonstaff physicians
   Disadvantages
   - High cost of construction, especially adjacent to a crowded medical center.

- Certificate of Need required by many states.
- Duplicates facilities and equipment.
- Difficulty converting ambulatory center space in case of a failed venture.

3. Hospital Satellite
   Advantages
   - Same as number 2 above.
   - Extends the hospital's market and opens a new revenue source.
   - Provides easier access, parking, and more convenience to patients by removing them from the congested hospital site.
   Disadvantages
   - Similar to number 2 above.
   - Physicians and citizens in the area may view the center in a hostile light for its imperialistic expansion.
   - Increased logistical problems for the unplanned patient admission to an inpatient setting. Detrimental care could result from a lack of access to quick hospital emergency backup.
4. Freestanding Autonomous
   Advantages
   - Same advantages as number 3 above.
   - Increased patient[21] and physician satisfaction result from the cheerful atmosphere and decreased governance of a non-hospital-owned establishment.
   - Further cost savings from reduced administrative overhead is passed on to patients. This is especially true of physician-owned centers.[22,23]
   Disadvantages
   - Similar to number 3 above.
   - Capital investment and ownership issues may be brought to the forefront as further limitations on physician ownership and referral are added to Stark Laws before Congress.

BUILDING THE TEAM

While there are a number of compelling factors that can lead to the development of a novel outpatient surgery program, this decision should be made carefully. Planning a new surgical center should involve a host of clinical and administrative staff. Once the executive decision to build an ASC is made and its particular mission or philosophy is chosen, a development team should be formed to carry out sundry tasks. The individuals comprising the development team will have a good deal of work cut out for them. If the group building the ASC is hospital-based, they have the distinct advantage of the talent already employed within their institution. The building committee needs only to be drawn from the ranks of employees and to rally selected members from all three branches of the hospital—the trustees, administrators, and medical staff—into a unified team. The contribution to the hospital team from the medical staff will involve surgeons from different ASC utilizing specialties, anesthesiologists, and chiefs of hospital departments of laboratories, radiology, and medicine. Nursing services can contribute their directors of nursing services, of outpatient nursing, of ambulatory services as well as their operating room (OR) supervisor. Hospital administration will need to supply the chief executive officer, the business manager, the chiefs of engineering and of the billing office, and the administrators of ambulatory services, of admissions, and of public relations. Hospital governance should furnish chairmen from the hospital trustees and the committees of planning, finance, and buildings and grounds. While the development team has the strength and experience of all pertinent members of the hospital team, its size prohibits it from making rapid executive decisions.[2]

For this reason a steering committee needs to be appointed, which should include a few surgeons, a few anesthesiologists, the administrator of ambulatory services, the nursing supervisor of ambulatory services, and the business administrator. This group needs to educate itself about current ambulatory surgery trends and anticipate future demands. It should review current literature, attend meetings, and, perhaps most important of all, visit other ASCs to see them in action.[24] This group will ultimately make command decisions regarding the autonomy of the ASC to decide privileges and permitted surgeries, as well as its hours of operation, staffing, record keeping, and billing. Such decisions are later submitted for discussion and ratification by the whole development team.[2]

In the development of an autonomous ASC the leadership is disadvantaged by its lack of organizational knowledge and a setting from which to work. The leadership is, however, simultaneously unhampered by administrative regulation, organizational tradition, or preordained long-term plans. For reasons of financial backing, the development team should hopefully involve enough numbers of surgeons to require a separate steering committee of seven to nine members. The steering committee should involve members with experience in construction, finance, and working with governmental bodies. Legal assistance should be obtained early to avoid costly juridical oversights and to allow the legal team to perform organizational tasks such as procuring architects, contractors, and financial services and soliciting government approval. Appointment of subcommittees to obtain Certificate of Need or CON (if necessary), financial backing, and to choose the site for construction are then needed. Obviously, physicians who have helped with governmental health planning, served on a bank's board of trustees, or who have had extensive real estate dealings are ideal candidates for these groups. While it cannot be overemphasized how slow and frustrating the process of obtaining CON can be, nonetheless, all groups should work simultaneously toward their ends. Once these ends are achieved, the steering committee or a *de novo* building committee needs to bid out the building's construction and oversee its completion. Finally the assemblage at large should elect a board of directors, which appoints a medical director. The position of medical director is often filled by an anesthesiologist.[25] The board also needs to determine autonomy for selection of types of surgeries, address hours of operation, medical record keeping, required preoperative labs, necessary patient follow-up, and ASC privileges.[2] Extending "operating" instead of "staff" privileges to surgeons negates their need to sit through staff meetings.[3] The fact that surgeons have privileges in nearby hospitals cancels out the need for transfer agreements between the ASC and a hospital.[26]

ASC PHYSICAL DESIGN

Attempting to positively influence ambulatory surgery clientele can be a difficult task owing to their high expectations.[27] These expectations definitely include a friendly staff in an attractive setting, with sufficient comfort-providing amenities. As such, many ASCs place great emphasis on the secretary who greets patients upon their arrival. While not minimizing this role or its impact, it is clear that lasting impressions are engendered earlier and are influenced by physical plant design. The aesthetic qualities of the building as well as the organization and layout of its components are influential in forming patient opinion of the ASC and in marketing the ASC to future patients.

Upon their arrival, patients first exit their vehicles and walk into the center. For this reason, when designing a center, the importance of ample, close, landscaped, or even covered parking cannot be overemphasized.[28] Regardless of whether the surgical center is hospital affiliated or free-standing, nobody wants to walk a great distance (through rain or snow) from the car to the door.

After parking allocation, attention must be turned to ingress and egress from the ASC. Starting with the patient entry door itself, building code dictates that it be wheelchair-accessible and common sense dictates that it be automated to aid the elderly or injured.

Thought should next be given to the flow of patient traffic, as poorly designed patient traffic patterns can easily generate a negative impression. Traffic patterns throughout the entire ASC will ultimately help determine the center's efficiency, safety, and aesthetic. The first autonomous ASC opened by Reed and Ford was visionary in its recognition of this concept. Two key ideas that it embodied have been utilized in the planning and construction of other centers throughout the world. These state that patients presenting for preoperative screening purposes should not circulate through areas reserved for clinical activity and that patients receiving surgery should never retrace their steps. These concepts prevent the mingling of presurgical, preoperative, and postoperative patients, which in turn minimizes preoperative patient anxiety, affords greater patient privacy and dignity, reduces staffing confusion, and avoids interruptions in clinical activities.[20]

With these guidelines in mind, the patient entry should be separate from the staff entrance to avoid the mixing of patients and staff in hallways. This also preserves the privacy of staff conversations, prevents patients from feeling "in the way," and satisfies ASC physicians. If possible to incorporate in the design, there should also be a patient exit separate from the entrance to ensure the continued separation of pre- and postoperative patients. Also, wheelchair storage should be out of view of the entrance to avoid confronting preoperative individuals with symbols of infirmity and illness.[29] A bench near the exit provides a place for patients to rest while their escorts retrieve the car.

After they pass through the door, the entrance and waiting area embody the next patient experience. Sufficient, clear, and concise signs should welcome patients to the reception desk and accompany them on their journey through the ASC. This helps alleviate the stress that is engendered when any patient feels lost or disoriented. Aided by a dynamic and customer-oriented receptionist, positive first impressions of the ASC continue to form. Because the family exposure to the ASC may be limited to only the reception and waiting areas, impressions formed here become the word of mouth that helps shape public opinion of the center.

Selection of building materials and an architectural style for the reception and waiting areas lays the foundation for a less stressful surgical experience. The overall design should minimize similarities to inpatient settings. The combination of natural light, colorful surroundings, music, artwork, and plant life can exude a sense of calm and confidence while at the same time blunting any sense of hospital-like sterility. Some successful ASCs have even incorporated thematic styles of architecture and décor. While some simulate a plush physician's office environment, others venture into a health park concept, complete with waterfalls and entertainment, or embrace a more residential quality that simulates the patient's home setting.[24] Regardless of theme or style, the physical appearance of the ASC will indeed help mold initial opinion and lasting impressions of the center.

Three distinct areas—the business office, the family waiting area, and patient preoperative holding—will need to be closely situated to the reception area. Apart from welcoming and identifying arriving patients, issues of insurance and payment will also occasionally arise. For this reason a business office should be directly accessible from the reception area. The layout of the business office should allow for confidential money matters to be discussed without embarrassing the patient.

For the comfort of the patient's family, their waiting area should be directly adjacent to the reception area and should be built sufficiently large to prevent the stress associated with overcrowding. Adapting inpatient "per person occupancy" space requirements allocates a minimum of 20–25 net square feet for waiting areas.[30] Because some patient and family anxiety is to be expected, rest rooms should be immediately available near the waiting area. Of note, preventing the rest room door from opening directly into the waiting room preserves some degree of patient privacy and dignity. Another consideration for the waiting area is a stocked kitchen area to keep family members at ease while their loved ones are in the operating suites.[31] The location of this waiting room should ultimately be near to the PACU, adjacent to physician-family consult suites, potentially near to the (outpatient) pharmacy window, and directly and immediately adjacent to parking. It should also be of sufficient distance from the staff lounge and the operating suites that the noise of staff merrymaking, the clang of orthopedic hammering, and the aroma of electrocautery are not enjoyed by all.

After checking in, patients proceed from the reception area or family waiting area to the patient preoperative holding area. Construction of cubicles instead of utilization of suspended curtains enhances the auditory and visual privacy of this area. A curtain across the entrance permits privacy but still allows response to a patient in distress. Also, utilization of the preoperative bedspace as a patient changing area enhances privacy and dignity. Patient belongings should be collected, labeled, and stored for safekeeping, preferably near the PACU. Continuation of the use of artwork—perhaps on the ceilings in lieu of wall hangings—and nonwhite wall colors can help maintain a reduced level of preoperative patient anxiety. Perioperative music too can be of assistance in this regard, as it has been shown to decrease cortisol blood levels from presurgical stress,[32] significantly improve perceptions of postsurgical recovery,[33,34] and modestly reduce perceptions of pain through distraction.[35] Speaker systems and different stations to accommodate musical preferences should therefore not be overlooked. Finally, if the nervous preoperative bladder does make its presence known, bathroom access will be appreciated by the patients.

The number of preoperative holding area beds should be at least as numerous, if not slightly greater in number, as the operating rooms. Their physical location should approximate that of the operating rooms and pharmacy, and be relatively close to, but separate from, the PACU. These considerations will enhance efficiency of patient transport, patient premedication, and keep anesthesiologists in proximity to preoperative and postoperative patients. Each preoperative cubicle should be able to accommodate a gurney with three additional feet on either side. Cubicles should also be equipped with standard American Society of Anesthesiologists (ASA) monitoring capabilities, oxygen, wall suction, and terminals for electronic medical record keeping if applicable. These features will allow anesthesiologists to sedate patients and record the performance of preoperative central neuraxial or peripheral nerve blocks. The ability to dim the lights after such procedures allows patients to nap comfortably prior to proceeding to the OR.

Building on the theme of Ford and Reed regarding patient separation, thought should be given to the separation of children from adult patients in order to alleviate stress for both parties. As described later, consideration can be given to the formation of a combined pediatrics preoperative holding and PACU room.

While attention to the needs of the patient is paramount in the construction of an ASC, the requirements of the staff should not be overlooked. For example, the need for male and female locker areas, each with a toilet and a shower, is a requirement of Medicare guidelines.[29] The most demonstrable benefit of a locker area to the ASC may be the reduction of infection rates by cutting down on the trafficking of scrub-borne insects into the ORs from outside the center. Adequately sized lockers, bright wall finishes, and full-length mirrors would also be appreciated by staff. Likewise, an area for scrub storage should not be overlooked.

Another required area is a staff lounge or break area. This lounge should be accessible to the ORs rooms and at the same time an adequate distance from patient and family areas to allow for the often noisy staff camaraderie to proceed without tarnishing the professional image of the ASC. Many of the same amenities provided in the family waiting area would also be appreciated by the staff, such as appliances to refrigerate, cook, or reheat meals and to clean dishes.

Attention should next be turned to the design of operating rooms, beginning with quantity. Choosing an improper number of ORs is an expensive engineering debacle, as overestimating the number will only increase overhead costs and rent for the ASC. Equally important, however, is avoidance of underbuilding the ASC such that a costly renovation might need to be made just a few years into the ASC's operation. Assuming a sufficient number of surgeries will be performed to maintain viability and growth, the number of ORs can be matched to expected caseload. A good estimate of cases done per OR is between 1000 and 1500 per annum,[36] but caseload throughput will depend primarily on the duration of procedure and OR turnover time and secondarily on delays during which patients are readied for and recovered from surgery. As the ASC establishes itself and matures, caseload typically increases by about 10% a year over a 5-year period.[29] Estimating the number of cases at 5 or 6 years and the average number of hours per case allows for a good estimate of OR number according to the formula[37] in Figure 4-7.

Besides OR number, OR size will also have to be determined. While 300 ft² may prove sufficient for a procedure room, minimum standard size of ambulatory surgery ORs is deemed by Medicare to be 360 ft². A variance can be granted by the state legislature if a description of intended usage shows the 360 ft² requirement to be excessive. Ultimately, the decision to build ORs smaller than Medicare recommendations or to expand them to a more typical hospital-sized OR of 400 ft² depends on the intended caseload and on the amount of equipment and technology to be built into the room.[30] When empty, a 360 ft² OR can seem sufficient. However, the height and placement of gas lines and storage units can rob the room and, more important, the anesthesiologist of needed space for patient care. Even the seemingly insignificant detail of the direction that OR doors open can make a difference in an emergency.[24]

Operating room design should likewise allow for the incorporation of modern technology, which serves as a boon for ASC physician recruitment. The most advantageous system for a surgeon is one that would be able to receive and store outside radiographs, mammograms, cat scans, and MRIs and subsequently display the images onscreen during the case. Incorporating voice activation capabilities would allow for seamless sterile manipulation of displayed images and permit robotic camera control for laparoscopies. On the flip side of the surgical drapes or blood-brain barrier, the anesthesiologists could incorporate computerized anesthesia records. Local area networking would permit data entry to follow the patient from preoperative areas through to their discharge from the PACU. Interfaced monitors in preoperative holding area and PACU displaying a real-time OR overview would facilitate preparedness to send for or receive the next patient. Downloading the record into the billing office could capture costs of pharmaceuticals and anesthesia supplies used, anesthesia time, and procedures for professional charges as well as surgical Current Procedural Terminology (CPT) codes to accurately submit a bill to the patient's insurance provider within minutes of departure from the PACU. Computer systems could also provide access to multiple protocols, from appropriate antibiotic regimens to treatment of malignant hyperthermia.

The physical appearance of the OR may prove to have some value in influencing surgical outcome. Allowing for natural light and the use of nontraditional bright wall colors can decrease patient as well as staff stress levels. One author even suggests a color specifically for ORs—light blue.[37] While color and the phototherapy of natural light can help reduce patient anxiety and improve staff mood, it should be remembered that the ability to darken a room is needed by ophthalmologists and can decrease glare and physician eyestrain in endoscopic cases.

As far as the location of the ORs is concerned, they should be close to the preoperative holding area and directly neighboring the PACU. They should be next to the storage of sterile supplies, the location of sterilizers, storage space for OR equipment, and close to garbage collection. This arrangement will decrease OR turnover times. They should also be close to the staff locker rooms and lounge facilities for staff convenience.

A final item impacting operating rooms is the decision to build ample storage, an important ASC commodity that is unfortunately always the first item to be sacrificed on a tight budget. Sacrificing the storage areas by necessity turns the ORs and hallways into storage areas, which can make for an unsightly and unorganized appearance, cause mishandling of sterile goods, and damage expensive equipment.[24]

After choosing and equipping the number of operating rooms, determining a proper number of PACU beds is another economic decision. It is important not to underbuild this area, as a bottleneck here will grind OR efficiency to a halt. Overall "per person" space requirements of 75–100 net ft² are needed for recovery areas,[24] and recommendations for bed numbers vary in the literature from 1.5 to 3 beds per OR.[20,24] The decision will be influenced primarily by the time taken by patients before being discharge-ready and secondarily by the speed with which patients stream from the OR to the PACU. Time until patients are discharge-ready will further depend on the typical mode of anesthesia employed and subsequent sequelae of postoperative nausea and vomiting (PONV) and pain. Representing one end of the spectrum, a center that primarily employs methodologies of peripheral nerve block with light intraoperative sedation will most easily accommodate high PACU throughput and turnover. The decision to add a phase II PACU or a 23-hr observation area will also decrease the needed number of phase I beds. Alternatively, ASCs that opt for automatic phase I PACU bypass or that construct a PACU with no phase II area can opt to build a recliner area to facilitate PACU bed turnover and help to transition patients toward discharge. If the recliners can be incorporated into a theater-like environment, some of the awkwardness of seating strangers together can be alleviated. Concurrently discharge instructions can be reinforced and patients can relax in front of a selected video presentation.

$$\frac{\text{\#Procedures/year}}{\text{\#Operational days/year}} \times \frac{\text{Average hours/procedure}}{\text{\#Hours/day}}$$

Figure 4-7 Projected number of needed operating rooms.

The location of the PACU is another decision that will affect safety, efficiency, and customer satisfaction. The PACU should be directly adjacent to the OR to minimize the risk of sequelae from iatrogenic respiratory insufficiency and to reduce the number of steps taken by the surgical team between cases, that being a factor in turnover time and efficiency. It should also be close to the family waiting area to easily reunite patients with their escorts. The relationship between PACU and the parking facility will impact patient satisfaction, in direct proportionality to the distance the patient has to travel to his/her their vehicle. Another distance to consider is that from PACU and/or family waiting area to the pharmacy, if the pharmacy will partake in filling outpatient pain prescriptions.

As to the size of the PACU rooms, they should be able to accommodate a stretcher with 3 ft of free space on either side. Attention to visual and acoustic privacy will serve to enhance patient solace, but this consideration must be balanced, of course, with concerns of patient safety, which can be somewhat ameliorated by centralized telemetry. Attention to the number and location of handicapped-accessible bathrooms will improve convenience. The personal belongings of patients relinquished for the OR should be stored securely near or in the PACU. This will facilitate the concept of patient dignity by reuniting patients with some of their (most) personal belongings and will also serve to speed discharge times.

The issue of separation of adult and pediatric patients resurfaces in the design of the ASC PACU and raises a host of issues. From an adult perspective on recovery, almost nothing is less comforting than being parked next to someone else's screaming child. From a child's perspective, almost nothing is more frightening than being wheeled past a multitude of strangers, some of whom have bandaged faces or freshly amputated extremities. While it is paramount to pediatric comfort to reunite them as soon as possible with their parents, this could compromise the Health Insurance Portability and Accountability Act of 1996 (HIPAA) requirements for patient privacy and confidentiality. Finally, children will fare better in a location specially designed and staffed for them,[38] which allows in turn for the location of rocking chairs near cribs and application of cartoon characters to the wall.[15] Accommodating these diverse needs requires a separate pediatric recovery area. The major disadvantage to the ASC is the cost of this space allocation. Pediatric volume would have to be high enough on a daily basis to warrant this sort of outlay. An alternative solution employed by the Surgicenter of Phoenix, Arizona is to combine the pediatric preoperative and PACU into the same room adjoining the main (adult) PACU. Admitting the patient and parents into this area and allowing parents to remain here during their child's procedure minimizes the time of separation.[10]

The PACU will certainly suffice for recovery from most of the outpatient surgeries being performed today. However, some ASCs today are accepting patients previously deemed unfit for ambulatory surgery. This growing and challenging outpatient surgical group includes patients with little or no social support network, those with multiple comorbidities, and those who present for outpatient surgery of a more aggressive nature. Thus, while not con-demning the aging widow or the otherwise-fit total joint recipient to an inpatient surgery experience, these patients are also not likely to be street-ready an hour after their wounds are dressed in the OR. For these individuals a 23-hr observation unit becomes a viable option. The overnight recovery area allows the anesthesia team to continue regional analgesia techniques through the fist night after surgery and to verify success of catheter infusions for continuous peripheral nerve blocks. It allows the surgeons to verify dry surgical sites and to discontinue surgical drains. Those with little at-home support can be tended to for a day and those with complex medical issues can be tuned up prior to their release.

From a practical perspective, constructing the observation unit's beds in multiples of four will minimize overnight nursing staffing costs. Placing the unit in a quiet corner of the building convenient to PACU and to patient parking facilitates both patient rest and discharge.

Moving away from patient-focused areas of the ASC, an on-site pharmacy may be required. The pharmacy board in most states requires that one be established for the storage and distribution of opioids.[24] Locating this component in an area accessible to preoperative holding area, PACU, and the family waiting area permits anesthesia and nursing staff to easily obtain needed antibiotics and opioids before and after surgery. It also allows the pharmacy to fill outpatient prescriptions as a convenience to patients.

Finally, clerical offices can be located in any nonsterile space where conversations cannot be overheard by patients, although placing them near the business office will benefit interoffice communication. Approximately 90–100 net ft^2 will be needed for office areas.[24] In addition to computer terminals at each work area, two FAX lines will be needed for sending and receiving patient information and instructions.

Apart from the visible physical components of the ASC, wiring the telecommunications system also requires careful consideration. The center will require dedicated voice lines in the preoperative, recovery, and administrative areas as well as two lines for the ORs (anesthesia phone plus other.) An intercom system on top of the phone system is also needed.[20] If a computerized patient record will be used, LAN access should be wired into presurgical exam rooms, preoperative bed spaces, the ORs, and PACU beds. A terminal in the business office to aid with billing will also be required.

Incorporation of a toll-free 24-hr hotline can resolve many patient and physician questions or conflicts. Staff fielding questions can answer questions about patient bills or direct them where to park. Additionally they can assuage physician concerns about equipment availability for specific procedures. The toll-free capability can allow out-of-state physicians to easily find out about available services and to refer patients.[28]

Designing the center such that medical gases and supplies can be delivered to and waste removed from the ASC during regular business (and delivery) hours without disrupting operations is also prudent. An area of the center will also be needed to store emergency generator equipment in case of a power outage.

With the design needs of a functional ASC and their multiple interrelationships, it is no wonder that important

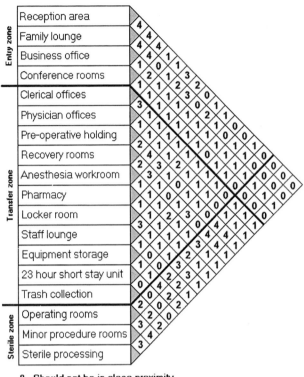

0 - Should not be in close proximity
1 - Could be in close proximity
2 - Desirable to be in close proximity
3 - Must be in close proximity
4 - Must be directly adjacent

Figure 4–8   ASC proximity matrix.

details can be overlooked. In an attempt to avoid planning errors and to minimize the number of blueprint modifications that your architect must draft, a proximity matrix can be a useful tool.[30] The proximity matrix, as adapted from the work of M.J. Berkoff and shown in Figure 4-8, assists in analyzing and prioritizing physical relationships within the surgical center.

After considering the components necessary for a functional ASC and looking at the actual square footage needed, cost and utility are the prominent vying concerns. Because of similar physical needs to acute-care hospitals, ASC construction costs are probably also over $100 (1981 prices) per square foot. The necessary infrastructure of medical gas pipelines, backup electric generators, electric line isolation, advanced telecommunications systems, and specialized heating, cooling, and ventilation systems comprises nearly half of this expenditure.[30] Cognizance of applicable regulations and building codes is an absolute engineering prerequisite. For example, the National Fire Protection Association Life Safety Code 101 demands construction of a 1-hr resistant firewall separating the ASC into at least two smokeproof compartments and separating the ASC vertically and horizontally from other tenants. It is easy enough to factor this firewall in early on, but very difficult and expensive to incorporate once construction has begun.[29] Engineers should be familiar with the local and statewide requirements and those of the Department of Health and Human Services, Joint Commission on Hospital Accreditation (JCHAO), Medicare, and Medicaid.

While initial construction costs may exert a large influence over the final building design, one should not unduly reject greater up-front costs engineered toward longer-term savings. For example, while a two-story ASC may minimize the costs of expensive roofing, foundation footings, and required land holdings, it may prove more expensive if it also requires duplication of staffing on both floors. The operational costs of staffing, energy use, and building maintenance comprise 80% of hospital costs. Value engineering tries to minimize the impact of these factors.[30]

Before finalizing decisions on building structure, a thought should be given to the possibilities of a joint construction venture. Such projects can help the ASC establish itself in a unique niche that allows it to garner market share. An example of such a venture would be to house an orthopedic ASC with a rheumatology clinic to create an arthritis center.[28] Another idea would be to combine an orthopedic ASC with a rehabilitation unit. This would permit the surgical performance of outpatient total joint replacements under anesthesia-managed continuous peripheral nerve block catheters with discharge to the outpatient care of physical therapists.

Regardless of final decisions regarding physical layout, when planning ASC construction it is advantageous to build quickly to beat inflation. Construction costs have increased annually at about a 9% rate.

Once a workable physical design has been achieved, attention can now be turned to methods of achieving ideal function within this design.

BUILDING SAFETY INTO THE AMBULATORY SURGERY CENTER

The overall data for ambulatory surgery indicate that it is quite safe. A study of 500,000 Medicare patients undergoing outpatient procedures from 1994 to 1999 had an overall mortality rate on the day of surgery of 2.4 per 100,000. Most of these deaths were from office-based liposuction procedures. Corrective action has since been taken to assure that tumescent liposuction is now performed in an appropriate setting.[39] Positive softer endpoints have also reached the press, such as the risk of infection in an outpatient center being consistently less—only 35% of that for inpatient surgeries.[11,40] The need to transfer outpatients to a hospital for any reason has also remained low, with rates ranging from 0.12% to 0.37%.[3,26,39,41]

Unfortunately, the bulk of adverse outpatient events that have occurred are due to medical error and are ultimately preventable. Fortunately, these can be easily prevented by adopting safety-based protocols and practices.

Physicians who believe that safety depends primarily in acceptance of individual responsibility and that adverse events are usually the result of individual error will not readily perceive opportunities to improve safety by improving processes and systems or by fostering greater teamwork and shared responsibility and authority.[11]

To ensure that "never events," as defined by the American Medical Association's National Quality Forum, never occur, adherence to the following guidelines is recommended[39]:

1. Become accredited and use accrediting standards to review and strengthen your safety program.
2. Initiate a quality improvement (QI) program to investigate root causes of problems when they occur. Record and analyze pre- and postcorrection data to document that an improvement and not busywork has occurred.[42]
3. Reinforce staff education through lectures or mock codes (discussed below).
4. Invite your malpractice insurer for an annual audit.
5. Utilize information technology; consider an electronic medical record; and put in place decision support systems to insure compliance with standard-of-care guidelines.[11]
6. Provide printed (and translated as necessary) medication instructions whenever possible as roughly 50% of all outpatient medication errors result from differences in physician expectations and patient understanding.[11]
7. Even if not JCAHO accredited, consider the seven JCAHO safety goals, effective January 1, 2004[43]:

   • Improve the accuracy of patient identification and include a presurgical incision "timeout."
   • Eliminate wrong-site, wrong-patient, and wrong-procedure surgery. Utilize a preoperative checklist referencing medical records *and imaging studies*. Involve the patient in surgical-site marking.
   • Reduce the risk of health-care-acquired infections by complying with Centers for Disease Control and Prevention (CDC) hand hygiene guidelines.
   • Improve infusion pump safety with pumps that ensure free flow.
   • Improve the safety of using high-alert medications and standardize concentrations.
   • Improve the effectiveness of communication among caregivers regarding verbal orders and written abbreviations.
   • Assure the effectiveness of clinical alarm systems with regular testing and checking that alarms are audible.

8. Comply with the Accreditation Association for Ambulatory Health Care (AAAHC) requirement to retain a physician or dentist qualified in resuscitation techniques on site until all patients operated on that day have been discharged.
9. Ensure that outpatients have an escort for a ride home as even normalization of psychomotor function after sedation with any agent belies ongoing electroencephalogram (EEG) impairment.[44]
10. Make a postoperative phone call to affirm outpatient wellness after discharge.[45]

When complications such as the unanticipated difficult airway, cardiopulmonary arrest, or an episode of malignant hyperthermia do occur, surviving them will depend as much on ASC staff preparedness as any other factor. Certain mechanical steps taken by the ASC, such as the purchase of fiberoptic airway carts, tracheostomy trays, defibrillators, and dantrolene, will help erect a safety net. However, it is the ongoing training of all ASC personnel that will help them recognize emergent situations, respond appropriately, and marshal resources efficiently in a time of crisis. Certification in and refreshment every 2 years of life support protocols as well as familiarity with emergency equipment are necessary, but even after 6 months, information will be forgotten and proficiency decreased.[46] The best way to keep this information fresh and germane to the ASC environment is to practice mock codes. The codes can cover a wide range of scenarios, from the three above to hypertensive crisis with cerebrovascular accident, intraoperative laser burns, pediatric laryngospasm, anaphylaxis, tension pneumothorax, grand mal seizure, profound vasovagal reaction, or massive hemorrhage with need for emergent transfusion. These codes should be scheduled for a time when there is minimal nonstaff presence in the ASC and should occur at least semiannually if not quarterly.[47] Including the local emergency medical services in the mock code will guarantee that they know which entrance to use for the facility, as well as its layout.[39] The more frequent these drills, the better prepared the staff and safer the ASC patients will be.

While the approximate 10% incidence of outpatient symptomatic vasovagal reactions may make this the most common complication with which ASCs need to contend,[48] disastrous external events can also impact ASC function. Both the AAAHC and JCAHO have standards for ASC preparedness for disasters or bioterrorism. Nearly every state has passed an emergency powers act giving public health officials the power to utilize all health care facilities for a disaster response. An ASC could possibly be used as an overflow site, an isolation unit, a care facility for noncritical hospital patients, a testing facility for potential bioterrorist agents, or even as a morgue. ASC staff may be diverted to help staff other facilities. Regardless, the ASC should know how to take care of its own in case of external exposure to biologic, chemical, or radiation attack. The National Institute for Occupational Safety and Health has published a guide on how to plan for and protect buildings from such an attack.[49] The most common protective roles that ASCs would play in such an instance would be to either "shelter in place" or to evacuate. To "shelter in place" in the event of an external toxic exposure would involve keeping employees and patients inside the building and closing off air-conditioning and fresh-air exchanges. Battery-operated radios and cell phones would be needed to comply with civil instruction for an organized evacuation of the ASC.[50]

BUILDING EFFICIENCY INTO THE AMBULATORY SURGERY CENTER

While patient safety is an inseparable concern from ASC function, efficient operations are also integral to its success. An area that combines these two concerns is preoperative laboratory testing. Historically, patients have been subjected to a battery of unnecessary tests, which served only to increase health costs or even cause needless anxiety from false-positive results. ASC anesthesiologists should take leadership roles in determining appropriate testing and in communicating these to surgeons. Selecting tests based on patient medical history and physical exam and requiring a pregnancy test of all women of childbearing age seems both sufficient and appropriate.[51]

Other issues routinely attempt to disturb the smooth flow of the day's events. First among these, of course, is the topic of patient no-shows that result in large periods of operating room downtime. Many centers currently utilize a reminder phone call the evening prior to surgery. A potential problem with this technique is that voice messages are often left in lieu of a conversation with the patient. This does not provide reassurance of attendance, and in the case of a forgotten appointment with need to reschedule, does not afford the ASC time to fill the vacancy. This practice also wastes patient and ASC time if medical error (such as continuation of anticoagulants or instability of diabetes) that would otherwise preclude outpatient surgery is not discovered. A viable alternative involves contacting patients 2 weeks before surgery, even by dispersing a health questionnaire with a prepaid return envelope, and calling nonresponders 1 week prior to surgery. Patients thus reached should achieve a 97.2% attendance. Patients contacted by neither method, on the other hand, should likely be canceled, as their attendance is a dismal 24.2%.[52]

The second most likely cause of delay involves patient paperwork. It is a JCAHO requirement that a history and physical examination be placed on the chart prior to the commencement of surgery. A dictated and not yet transcribed report does not suffice. Abiding by this hard-and-fast rule can become a headache if surgeons are not compliant with this prerequisite. Having a deadline for complete preoperative paperwork of 48 hr prior to surgery, requiring the attending surgeon to manually write out an absent history and physical, or comparing the tardy surgeons' compliance anonymously to their colleagues may help, but the sole ingredient that has been uniformly successful has been the backing of this regulation by the senior medical staff.[53]

Expounding on the search for efficiency, the scheduling of operating room cases is another area of consternation. In the area of the OR schedule, it is clear that efficiency does not equate with 100% utilization. Indeed, depending on the aims of the management, an ASC can simultaneously achieve only two out of three commonly sought-after goals:

1. Achieving a set and predictable number of working hours for staff.
2. Caring for all patients that surgeons bring to the OR on any given day.
3. Maintaining a high-enough margin (revenue less variable costs) to sustain growth.

Choosing to maximize revenue while limiting the number of cases to those fitting within a budgeted amount of time has several advantages to the ASC. First, the staff remains happy because they rarely have to work overtime. This also saves the ASC from having to pay employees time-and-a-half and to replace burned-out staff. Second, patients have the ability to choose the date of their surgery, which helps them retain some autonomy and improves their satisfaction. Next, purposefully underestimating the duration of cases is a financial disadvantage to the ASC and its surgical investors. By preventing cases from running over and delaying the next one, patient satisfaction again remains high. This overall strategy also provides incentive to surgeons to fill their block time with high-revenue-producing cases and release any unused hours.[54]

Achieving efficient scheduling of the OR requires the matching of estimated to actual case times. It has been demonstrated that relying solely on historical case times is fraught with inaccuracy.[55] To improve the precision of posted times, given that the surgeon, surgical procedure, and anesthesia type are the same, adjusting a historic time up or down by 10% based on predicted difficulty has proven beneficial.[56] Computerized assistance in management of surgical block times has also been of benefit.

A final area of OR efficiency relates to OR setup and turnover times. Using knee arthroscopy as an example, the median studied ASC setup time was 20 min with the top achievers setting up in 9 min. The median cleanup time was 13 min with the best achievers doing so in 5 min. In order to perform as a top achiever, centers sent dirty instruments out of the room prior to patient egress, with the instrument technician returning to help the scrub nurse and circulator with turnover. Prior to the end of a case, the supplies and instruments for the next case were left on a prep table outside the OR by the instrument technician.[23]

Heading from the OR to the PACU raises the question of patient safety and "fast tracking." While leaving the decision to bypass phase I recovery beds in the hands of the anesthesiologists, ambulatory surgery centers that instituted fast tracking were able to do so in 42% of general anesthetics and 80% of MAC anesthetics. Typical PACU bypass criteria are:

- Awake, alert, oriented
- Vital signs stable
- No active bleeding
- Minimal pain
- Minimal nausea, no vomiting
- If used, clinically reversed neuromuscular blockade
- Oxygen saturation of 94% or baseline while on room air for 3 min or more.

Fast-track capabilities were better with desflurane than sevoflurane than propofol with percentages of 90, 75, and 26, respectively. Annualized savings of up to $158,000 can be realized with shortening total recovery time by 1 hr.[57] A prerequisite to bypassing stage I recovery, of course, is avoidance of PONV. Fast tracking aside, the avoidance of PONV alone has profound effects on efficiency and economics of postsurgical care. The cost of one outpatient experiencing PONV has been estimated by various authors to range in time from 14 to 35 additional minutes and in money from $415 to $1040, with an annual cost to an ASC of up to $284,000.[58,59] Clearly, the mode of anesthesia utilized and the prevention of PONV can have profound effects on ASC performance.

A final thought on improving efficiency relates to staff motivation. A valuable methodology of aligning their goals with those of the ASC involves a plan of employee profit sharing as a reward for exemplary performance. Tying employee performance to concrete goals can demonstrate ASC successes on a monthly basis. These goals can vary from the number of phone calls answered in the first three rings to keeping the supply cost of a case lower than the budgeted amount to meeting a quarterly volume of surgical cases. Centers with more than $200,000 in annual profits will typically pool 2–5% of net income for distribution to employees.[60] Distribution methodologies can be varied, but often involve peer review, an assessment of attitude and quality of work, and employee longevity. In addition to motivating workday efficiency, this can also prove to be a valuable tool for staff retention.[61]

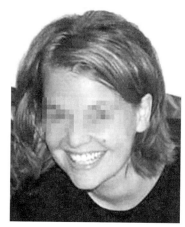

Figure 4-9   The first outpatient recipient of a total knee prosthesis.

THE FUTURE OF AMBULATORY SURGERY

The only consistent observation regarding prior authors' predictions of the future of ambulatory surgery is that their predictions have fallen far short of reality. As in the past, advances in both anesthesia and surgery have permitted the performance of previously considered "major surgeries" in an outpatient setting. The future undoubtedly holds more of the same with advances in robotic-assisted surgery and the development of nanotechnology. Recent news clips promise that endoscopies and colonoscopies as we know them will cease to exist, with future patients able to swallow pill-sized cameras that record and transmit images of the entire digestive tract. Hospital ASCs may be able venture into same-day cardiac surgeries with advances in robotics and minimally invasive techniques. Novel anesthetic drugs will likely further reduce side effects of surgery with the release of peripheral opioid antagonists, nondepolarizing neuromuscular blocking agent neutralizers, micelle suspended local anesthetic depot delivery systems, and environmentally friendly rapid emergence anesthetic gases, all of which are already involved in clinical study.

Regardless of future technologic innovations, the near future of ambulatory surgery will most likely see incorporation of already existing technologies into standard practice. For instance, standardization and utilization of the electronic medical record promises improved patient safety and permits greater perioperative vigilance by anesthesia providers. Employment of wireless monitoring systems, already existent in Europe, will add convenience and time savings when moving patients from one environment to another. Improved training in and practice of peripheral nerve blockade techniques by anesthesiologists will decrease the need for general anesthesia and of PONV and increase the performance of previously pain-prohibitive surgeries on an outpatient basis.

Indeed, on June 24, 2003 the first outpatient total knee replacement in the history of medicine was performed at Duke University Medical Center's ASC (Fig. 4-9). The patient received continuous peripheral nerve blocks and was ambulating in the care of physical therapists on postoperative day 1 with minimal discomfort. Such advances, together with ideally structured and functioning ASCs, will continue to attract outpatients for surgery and likely increase outpatient surgical rates toward 80%. The future of ambulatory surgery is indeed hard to predict. One certainty, however, is that its successes will continue to surprise us all.

REFERENCES

1. Clower WT, Finger S. Discovering trepanation: the contribution of Paul Broca. Neurosurgery 2001;49(6):1417–25; discussion 1425–26.
2. Davis JE. The major ambulatory surgical center and how it is developed. Surg Clin North Am 1987;67(4):671–92.
3. Reed WA. The surgicenter experience. Contemp Surg 1982; 20(1):66–67, 71, 74 passim.
4. Nicoll JH. The surgery of infancy. Br Med J 1909;2:753–56.
5. Waters RM. The downtown anesthesia clinic. Am J Surg (Anesthesia Suppl) 1919;33(7):71–73.
6. Butterworth Hosp News, Grand Rapids, MI, 1961.
7. Cohen DD, Dillon JB. Anesthesia for outpatient surgery. JAMA 1966;196(13):1114–16.
8. Levy ML, Coakley CS. Survey of in and out surgery—first year. South Med J 1968;61:995–98.
9. Anonymous. Nation's first freestanding surgery center still strong. OR Manager 1995;11(7–8):15–16.
10. Burden N. Ambulatory surgery in Phoenix. J Post Anesth Nurs 1986;1(3):195–201.
11. Hammons T, Piland NF, Small SD, Hatlie MJ, Burstin HR. Ambulatory patient safety: what we know and need to know. J Ambul Care Manage 2003;26(1):63–82.
12. Hospital Cost Trends. In: BCBShealthissues.com, June 19, 2003.
13. Sinclair G, President Elect, American Society of Anesthesiology, Personal conversation, 12/15/2003.
14. Parsons RJ, Tonkinson RE, Jr. Conducting a feasibility analysis for freestanding ambulatory surgery centers. AORN J 1986;44(6): 1026–33.
15. Bowles CF. Ambulatory surgery: considerations in planning. Med Group Manage 1981;28(1):60–62, 64, 66 passim.
16. Cryan B. Hospital Costs in Rhode Island—October 1999. In: Rhode Island Department of Health: Publications, October 2001, http://www.healthri.org/publications/list.htm (accessed October 2003).

17. SHAPE: Statewide Health Assessment Planning and Evaluation Study. In: shaperi.com, November 18, 2002, http://www.shaperi.org/shapereport.htm (accessed October 2003).

18. Richards PB. Ambulatory surgical center: developing a health care opportunity. Coll Rev 1996;13(1):51–89.

19. O'Donovan TR. Ambulatory surgery update: pros and cons of basic program models. Same Day Surg 1980;4(8):69–71.

20. Snyder DS, Pasternak LR. Facility Design and Procedural Safety. In: White PF (ed.) *Ambulatory Anesthesia and Surgery*. Philadelphia: WB Saunders, 1997. pp. 61–76.

21. Pica-Furey W. Ambulatory surgery—hospital-based vs freestanding: a comparative study of patient satisfaction. AORN J1993;57(5):1119–27.

22. Anonymous. Diminishing returns for larger ASCs. OR Manager 2002;18(4):34.

23. Anonymous. Smaller amb surgery facilities perform better, surveys find. Data Strateg Benchmarks 2002;6(3):44–46.

24. Fellows GE. Ambulatory surgery design: a consultant's perspective on facility planning. AORN J 1987;45(3):708–24.

25. Hattox J. Director offers step-by-step guide for independent units. Same Day Surg 1981;5(8):97–100.

26. Knapp MR. The Wichita Minor Surgery Center: perspective of the independent, free-standing surgery center. J Ambul Care Manage 1981;4(3):75–84.

27. Anonymous. Survey shows outpatients have high expectations. Healthc Benchmarks 1997;4(9):134–35.

28. Mathias JM. Building a successful ambulatory surgery program. OR Manager 1993;9(2):22.

29. Marasco JA, Marasco RF. Designing the ambulatory endoscopy center. Gastrointest Endosc Clin North Am 2002;12(2):185–204, v.

30. Berkoff MJ. Planning and designing ambulatory surgery facilities for hospitals. J Ambul Care Manage 1981;4(3):35–51.

31. Anonymous. Patients' needs guide to redesign. OR Manager 1998;14(6):12–13.

32. Miluk-Kolasa B, Obminski Z, Stupnicki R, Golec L. Effects of music treatment on salivary cortisol in patients exposed to pre-surgical stress. Exp Clin Endocrinol 1994;102(2):118–20.

33. Heitz L, Symreng T, Scamman FL. Effect of music therapy in the postanesthesia care unit: a nursing intervention. J Post Anesth Nurs 1992;7(1):22–31.

34. Shertzer KE, Keck JF. Music and the PACU environment. J Perianesth Nurs 2001;16(2):90–102.

35. Nilsson U, Rawal N, Enqvist B, Unosson M. Analgesia following music and therapeutic suggestions in the PACU in ambulatory surgery; a randomized controlled trial. Acta Anaesthesiol Scand 2003;47(3):278–83.

36. Earnhart SW. What's best mix of procedures for ASC? OR Manager 2002;18(7):26–27.

37. Goodspeed SW, Earnhart SW. Planning, developing, and implementing a freestanding ambulatory surgery center. Health Care Strateg Manage 1986;4(2):18–22.

38. Anonymous. Advice from the pros: tips for your same-day unit. Same Day Surg 1978;2(10):156–57.

39. Anonymous. What's being done to make ambulatory surgery safer? OR Manager 2003;19(3):30–35.

40. Hugar DW, Newman PS, Hugar RW, Spencer RB, Salvino K. Incidence of postoperative infection in a free-standing ambulatory surgery center. J Foot Surg 1990;29(3):265–67.

41. Natof HE. Complications associated with ambulatory surgery. JAMA 1980;244(10):1116–18.

42. Anonymous. "Close the loop" in QI for ASCs. OR Manager 2000;16(3):17, 20.

43. 2004 National Patient Safety Goals. In: jcaho.org. 2003. http://www.jcaho.org/accredited+organizations/patient+safety/04+npsg/04_npsg.htm (October 2003).

44. Anonymous. Fail-safe discharge: patients with no ride home. OR Manager 1997;13(8):14–15.

45. Anonymous. What must ASCs do about practice guidelines? OR Manager 2002;18(4):25.

46. Schwid HA, O'Donnell D. Anesthesiologists' management of simulated critical incidents. Anesthesiology 1992;76(4):495–501.

47. Figley E, Burden N. Preparing for the unexpected in the ambulatory surgery unit. J Post Anesth Nurs 1991;6(2):117–20.

48. Pavlin DJ, Links S, Rapp SE, Nessly ML, Keyes HJ. Vaso-vagal reactions in an ambulatory surgery center. Anesth Analg 1993;76(5):931–35.

49. Mead KR, Gressel MG. Guidance for Protecting Building Environments from Airborne Chemical, Biological, or Radiological Attacks. In: CDC: National Institute for Occupational Safety and Health; 2002.

50. Anonymous. What's the ASC's role for mass casualties? OR Manager 2002;18(11):23–25.

51. Mathias JM. Assess first, test later, centers say. OR Manager 2001;17(5):26–28.

52. Basu S, Babajee P, Selvachandran SN, Cade D. Impact of questionnaires and telephone screening on attendance for ambulatory surgery. Ann R Coll Surg Engl 2001;83(5):329–31.

53. Anonymous. The paper chase: getting H&P on patient's chart before surgery. OR Manager 2002;18(5):1, 10.

54. Dexter F. Efficient scheduling of OR cases. OR Manager 2000;16(3):27–28.

55. Zhou J, Dexter F, Macario A, Lubarsky DA. Relying solely on historical surgical times to estimate accurately future surgical times is unlikely to reduce the average length of time cases finish late. J Clin Anesth 1999;11(7):601–5.

56. Dexter F, Traub RD. How to schedule elective surgical cases into specific operating rooms to maximize the efficiency of use of operating room time. Anesth Analg 2002;94(4):933–42, table of contents.

57. Anonymous. "Fast tracking" of patients through PACU: is it safe? OR Manager 1998;14(6):1, 8–9.

58. Carroll NV, Miederhoff PA, Cox FM, Hirsch JD. Costs incurred by outpatient surgical centers in managing postoperative nausea and vomiting. J Clin Anesth 1994;6(5):364–69.

59. Sanchez LA, Hirsch JD, Carroll NV, Miederhoff PA. Estimation of the cost of postoperative nausea and vomiting in an ambulatory surgery center. J Research Pharm Econ 1995;6(2):35–44.

60. Zasa RJ, Pierson MR. 10 key factors to improve operations in ambulatory surgery centers. MGMA Connex 2002;2(5):62–68.

61. Anonymous. What's the best way to reward staff? OR Manager 2002;18(12):22–24.

Ambulatory Perioperative Nursing and Patient Education

CYNTHIA VINCENT

INTRODUCTION

Perioperative nursing in the ambulatory surgery atmosphere requires concise and accurate education to patients and their families/significant others. The education begins prior to the patient arriving for surgery, which will reduce patient anxiety and stress. Nurses who administer quality patient care throughout the perioperative process follow standards of practice. Education postoperatively must be administered in different modes, with a short window of time to deliver the instructions. Patient satisfaction is high when the education is administered effectively both preoperatively and postoperatively. A plan of care for the ambulatory surgery patient is a necessity, facilitating consistent quality patient care. Patients should be discharged from phase 1 and phase 2 recoveries when they meet discharge criteria based on standards of nursing practice. An extended recovery period following ambulatory surgery may be required by some patients.

Preoperative Nursing and Patient Education

Patient education can begin from the moment the surgery is scheduled in the physician's office. The perianesthesia nurse has the opportunity to administer teaching prior to the patient preadmission interview. Patient-centered surgical brochures with the educational needs of the preoperative patient addressed are the initial phase of teaching. Physician office staff can give this information to patients when they are scheduling surgery.[1]

Anticipation of patient needs and education can be completed primarily with a preoperative phone call to the patient or parent/guardian. Ambulatory surgery patients are communicating their preferences to health care providers of the need and desire for preoperative teaching before they are admitted for surgery. It does not matter where the ambulatory environment is, in a physician's office, inside hospitals, or in freestanding ambulatory surgery centers. These patients are still requiring information regarding the preoperative phase desiring to learn about their impending surgical experiences prior to admission. It was found that patients thought it is most important to know when events and procedures would occur and least important to know about the preoperative nursing care they would receive.[2] Patients appreciate the knowledge in advance to plan for their surgical experience, including planning on who will take them home and assist them with their care postoperatively.

Patients have many fears regarding surgery, including fear of death, anesthesia, and pain. To manage stress, patients can utilize a mechanism entitled coping. "Coping is a process of constantly changing cognitive and behavioral efforts to manage specific external and/or internal demands that are appraised as taxing or exceeding the resources of the person. Coping can be either problem-focused or emotion-focused. The greater the threat, the more primitive defensive emotion-focused coping is used." When a stressor can be changed it is perceived as problem-focused. Making life more bearable is part of the emotion-focused coping method. Preoperative teaching gives the patient the ability to utilize coping mechanisms to prepare for and experience the surgery. In addition, preoperative education reduces anxiety and stress for the patients. It has been found that patients assessed as having mild stress receive the most complete teaching. The stress increases as the teaching received by the patient decreases. There has to be a balance between too much and too little information given. Alleviating stress through preoperative teaching is essential for the patient plan of care.[3]

It has been found in previous studies that preoperative teaching decreases complications, increases patient satisfaction, shortens the length of hospitalization, and promotes psychologic well-being.[4] Preoperative teaching will usually consist of the following contents:

- location of surgical facility,
- time to arrive on the day of surgery,
- instructions on not eating or drinking after a specified time,

- no alcohol or smoking the night before surgery,
- allowed medications preoperatively,
- special instructions for diabetics,
- specific instructions related to their surgery for the preoperative phase, and
- expectations of postoperative care including any devices anticipated, such as: crutches or a walker.

Informing patients that they must have a responsible adult to drive them home and care for them for 24 hr following surgery is imperative to patient safety and to facilitate timely discharge. Many nurses will take this opportunity to interview the patient for medical and health history. This information may be reviewed by an anesthesiologist and utilized to determine whether the patient will need a preoperative testing appointment.

American Society of Anesthesiologists (ASA) standards are utilized to classify the patient health history. Published on the ASA website is the Physical Status Classification System:

P1   A normal healthy patient;

P2   A patient with mild systemic disease;

P3   A patient with severe systemic disease;

P4   A patient with severe systemic disease that is a constant threat to life;

P5   A moribund patient who is not expected to survive without the operation;

P6   A declared brain-dead patient whose organs are being removed for donor purposes.[5]

Patients who are classified as ASA Class I or II are healthy enough not to require preoperative testing but may need preoperative laboratory screening performed the day of surgery preoperatively. Anesthesiologists have set standards for required preoperative screening for patients with several comorbidities. This allows nurses to be able to inform patients what to anticipate for preoperative screening.

On the day of surgery preoperative teaching focuses on what the patient can expect through the perioperative experience, initiation of an intravenous access for patients not having local anesthesia, surgical skin prep if ordered by the surgeon, and any preoperative orders such as laboratory testing, X-rays, and electrocardiograms. The type of anesthesia will be discussed between the patient, family/significant other, and anesthesiologist. Nurses instruct the patient on the use and purpose of pain scales (visual or numeric scales) utilized to identify levels of pain pre- and postoperatively. For patients receiving regional anesthesia it is important for the nurse to instruct the patient and family on the protection of the limb from injury, which may be insensate to weight bearing, pain, heat, or cold following surgery.

Signs and symptoms of local anesthetic toxicity are reviewed with the patient prior to administration of continuous peripheral nerve blocks. "Symptoms of toxicity are manifested primarily through the cardiovascular and central nervous systems. Symptoms progress from:

- tachycardia and hypertension from the epinephrine;
- ringing in the ears;
- metallic taste in the mouth;
- numbness of the lips;
- twitching of the eyes and lips leading to seizures; to
- cardiovascular, respiratory, and central nervous system depression (e.g., loss of consciousness) if allowed to continue without treatment."[6]

Patients are informed of when to anticipate the motor function return followed by the sensory blockade resolving. The initial teaching of proactive pain management is essential for patients as soon as possible.

Standards of Care

Upon admission to the surgical facility the patient is assessed by a nurse including obtaining vital signs and pain level preoperatively. Assessment data collection provides nursing with information for the patient plan of care. Preoperative plan of care can be initiated during the preoperative phone call or the preoperative testing visit. Preoperative physician orders are accomplished. An intravenous access is initiated. Patients to receive regional anesthesia in the preoperative holding area will be placed on standard ASA monitors for sedation to begin prior to the block. Nurses need to be available to assist the anesthesiologist and monitor the patient during this procedure.[7]

Postoperative care of the patient is administered following Joint Commission Accreditation of Healthcare Organizations (JCAHO) and American Society of Perianesthesia Nurses (ASPAN) guidelines. ASPAN staffing guidelines are based on patient classification with nurse:patient ratios. Patients in immediate postanesthesia care are in phase 1 and are transitioned to phase 2 level of care, extended recovery, or observation status.

According to ASPAN guidelines on the discharge assessment from phase 1 level of care, the patient will be evaluated and not limited to:

1. Airway patency, respiratory function, and oxygen saturation.
2. Stability of vital signs.
3. Hypothermia resolved.
4. Level of consciousness and muscular strength.
5. Adequate pain control.
6. Mobility.
7. Patency of tubes, catheters, drains, and intravenous lines.
8. Skin color and condition.
9. Condition of dressing and/or surgical site.
10. Intake and output.
11. Comfort.
12. Anxiety.
13. Child-parent/significant others interactions.
14. Numerical pain score, if used.[7]

Discharge Assessment for phase 2 of recovery according to ASPAN will evaluate:

1. Adequate respiratory function.
2. Stability of vital signs.
3. Hypothermia resolved.

4. Level of consciousness and muscular strength.
5. Ability of ambulate consistent with baseline/procedural limitations.
6. Ability to swallow.
7. Minimal nausea/vomiting.
8. Skin color and condition.
9. Adequate pain control.
10. Adequate neurovascular status of operative extremity.
11. Ability to void as indicated.
12. Patient and home care provider understand discharge instructions.
13. Written discharge instructions given to patient/accompanying responsible adult.
14. Verify arrangements for safe transportation home.
15. Provide additional resource to contact if any problems arise.
16. The professional perianesthesia nurse will complete a discharge follow-up to assess and evaluate patient status.[7]

Fast-tracking in ambulatory surgery refers to bypassing the postanesthesia care unit (PACU) I (phase 1 of recovery). This concept is received positively when patients have a more rapid recovery as a result of being less deeply sedated. The patient will go from the operating room (OR) directly to PACU II (phase 2 recovery) awake, alert, meeting the discharge criteria from phase 1 recovery. This is a patient satisfier as well as a cost savings for the surgical facility. For a successful fast-tracking program the team of practioners, including surgeon, anesthesiologist, certified registered nurse anesthetist (CRNA), and staff nurses, need to be on board with the concept. The use of newer, shorter-acting anesthetic and adjunctive drugs may provide important benefits to the patients, having decreased side effects from medications and the ability to perform normal life activities sooner. An additional cost savings can be seen with nurses being cross-trained to work in the OR and the PACU II areas or PACU I and PACU II.[8,9]

It is crucial that patients are educated to the fast-track concept prior to surgery, preparing them for a short recovery period without feeling like they are being rushed home following surgery. Fast-tracking is based on patients meeting specific criteria rather than being based on a procedure that is performed. Patients with a significant medical history will require the need of PACU I recovery. Patients who have received spinal or epidural anesthesia will need monitoring in PACU I until they meet the appropriate discharge criteria.[8,9]

Fast-tracking may be utilized in a different fashion when the step-down unit (PACU II) is already burdened with patients. Studies have been performed to evaluate the effectiveness of fast-tracking outpatients to home directly from the PACU, determining the potential impact on the amount of time required for discharge of the patient in this manner. It was found that this method of fast-tracking was a means to "free up" space in the PACU and in the day surgery unit. To facilitate this process a responsible adult needs to be readily available to allow prompt discharge of the patient when he/she meets discharge criteria. Other considerations are to have a patient bathroom in close vicinity, curtains or screens to provide privacy, a mechanism for storing patient belongings, and the availability of dedicated nurses cross-trained in PACU I and PACU II. It is important to have a good working relationship between perioperative nurses and the anesthesia team for a cohesive fast-tracking program.[10]

Time required to promote the patient to achieve a state of home-readiness after ambulatory surgery and feel satisfied with his/her care is influenced by a wide variety of surgical and anesthetic factors. However, the major contributing factors for discharge delay after ambulatory surgery are nausea, vomiting, pain, dizziness, and prolonged sympathetic and/or motor blockade (not anticipated).[8] Some nerve blocks are purposefully administered to last for 12–18 hr, during which the nurse teaches the patient how to manage the limb that is blocked. These particular patients usually do not experience nausea and vomiting or pain requiring medication relief since the surgical site is insensate.

Some patients require extended recovery following outpatient surgery. The most common reasons for extended recovery are pain control, nausea and vomiting, and observation for bleeding at the surgical site. The goal is to develop a plan of care to meet the patient needs and discharge him/her in less than 24 hr as soon as discharge criteria from PACU II are met.

Postoperative Teaching

Patients and their families/significant others are instructed on the anticipated length of surgery and when to expect to see the patient again. As soon as the patient is in stable condition in the PACU, he/she is usually allowed visitors. Having the responsible adult at the bedside who will be caring for the patient when he/she is discharged is ideal but not always possible. It is advantageous to give postoperative instructions to the patient and the responsible adult to care for the patient at the same time. Questions can be answered for the patient and family member/significant other while reviewing the postoperative instructions.

Simply handing written instructions to a patient and family member is not adequate to meet their needs. It is the role of the perioperative nurse to translate the written instructions in a thorough manner that promotes understanding and ease of compliance in the home environment. The perioperative nurse must take into consideration the patient's learning needs (knowledge deficits, if any) and psychologic needs (emotional state).

Postoperative instructions usually consist of:

- activity level and lifting restrictions if needed,
- diet restrictions or advancing diet as tolerated,
- bowel movements and reasons for constipation,
- resumption of sexual activity,
- monitoring urine output (making sure the patient can void 6 hr postoperatively),
- driving or operating heavy machinery restrictions,
- pain control modes and use of medication,
- wound or dressing care, signs of infection,

- drain care if present,
- bathing and keeping surgical area dry,
- use of devices as ordered (cold therapy device, crutches, walker, sling), and
- return to work/school.

Postoperative patient education is a precursor to high satisfaction for patients and family members.[11]

Patients who have received peripheral nerve blocks will need specific instructions about care of the insensate limb. Explanation on the inability to use the extremity and protection of the extremity will be discussed and written for the patient. Stressing no weight bearing on the lower extremity that is blocked and the use of crutches or a walker is necessary.

SUMMARY

After demonstration and instruction of use, return demonstration for patients being discharged with devices is another mode of education. The patient will have more confidence in caring for him/herself when they can utilize the device being sent home with them.

Perioperative nursing and patient education is very influential to the successful surgical experience for patients. Ambulatory surgery has limited time to implement the patient plan of care in an efficient manner. The perioperative health care team members must collaborate to accomplish patient satisfaction with ambulatory surgery.

REFERENCES

1. Barnes S. Preparing for surgery: providing the details. J Perianesth Nurs 2001;16(1):31–32.
2. Brumfield VC, Kee CC, Johnson JY. Preoperative patient teaching in ambulatory surgery settings. AORN J 1996;64(6):941–52.
3. Garbee DD, Gentry JA. Coping with the stress of surgery. AORN J 2001;73(5):946, 949–51.
4. Oetker-Black SL, Teeters DL, Cukr PL, Rininger SA. Self-efficacy enhanced preoperative instruction. AORN J 1997;66(5):854–64.
5. ASA physical status classification system. Available at: http://www.asahq.org/clinical/physicalstatus.htm.
6. Murauski JD, Gonzalez KR. Peripheral nerve blocks for postoperative analgesia. AORN J 2002;75(1):134, 136–40, 142–51, 153–54.
7. Miller K, Sullivan E, Allen J, Cannon K, Clifford T, Flanagan K, et al. Standards of perianesthesia nursing practice. Cherry Hill, NJ: American Society of PeriAnesthesia Nurses, 2002, pp. 27–31.
8. Watkins AC, White PF. Fast-tracking after ambulatory surgery. J Perianesth Nurs 2001;16(6):379–87.
9. Sullivan EE. How to fast-track safely. Outpatient Surg Mag 2001; 11(2):18–23.
10. White PF, Rawal S, Nguyen J, Watkins A. PACU fast-tracking: an alternative to "bypassing" the PACU for facilitating the recovery process after ambulatory surgery. J Perianesth Nurs 2003;18(4): 247–53.
11. Fox VJ. Postoperative education that works. AORN J 1998;67(5): 1010–17.

Preoperative Evaluation of Ambulatory Surgery Patients

ANGELA M. BADER

INTRODUCTION

Surgical centers vary in their procedural scheduling of ambulatory surgical patients. Some centers, such as Brigham and Women's Hospital in Boston, mix both ambulatory and admitted patients in their operating rooms (ORs). Other centers, such as Duke University in Durham, find greater efficiencies in scheduling these ambulatory patients in a freestanding ambulatory procedure center. Regardless of the choice of scheduling, the same level of preoperative assessment and organization is required to ensure that all medical and nonmedical issues are addressed. In this way, procedures can be done in the safest and most efficient manner. In an era of diminishing health care resources and increasing customer demands from patients, surgeons, and health insurance organizations, efficient and effective organization and utilization of the preoperative clinic is essential. The goal is to provide high-quality assessments that will optimize outcomes, utilizing a value-based, patient-centered focus. This chapter will discuss the various aspects that this involves, including structural organization, personnel stratification, and clinical assessments and guidelines.

ORGANIZATIONAL STRUCTURE OF AN AMBULATORY PREOPERATIVE ASSESSMENT CLINIC

Defining Goals and Expectations

It is important to understand that the structure of the ambulatory procedure preoperative clinic will be very different depending on the particular institution. Although all patients require the same level of assessment and chart organization, this does not equate to all patients seeing the same type of providers or even having a physical visit to the clinic. Therefore, the first step is to define the needs of the particular institution.

It is a useful exercise to look at several weeks' worth of OR schedules to generate statistics regarding number and type of cases by surgical service. Generating information regarding acuity level of these cases is also extremely useful. Decisions regarding the acuity level that will be acceptable in the ambulatory center will vary based on the available resources. Include non-OR cases, such as endoscopy or radiology, that require anesthesia if these need to be part of the staffing plan. Adding to these data information about projected surgical volume for future fiscal years will make the projections more in line with institutional expectations.

Once these data are obtained, identification of assessments to be performed is the next step. Preoperative assessment according to Joint Commission on Accreditation of Healthcare Organizations (JCAHO) guidelines requires the following:

1. Surgical history, physical examination, and consent
2. Anesthesia assessment and consent
3. Nursing assessment
4. Laboratory testing, electrocardiograms (ECGs) and X-rays when required.

Each of these assessments has specific required elements. According to the JCAHO, the surgical history and physical examination must be dated within 30 days of the procedure. None of the other assessments or tests has dating requirements, according to the JCAHO or any other professional societies. Some insurance organizations have dating requirements that influence reimbursements. Most institutions have established standards and guidelines in this regard that are in line with comparable surgical centers.

Decisions then need to be made regarding which of these assessments will be done in the clinic, which will occur at other locations, and what flow plans can be developed to ensure that all information is collected, reviewed, and sent to the OR in a timely fashion.

The following factors need to be considered in plan development:

1. Space available for preoperative assessment;
2. Development of staffing plan for both clinical and nonclinical staff based on space available and assessments to be performed on site;
3. Development of scheduling system for patient evaluation based on volume and acuity level, as well as type of provider;
4. Development of algorithms and pathways with surgical office staff to ensure that necessary information is available at the time of the patient's visit;
5. Development of phone screen systems for appropriate patients;
6. Fostering efficiency and improving staff interactive skills to improve patient satisfaction with process;
7. Developing feedback systems to monitor effect on OR; cancellation and delay rates, patient satisfaction, and clinic efficiency;
8. Facilitating specific surgical needs and improving surgeon satisfaction with the preoperative process;
9. Definition and appointment of a preoperative clinic director;
10. If appropriate for your institution, including planning for resident involvement and residency education in preoperative assessment.

Presenting a Plan

In an era of diminishing resources, hospital administration may be reluctant to commit resources to the preoperative clinic. However, maximum OR utilization and efficient turnover times can only occur if proper patient preparation has been done. In a time when the acuity level of patients coming for ambulatory procedures is increasing, appropriate patient evaluation is essential for the operating suite to function smoothly. Any delay, whether due to missing test results, absent surgical consents, or abnormal ECGs that have not been addressed, can lead to costly unused OR time while the issue is resolved or another patient is moved into the now-vacant OR time slot. When presenting such a plan to surgical, anesthesia, and administrative departments, the benefits should include financial savings as well as increases in patient and surgeon satisfaction. As the preoperative clinic is not a significant revenue-generating area, administrators need to realize that the major cost savings will be seen in improved OR efficiencies and room utilization, particularly in percent utilization of ORs in prime time hours.

Anticipated Cost and Related Savings

1. Reducing unreimbursed or excessive laboratory testing: In the current era of managed care, capitation as well as Health Care Financing Administration (HCFA) restrictions on laboratory testing motivate hospital staff to reduce unnecessary and unreimbursed testing. Numerous studies have shown that screening presurgical laboratory testing in the absence of clinical indications failed to influence perioperative management.[1-4] Proper International Classification of Diseases, Ninth Revision (ICD-9) coding is essential to ensure that laboratory testing is appropriately reimbursed. Since 1996, HCFA will not reimburse for testing without appropriate ICD-9 coding and coding of approved comorbidities. A preoperative clinic will help to provide protocols and therefore consensus among surgeons and anesthesiologists about which laboratory tests are really necessary. Comorbidities can be properly documented. The clinic providers can be authorized to cancel unnecessary testing. At the Brigham and Women's Hospital, the preoperative clinic laboratory ordering form includes the ICD-9 codes and appropriate comorbidity conditions, helping to ensure Medicare compliance and appropriate reimbursement.

2. Reduction in costs due to cancellations or delays: Many causes for cancellations, both medical and nonmedical, can be reduced by the appropriate functioning of a preoperative clinic. For example, recent data from the University of California calculated their ambulatory surgery cancellation rate of 287/2173 as follows: patient ill or absence of preoperative fasting—28%; no show—22%; needed further workup—17%—all causes that could have been reduced by appropriate patient education and evaluation preoperatively.[5]

3. Higher reimbursement due to improved documentation: At the Brigham and Women's Hospital, the vast majority of presurgical histories and physical examinations are done in the preoperative clinic. These histories and physical examinations tend to be far more detailed and inclusive of comorbidities, to ensure appropriate reimbursement based on Diagnosis Related Group (DRG) coding of comorbidities.

4. Generation of revenue via facility fees: Many institutions, including the Brigham and Women's Hospital, bill a standard fee for use of the preoperative clinic. Although billing far exceeds reimbursement in this area, the collected revenue can at least in part offset the cost of the clinic. For example, data from the University of Florida show that this institution bills a facility fee of $140 per preoperative clinic visit, with a collection fate of 23% of billings in outpatient surgery patients, yielding a net revenue of $238,980 on billings of $1,176,000.[1]

Efficient Manpower Usage

A recent service excellence project at Brigham and Women's and Faulkner Hospitals in Boston concluded that significant increases in patient satisfaction as well as in overall clinic efficiency could be achieved by striving to limit the number of providers that each patient sees. This also eliminates redundant questioning and duplicate paperwork.

Therefore, one of our current manpower goals at the Brigham and Women's Hospital is to utilize nurse practitioners to perform the required preoperative surgical, anesthesia, and nursing assessments. The patient would therefore be seen by one nurse practitioner and then have a laboratory technician come into the room to perform blood testing and ECGs if necessary. This goal also includes leaving the patient in one room and having all practitioners come to the patient. This also eliminates the need for the patient to undress and dress twice, which is required if the history and physical examination and the ECG are done by providers in different rooms.

There is also a smaller group of patients at the Brigham and Women's Hospital who have their surgical history and physical examination performed by either their surgeon or their primary-care physician (PCP). These patients are seen in the preoperative clinic by an anesthesia resident and a nurse. Each surgical center needs to make the decision regarding where the various elements of the preoperative evaluation will be done and by whom; this may require negotiations between hospital administration, surgery, anesthesia, and nursing. The ultimate goal is to ensure that adequate, medically appropriate evaluations are done so that all medical issues are addressed, patient safety and well-being is optimized, and coding for appropriate reimbursement is expedited.

Facilitation of Specific Surgical Needs

Establishment of an effective preoperative clinic provides a mechanism whereby surgeons can have needs for specific groups of ambulatory patients addressed. For example, at the Brigham and Women's Hospital there are a group of ambulatory surgery patients coming from the Dana Farber Cancer Institute for central venous access placement. These patients would not normally qualify as phone screen patients owing to the complexity of their illnesses. However, these patients have extensive histories known to the Farber and additional evaluation at the Brigham seemed redundant. Therefore, a second phone screen system was initiated in which these patients are assessed via phone with a separate checklist. Medical information, ECG, and laboratory results are obtained from the Farber, the nursing assessment and education is done as part of the phone call, and a physical visit to the preoperative clinic is eliminated.

An important specific surgical need that is addressed in the preoperative clinic is patient and family education. The surgeon may have little time in his or her office to go into extensive details regarding the hospitalization and recovery periods. Nurses in the preoperative clinic take time with patients and their families to review all of this information, provide instructions, and ensure that all of these issues are addressed prior to the procedure. This also expedites the process on the morning of surgery. The nursing assessment and patient education have already been performed and documented and all of the patient and family questions have been answered. This work is completed on the phone for patients who are triaged to not need a physical visit to the clinic.

Policy and Procedure Alignment

The establishment of a preoperative clinic provides a structure that allows for policy development. This promotes alignment within the anesthesia group and between the anesthesia, surgery, and nursing departments. Protocols can be established to ensure appropriate transmission of information throughout the preoperative period.

Unfortunately, the literature available regarding appropriate evaluation, risk assessment, and outcome does not provide clear guidance. Uniform clinical goals can be established via communication and conferences. Policies and guidelines should be clear, available in written form, and distributed throughout the department. Alignment of policies and goals is essential so that patients assessed in the preoperative clinic are not delayed or canceled by an anesthesiologist or surgeon on the day of operation.

At the Brigham and Women's Hospital, patient evaluations in the clinic are generally booked by a surgeon's secretary through a central system after registration and insurance precertification have been performed. The patient is given an Internet address so that he/she can submit information in a secure fashion, which is received and reviewed by the preoperative clinic. Based on this information, the patient may be triaged to a phone screen. Also, information from outside providers described in this online assessment (stress tests, echocardiograms, etc.) can be obtained prior to the patient's clinic visit. This Internet process will be described in detail below.

The secretary also has the option of booking a visit or a phone screen assessment. Algorithms for determining which patients can be phone-screened have been provided to the surgeons' office staff and will be described below. The surgeon's office staff then sends a packet to the preoperative clinic, which contains the surgeon's office note, history, and physical examination if done by surgeon, and laboratory testing orders. Packets are requested in the preoperative clinic 72 hr prior to the patient's visit so that a chart can be compiled. The surgeons and their office staff are aware that prolonged clinic visit times, patient dissatisfaction, poor patient care, and potential cancellation of the procedure may result if this information is not available.

Patient appointments are scheduled via computer program, which has been developed so that patients are evenly distributed throughout the day by provider. At the Brigham and Women's Hospital, we currently see approximately 90 patients per day; an additional 10–20 patients per day are evaluated without a physical visit. Communication via this scheduling program with the medical records department allows the patient's old chart to be available at the time of the appointment. Unscheduled patients are discouraged, as no information will generally be available. Unscheduled patients will also increase overall patient waiting time for the scheduled patients.

As described above, patients are seen by either a nurse practitioner and a laboratory technician or an anesthesia resident, nurse, and laboratory technician. An attending anesthesiologist is available on site and reviews all abnormal ECGs before the patient leaves. This ensures that no unresolved issues remain and also provides an opportunity for resident education when the abnormalities and plan are discussed. Other laboratory data are not available for several hours. These data are printed out and filed in the chart by the next morning. All patient charts are then reviewed by a nurse practitioner so that any abnormalities or unresolved medical issues can be addressed. The nurse practitioner fills out a "surgical checklist," which is the first sheet in every chart sent to the OR. The presence and correctness of all appropriate paperwork, laboratory results, ECGs, and consents is noted so that all issues can be quickly reviewed without randomly searching through paperwork. Any unresolved problems are identified by the nurse practitioner and resolved before the chart is sent to the OR.

The surgeons' offices have received general guidelines as to which patients may be evaluated via phone screen and do not need an appointment. American Society of Anesthesiologists (ASA) physical status class I and II patients without known cardiac problems who do not require laboratory testing in the clinic and who have had a surgical history and physical examination performed in the surgeon's office are not required to come to the preoperative clinic and can be evaluated via Internet/phone screen. All laboratory testing except for type and screens is accepted from outside facilities. The paperwork from the surgeon's office is sent to the clinic as usual in the patient's packet. The surgeons' office staff schedules the patient through the same central computer program system but schedules the patient as a "phone screen" instead of an appointment. A computer printout of these "phone screen" patients is then printed out in the clinic. When this printout and the surgeon's packet containing the history and physical examination are received, the patient receives a telephone screen by a preoperative clinic nurse, which is placed in the patient's chart, assembled, and filed as usual. Any patient in whom the telephone interview reveals an area of concern is discussed with the attending anesthesiologist and may be scheduled to appear for an appointment. Since institution of this program, less than 1% of phone screen patients have needed appointments and there have been no OR cancellations as a result of inadequate phone screen interviews.

The preoperative nursing assessment is done during this phone call with the nurse, eliminating the need to perform this assessment on the day of surgery. This decreases the OR turnover time for these cases, which are usually short day surgical procedures. Patients also receive preoperative instructions, preoperative fasting orders, and instructions regarding which medications should be taken on the morning of surgery. This eliminates problems with phone screen patients arriving on the day of surgery without having followed appropriate preoperative fasting and medication guidelines.

All preoperative clinic personnel are instructed to notify the anesthesia and OR scheduling office via e-mail with particular patient issues of which the assigned anesthesia team should be aware. These issues may include potential difficult intubation, severe cardiac compromise, Jehovah's Witness patients, pregnant patients coming for nonobstetric surgery, latex allergy, among others. Identifying these issues aids with OR scheduling, ensures appropriate equipment is available, and aids in departmental uniformity regarding anesthesia care. Infection control issues can be identified early and appropriate room assignment facilitated.

DEFINING MANAGEMENT ROLES IN THE PREOPERATIVE CLINIC

The preoperative clinic provides a vehicle through which the hospital can promote its mission of patient-focused care. A successful preoperative clinic visit will foster in the patient a sense of confidence in the hospital and health care providers and put the surgical experience in a positive light. A disorganized, inefficient, incomplete visit during which a sense of concern for the patient is not expressed will result in low patient satisfaction and loss of confidence in the hospital and the surgical process. It is essential to stress the importance of patient-centered interaction and an attitude of competence, compassion, and caring with all members of the clinic team. Front-line service has a strong influence on the patient's perception of a hospital's performance.

The team concept is fostered by uniting all clinic personnel, including all types of clinical providers as well as support staff, under a single administrative team. It is difficult to foster the team concept of a patient-oriented service line in a preoperative evaluation clinic in which multiple lateral providers work via different reporting lines and consider their roles in a unifunctional manner. Our preoperative clinic holds regular staff meetings attended by all members who work in the unit. These meetings foster a team approach to problem solving and generate a positive feeling regarding the unit's mission that can be transmitted to the patients. All personnel roles in the clinic are essential to the success of the overall mission.

The preoperative clinic is a self-contained area staffed with surgical, anesthesia, nursing, support staff, and laboratory personnel so that the patient can usually receive all preoperative evaluations required in a single location. A collaborative effort and management structure among the departments of anesthesia, nursing, and hospital administration is required. At the Brigham and Women's Hospital, an anesthesiologist serves as director of the clinic. This director reports to both the hospital vice president for surgical services and the chairman of the department of anesthesiology. A nonclinical administrative manager and support staff report to the anesthesiologist serving as director. Although nursing reporting lies with the OR nurse manager, the day-to-day clinical roles of the nurses in the preoperative clinic are defined by the director in conjunction with the OR nurse manager. Staffing and budget issues for the clinic, including the majority of the clinic nursing budget, are made by the director in conjunction with the nurse manager, and approved by the vice president for surgical services. Laboratory technicians are on site in the preoperative clinic, although they report through a different supervisor and are included in the budget for laboratory administration.

The establishment of the role of a director of the preoperative clinic provides a number of advantages:

1. A clinician with expertise in the area of preoperative assessment is in a position to establish systems, algorithms, and clinical protocols to improve efficiency of the preoperative clinic and the OR.
2. The director is available to serve as a liaison between anesthesia, surgery, nursing, and hospital administration to resolve preoperative issues.
3. The director provides accountability. Systems can be established to provide feedback regarding effectiveness of the preoperative services provided.
4. The director, together with the clinic management team, can perform long-term planning for the clinic as

far as budget and staffing based on projected surgical volume and acuity levels.

5. The director can formulate time lines with the clinic management team, anesthesia, surgery, nursing, and hospital administration to achieve improvements in patient satisfaction, develop clinical pathways, and attain continued improvements in providing preoperative services.

6. The director is responsible for ensuring educational opportunities so that all clinic providers maintain preoperative assessment competencies.

Because the major role of the preoperative center involves clinical decision making, the anesthesiologist seems particularly suited by training to play a key role in the organization and direction of these centers. Specific expertise regarding clinical assessment, appropriateness of preoperative testing, and effective preoperative management should allow the development of integrated and efficient patient evaluation. Unfortunately, few anesthesiologists demonstrate both the interest in the preoperative area and the administrative skills needed to successfully take on this role. As described below, a generational change in mindset of the anesthesiologist is required. The ability to negotiate with hospital administration, nursing, and surgery to define and support the role of the anesthesiologist in preoperative assessment in each particular institution is necessary.

INCREASED PATIENT SATISFACTION VIA PATIENT-FOCUSED PREOPERATIVE ASSESSMENT

The preoperative clinic provides a vehicle through which the hospital can promote its mission of patient-focused care. A successful preoperative clinic visit will foster in the patient a sense of confidence in the hospital and health care providers and put the surgical experience in a positive light. A disorganized, inefficient, incomplete visit during which a sense of concern for the patient is not expressed will result in low patient satisfaction and loss of confidence in the hospital and the surgical process. It is essential to stress the importance of patient-centered interaction and an attitude of competence, compassion, and caring with all members of the clinic team. Front-line service has a strong influence on the patient's perception of a hospital's performance.

Uniting all clinic personnel, including all types of clinical providers as well as support staff, under a single administrative team fosters the team concept. It is difficult to foster the team concept of a patient-oriented service line in a preoperative evaluation clinic in which multiple lateral providers work via different reporting lines and consider their roles in a unifunctional manner. Our preoperative clinic holds regular staff meetings attended by all members who work in the unit. These meetings foster a team approach to problem solving and generate a positive feeling regarding the unit's mission that can be transmitted to the patients. All personnel roles in the clinic are essential to the success of the overall mission.

The patient's family members are encouraged to be present during all interviews and their concerns are addressed as well. Courteous behavior, a professional appearance, and expressions of genuine concern are fostered. All personnel are instructed to address the patient by name, to introduce themselves professionally, and to conduct the interview with the patient in a respectful and empathetic manner. Although our providers must see large numbers of patients within significant time constraints, the concern and caring perceived by the patients is reflected in the high ratings our unit receives in patient satisfaction surveys even during these short visits. Although our patient satisfaction surveys demonstrate opportunities for improvement in efficiency of the process, the scores for clinical care provided are uniformly extremely high.

EDUCATION IN PREOPERATIVE ASSESSMENT

To successfully take on management roles in the preoperative assessment of ambulatory surgery patients, a generational change in mindset of the anesthesiologist is required. Evidence suggests that this is only very slowly occurring. Anesthesiologists are often reluctant to take on clinical roles outside the OR and may feel uncomfortable in situations involving extensive patient interaction. Until recently, residency programs have been severely lacking in emphasis on the importance of patient assessment skills as well as the importance of administrative and organizational skills, leaving few anesthesiologists with the competence and commitment to take on major roles in this area. Surgeons vary in their ability to manage preoperative risk assessment issues; some may not perceive the implications of concurrent medical issues or the importance of obtaining appropriate information and test results from PCPs.

The role of anesthesiologists continues to expand outside the OR into areas of perioperative medicine; however, training programs may be inadequately preparing residents to effectively take on these roles. Evaluating patients in the preoperative clinic is often viewed by anesthesiologists as an undesirable assignment. We believe that there is insufficient training in both organizational and clinical aspects of perioperative assessment. Lack of exposure to this area during residency contributes to poor attitudes and ineffectiveness. We undertook a national survey to evaluate existing methods of residency training and departmental attitudes regarding preoperative evaluation.[6]

A three-page survey was sent to every accredited anesthesiology residency program in the United States. This survey addressed the areas of departmental preoperative curriculum, general structure of the preoperative clinic, and scheduling and supervision of residents in the preoperative clinic.

A total of 140 surveys were distributed and 116 responses were received (83% response rate), representing 3466, or about 82%, of current residents in training. Fifteen programs (11%) do not have a preoperative clinic. Residents never rotate through the clinic in 33% of programs with clinics. Thirty percent of programs report that less than 10% of anesthesia staff have any interest or expertise in this area (range 0–100). Less than half (45%) of programs have an established curriculum in this area. The prevailing feeling about departmental commitment and attitudes about this area were generally negative, as evidenced by written responses.

In conclusion, fewer than half of accredited anesthesiology residency programs have any formal curriculum in preoperative assessment and in 44% of programs residents have no contact with a preoperative clinic. This may account for the negative attitudes of anesthesiologists regarding preoperative evaluation, resulting in inability to resolve organizational and clinical issues. Exposure to both organizational and clinical aspects of this area may improve our effectiveness and attitudes.

However, for the preoperative clinic to run successfully, anesthesia residents are only one group of providers that require clinical and organizational education. A central plan and effort must be in place to ensure that all providers giving presurgical care, including nursing, anesthesia, surgical, and laboratory providers, are continually assessed and educated regarding competencies in preoperative assessments. In an effort to address this issue, education of all clinical providers should be considered a major part of the preoperative clinic's effort and vision.

At the Brigham and Women's Hospital, a 2-week resident rotation has been established, which includes a core curriculum in preoperative assessment given in 1-hr morning lectures each day of the rotation. Regular Wednesday staff meetings are held for all clinic providers to provide a format for updates, in-services, and competency maintenance in all areas of preoperative assessment. Seminars in customer service, team building, and increasing patient satisfaction are also given during this time period. All clinic providers, both clerical and clinical, are expected to attend.

COMMUNICATION WITH CONSULT SERVICES

The misused and unfortunately perpetuated concept of "clearance" prior to a surgical procedure needs to be rethought. Many surgeons and anesthesiologists incorrectly feel that "clearance" of complicated patients who have been followed extensively by PCPs or cardiologists outside the hospital can be provided instantly by referring a patient for consultation with an internist or cardiologist at the hospital who knows nothing about the patient and is evaluating him/her for the first time. This is a misguided concept, as all accessible appropriate information on the patient needs to be accessible at the time of the preoperative evaluation. Asking for "clearance" does not obviate the need to include this information and the input of the patient's primary health care providers in the preoperative assessment. In fact, failure to do so would constitute substandard patient care. Appropriate patient assessment utilizing an organization that provides mechanisms for including all relevant patient data will significantly reduce the need for formal consultation, as described below.

At the Brigham and Women's Hospital, we have significantly decreased the number of cardiology consultations requested despite an increase in both volume and acuity level of patients assessed. This is the result of several factors: first, a new emphasis on patient assessment in our training program. More important, the anesthesiologists who work in the preoperative assessment testing clinic (PATC) at our institution have developed expertise in functioning as consultants in the area of preoperative assessment, in communicating appropriately with the patient's existing primary care providers and outside cardiologists, and in obtaining and reviewing all appropriate information. We provide algorithms for cardiac evaluation and train our staff to be familiar with the literature available.[7] If the anesthesiologist does decide after a review of all available information on the patient that a patient requires a consultation with a cardiologist, the preoperative clinic clerical staff arranges this. Because of the emphasis placed on education of the anesthesia staff in the area of preoperative assessment and improved interdepartmental communication, consults obtained are phrased in a tone such that specific questions for the patient involved are answered. The cardiologist is not asked for a vague "clearance," but rather if further testing would be beneficial or if suggestions could be made regarding medical optimization prior to surgery. This greatly improves the usefulness of the consults obtained.

We have recently published data regarding the effect of alterations in procedures, education, and staffing in our PATC on reducing the number and improving the yield of cardiology consultations.[8] All anesthesiologist-requested cardiology consultations for patients undergoing elective noncardiac surgery from 1993 to 1999 were reviewed. This period corresponded to 3 years before and after a change in the clinic leadership, which resulted in more stringent consultation algorithms and the institution of a cardiac assessment and ECG interpretation educational program for all clinical staff. We found a significant decrease in number of consultations requested in the period after the changes were instituted, despite a documented increase in the surgical case-mix acuity. Of the consultations requested, a significantly greater percentage was felt by the cardiologist to require further cardiac testing. This would suggest that we were referring more patients who genuinely needed further evaluation and fewer in whom the consultation was unnecessary. A significant reduction in consultation request because of ECG abnormalities was also reported. Specifically, the number of consultations for ECGs that were interpreted by the consulting cardiologist as "unchanged from prior ECG," "normal," or "abnormality secondary to lead placement" was markedly decreased. However, the percentage of ECGs referred to cardiology and read as significantly abnormal showed a marked increase. There was no increase in overall cardiac complication rate postoperatively despite the decrease in overall consultations.

LABORATORY TESTING

Most care providers are well aware that the previous practice of randomly ordering batteries of test prior to surgical procedures was costly and inefficient, with little impact on patient management.[9,10] A review of 15 studies researching the utility of routine chest X-rays concludes this to be a practice reserved only for patients with clinical evidence of pulmonary disease or those undergoing intrathoracic surgery.[11] Urinalysis in asymptomatic patients rarely leads to beneficial changes in management.[12,13]

We have significantly decreased the amount of preoperative testing by streamlining our laboratory order form based on the literature available. The order form includes indications for testing so that guidelines can be followed by anyone using the form. In general, no laboratory testing is required for otherwise healthy males or nonpregnant females less than age 50. ECGs are required for all patients over age 50. Complete blood counts (hematocrit, white blood cell, and platelet) are required for all patients over age 60. Chest X-rays are done only in the patient with significant pulmonary disease, heart disease, or malignancy, or as a baseline prior to intrathoracic surgery. Urinalyses are performed only in cases of hardware insertion or suspected urinary-tract infection. All other laboratory testing should be based on concurrent medical conditions. These guidelines are fairly conservative; some other institutions have decreased requirements further depending on anticipated type of anesthetic and relative risk of surgical procedure.

COMPUTER-BASED PREOPERATIVE ASSESSMENT

Few institutions are currently utilizing the great potential inherent in computer- and/or Internet-based preoperative information systems. Although it would seem a natural progression to transition to computer-based systems for the collection, storage, and recall of preoperative information, several barriers can be postulated that may be the cause of the slow progress made in this area.

First, there is great concern regarding the confidentiality of patient information transmitted via the Internet. How will the information be entered? Who will be responsible for verifying its accuracy? How will it be stored? Who will have access to the information? How will security be maintained? How will this information be contained in the patient's OR chart? Great concerns about the confidentiality of computerized information have led some hospitals to feel reluctant to enter patient data in this fashion via an Internet-based technology. It seems ironic, however, that the security of a medical record on paper that is bound in a chart and can be left on shelves, in offices, or elsewhere where many personnel may have unauthorized access is not of even greater concern to these institutions.

Second, many institutions, particularly smaller institutions, may not have the information systems resources necessary to develop, implement, and maintain such computerized data. A significant commitment is necessary on the part of the institution, and with limited programming resources, this area may not be seen as a priority.

Third, successful development of a computerized preoperative process requires close collaboration among experts in the various areas involved—programming, anesthesia, surgery, and hospital administration. A project manager should be chosen who is familiar with the entire preoperative processes and what the eventual goals should be. We have published our experience in the area of the anesthesiologist's interest in the preoperative clinic.[6] This would indicate that few hospitals have anesthesiology departments with a great deal of interest in the preoperative process and that many residents finish their training with little exposure to this area. Anesthesiologists in general seem less willing to take on administrative roles in the preoperative clinic, particularly where no additional reimbursement to their department may be involved.

Fourth, patients and health care professionals may be somewhat reluctant to switch from standard methods of giving and recording patient information to a system that is much more based on technology. They may feel that the learning curve is too great, that it may interfere with current work styles, and that access to computer terminals in their institutions is still too limited in patient care areas. They may feel that patients will dislike having providers typing on a computer keyboard while interviewing them, and that this may increase the distance between provider and patient. An additional concern is that patients, particularly those in the older age groups, may be reluctant to use or be unfamiliar with Internet technology. However, use of the Internet will only continue to expand over the next few years, and even patients in the older age groups are likely to become more familiar with this medium.

A final consideration that may be presenting some concern as these information systems are developed is the ongoing process of development of federal regulation. The federal government is currently in the process of developing rules and regulations regarding standards for privacy of individually identifiable health information. These regulations are developments of the Health Insurance Portability and Accountability Act (HIPAA) of 1996. Institutions may be concerned about developing systems that may not be in compliance with these standards or may be unsure of what current regulations require.

In response to the need to provide an easily accessible, Internet-based vehicle for preoperative assessment, the author has developed a commercially available website (www.smartsleep.com).[14] Through this site, patients can fill out a questionnaire regarding their preoperative medical history, which is then submitted via a secure connection to the hospital at which the patient will be having his/her surgery. The application is licensed by the hospital, the domain name is distributed to the hospital's presurgical patients, and a permanent, secure database of all preoperative surgical information is then available to selected providers at that hospital via password access. Data can be entered wherever Internet accessibility is present. Patient and procedure-related educational information that is hospital-specific can also be distributed via this website. A demonstration module of the capability of this website when utilized by a particular hospital is available at www.smartsleep.com/demo.

The Brigham and Women's Hospital has seen several major benefits from the use of this Internet-based system. Patients are able to provide information regarding their PCPs, specialists, and medical conditions that can be reviewed in advance of the clinic visit. Previous testing done at outside institutions can be retrieved prior to the patient visit. For example, cardiac tests such as echocardiograms, stress tests, and catheterizations can be obtained and reviewed before the patient arrives. Previously, the patient would have to wait in the clinic while information necessary for the preoperative evaluation was retrieved. Also, after review of the Internet submission some patients could be triaged to a "phone screen" group and the physical visit eliminated, resulting in increased patient satisfaction and more efficient use of clinic resources. Finally, a permanent database is created on the presurgical patients, and available to all appropriate providers in a password-protected manner.

Some institutions and providers may be concerned that patient responses during an automated interview would differ from those obtained during a verbal interview. Data in the literature would indicate that this is not the case.[15] Suggested laboratory testing based on history did not differ between groups of patients using "Health Quiz" to provide information regarding their history and those questioned orally during an interview. Patients from differing socioeconomic backgrounds responded similarly to both automated and oral presentation of questions.

SUMMARY

The current challenge of preoperative evaluation is to perform value-based, efficient and effective preoperative assessments, which result in maximum OR efficiency. In an era of diminishing health care resources, efficient organization and utilization of those resources available in the preoperative clinic will result in cost savings via reductions in OR delays and cancellations. Effective organization can also reduce laboratory testing and the use of outside consultation. Fostering a patient-centered focus in the preoperative clinic can reap the additional benefits of increased patient satisfaction and confidence in the hospital and health care providers.

REFERENCES

1. Gibby GL. How preoperative assessment programs can be justified financially to hospital administrators. Int Anesth Clin 2002;40: 17–30.
2. Roizen MF. Cost-effective preoperative laboratory testing. JAMA 1994;271:319–20.
3. Golub R, Cantu R, Sorrento JJ, et al. Efficacy of preadmission testing in ambulatory surgical patients. Am J Surg 1992;163:565–70.
4. Power LM, Thackray NM. Reduction of preoperative investigations with the introduction of an anaesthetist-led preoperative assessment clinic. Anaesth Intens Care 1999;27:481–88.
5. Shah NK, Lim M, Trautloff T, et al. Incidence and reasons for cancellation of cases in an ambulatory surgery center. Anesthesiology 1999;91:A34.
6. Tsen LC, Segal S, Pothier M, Bader AM. Survey of residency training in preoperative evaluation. Anesthesiology 2000;93:1134–37.
7. Fleisher LA. Evaluation of the patient with cardiac disease undergoing noncardiac surgery: an update on the original AHA/ACC guidelines. Int Anesth Clin 2002;40:109–20.
8. Tsen LC, Segal S, Pothier M, Hartley LH, Bader AM. The effect of alterations in a preoperative assessment clinic on reducing the number and improving the yield of cardiology consultations. Anesth Analg 2002;95:1563–68.
9. Roisen MF. More preoperative assessment by physicians and less by laboratory tests. N Engl J Med 2000;342:204–5.
10. Narr BJ, Warner ME, Schroeder DR, Warner MA. Outcomes of patients with no laboratory assessment before anesthesia and a surgical procedure. Mayo Clin Proc 1997;72:505–9.
11. Lutner RE, Roizen M, Stocking CB, et al. The automated interview versus the personal interview: do patient responses to preoperative health questions differ? Anesthesiology 1991;75:394–400.
12. Narr BJ, Hansen TR, Warner MA. Preoperative laboratory screening in healthy Mayo patients: cost effective elimination of tests and unchanged outcomes. Mayo Clin Proc 1991;66:155–59.
13. Mancuso CA. Impact of new guidelines of physicians' ordering of preoperative tests. J Gen Int Med 1999;14:166–72.
14. Bader AM. Computer-based preoperative assessment. Int Anesth Clin 2002;40:193–99.
15. Tape TG, Mushlin AI. The utility of routine chest radiographs. Ann Intern Med 1986;104:663–70.

Running a Perioperative Ambulatory Acute Pain Service: A Physician's Perspective

EUGENE R. VISCUSI • MICHAEL KERNER • MICHAEL SIMON-BAKER

Ambulatory surgery continues to grow at a rapid rate. Increasingly complex procedures are now being performed in ambulatory settings. Pain control is key to the success of outpatient procedures and is often the rate-limiting step determining whether a procedure can be undertaken in the ambulatory setting. Delayed discharge, unplanned admission, and readmission after discharge are directly linked to adequacy of pain control.[1] Adequate ambulatory pain control enhances recovery and return to normal function. Unfortunately, as is true in most areas of pain management, there is evidence to suggest we should be doing considerably better.

In theory, an ambulatory acute pain service has the same goals as an inpatient service: enhanced pain control, reduction in side effects, better surveillance of patients, and patient and family education. The final outcome should be faster recovery and return to normal daily function. Because observation is limited after discharge, the analgesic plan must be well thought out and agreed upon by patient, surgeon, and anesthesiologist. A careful system of follow-up must be maintained. Great care must be taken to match the technique to the patient and procedure. The most aggressive outpatient pain management techniques have an inherent risk. Not all patients are suitable for these techniques, especially if they are unwilling or incapable of following all discharge instructions.

Pain management, whether ambulatory or inpatient, is best provided with a multimodal approach. Utilizing a variety of analgesics reduces the reliance on opioids alone and should therefore reduce opioid-related side effects. Further, combining agents that work by different mechanisms and at different sites enhances overall success in pain management. Analgesics useful in the outpatient setting include opioids, local anesthetics, nonsteroidal anti-inflammatory drugs (NSAIDs), cyclooxygenase-2 (COX-2) selective inhibitors, and acetaminophen. Local anesthetics can be infiltrated into wounds or infused through catheters, used in single injection or continuous peripheral nerve blocks, or instilled into joint spaces. Antiemetics are also standard as part of these regimens.

The following discussion will present the available techniques and their risks and benefits along with the current evidence to support use. Approaches to follow-up will be described.

MULTIMODAL ANALGESIA

The goal of multimodal analgesia is to balance a combination of multiple drugs during both preoperative, intraoperative, and postoperative moments to minimize unwanted side effects and assure a more successful analgesic result. These drug combinations, working by various mechanisms of action, generally have a synergistic effect so that a smaller amount of a single agent can be used to improve relief of pain, result in fewer side effects, possibly decrease cost, and increase overall patient satisfaction.[2–4] The multimodal approach also takes advantage of the known mechanisms involved in acute postoperative pain. Postoperative pain is primarily due to injured tissues, sensitized nociceptors, and the initiation of central pain pathways; the use of each specific drug can target a particular type of pain mechanism. In addition, the preoperative administration of these drugs may further decrease the overall intraoperative need for analgesia, leading to an easier and earlier recovery from ambulatory surgery. The drugs used for this balanced analgesia include four general types: opioids, NSAIDs, COX-2 selective inhibitors, and local anesthetics.

Opioids

Although opioids are indicated for moderate to severe pain in the ambulatory setting, in many cases they should not be relied upon as the primary analgesic.[5] Opioids are useful for rescue purposes to relieve extreme pain, suffering, and harmful physiologic effects, such as myocardial ischemia and, at times, nausea and vomiting due to acute pain.[3,6] Opioids act to modify both central and peripheral nociception in the brain and spinal cord, but their major undesirable effects postoperatively are a direct extension of the mechanism of central nervous system (CNS) action. Though opioids have a safe track record with relatively no toxicities, their central mechanism of action may produce unwanted side effects, including nausea, vomiting, sedation, constipation, and occasionally respiratory depression.[7,8] Treating these side effects is more challenging when patients are no longer in the hospital. If opiates are deemed necessary, they are best titrated to patient comfort to reduce side effects that may negatively affect recovery. Limitations to their use are due, again, to their central action, often initiating nausea, vomiting, dysphoria, sedation, constipation from reduced gastrointestinal motility, and confusion, especially in the geriatric patient population.[6,10–12]

Intravenous (IV) opioids commonly used during surgery and prior to discharge include fentanyl, alfentanil, remifentanil, morphine, meperidine, and hydromorphone. Claxton et al. compared equipotent doses of morphine and fentanyl in patients after ambulatory surgical procedures and reported that the incidence for postoperative nausea and vomiting (PONV) was markedly higher for morphine use.[13] However, they noted that pain scores were higher in the postanesthesia care unit (PACU) for patients who received fentanyl and that their oral opioid requirements were greater soon after. Fentanyl in equivalent dose has a longer duration of respiratory depression compared to alfentanil with a similar or longer recovery time.[8,13,14] Remifentanil has markedly less postoperative respiratory depression because of its short context-sensitive half-time, and can be disadvantageous if not combined with local anesthetics or longer acting opioids for painful procedures.[8,9] Michaloliakou et al. examined a preoperative multimodal analgesia with both meperidine and ketorolac given intramuscularly 45 min prior to induction for patients undergoing laparoscopic cholecystectomy. They reported a sixfold reduction in postoperative pain versus placebo in the PACU, with marked reduction in PONV, and earlier discharge from the PACU.[2] Tramadol, used widely in Europe for postoperative pain, is a weak-acting opioid agonist that also inhibits reuptake of both 5-hydroxytryptamine (5-HT) and norepinephrine.[14–17] It has limited use in the PACU because it is available in the United States only as an oral preparation[15] but is widely used in Europe as an IV agent. Tramadol has an analgesic profile comparable to meperidine with markedly less respiratory depression than opioid agonists.[16] Oral opioids commonly used include oxycodone, hydrocodone, and codeine, often in combination with acetaminophen.

Nonsteroidal Anti-inflammatory Drugs

Well known for treating nonsurgical arthritic pain, NSAIDs have become an integral part of multimodal analgesia and are among the most frequently used drugs to reduce postoperative pain. IV ketorolac is widely used for its opioid-sparing effect and associated reduction of PONV.[5,18] Injury

to tissue occurs during surgery not only at the site of injury (primary hyperalgesia), but also in adjacent intact tissues (secondary hyperalgesia). In addition to the central afferent pain signals produced from tissue injury, inflammation at the site of surgery causes the synthesis of new prostaglandins from the cyclooxygenase pathways (COX-1 and COX-2), resulting in the sensitization of peripheral nociceptors and reduction in nociceptive threshold.[19,20] The NSAIDs effectively block both cyclooxygenase pathways nonselectively and inhibit the formation of prostaglandins. Administration of NSAIDs preoperatively is aimed at minimizing this pathway to halt the induction of prostaglandins from COX-2 before incision. COX-2, generally found in low concentration, is induced by painful stimuli that cause inflammation and is therefore blocked by NSAIDs.[19] However, COX-1 is constantly present in many tissues, including kidneys, stomach, and platelets, and is involved in the function of their routine cellular activity. When inhibited, it is responsible for most of the undesired side effects of NSAIDs, such as bleeding (both operative and gastrointestinal), renal tubular dysfunction, gastritis, and gastric ulcers.[20]

Many reports have compared the analgesic efficacy of NSAIDs to that of opioids. Ketorolac, when used in balanced analgesia for ambulatory surgery, enhanced postoperative analgesia and patient well-being.[21] When ketorolac is substituted for opioids, patients have less PONV, are more alert, advance to oral diet more rapidly, and are released from the PACU earlier.[21,22] Oral and rectal administration of other NSAIDs has similar outcomes.[23] In addition, Rosenblum et al. compared premedication with 800 mg of oral ibuprofen versus 70 µg of IV fentanyl, resulting in longer-lasting analgesia with ibuprofen.[24] Obviously, there is a role for NSAIDs in ambulatory surgery; however, they should be used cautiously both for patients with preexisting disease, such as gastrointestinal disease or renal impairment, and for surgical procedures at higher risk for bleeding.

Cyclooxygenase-2 Selective Inhibitors

COX-2 selective inhibitors (e.g., rofecoxib, celecoxib, valdecoxib, parecoxib) have an improved side effect profile over traditional NSAIDs and have a role in ambulatory surgery as a nonopioid supplement to balanced analgesia. As they selectively inhibit COX-2, there is reduced gastrointestinal bleeding and irritation and no antiplatelet effect. Surgical trauma induces COX-2 and the prostaglandin pathway.[5] Prolonged trauma lowers the threshold of peripheral nociceptors, producing peripheral sensitization, and also induces changes in central afferents, further exciting spinal neurons, causing central sensitization. With this injury, a "wind-up" effect of both central and peripheral hypersensitivities amplifies pain in the postoperative period.[5,19] Furthermore, the COX-2 enzyme is expressed centrally in both brain and spinal cord and is induced by continued noxious stimuli.

Preoperative dosing of COX-2 selective inhibitors may inhibit both central and peripheral hypersensitization. Reuben et al. compared premedication using 50 mg of rofecoxib 1 hr before surgery versus 50 mg 15 min after surgery, finding that premedicated patients required less opioids after 24 hr, had longer analgesic duration prior to opioid rescue, and lower overall pain scores.[25] Reuben et al. showed that postoperative rofecoxib provided more effective analgesia than celecoxib, and Issioui et al. showed it was both more effective and provided more prolonged analgesia than acetaminophen.[26] In addition, a small study examined an IV COX-2 selective inhibitor, parecoxib, looking at postoperative opioid-sparing effects. Though the study followed nonambulatory patients with IV opioid patient-controlled analgesia (PCA) abdominal surgery, they found quite a significant reduction in opioid consumption over 24 hr with almost all sparing effects occurring in the first 6 hr.[27] Furthermore, preliminary findings in animal models have shown parecoxib to be comparable in analgesic efficacy to ketorolac.[28] COX-2 selective inhibitors have a safety and efficacy profile well suited for short-term use after ambulatory surgery. Delayed bone growth and bone healing require further human study but currently do not appear to be a contraindication in this setting.

Acetaminophen is an effective nonopioid analgesic especially when dosed at regular intervals. Acetaminophen exhibits opioid-sparing qualities but lacks the peripheral anti-inflammatory action of NSAIDs and COX-2 selective inhibitors. Because it does not inhibit platelets, it remains a standard therapy, often in combination with opioids. The proposed mechanism of action is a central COX-3 pathway.

Because COX-2 selective inhibitors can be dosed once or twice daily, they offer convenience and sustained analgesic and anti-inflammatory action when compared with traditional NSAIDs and acetaminophen. This may enhance compliance and the quality of analgesia.

LOCAL ANESTHETICS

Preemptive Analgesia

Recent advances in anesthetic and surgical techniques combined with escalating health care costs, have resulted in an increasing number of surgical procedures being performed in an ambulatory surgery setting. Many extremely painful procedures can now be performed in the ambulatory setting with aggressive postoperative pain control techniques. The intensity of early acute postoperative pain may be an important predictor of the development of chronic pain. For example, chronic pain can be a problem after open inguinal hernia repair.[29]

Preemptive analgesia is an antinociceptive treatment that prevents establishment of altered processing of afferent input that amplifies postoperative pain. Crile formulated the concept of preemptive analgesia on the basis of clinical observations. He postulated that the use of regional blocks, in addition to general anesthesia, could prevent intraoperative nociception and the formation of painful scars, caused by changes in the CNS during surgery. Preemptive analgesia has been defined as treatment that:

1. Starts before surgery;
2. Prevents the establishment of central sensitization caused by incision injury (covers only the period of surgery);

3. Prevents the establishment of central sensitization caused by incision and inflammatory injuries (covers the period of surgery and the initial postoperative period).[30]

Thus, preemptive analgesia involves the delivery of analgesic therapy that precedes, adequately blocks, and outlasts the nociceptive stimuli that accompany tissue injury. The aim is to prevent the peripheral and central sensitization that occurs in response to painful stimuli, while leaving the physiologic pain responses intact.[31]

Preemptive analgesia remains controversial. While some studies clearly show benefit, others remain unimpressive. Preemptive analgesia is likely influenced by many variables in the true clinical setting. When regional anesthesia is concerned, complete intraoperative blockade is probably necessary to observe a preemptive effect. Even in the presence of aggressive postoperative pain management, preemptive analgesia may decrease postoperative pain during hospitalization and long after discharge. A block of sufficient duration is another requirement for positive clinical outcome of preemptive treatment.[31] The effects of preemptive analgesia can also be applied to the ambulatory patient.

Techniques

Safety, rapid recovery, and minimal postoperative problems are essential in selecting surgical procedures and anesthesia techniques for day case surgery. The nature, technique, extent, and duration (> 90 min) of surgery along with the choice of anesthetic technique can affect the incidence of postoperative morbidity at home.[30]

A number of regional anesthetic techniques are available for same-day surgery patients. These techniques involve little physiologic trespass, compared with general anesthesia, making them well suited to high-risk elderly patients. Techniques include intravenous regional anesthesia (IVRA), wound infiltration, intra-articular, and peripheral nerve blockade.

IVRA is one of the most common regional techniques. It is best suited for cases of short duration, usually less than 45–60 min involving the distal extremities. Good surgical anesthesia can be achieved rapidly after the injection of local anesthetic. Recovery is rapid with block resolution beginning immediately after the release of the tourniquet. No other regional anesthetic technique provides such a control over the onset, duration, and recovery of block. However, this technique has some problems. There is pain associated with the use of a tourniquet and potential life-threatening local anesthetic toxicity should the tourniquet fail. IVRA's restriction to use on only a distal extremity is also considered a disadvantage to some practitioners.[29]

Local analgesia placed into a surgical wound has limited benefit and does not appear to fulfill the preemptive analgesia requirement. Timing of wound infiltration is important. Some investigators have shown that wound infiltration can provide some prolonged postoperative analgesia. When preemptive analgesia was studied by comparing preincision versus postincision treatment groups, many authors found no difference in the pain outcome, while others reported statistically significant, but clinically modest, benefits with preincision analgesia.[30] For example, Kelly et al.[32] found the demand for additional postoperative analgesics was higher, and occurred earlier, in those patients who received postincision lidocaine infiltration compared to those who received preincision lidocaine.

Klein et al. infiltrated wounds of patients following total abdominal hysterectomy with a single dose of 40 mL of 0.25% bupivacaine with epinephrine 1:200,000 between the muscle and subcutaneous layers during the surgical wound closure. This did not reduce PCA morphine consumption or pain scores for the first 48 hr.[32] To increase the duration of analgesia afforded by the instillation of local anesthetics into the wound, a number of devices are now available to provide a constant delivery by a catheter placed directly into the surgical wound. Zohar et al. attempted to determine the analgesic efficacy of in-hospital patient-controlled bupivacaine wound instillation after total abdominal hysterectomy with bilateral salpingoooophorectomy. A catheter to instill local anesthetic was placed above the fascia with the catheter tip at the midpoint of the incision. The PCA device was programmed to deliver 9 mL of 0.25% bupivacaine with a lockout time of 60 min and no basal infusion. The instillation was performed over a 5-min period. The results indicated a decrease in opioid requirement, decreased incidence of nausea, and less antiemetic drug administration.[33] In the published study of Klein et al., intra-articular analgesia with a continuous infusion of 0.5% ropivacaine infusing at 2.0 mL/hr into the shoulder joint provided improved analgesia when compared with a brachial plexus block with long-acting amide local anesthetic alone.[34]

This technique, now utilizing disposable elastometric pumps, is now a standard technique for many ambulatory procedures. Studies demonstrate that the pain control obtained by wound instillation can vary. It can be very dependent on catheter placement and drug delivery. Local anesthetic can leak from the insertion site, which may cause concern to the patient.

Some surgeons prefer intra-articular injection of local anesthetic for postoperative analgesia. Intra-articular drug administration has gained popularity because of its simplicity and efficacy in achieving anesthesia for diagnostic and operative arthroscopy.[29] Patients undergoing ambulatory anterior cruciate ligament repair of the knee receiving a combination of selective pre- and postsurgical local infiltration of the knee with bupivacaine (0.25%) containing epinephrine (1:200,000) had reduced postoperative analgesic requirements by more than 50% within the first 4 hr postoperatively, compared with intra-articular instillation at the end of surgery alone. Other benefits included the time to readiness for discharge being approximately 30 min earlier, as well as a decrease in incidence of adverse effects. Interestingly, there was no decrease in postoperative pain in the first 24 hr.[35]

Adequate analgesia after knee arthroscopy not only adds to a patient's acceptance of this procedure on an outpatient basis, but may also affect the recovery profile and discharge time from the hospital. Bupivacaine is considered by many to be the ideal drug to achieve postarthroscopy analgesia of the knee. It is used in combination with a variety of other intra-articular analgesics such as ketorolac, morphine, and clonidine. Conversely, several studies have failed to show a benefit to intra-articular instillation of bupivacaine. Despite these reports, the use of bupivacaine as part of postarthroscopic analgesic regimes is widely accepted and generally regarded as clinically useful.

Absorption of local anesthetics from the postoperative intra-articular surface is unpredictable and systemic toxicity has been reported with bupivacaine in doses below 100 mg. Blood levels following injection into the knee joint of 30 mL of 0.5% bupivacaine are < 480–650 µg/mL with peak level occurring at 20–43 min after injection. These levels are 8–10 times less than those reported to cause convulsions in humans. There are reports of bupivacaine toxicity occurring during knee arthroscopy involving the more vascular structures of the knee.[36]

Ropivacaine, in contrast to bupivacaine, has inherent vasoconstrictor properties that may affect its uptake. Convery et al. showed peak plasma concentrations of both agents can be within the acceptable safety ranges when injected into the knee joint.[37]

In ambulatory surgery patients, regional or peripheral nerve block techniques are preferable methods of preemptive analgesia. Regional anesthesia can reduce or avoid the hazards and discomforts of general anesthesia, including sore throat, airway trauma, and muscle pain.

A controversial issue in day surgery is whether regional anesthesia offers significant benefits over general anesthesia for ambulatory surgery. Published data are conflicting. All general and regional anesthesia techniques have advantages and disadvantages. In a study comparing spinal, epidural, and propofol anesthesia for knee arthroscopy, propofol anesthesia was associated with the shortest stay in the operating room but the greatest postoperative pain and drug costs. Mepivacaine epidural block resulted in the longest stay with the most prolonged postoperative analgesia. Spinal anesthesia was the least expensive, but one patient developed postdural puncture headache. Acceptance of a given technique by surgeon and patient, and the expertise of the anesthesiologist, are crucial to making regional anesthesia work efficiently in an ambulatory surgery center. It is essential that each unit audits its own complication rates, recovery room times, and patient opinions to determine the relevance of regional or general anesthesia. Day surgery performed under local anesthesia is often the simplest, safest, and cheapest. Having the ability of regional anesthesia to provide a predictable intra- and postoperative course can aid in a smooth transition from surgery to recovery with anticipated early discharge. This is in contrast to the use of general anesthesia with the associated risks of delayed discharge due to complications, most commonly nausea, vomiting, and uncontrolled pain. Unanticipated admission for nausea, vomiting, and pain are almost exclusively a problem in patients receiving general anesthesia and opioids.[29] These remain key cost drivers in the ambulatory setting.

There are, of course, some disadvantages to regional anesthesia. It may take longer and require active cooperation of the patient and surgeon. Performance of the block may be associated with minor discomfort along with local-anesthetic- and block-specific complications. Further, not all patients are suited for regional anesthesia. There are contraindications to the use of regional anesthesia, such as patient refusal, localized infection, or anticoagulation. Heavy sedation may be required for the anxious patient, which may negate some of the positive nonsedating aspects of regional anesthesia. Remedies for a failed block range from supplemental local anesthetic provided by the surgeon, to conversion from a regional anesthetic to a general anesthetic.[29]

Several concepts will help the practitioner perform regional anesthesia in an efficient manner. The chosen technique should be appropriate for the intended surgery. The selected local anesthetic should provide analgesia well into the postoperative period. In patients undergoing surgery using regional anesthesia, patient education should begin during the preoperative clinic visit. This helps to improve patient acceptance of the use of regional anesthesia. Audiovisual material and information pamphlets are helpful tools, giving patients time to make an intelligent decision and to be psychologically prepared for the block. Patient education will also help to allay apprehension about being awake during the surgery and to address the fear of pain during the block.

The timing of the block placement is important. Special block rooms outside operating rooms (ORs) should be available to handle the high volume and turnover of patients as well as the ability to perform the blocks well in advance of the scheduled surgery start time to allow sufficient "soak" time for the local anesthetic. This allows the physician time for the block to become established. If sufficient time has passed and the peripheral nerve blockade is not sufficient for surgery, the practitioner will then need to decide whether to proceed with a rescue block or convert to a general anesthetic before the patient arrives in the OR.

Both bupivacaine and ropivacaine appear to be efficacious as long-acting local anesthetics. Opioid and nonopioid adjuncts have been added to local anesthetic solutions in an attempt to improve or prolong analgesia. Although several studies have reported that analgesia lasts longer when opioids such as morphine, sufentanil, and buprenorphine are added to local anesthetics, other studies found no advantages. Clonidine, 0.5 μg/mL, is reported to prolong anesthesia and analgesia. However, at higher doses, 300 μg can cause sedation and hypotension that are undesirable in ambulatory surgery patients. Many practitioners prefer to use "plain" local anesthetic without such additives.

Ropivacaine, a long-acting amide local anesthetic, is chemically related to bupivacaine but it has less cardiac and CNS toxicity. It produces cutaneous vasoconstriction that restricts systemic absorption of the drug and increases its duration of action. Further, ropivacaine has anti-inflammatory activity that may further reduce pain and increase its duration of action. At the end of major shoulder surgery, Horn et al. injected 30 mL of 0.75% ropivacaine into the wound; 10 mL of the solution was injected subcutaneously and 20 mL was injected into the wound drain, which was then clamped for 10 min. Unbound ropivacaine plasma concentrations peaked after 15 min at 0.08 ± 0.09 μg/mL; the maximum blood concentration was 0.30 μg/mL compared to a toxic threshold of 0.60 μg/mL.[38]

Many studies with regional anesthesia have been supportive of the preemptive effect. Femoral nerve blocks with bupivacaine, although supportive of a preemptive effect, is a one-time intervention, which limits its possible efficacy to the immediate postoperative period.[31] Ilioinguinal and iliohypogastric nerve blocks for inguinal hernia repair, although supportive of preemptive effect, did not prevent the afferent input firing of inflammatory phase that follows the immediate 24-hr postoperative period. Comparing hernia repair under general anesthesia alone, general with bupivacaine infiltration, and spinal anesthesia, local anesthetic significantly reduced the intensity of all types of postoperative pain. This effect was particularly evident with constant incision pain that disappeared almost completely 24 hr after surgery. Spinal anesthesia was less effective than local infiltration presumably because of its shorter duration of action.[31]

Postoperatively, fast-track discharge criteria should be established to minimize patient recovery and discharge times. Discharge should be criteria-based, not time-based, to avoid unnecessary delays. Patients generally leave the ambulatory surgery center before the regression or resolution of the block. The limb with residual motor and sensory block should be protected appropriately until complete resolution of the block. Patient education is critical in this area to avoid injury and potential litigation. A telephone follow-up the following day monitors effectiveness of pain control, patient satisfaction, as well as any postsurgical complications.

There are several risks related to catheter delivery of local anesthetics for continuous peripheral nerve blocks that the practitioner must keep in mind. A major safety concern is that local anesthetic accumulation may result in blood concentrations larger than accepted toxic levels. Therefore, infusion volume and lockout time must then be reduced, limiting patient analgesia. Catheter-associated infection and delayed wound healing is also a concern. There seems to be little association between local anesthetic wound instillation, neurotoxicity, or catheter-related infection in the clinical setting. Local anesthetics are myotoxic. Although experimental, myotoxic responses are both intense and reproducible. In the clinical setting, local anesthetic myotoxicity seems to be rare probably because local anesthetic-induced analgesia and anesthesia is achieved at a dosage insufficient to produce clinically recognizable myotoxicity. Optimal site of drug administration (above or below the fascia) and the optimal volume and drug concentration play a role in success. Use of a single instillation catheter as part of an elastometric pump, which provides a limited volume of anesthetic, may be unable to provide adequate coverage for longer incisions. Adding a patient control mechanism to the pump requires intact mental and psychomotor function.[39]

A number of recent studies using perineural catheters to infuse local anesthetic have demonstrated safety and efficacy in the ambulatory setting. Yet, this is a relatively new technique with a limited body of evidence-based data. Further studies will need to evaluate the various aspects of this technique. Although some centers routinely employ this technique, many others are opposed to sending patients home with such devices. Because of the inherent risks stated above, patient selection is critical to ensure safety when patients are at home without the safety net of direct observation. Hence, a center that embarks on this program must ensure adequate monitoring protocols for the home-bound setting and 24-hr physician availability in the event of problems. As is true with inpatient acute pain services, initiating the technique is a small part of ensuring safety and efficacy of a given management approach.

Various portable electronic and nonelectronic infusion pumps are available to provide home infusion of local anesthetics. Proponents of the electronic pump believe that this device offers accuracy, consistency, flexibility, and reliability. They provide increased duration of action at reasonable cost. Electronic pumps allow the user to adjust infusion rates to optimize analgesic quality and duration. Electronic pump advocates argue that the temperature-dependent flow-restrictor device on the nonelectronic pump is too dependent on the patient's skin temperature, making this device inaccurate. The electronic pump permits patient-controlled regional anesthesia (PCRA), allowing bolus dosing for breakthrough pain management. Electronic pumps use external reservoirs, permitting volumes as large as 1000 mL. This is greater than the typical nonelectronic pump volume of 300–550 mL. The increase in pump volume therefore permits longer duration of block.

Nonelectronic pumps are exclusively single-use devices. Electronic pumps are generally reusable with a disposable cassette. Therefore, the patient must either return the pump to the surgery center or return the pump in a hospital-addressed, stamped, padded envelope. Only electronic pumps have alarms that may alert the patient to catheter occlusion.

Proponents of the nonelectronic, elastometric pump believe the simplicity of the device is better suited for ambulatory patients. They believe that a properly placed catheter does not require flow modifications and the patient's care will not be limited by electronic problems common with an electronic pump. Some patients, such as the elderly, the anxious, or the technically naive, may be less likely to manage PCRA successfully. Misuse of the electronic pump controls could lead to inadequate analgesia or, worse, toxic local anesthetic levels. Financially, advocates of the nonelectronic pump cite a lower mean cost per patient. Of course, the nonelectronic pump lacks the cost involved in reprocessing and resterilizing a reusable pump, not to mention the potential that reusable pumps might not be returned.

When should the local anesthetic be injected—before or after the catheter placement? Some practitioners will inject the entire volume of local anesthetic first. They contend that should the catheter fail, at least the patient will have a surgical block. However, this leaves the catheter untested until the primary block resolves. Catheter failure may not be detected until the patient has pain long after discharge. Also, an intravascular catheter might not be detected, leading to toxicity. Ayers and Kennedy[40] describe a technique of first injecting 3–4 mL of local anesthetic through the needle followed by catheter placement and further dosing. Using this technique, catheter placement can be verified prior to patient discharge. Stimulating catheters are also available that permit confirmation of catheter location by motor stimulus. This assures catheter placement prior to administration of local anesthetic. Some practitioners feel that surgical blocks are more reliable if injected first through the needle. Although there is information in the literature, the answers to these questions as well as the best approach to managing the infusion will require further studies.

Many issues need to be addressed when an ambulatory patient leaves the hospital with an indwelling catheter. Some of the issues are applicable to all catheters and some specific to the type of infusion device. All these issues need to be addressed in an easily understandable, written form for the patient to take home. This information should include how to protect the limb and joint as well as how to care for the catheter leaks, kinks, and disconnections. Inadequate pain control, signs of local anesthetic toxicity, infection, or nerve irritation also needs to be addressed.[29] There should be a plan for rescue analgesia should the catheter prove inadequate. As discussed previously, a multimodal approach will enhance the results obtained from this technique. Patients should be prepared for the possibility of fluid leaks and accumulation at the site of catheter insertion. The patient should be provided with a contact number for 24-hr coverage.

A visiting nurse could do catheter inspection, care, and problem solving. The nurse would likely be less expensive than a hospital admission for additional days of pain relief. The patient will still need to be able to contact someone 24 hr a day, 7 days a week in case of an emergency. Removal of the anesthetic catheter should be no different than the removal of a surgical drain by a general surgery patient. Whoever removes the catheter (including the patient) should be alerted to examine the tip to ensure complete removal. It should be saved for inspection if there is any doubt on the patient's part. Many centers require that the patient return for catheter removal by a health care provider. Visiting nurses could also perform this function.

Some institutions use follow-up phone calls at 24 hr, 7 days, and 3 weeks postoperatively to gather data on their successes, failures, and complications.[41] Chelly et al. prefer to evaluate each perineural catheter at least once a day to verify adequate sensory blockade and that the site is clear and not leaking fluid or showing signs of inflammation or infection. Transferring the responsibility for the care of these catheters to the patient seems inappropriate to some practitioners. Chelly et al. suggest several telephone calls from a trained health care professional and follow-up visits as the minimal involvement that should be undertaken by practitioners.[41] Their institution will also call the patient the day of and a week after surgery to verify absence of complications and verify the quality of postoperative pain control.

Infusion of local anesthetics in an ambulatory setting is an emerging technology. Many questions remain. Ideal location of catheter placement for a given block, how the catheter should be placed, and timing of local anesthetic injection remain unanswered. Anesthetic concentration and duration of catheter placement are also variable. Answers to these questions and long-term follow-up for complications will help develop evidence-based guidelines for regional anesthesia.

PATIENT FOLLOW-UP

A common thread in much of the above discussion advocates attention to patient follow-up. Each ambulatory surgery center must undertake the development of protocols for patient surveillance following discharge, much as an inpatient acute-pain service functions. These protocols should be designed in consideration of the issues pertinent to the particular center. These include types of procedures, skills of the anesthesiologist, surgeon involvement, patient populations (age, education, family support), and average commuting distance for patients. Some centers provide local accommodations (in a hotel) to facilitate follow-up.

Telephone checks are the most common form of follow-up, which should be minimally on the first postoperative day. When catheter delivery is employed, a phone call after removal is helpful to check for complications and answer questions. Knowledgeable nurses can handle these phone calls, but a physician must always be available for patient problems. A nurse or physician must be available at all times by phone in the event the patient has uncontrolled pain or a complication. There is no current standard for telephone follow-up; rather, frequency should be dictated by the above factors. A center lacking the resources for follow-up may be limited in the techniques it can provide.

Visiting nurses can provide a high level of attention for homebound ambulatory patients. Centers performing complicated and painful procedures (that might otherwise be inpatient surgery) can benefit from this service. Nurses can provide daily (if necessary) observation for pain control and surgical or anesthetic complications. A follow-up call is in order for all postoperative patients. It is of benefit when the anesthesiologist can undertake this, but this can be performed by the surgeon. In any event, the anesthesiologist must evaluate anesthetic or pain management complications. Table 7-1 lists the essential phone contact questions.

KEEPING TRACK OF SUCCESSES AND FAILURES

Measuring outcome is the key to success. Without knowledge of results, it is impossible to improve care and justify added expenses. Quality indicators include patient satisfaction, a survey of pain assessments, and number of readmissions because of pain. It is useful to keep track of technical failures to measure success with particular techniques. Surgeon satisfaction, key to marketing, can be a valuable indicator. Complications should, of course, be carefully reviewed as a means to improve care and reduce adverse events. See Table 7-2.

SUMMARY

As increasingly complicated and painful procedures are performed in the ambulatory setting, pain control tech-

Table 7-1   24-Hour Follow-up Questionnaire

1. If 0 is no pain and 10 is the worst pain imaginable, how would you rate your average pain during the last 24 hr?
2. Have you had discomfort any place other than the surgical site? Where?
3. Has pain interfered with sleep or prevented you from performing basic activities?
4. If 0 is no nausea and 10 is the worst nausea imaginable, how would you rate your nausea during the last 24 hr?
5. Describe how you are using your pain medications.
6. (If patient has a catheter system). Do you have any problem at the catheter site: clear or bloody drainage, swelling, and tenderness?
7. Would you have the same kind of anesthesia, pain management in the future? Why?

Table 7-2   Outcome Measures

- Pain scores
- Rate of readmission
- Adverse events:
  - Nausea, vomiting, orthostasis, excessive sedation
- Patient satisfaction
- Incidence of technical failures
- Serious adverse events:
  - Local anesthetic toxicity, bleeding, or infection related to pain management
- Surgeon satisfaction

niques will become more aggressive. This is best served by a multimodal approach incorporating local anesthetics, nonopioid analgesics, opioids, and nonpharmacologic techniques (cold therapy, relaxation). Continuous-drug-delivery systems are beneficial for constant severe pain but require skill to place and a system of patient follow-up. Analgesic techniques should be carefully matched to the patient, procedure, surgeon, and anesthesiologist. Key outcome measures should be tracked to improve patient care.

REFERENCES

1. Pavlin DJ, Chen C, Penaloza DA, et al. Pain as a factor complicating recovery and discharge after ambulatory surgery. Anesth Analg 2002;95:627–34.
2. Michaloliakou C, Chung F, Sharma S. Preoperative multimodal analgesia facilitates recovery after laparoscopic cholecystectomy. Anesth Analg 1996;82:44–51.
3. Shipton E. *Pain Acute and Chronic*. New York: Oxford University Press, 1999.

4. Erikson H, Tenhunen A, Kortilla K. Balanced analgesia improves recovery and the outcome after outpatient tubal ligation. Acta Anaesthesiol Scand 1996;40:151–55.

5. White P. The role of non-opioid analgesic techniques in the management of pain after ambulatory surgery. Anesth Analg 2002;94:577–85.

6. Chung F, Ritchie E, Su J. Postoperative pain in ambulatory anesthesia. Anesth Analg 1997;85:808–16.

7. Philip B, Scuderi P, Chung F, et al. Remifentanil compared with alfentanil for ambulatory surgery using total intravenous anesthesia. Anesth Analg 1997;84:515–21.

8. Sa Rego M, Watcha M, White P. The changing role of monitored anesthesia care in the ambulatory setting. Anesth Analg 1997;85:1020–36.

9. White P, Coe V, Shafer A, et al. Comparison of alfentanil with fentanyl for outpatient anesthesia. Anesthesiology 1986;64:99–106.

10. Fernandez-Galinski D, Rue M, Moral V, et al. Spinal anesthesia with bupivacaine and fentanyl in geriatric patients. Aneth Analg 1996;83:537–41.

11. Bekker AY, Berklayd P, Osborn I, et al. The recovery of cognitive function after remifentanil-nitrous oxide anesthesia is faster than after an isoflurane-nitrous oxide-fentanyl combination in elderly patients. Anesth Analg 2000;91(1):117–22.

12. Cook D, Rooke A. Priorities in perioperative geriatrics. Anesth Analg 2003;96:1823–36.

13. Claxton A, McGuire G, Cruise C, et al. Evaluation of morphine versus fentanyl for postoperative analgesia after ambulatory surgery procedures. Anesth Analg 1997;84:509–14.

14. Scott L, Perry C. Tramadol: a review of its use in perioperative pain. Drugs 2000;60:139–76.

15. Dayer P, Desmueles J, Collart L, et al. Pharmacology of tramadol. Drugs 1997;53 (Suppl 2):18–24.

16. Lewis K, Han N. Tramadol: a new centrally acting analgesic. Am J Health Syst Pharm 1997;54:643–52.

17. Radbruch L, Grond S, Lehmann K. A risk-benefit assessment of tramadol in the management of pain. Drug Safety 1996;15:8–29.

18. Smith I, Shively R, White P. Effects of ketorolac and bupivacaine on recovery after outpatient arthroscopy. Anesth Analg 1992;75:208–12.

19. Reuben S, Bhopatkar S, Maciolek H, et al. The preemptive analgesic effect of rofecoxib after ambulatory arthroscopic knee surgery. Anesth Analg 2002;94:55–59.

20. Gilron I, Milne B, Hong M. Cyclooxygenase-2 inhibitors in postoperative pain management. Anesthesiology 2003;99:1198–1209.

21. Jimenez M, Catala E, Casas J, et al. Analgesia of postoperative pain in ambulatory surgery. Rev Esp Anesthesiol Reanim 1995;42:125–31.

22. Ding Y, White P, et al. Comparative effects of ketorolac, dezocine, and fentanyl as adjuvants during outpatient anesthesia. Anesth Analg 1992;75:566–71.

23. Raeder J, Steine S, Vatsgar T. Oral ibuprofen versus paracetamol plus codeine for analgesia after ambulatory surgery. Anesth Analg 2001;92:1470–72.

24. Rosenblum M, Weller R, Conard P, et al. Ibuprofen provides longer lasting analgesia than fentanyl after laparoscopic surgery. Anesth Analg 1991;73:255.

25. Rueben S, Connelly N, et al. Postoperative analgesic effects of celecoxib or rofecoxib after spinal fusion surgery. Anesth Analg 2001;91:1221–25.

26. Issioui T, Klein K, White P, et al. Cost-efficacy of rofecoxib versus acetaminophen for preventing pain after ambulatory surgery. Anesthesiology 2002;97:931–37.

27. Tang J, Li S, White P, et al. Effect of parecoxib, a novel intravenous cyclooxygenase type-2 inhibitor, on the postoperative opioid requirement and quality of pain control. Anesthesiology 2002;96:1305–9.

28. Talley J, Bertenshaw S, Brown D, et al. N- [(5-methyl-3-phenylisoxazol-4-yl)-phenyl]sulfonyl] pronpanamide, sodium salt, parecoxib sodium: a potent and selective inhibitor of COX-2 for parenteral administration. J Med Chem 2000;43:1661–63.

29. Rawal N. Analgesia for day-case surgery. Br J Anaesth 2001;87:73–87.

30. Kissin I. Preemptive analgesia. Anesthesiology 2000;93:1138–43.

31. Kelly D, Ahmad M, Brull S. Preemptive analgesia II: recent advances and current trends. Can J Anesth 2001;48:1091–1101.

32. Klein JR, Heaton JP, Thompson JP, et al. Infiltration of the abdominal wall with local anesthetic after total abdominal hysterectomy has no opioid-sparing effect. Br J Anesth 2000;84:248–49.

33. Zohar E, Fredman B, Phillipov A, et al. The analgesic efficacy of patient-controlled bupivacaine wound instillation after total abdominal hysterectomy with bilateral salpingo-oophorectomy. Anesth Analg 2001;93:482–87.

34. Klein SM, Nielsen KC, Martin A, et al. Interscalene brachial plexus block with continuous intraarticular infusion of ropivacaine. Anesth Analg 2001;93:601–5.

35. Butterfield N, Schwarz SK, Ries CR, et al. Combined pre- and postsurgical bupivacaine wound infiltrations decrease opioid requirements after knee ligament reconstruction. Can J Anaesth 2001;48:245–50.

36. Liguori GA, Chimento GK, Borow L, et al. Possible bupivacaine toxicity after intraarticular injection for postarthroscopic analgesia of the knee: implications of the surgical procedure. Anesth Analg 2002;94:1010–13.

37. Convery P, Milligan K, Fee JPH. Comparison of the uptake of ropivacaine and bupivacaine from the knee joint. Br J Anaesth 1999;83:111–12.

38. Horn EP, Schroeder F, Wilhelm S, et al. Wound infiltration and drain lavage with ropivacaine after major shoulder surgery. Anesth Analg 1999;89:1461–66.

39. Fredman B, Shapiro A, Zohar E, et al. The analgesic efficacy of patient-controlled ropivacaine instillation after cesarean delivery. Anesth Analg 2000;91:1436–40.

40. Ayers J, Kennedy FK. Continuous lower extremity techniques. Tech Reg Anesth Pain Manag 1999;3:47–57.

41. Chelly JE, Greger J, Gebhard R, et al. Ambulatory continuous perineural infusion: are we ready? Anesthesiology 2000;93:581–82.

Perioperative Pain Management in the Ambulatory Setting: A Nursing Perspective

JEANELLEN NEWKIRK • BRETT DICKINSON • ELAINE NICHOLS

NURSES' ROLE IN CARING FOR AMBULATORY SURGERY PATIENTS

Interventions provided by the nursing staff throughout the ambulatory surgery experience directly influence a patient's pain management and outcomes. The Joint Commission on the Accreditation of Healthcare Organizations (JCAHO) requires all patients to be provided the basic right of pain management.[1] Findings by the Committee on Quality of Health Care in America reveal that this right to physical comfort and pain management is not being met.[2] The American Society of Perianesthesia Nurses (ASPAN) conducted a research study in 2001 that supported these findings. ASPAN noted that nurses identified the patient's desired level of pain 21% of the time in the preoperative phase. The highest level of pain assessment was during the admission process ranging from 40 to 75%.[3] With this information in hand, it is essential for ambulatory surgery nurses to commit to the highest standards and best practices available when managing a patient's postoperative course.

A nationwide trend is occurring to perform surgical procedures on an outpatient basis. Ambulatory surgery now constitutes 60–70% of surgical procedures performed, yet 80% of patients still report moderate to severe pain postoperatively.[4] Advancements in anesthetic agents and anesthesia techniques have led to a broader spectrum of procedures to be performed safely in an ambulatory setting. However, performing these more complex procedures brings new challenges to nurses to meet the needs of this patient population in a timely manner. Early and effective treatments for pain and nausea decrease the amount of time spent in the postanesthesia care unit (PACU), while increasing patient satisfaction. Adequate and effective postoperative pain management for home care must be reviewed and stressed with the patient and his/her caregiver. This chapter will address these issues from the nursing perspective in the management of an ambulatory surgical patient.

PREOPERATIVE AND INTRAOPERATIVE PAIN MANAGEMENT

A variety of patient populations have surgical procedures performed in an ambulatory surgical setting. The largest portion of procedures is conducted on orthopedic and general surgery cases. Other surgical services utilizing outpatient facilities include gynecology, urology, plastics, eye, dental, and otolaryngology—head and neck. The nurse provides the direct care and observation for each patient from the preoperative holding area to the time of discharge. It is valuable for preoperative nurses to communicate any significant findings or concerns to the operating room (OR) and PACU nurses. This will assist with the coordination of patient care and allow for a less complicated recovery phase. Postoperative pain management actually begins preoperatively. Preoperative teaching must include the patient and the caregiver, as well as their expectations for relief of pain. It is not realistic to believe that there will be no postoperative pain. Misconceptions must be clarified. The nurse should document the patient's rating of current pain level and location prior to any interventions in the preoperative area. This provides a baseline for a preexisting level of pain and will serve as a reference point to monitor effectiveness of interventions.

Patients should be encouraged to participate in their pain management, with emphasis placed on preemptive analgesia and integration of relaxation techniques to achieve adequate pain control. Many patients have access to the Internet and use the World Wide Web as a source of health care information. Patients who consider themselves well informed and have an understanding of the surgical procedure and postoperative pain management are more likely to have a positive outcome. Acquisition of pain management information prior to surgery allows patients time to plan, consider options, and identify and seek answers to specific questions.[5] The nurse functions as a resource to validate the accuracy of information obtained from the Web. Acupuncture, hypnosis, supplements, herbs, and homeopathic medications are viewed as complementary and alternative medicine. Certain herbs when combined with anesthesia can increase the risk of bleeding, hypertension, or prolong the effect of anesthesia.[6] It is important for the nurse to provide education to the patient on the risks and interactions of anesthesia and alternative medicine. Ideally, preoperative screening nurses will identify the use of alternative medicine and document and share the findings with the anesthesiologist, thereby protecting the surgical patient from harm.

Reports have shown that the administration of an oral cyclooxygenase-2 (COX-2) inhibitor before a surgical case can lessen the severity of postoperative pain.[7] Some orthopedic surgeons are providing patients with a prescription for rofecoxib to take in the morning prior to arrival for outpatient surgery. When possible it is beneficial to have prescriptions filled prior to surgery. Patients who receive their prescriptions during a preoperative clinic visit are able to have them dispensed and available when needed. This will alleviate the burden of feeling rushed to get home before anesthesia has worn off and the onset of pain. Many patients do not live in close proximity of the facility and some will even travel from out of state. Several ambulatory surgery centers (ASCs) are now providing an outpatient pharmacy on-site to assist in meeting this need. By addressing access to postoperative pain medication, reduction of surgical-related stress can be achieved. Reducing the overall anxiety related to the procedure promotes adequate pain and nausea control postoperatively. A well-prepared patient and caregiver will have overall high levels of satisfaction promoting the surgical procedure in the ambulatory setting as a positive experience.

Intraoperative pain management also improves postoperative pain perceptions. When general anesthesia (GA) is used, there is a need to monitor and access the patient frequently as he/she will not be able to provide verbal feedback relating to pain. If the patient does not awaken from anesthesia in severe pain, it is much easier to provide effective pain interventions in the PACU. Studies have shown that the administration of intraoperative ketorolac diminishes the need for postoperative opioids.[8] This is thought to be related to reduction in tissue inflammation at the surgical site. Administration of intraoperative antiemetics, such as ondansetron, markedly diminishes the incidence of nausea and vomiting after GA.

POSTOPERATIVE PAIN MANAGEMENT

Postoperative pain management is part of a complex treatment plan, as the cause of pain is multifactorial. Acute pain from surgery has three major components: (1) tissue injury, (2) nociceptor sensitization, and (3) activation of central pain pathways.[9] These factors must be taken into account to adequately manage postoperative pain. The path that is taken to manage postoperative pain is partly dependent on the type of anesthesia used for the surgical procedure. However, some basic principles remain the same. The airway and adequate oxygenation are of the utmost importance and these must be effectively managed prior to aggressive pain management. Once the patient is responsive enough to admit to pain either verbally (talking, moaning, grimacing) or by change in vital signs (elevated systolic blood pressure, tachycardia, tachypnea), early and aggressive treatment is indicated. A three-phase pain management approach is utilized: (1) short-onset intravenous (IV) opioid, (2) intermediate-duration opioid for more severe pain, and (3) initiation of oral (PO) analgesics.[10] Fentanyl, 25 µg IV every 3–5 min, up to a maximum of 100 µg, has the benefit of rapid effectiveness with fewer side effects. Fentanyl is quickly metabolized, necessitating more frequent administration. Morphine sulfate, 2–3 mg IV every 5 min, up to a maximum of 10 mg, may also be used. Morphine takes slightly longer to be maximally effective but the pain management tends to last longer. Some studies have shown that there is an increased and extended nausea when morphine is used instead of fentanyl. This may be due to an effect on the vestibular apparatus.[11] Either or both of these medications are usually effective for the opioid-naive patient. In patients with refractory pain, hydromorphone, 0.5 mg IV every 5–10 min, to a maximum of 2 mg, may be necessary. Intravenous nonsteroidal anti-inflammatory drugs (NSAIDs) should be given unless already given intraoperatively or are contraindicated. Contraindications include asthma, peptic ulcer disease, or bleeding disorders. The patient who has exercise-induced asthma and has not required emergency room visits for recent treatment may be a candidate for IV NSAIDs under the guidance of an anesthesiologist. Once the patient is tolerating oral fluids, convert to oral analgesics and continue to promote comfort measures to reduce pain.

Postoperative nausea and vomiting (PONV) is a major cause of dissatisfaction for ambulatory patients. A reciprocal pattern is formed where pain can cause PONV and PONV can worsen pain; so it must be effectively treated. Prevention is fairly effective when ondansetron is administered within the last 15 min of the surgical procedure.[12] The patient should be placed in a decreased-environmental-stimuli area and instructed to avoid rapid movements and ensure adequate hydration. It is helpful to prevent PONV with adequate antiemetic prophylaxis, to include: ranitidine, ondansetron, droperidol, metoclopramide, and/or dexamethasone. Promethazine is frequently more effective when used in small IV doses (6.25 mg) in the early postoperative phase. Refractory PONV may respond well to droperidol, 0.625 mg IV once, but requires additional monitoring time after administration. Conversion to oral antiemetics may be necessary prior to discharge home.

The increased use of regional anesthesia, especially peripheral nerve blocks, has broadened the scope of ambulatory surgery. A variety of surgical procedures and patient populations can now be cared for in the ambulatory setting. These patients receive much less opioids, are able to maintain their airways unassisted, and have excellent post-operative pain control, making them an ideal choice of anesthesia for any patient population but especially the elderly and high-risk patients.[13] Pain management after a regional block is slightly different, as these patients are frequently alert and pain-free upon arrival to PACU. It is important to maintain comfort measures and institute safety measures to the affected extremity, as the patient will be unable to assist. Use pillows or foam cradles to elevate and provide padding to the blocked extremity. Ice packs or a cryotherapy system should begin as soon as possible to decrease inflammation and promote peripheral pain management. Many ASCs have the cryotherapy unit applied in the OR to the operative site upon completion of the case.

Once the patient is tolerating oral fluids well, the multimodal analgesia approach should begin with the use of acetaminophen, 650 mg PO, and NSAIDs (IV or PO) every 6 hr (around the clock). Oral opioids may then be administered in addition to the above medications as needed. If the patient develops postoperative discomfort in the PACU, the anesthesiologist may chose to reblock the extremity if indicated to obtain effective analgesic levels.

A perineural indwelling catheter may prolong analgesia as well. Patients undergoing surgery under continuous peripheral nerve blocks receive a postoperative infusion of 0.2% ropivacaine either in the overnight unit or via disposable pump in the home setting. The catheter is tested after surgery with a test dose of 0.5% ropivacaine with epinephrine 1:400,000 prior to infusion initiation. Breakthrough pain can occur in these patients, requiring aggressive and early intervention, as previously discussed. The anesthesiologist should also evaluate the patient to determine whether additional local anesthetic boluses or IV opioids are indicated.[14]

Patients recovering from GA require a slightly different approach to pain management. Comfort measures are delivered in a calm, efficient manner to diminish the patient's anxiety. A warmed blanket to the abdomen after gynecologic procedures and cryotherapy to sites of orthopedic procedures can be helpful as adjuvant therapies to control pain. Splinting techniques with the use of pillows to assist in supporting the injured muscles at the surgical site are taught to the patient. It is important to begin aggressive pain management as previously discussed with IV opioids and IV NSAIDs if not already given in the OR or contraindicated. It is equally important to aggressively treat PONV, as previously discussed. Once the immediate pain and/or PONV crisis has been managed, the patient should be converted to oral analgesics and antiemetics. These should be administered, if indicated, prior to discharge, as it may take several hours to fill the prescriptions. Oxycodone, 5–10 mg PO, is the most common oral opioid, with promethazine, 25 mg PO, as the most common antiemetic prescribed.

The patient and caregiver must be instructed in extended postoperative pain management for home care. It is important to stress the effectiveness of the multimodal analgesia approach with acetaminophen and NSAIDs every 6 hr (around the clock), as well as use of opioids for breakthrough pain. The side effects of these medications are included in the postoperative teaching when patients are also instructed to take medications with food. Appropriate comfort measures are also included as part of the discharge teaching. A 24-hr follow-up phone call from a registered nurse (RN) offers assistance with patient's comfort level. It also provides a forum for additional teaching about adequate pain management and encouragement to modify the current plan based on the patient's needs.

EXTENDED CARE PAIN MANAGEMENT

Some patients undergoing a surgical procedure in an outpatient facility are not ready to go home within a few hours of surgery. An extended-care area is set up to provide 23-hr monitoring of the patient while maintaining an outpatient status. These units are staffed with RNs with an industry standard of 1:4 nurse–patient ratios. American Society of Anesthesiologists (ASA) physical status II and III patients are the most common population staying in the extended recovery area. Nurses' input will assist the ASC medical director in making an appropriate decision on the disposition of ASA IV patients. Each ASA IV patient is looked at upon an individual basis regarding the level of care and resources required to safely be monitored in the overnight area of the ambulatory surgery center.

The extended-care area is usually designed to care for patients receiving continuous regional anesthesia (e.g., continuous peripheral nerve blocks, epidural blocks), requiring observation for postoperative bleeding, monitoring for airway competency, acute pain management, and PONV treatment. Occasionally a patient meets criteria to stay overnight due to advanced age or a long-distance travel to home combined with unavailability of home care providers. In these situations the staff needs to involve home health, social workers, and family members to arrange for the patient's care and safety upon discharge.

Certain types of surgical procedures will require the use of GA, for example, endoscopic sinus surgery. General anesthesia is also used if a patient is not a candidate for a regional block (i.e., preexisting peripheral nerve injury or infection at the block site). The patient undergoing GA tends to be at greater risk for PONV if oral pain agents are introduced too soon after surgery. This patient population is the most common to receive an IV opioid patient-controlled analgesia (PCA) (Fig. 8-1). The patient is converted in the early morning to oral agents; preferably at 6 A.M. the IV opioid PCA is discontinued and oxycodone, 5–10 mg PO, is administered. This allows the oral pain medication to be in effect while the patient is dressing, performing activities of daily living (ADL), and preparing for discharge by 9 A.M.

The management of patients with single-injection peripheral nerve blocks consists of protecting and elevating the operative extremity along with early use of cryotherapy, acetaminophen, and NSAIDs (Fig. 8-2).

The use of regional anesthesia allows patients with multiple comorbidities to undergo ambulatory surgery. A patient with a significant cardiac history or severe pulmonary disease is not well suited for the stress of endotracheal in-

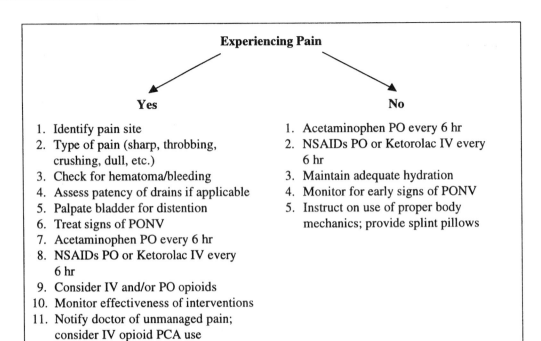

Figure 8-1   Pain algorithm for general surgery.

tubation or GA. Regional anesthesia offers the perfect solution to conduct ambulatory surgery on this patient population. When indicated, these patients can stay in the extended recovery area to be observed closely by nurses. The rapid intervention by the nurses will prevent a pain episode from developing into a crisis and subjecting a high-risk patient to undue stress.

Although continuous perineural infusions of ropivacaine are routinely initiated in the PACU, they may be started in the extended-stay area. Ropivacaine at 0.2% concentration is started either with or without a bolus dose, depending on the doctor's order. The doses of local anesthetic infused along with patient's pain scores are recorded

on a flow sheet every 4 hr. If a patient is having breakthrough pain rated ≥ 4 using a verbal analog scale (VAS) with a numeric range of 0–10, treatment is started immediately. If the patient is not yet tolerating oral fluids, pain is treated with IV opioids and IV NSAIDs (Fig. 8-3). Effectiveness of the pain medication is assessed continually until the pain is controlled to the patient's comfort level. Occasionally, patients experience episodes of breakthrough pain during block resolution (transition phase from anesthesia to analgesia). It is the responsibility of the nurse to assess this pain and to medicate the patient in a timely manner using the multimodal analgesia approach. For example, if the patient's pain VAS scores escalate from

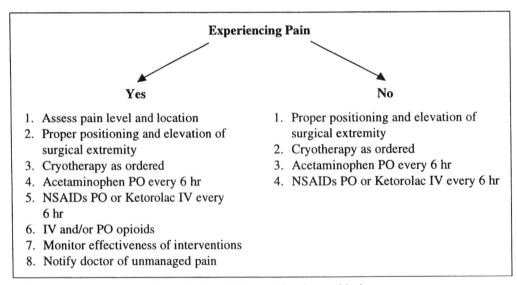

Figure 8-2   Pain algorithm for regional anesthesia: Single-injection peripheral nerve block.

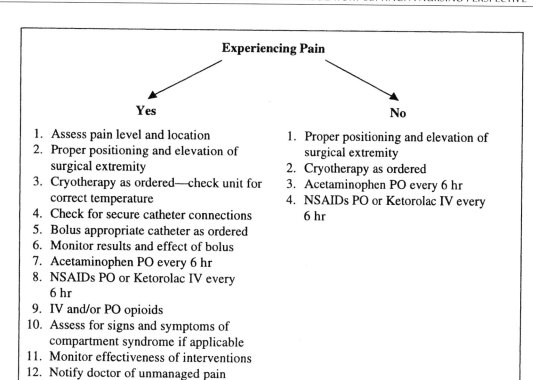

Figure 8-3   Pain algorithm for regional anesthesia: Continuous peripheral nerve block.

0/10 to 10/10 within 10 min, the RN must reassure the patient that the pain will be under control rapidly. This is an effective approach for the nurse to acknowledge the pain, provide a calm environment, and reassure that interventions are being performed. The most commonly used IV opiods in this area are morphine, fentanyl, or hydromorphone. During a crisis, pain relief is assessed at a minimum of every 10 min. If the additional local anesthetic perineural bolus and IV opioids are not effective in resolving breakthrough pain episodes, the on-call anesthesiologist is consulted regarding the potential use of an IV opioid PCA.

A clear benefit of optimal postoperative pain management is the ability to have early mobilization after surgery. Movement and ambulation will increase circulation, resulting in an increasing oxygenation of tissue. Earlier activity after surgery can reduce atelectasis, deep-vein thrombosis, or pneumonia, which may occur with prolonged immobilization and insufficient respirations.[15] The use of regional blocks has permitted patients to participate sooner in aggressive physical therapy and rehabilitation programs, which enhances overall patient outcomes.[16] When indicated by the orthopedic procedure performed, continuous-passive-motion (CPM) machines can be implemented the first postoperative night to enhance patient mobility. All of these interventions to restore function can be accomplished when a patient's pain control is properly managed.

Now that the surgical procedure is complete, it is important to reassess the patient's expectations for and understanding of pain management overnight and when he/she goes home. The nurse posing the simple question to the patient, "what is your expectation of pain management?" is extremely helpful. Some patients are young, healthy athletes undergoing a first-time orthopedic procedure and others are chronic pain patients having a joint replaced for rheumatoid arthritis. This broad range of patients necessitates the tailoring of a plan of care for pain management to each individual. What worked yesterday on one patient, who had a similar procedure, may not be effective in today's case. Each patient possesses a unique personality and will vary in his/her own pain perception. Postoperative patients range from being intolerant of any form of minor discomfort to surprising self-control or those who consider pain to be a normal part of life.[17] Educating patients before a pain crisis reduces the apprehension they feel if they do experience breakthrough pain. Patients are encouraged to notify the RN with the first signs of breakthrough pain, and it is explained to the patient the benefit to treat pain in the early stages and not when pain is at a high level. This becomes particularly important when treating the elderly or a patient from a different cultural background. Some elderly patients make the statement that they "didn't want to be a bad patient" and will not call for medication in the early phases when it can be the most effective. The cultural and language barriers in health care are becoming more significant in pain management situations. An example is the Hispanic male patient who will not request pain medication and attempts to be courageous. The relationship of pain management, cultural variables, and patient satisfaction in ethnic groups has not fully been addressed or researched.[18] If the nurse is faced with a language barrier that is impeding care, it is his/her responsibility to arrange for an interpreter to be onsite and meet this fundamental patient need.

Table 8-1   Contributing Factors to Consider When Assessing Postoperative Pain

Contributing Factor to Postoperative Pain	Nursing Intervention
1. Bladder distension	1. No void 6 hr postoperative, obtain order for in-and-out catheterization. If greater than 400 mL returned, leave indwelling Foley catheter.
2. Volume depletion	2. Maintain IV fluids, crystalloid boluses as ordered.
3. Hematoma/bleeding	3. Report excessive bleeding to surgeon; maintain drain patency with minimum every-4-hr drain stripping.
4. Constrictive dressings	4. Where permitted, provide padding for comfort; if warranted, obtain order from surgeon to loosen dressing.
5. Tobacco/ETOH withdrawal	5. Provide nicotine patch/use of lorazepam if needed.
6. Anxiety	6. Reassurance, calm environment, resume home antianxiety medication if previously taken, use of lorazepam if needed.
7. Postoperative nausea and vomiting	7. Encourage patient to notify at onset of nausea for treatment; anticipate history of motion sickness or PONV; premedicate prior to first OOB and activity; maintain adequate hydration.
8. Chronic pain	8. Resume patient's home medication routines as soon as possible, elicit patient input on positioning for comfort.
9. Migraines	9. Consider caffeine withdrawal from NPO status; may respond to coffee or a caffeinated beverage. If not effective, obtain order for IV caffeine (100 mg) and NSAIDs.

When a patient is not responding to pain management interventions, the nurse should consider what other causes might be involved (Table 8-1). Effective measures to prevent or decrease postoperative pain other than medications are proper positioning of the blocked limb, protecting the limb from harm, and ensuring that the patient is correctly aligned in bed. At times patients experience discomfort at the insertion site of single-injection or continuous peripheral nerve blocks. An ice pack to this area usually eliminates the need to medicate the patient for this discomfort. Finding the root cause of the discomfort may not always be the immediate surgical pain but any number of mitigating factors. Treating the underlying issues in conjunction with postoperative pain is the best approach to achieving optimal relief for the patient.

A practice established in the author's facility extended-stay area is to maintain crystalloid IV fluids at a rate of 125 mL/hr unless there is a contraindication to additional fluid. The maintenance of IV fluids facilitates recovery by decreasing PONV, dizziness, and orthostatic hypotension in the morning of postoperative day one when patients are ready to go home.

Patients must absorb a large amount of information in a short period of time when undergoing ambulatory surgical procedures. Nurses prefer to direct the postoperative education toward the patient and involve the family members or significant others. Signs and symptoms of potential complications are explained to patients and families along with providing preprinted handouts of reviewed instructions.

Contact information for obtaining access to a nurse or physician is also reinforced. Questions run the gamut from expressing concerns on how to climb stairs with an insensate lower extremity to the proper technique of stripping a Jackson-Pratt drain. The nursing staff must help the patient understand the discharge information in terms they will comprehend. The most important discharge teaching involves the need to comply with multimodal pain management regimens prescribed by physicians. Nurses should work closely with physicians to ensure that patients have all the information needed to have a successful recovery with minimal postoperative pain.

SUMMARY

Perioperative nurses will continue to be key players in directing patient care and outcomes in all aspects of the ambulatory surgical experience. Throughout the continuum of care the nurse is responsible for implementing the appropriate course of treatment toward optimal patient comfort. Inadequate pain control is no longer an acceptable or a tolerable practice. Standardization of pain management approaches, guidelines for nursing practice and ongoing feedback on performance are crucial elements to enhance the quality of pain control.[19]

Rawal proclaims, "The solution to the problem of inadequate postoperative pain relief does not lie so much in the development of new techniques, but rather in the establishment of a formal organization."[20] The formation of pain guidelines and evidence-based practice are resources available to facilitate the nurses' management of postoperative pain. Ultimately, adequate postoperative analgesia in the ambulatory surgery setting provides earlier mobility, a shortened stay, reduced costs, and better patient outcomes, which lead to patient's satisfaction.

REFERENCES

1. Joint Commission on Accreditation of Healthcare Organizations. *Comprehensive Accreditation Manual for Behavioral Health Care (CAMBHC) Pain Assessment and Management Standards 2001–2002.* Oakbrook Terrace, IL: JCAHO, 2002, pp. 1–14.

2. Committee on Quality of Health Care in America (Institute of Medicine). *Crossing the Quality Chasm.* Washington, DC: National Academy Press, 2001, pp. 49–50.

3. Krenzischek D, Wilson L. An introduction to the ASPAN Pain and Comfort Clinical Guideline. J PeriAnesth Nurs 2003;18(4):228–30.

4. Chung F, Ewan R. Postoperative pain in ambulatory surgery. Anesth Analg 1997;85(4):2.

5. Goldsmith D, Safran C. Using the Web to reduce postoperative pain following ambulatory surgery. AMIA Fall Symposium 1999. Available from http://www.ics.uci.edu/~pratt/courses/goldsmith.pdf. Accessed August 24, 2003.

6. Carol N. Complementary and alternative medicine use by surgical patients. AORN 2002;76(6):1013–21.

7. Pavlin DJ, Chen C, Penzaloza D, et al. Pain as a factor complicating recovery and discharge after ambulatory surgery. Anesth Analg 2002;95(3):627–34.

8. Williams J, Wexler G, Novak P, et al. A prospective study of pain and analgesic use in outpatient endoscopic anterior cruciate ligament reconstruction. Arthroscopy 1998;14(6):613–16.

9. Michaloliakou C, Chung F, Sharma S. Preoperative multimodal analgesia facilitates recovery after ambulatory laparoscopic cholecystectomy. Anesth Analg 1996;82:44–51.

10. Kapur P. Postanesthesia care unit challenges. Anesth Analg 2001; 92:64–69.

11. Claxton A, McGuire G, Chung F, et al. Evaluation of morphine versus fentanyl for postoperative analgesia after ambulatory surgical procedures. Anesth Analg 1997;84:509–14.

12. Chen X, Tang J, White P, et al. The effect of timing of dolasetron administration on its efficacy as a prophylactic antiemetic in the ambulatory setting. Anesth Analg 2001;93:906–11.

13. Murauski J, Gonzalez K. Peripheral nerve blocks for postoperative analgesia. AORN Online 2002;75:134, 136–40, 142–51, 153–54.

14. Klein S, Nielsen K, Greengrass R, et al. Ambulatory discharge after long-acting peripheral nerve blockade: 2382 blocks with ropivacaine. Anesth Analg 2002;94:65–70.

15. Cundy C. Post operative pain management: my free CE. 2002. Available from http://www.myfreece.com/Public/Course_Take.asp?CourseId=58. Accessed Aug 24, 2003.

16. Reuben S, Sklar J. Pain management in patients who undergo outpatient arthroscopic surgery of the knee. J Bone Joint Surg 2000; 82(12):1756.

17. Nicola A. Postoperative pain management: the virtual anaesthesia textbook 2000 April. Available from: http://www.virtual-anaesthesia-textbook.com. Accessed October 8, 2003.

18. Sherwood G, Starck P, Disnard G. Changing acute pain management outcomes in surgical patients. AORN 2003;77(2):378–79.

19. Bardiau F, Taviaux N, Albert A, et al. An intervention study to enhance postoperative pain management. Anesth Analg 2003;96(1): 179–85.

20. Rawal N. Acute pain services revisited: good from far, far from good? Reg Anesth Pain Med 2002;27:117–21.

What Outcomes Are Important in Ambulatory Anesthesia?

ANIL GUPTA   •   LEE A. FLEISHER

INTRODUCTION

With the rapid expansion in ambulatory surgery world-wide, there is an increasing focus on "outcome," which is relevant to both the caregiver and the caretaker. Not only are patients interested in knowing the risks and outcomes following ambulatory surgery, but even hospitals and insurance companies see this as an important aspect of continuing quality care for patients. Outpatient surgery has traditionally been viewed as inherently safe and only the most egregious bad outcomes have been reported, usually in the media. In addition, there has been minimal oversight of ambulatory surgery, particularly in those settings remote from the hospital. However, a regular forum for discussion of outcomes has recently evolved. The consequence of these developments is a process of "benchmarking" where quality of patient care can and is compared regularly between hospitals and ambulatory surgery centers (ASCs) in order to achieve and promote the highest levels of patient care. This is likely to expand further in the future as new tools emerge that can be used as a means for benchmarking of outcomes following ambulatory surgery.

Which outcomes are of interest following ambulatory surgery depends on who is being asked this question since there are stakeholders: the caretaker (patient), the caregiver (the hospital/ambulatory surgical unit), and the cost bearer (insurance provider). Although all parties have an interest in achieving the "best" outcome, there is a constant debate in recent years on the costs incurred to achieve "best" outcome. Strategies to reduce major morbidity in high-risk surgeries may be cost-saving in many situations by reducing hospital length of stay and utilization of intensive-care resources. For example, beta-blocker administration in major vascular surgery can be cost-saving by reducing perioperative myocardial infarction and death.[1] However, ambulatory surgery is associated with very low rates of major morbidity and mortality, and more common complications such as postoperative nausea and vomiting (PONV) may not be associated with the same level of medical costs. In such cases, can reduction in adverse events be achieved by increasing costs, and if so, what is the cost-benefit to the patient and the health care system? For PONV, reduction in its incidence can be achieved by a significant increase in costs, but the question arises: does the increase in costs justify the outcome of interest? One approach to the importance of such outcomes is to determine the willingness to pay on the part of the patient or family. In one recent study, the authors concluded that patients are willing to pay an extra $100 to reduce the risk for PONV.[2] This poses many interesting questions, which will be discussed later in this chapter.

This chapter will review the possible outcomes that may be of interest during ambulatory surgery and anesthesia and the means of assessing these outcomes, evaluate specific examples, and outline an approach to the cost benefit to the different parties in achieving these outcomes.

HOW IS PERIOPERATIVE RISK DEFINED AND STUDIED?

Several issues related to studying anesthetic risk can have an impact on the findings. There are multiple definitions of perioperative morbidity and mortality in the literature. In particular, the time frame in which a complication can be attributed to the surgery and delivery of anesthesia varies. As in-hospital stays have shortened, many events related to surgery may occur after discharge. This is particularly the case in ambulatory or short-stay surgery, in which recovery from anesthesia occurs at home. As we continue to monitor our patients for safety, it will be important to include follow-up beyond the traditional hospital setting. Many recent studies have included such an approach; although the traditional definition of 30-day outcomes may be too long in the ambulatory setting, i.e., for minor procedures, the rate of complications may return to baseline before the 30-day time period.

A major problem in any study of risk is the actual rate of complications in the population of interest. There are multiple sources of data for studying perioperative risk. Although some of the original studies utilized data from only a single or small group of institutions, such approaches may not be practical in the ambulatory setting for all but minor complications such as PONV. For example, the rate of anesthetic-related mortality described in the Confidential Enquiry into Perioperative Deaths was 1 in 185,000 patients.[3,4] Considering the current rate, any study would have to be enormous to detect anesthesia-related mortality. Such a study would require information from a large number of sites, or cover multiple years (or decades) from a single institution.[5]

An alternative approach is to identify bad outcomes and study them for patterns of errors. For example, Cheney and colleagues developed the American Society of Anesthesiologists (ASA) Closed Claims Study.[6] By obtaining the records of major events that led to legal litigation, they were able to identify factors that contributed to bad outcomes. Using such methodology, selected morbidity, which leads to litigation, can be identified. The limitation of this methodology is that the actual rates of complications are unknown; only the number of closed legal claims is known. Additionally, those cases that do not result in litigation are not included in the database.

With respect to inpatient surgery, several attempts have been made to establish large epidemiologic databases.[7–13] These databases are used for defining risk factors for poor outcome, benchmarking local to national complication rates, and as educational tools. Unfortunately, these databases have not focused on ambulatory surgery. In addition, such databases include a predominance of patients from academic or major medical centers, and do not include the data from smaller or community hospitals or freestanding facilities, where the majority of ambulatory surgery is performed in the United States. Although these databases may provide extremely important information to improve care, the ability to generalize the results to the nonacademic centers is unknown.

When extremely large sample sizes are needed, administrative databases may be among the most cost-effective approaches to this issue. Examples of administrative databases include Medicare claim files, private-insurance company claims, and hospital electronic records. These databases include a small number of data points on an extremely large number of subjects. For example, the Medicare database includes both financial data and International Classification of Diseases, Ninth Revision (ICD-9) (disease) and Current Procedural Terminology (CPT) (procedure) codes for each patient. They also include information regarding location of care and provider type. The Medicare claim files are now being extensively utilized to benchmark rates of mortality and major complications after coronary bypass surgery.[14] Hospitals can compare their rates to those of neighboring and competing hospitals, and may use these data as markers for quality of hospital care.[15,16] Care in outpatient settings can also be assessed, including procedures performed in offices using physician bills.

Unique Issues in the Outpatient Setting

The issue in evaluating morbidity and mortality after outpatient surgery in the modern era is that the complexity of both the procedures and the patients is steadily increasing. Although a given procedure may be associated with very low and acceptable morbidity in an outpatient setting if performed in relatively healthy individuals, insurance companies frequently generalize these findings to patients with increase in comorbidity. For example, tonsillectomy is associated with a 1-in-250 to 1-in-500 rate of emergency readmission for bleeding within 24 hr in healthy children.[17] Performing an outpatient tonsillectomy may be associated with increased morbidity in premature infants or those with obstructive sleep apnea.[18] It is important to determine whether this represents safe or unsafe practice and whether the rates of "morbidity" are acceptable as practices are diffused.

An alternative approach involves a national (or local) multiyear surveillance to determine the safety of a given procedure. As a baseline, morbidity should be defined as the need for admission or readmission after ambulatory surgery. This time horizon for readmission must be evaluated. Certainly readmissions within 24 hr are of greatest concern, but admissions within 1 week may still be related to perioperative care. The rates in outpatient centers must be benchmarked and compared to those of inpatient centers from this national database, and the primary cause for readmission must be determined. In this manner, a "safer" perioperative experience can be defined.

OUTCOMES OF INTEREST AND MEANS OF ASSESSING THEM (TABLE 9-1)

Major Complications

Mortality

The single most important but singularly uncommon outcome is death (mortality) following ambulatory surgery. In one study published more than 10 years ago on 45,000 patients undergoing ambulatory surgery, the authors found a very low risk of death (1 in 22,000) from all causes within 28 days after surgery.[19] The overall (crude) mortality rate in all patients undergoing surgery is approximately 1 in 2500,[20] which reflects on the 10-fold lower mortality in ambulatory surgery patients. This is due to a multitude of factors, including healthier patients, minor surgery, absence of emergency patients, or cesarean sections. Yet, many patients die following ambulatory surgery and these patients are sometimes not reported in the literature, suggesting that better methods for documentation are necessary to obtain correct statistics. One study on aesthetic surgery performed as an ambulatory procedure reported 95 uniquely authenticated fatalities in 496,245 liposuctions.[21] In this census survey, the mortality rate computed to 1 in 5224, or 19.1 per 100,000, which was much higher than that reported earlier, although lower than for inpatient procedures.

Table 9-1 Outcomes of Interest in Ambulatory Surgery

	Outcome of Interest
Patient (caretaker) perspective	Mortality and morbidity Home discharge Street fit Return to work
Hospital (caregiver) perspective	Mortality and morbidity Home discharge Re- or unplanned admission Costs of drugs and techniques
Insurance (care provider) perspective	Mortality and morbidity Length of hospital stay Return to work Total costs

Vila and colleagues found that adverse incidents occurred at a rate of 66 and 5.3 per 100,000 procedures in physician offices and ASCs respectively in Florida.[22] The death rate per 100,000 procedures performed was 9.2 in offices and 0.78 in ASCs. Thus, there was an approximately 10-fold increased risk of adverse incidents and death in the office setting. These authors concluded that if all office procedures had been performed in ASCs, approximately 43 injuries and six deaths per year could have been prevented.

Fleisher and colleagues determined the rates of death and admission within 7 days of 16 different surgical procedures in a nationally representative (5%) sample of Medicare beneficiaries for the years 1994–1999.[23] A total of 564,267 procedures were studied, with 360,780 in an outpatient hospital, 175,288 in an ASC, and 28,199 in an office. There were no deaths the day of surgery in the office, with 4 deaths in the ASC (2.3 per 100,000) and 9 in the outpatient hospital (2.5 per 100,000). Within 7 days of surgery, there were 10 deaths after surgery in an office (35 per 100,000), 43 deaths after surgery in an ASC (25 per 100,000), and 179 deaths after surgery in the outpatient hospital (50 per 100,000). Importantly, these data represent all-cause mortality and therefore cannot be compared to the confidential enquiry into perioperative deaths (CEPOD) data. Of note, the finding in these several studies that mortality is lowest on the day of surgery suggests that "anesthetic" clearance for outpatient surgery is associated with lower mortality than expected if these patients were not having surgery.

Morbidity

While mortality is rather uncommon, morbidity continues to be a problem. Patients expect to be able to come home soon after surgery and have an uncomplicated recovery. With the diffusion of outpatient surgery to patients with more complex comorbidities, the probability of sustaining a postoperative or postdischarge event such as a myocardial infarction, pneumonia, or infection has increased. One means of assessing the presence of morbidity is the need for direct admission or readmission after outpatient surgery. A recent analysis of Medicare claims demonstrated that the rate of outpatient mastectomy has increased from only two procedures reported to Medicare in 1986 to 10.8% of the mastectomies performed in this population in 1995.[24] The authors compared the rate of readmission within 7 days of surgery for those who had the procedure on an inpatient-versus-outpatient basis, adjusting for severity of disease. Simple mastectomies performed on outpatients had a significantly higher rate of readmission compared to 1-day stays with an adjusted odds ratio of 1.84. There were 33.8 readmissions per 1000 cases for 1-day length of stay compared with 24.2 readmissions for outpatients. There were significantly lower rates of readmission for 1-day length of stay for infections (4.1/1000 vs. 1.8/1000 cases), PONV (1.1/1000 vs. 0), and pulmonary embolism/deep vein thrombosis (1.1/1000 vs. 0). Similarly, modified radical mastectomies performed on outpatients had a significantly higher rate of readmission compared to 1-day stays with an adjusted odds ratio of 1.72. The authors suggest that patients who have the procedure on an outpatient basis may wait longer at home until seeking medical care and present with more advanced symptoms.

Twersky and colleagues studied 6243 patients who underwent ambulatory surgery over 12 consecutive months and reported 187 (2.9%) who returned to the same hospital, of which 1.3% were for complications.[25] Mezei and Chung reported 17,638 consecutive patients undergoing ambulatory surgery.[26] A total of 193 readmissions occurred within 30 days after ambulatory surgery (readmission rate 1.1%). In the previously described study of Medicare patients, the rate of admission to an inpatient hospital within 7 days was 0.9% in the office, 0.8% in the ASC, and 2.1% in the hospital.

Another approach to the assessment of complications is the use of surveys. The American Association for Accreditation of Ambulatory Surgery Facilities (AAAASF) mailed a survey to their members to determine the incidence of complications in an office.[27] The overall response rate was 57%. Of note, 0.47% of patients had at least one complication including bleeding, hypertension, infection, and hypotension, and 1 in 57,000 patients died. Assuming that only healthy individuals or very minor procedures are being performed in an office-based setting, a rate of mortality that is three times the current estimate for anesthetic-related complications is concerning. Further research and quality assurance mechanisms need to be in place before this practice is generalized. One of the problems inherent to an office-based setting is the inability to perform quality assurance reviews. For example, few, if any, surgeons or anesthesiologists would be willing to allow their "competitors" to review their complications unless mandated to perform such a review.

Minor Complications

Minor complications that are of interest in outcome are summarized in Table 9-2. Wu and colleagues reviewed the literature and identified postdischarge symptoms after out-

Table 9-2   Minor Complications That Affect Outcome Following Ambulatory Surgery

	Complications That Affect Outcome
Surgery-related	Postoperative bleeding Injury to tissues and organs Chronic pain syndromes Postdischarge complications
Anesthesia-related	Acute pain Postoperative nausea and vomiting Tiredness, drowsiness, amnesia Postdischarge complications
Hospital-related	Delay in discharge (administrative reasons)

patient surgery.[28] They found that the overall incidence of postdischarge pain was 45%, nausea 17%, vomiting 8%, headache 17%, drowsiness 42%, tiredness or fatigue 21%, myalgia 31%, and sore throat 37% and represented the most common symptoms. The presence of these symptoms may potentially impede resumption of normal daily activity and function, thereby affecting outcome. However, the extent to which these symptoms increase the burden on patients, their caregivers, or the society remains unclear. For many of these outcomes, their importance is best expressed by their influence on patient satisfaction and quality of recovery.

Quality of Recovery

Different tools are available for the assessment of recovery following anesthesia and surgery. The two instruments that have been validated in the outpatient setting include the Quality of Recovery (QoR-40) Questionnaire and the 24-Hour Functional Ability Questionnaire (24hFAQ). Quality of recovery after anesthesia is an important measure of the early postoperative health status of patients.[29] A 40-item questionnaire as a measure of quality of recovery (QoR-40; maximum score 200) was developed by these authors and was found to have good convergent validity between QoR-40 and the visual analog scale (VAS). The QoR-40 could be completed in < 7 min and was thought to be a good objective measure of quality of recovery after anesthesia and surgery. The 24-Hour Functional Ability Questionnaire (24hFAQ) was developed to measure final recovery and satisfaction 24 hr after surgery.[30] The content, construct, discriminant, and criterion (predictive) validities demonstrated the utility of this assessment instrument in the outpatient setting.

Using the QoR-40, Myles et al.[31] examined their database of 5672 adult patients to determine whether quality of recovery was associated with satisfaction with anesthesia and to identify the perioperative factors that might influence both these outcome measures. They found that a nine-item quality of recovery score ("QoR Score") was related to satisfaction with anesthesia: the overall level of satisfaction was high (97.2%); 2.1% were "somewhat dissatisfied" and 0.6% were "dissatisfied" with their anesthesia care. In addition, patients who experienced any of a number of perioperative complications had lower QoR scores. Myles also reported that patients recovering from day surgery have higher QoR scores than those recovering from minor surgery, and both have higher scores than those recovering from major surgery.[32] Patients with preexisting illness or those who develop postoperative complications have lower QoR Scores. Patient satisfaction is associated with higher QoR scores.

Using the 24hFAQ, Fleisher et al. found that remifentanil was superior to fentanyl for the four functional assessments evaluated: walking without dizziness, thinking clearly, concentrating, and communicating effectively.[33] More studies are in progress at the moment using these validated questionnaires for assessment of quality of recovery after ambulatory surgery.

Patient Satisfaction

Outcomes research has allowed for better analysis of the safety and efficacy of care given to patients.[34] Researchers have begun to focus their attention beyond mortality and morbidity as end points, and take into account patients' postoperative functional status and satisfaction as a way to assess the overall quality of patient care, specifically in the ambulatory surgery setting. Patient satisfaction is an important true outcome measure that remains inadequately studied. Previously, the lack of availability of objective methods to measure patient satisfaction may have been a problem. Quality assurance and benchmarking has resulted in the evolution of newer and better methods to assess patient satisfaction. Quality of recovery goes hand in hand with patient satisfaction as poor scores on QoR have resulted in lower patient satisfaction. The Patient Satisfaction Scale, which specifically focuses on patient satisfaction with nursing care, was assessed by Yellen et al.[35] Psychometric testing of the patient satisfaction scale resulted in a 15-item scale with three underlying dimensions, which could be used clinically. Another method under evaluation is the Evan questionnaire, with 25 questions that explores six areas, each one being marked out from 0 to 100, as in the VAS.[36] Many of the methods used to assess patient satisfaction suffer from lack of sensitivity and are consequently unable to differentiate minor differences between anesthesia techniques.

Postoperative Pain

Results from a national survey conducted recently by Apfelbaum and colleagues[37] suggest that postoperative pain continues to be undermanaged since as many as 86% of patients had moderate-severe pain and 59% patients experienced concern regarding postoperative pain, which appeared to be more common in the postdischarge period. Postoperative pain can delay discharge in addition to causing significant discomfort. Even if pain is controlled in the outpatient setting, it may be less well controlled once the intravenous agents have worn off, or the ride home and increased movement has exacerbated the pain. Using better methods to define a successful outcome for the patient in terms of improved pain relief, the concept of numbers needed to treat (NNT) has evolved in recent years. A drug with a low NNT (< 2) is said to be good for the relief of postoperative pain.[38] The focus in the ambulatory setting has been to develop agents that provide excellent pain relief and allow the transition to home. For example, the evidence available to date would suggest that acetaminophen combined with codeine, ibuprofen, or diclofenac is equally effective in relieving postoperative pain, and comparable to morphine, 10 mg, given intramuscularly. Other investigators have utilized regional anesthesia techniques to reduce postoperative pain. This is clearly an important and fertile area of study.

Postoperative Nausea and Vomiting

PONV has emerged as an important end point for outcome and something that patients would like to avoid after surgery. Over the last few years, more than 100 publications/year in peer-reviewed journals have devoted time and space to the management of PONV, thus highlighting its importance to the patient and the caregiver. Although giant strides have been taken toward its better management, PONV continues to be a problem to the patient. Multimodal management using a combination of drugs appears to be the answer to the problem of PONV in the future. However, cost is an important consideration here. The benefits offered to the patients using routine prophylaxis for PONV are probably marginal, and benefit, at best, one patient in five using single drugs. Thus, the increase in costs to the health care system may not be justifiable when it benefits only a few patients. The fact that patients are willing to pay an additional $100 to prevent PONV is interesting for the caregiver and is worthy of greater attention in future studies as a measure of outcome. Whether prevention is better than cure in this respect remains unclear because of cost-benefit analysis, but high-risk patients should certainly be offered preventive methods to reduce the risk for PONV.

Postdischarge Nausea and Vomiting

Increasingly, the postdischarge period is being discussed in the literature as an important but poorly studied period and there is now a greater stress on authors to provide data into this period. Postdischarge nausea and vomiting (PDNV) is one symptom that was shown by Wu et al. to be an important side effect requiring greater attention.[28] To assess the impact of treatment of PDNV using different drugs, Gupta et al. did a systematic review of the literature and found that prophylactic treatment of PDNV with ondansetron, 4 mg, or a combination of two drugs results in a significant reduction in PDNV when compared to placebo.[39] However, the NNT for ondansetron alone was 13 while that for combination treatment was five, which would favor the latter, particularly in high-risk patients. This study could be criticized in that only three studies were included in the combination-treatment group, and these patients received a combination of different drugs, resulting in some degree of uncertainty as to which combination is the most appropriate to avoid PDNV.

Other Minor Factors Affecting Outcome

Other outcomes of importance to the patient are tiredness and amnesia. Why are patients tired after the operation? This could be due to the residual effects of anesthesia, or the consequence of surgery. Unfortunately, tiredness after operations remains poorly studied, and although many studies have assessed this parameter, very few have actually studied it prospectively as an important end point following surgery. Cognitive dysfunction remains for up to 24 hr after anesthesia and minor surgery when compared to unoperated controls, and therefore driving a car within 24 hr after surgery is not recommended. The ability to drive a car after ambulatory surgery remains an important end point and a measure of outcome for some patients and is likely to increase in the future. Most studies on this outcome measure were done in the late 1970s when different anesthetic agents were used, and therefore the exact time span before driving should be permitted after anesthesia using modern agents remains unknown.

One further problem of importance to the patient and that may affect outcome is amnesia. Many drugs cause amnesia that is of varying duration. Benzodiazepines are particularly notorious in this respect and some that have active metabolites, e.g., diazepam, can give prolonged amnesia. Although there may be no physical effect or injury to the patient as a consequence of amnesia, it is distressing and can lead to other complications as a result of not following instructions given by the doctor or nurse at the time the patient is amnesic. Written and verbal instructions are therefore important to all patients undergoing ambulatory surgical procedures. Outcome is then likely to be much better for the patient.

Economic Outcomes

Finally, economic implications of ambulatory surgery are becoming increasingly important. Ambulatory surgery has been shown to be cost-saving compared to inpatient surgery. However, this assumes a low rate of unplanned admissions or readmissions. Therefore, any economic assessment should include these factors in the analysis. There are also significant costs borne by the patient and family associated with outpatient surgery. It is therefore important to understand how to evaluate these economic benefits of outpatient surgery and any strategies used to reduce the rate of "complications," including pain and PONV.

It is estimated that expenditures influenced (directly or indirectly) by anesthesia providers represent 3–5% of the total health care costs of the United States.[40] The technology assessment of various practices in anesthesiology with economic considerations will lead us to provide what is called *value-based anesthesia care*, i.e., the best patient outcome achievable at a reasonable economic input. In medical economic analysis, there are essentially three dimensions with different issues in each dimension that need to be considered in the analysis. Application of a particular method of economic analysis requires proper understanding of the appropriate terminology, and has been reviewed elsewhere.

When reviewing studies that include economic outcomes, it is important to understand how they are commonly reported. Therefore, definition of three important terms related to "cost" is warranted. Charge is the amount the hospital, the clinic, the physician, or the pharmacy attempts to recover (or bills) for providing a service. Payment is the amount actually paid by the individual or the third-party payor for the service. Cost of particular service is a function of resources consumed for that service. Types of relevant costs include direct, indirect, and intangible. *Direct costs* are organizing and operational expenditures in the delivery of medical care. These costs can be medical or nonmedical. *Direct medical costs* include those incurred by hospitalizations, drugs, physician and other relevant personnel, etc. A technique called *time-and-motion* method is often employed to determine the hospital costs, typically the direct costs of drugs. To estimate direct cost of a particular drug, this method involves measuring the time taken for the nurse to gather the materials, prepare, and administer the medication. Direct nonmedical costs include family and patient expenses that result from illness, such as those for food, transportation, family lodging, home help, etc. These direct nonmedical costs can be substantial, and are not usually covered in any significant degree by insurance companies and therefore are borne by patients. Although these costs are not usually included in analyses, these direct nonmedical costs should be included when pertinent to the perspective.

Indirect costs relate to the cost of loss of income (lost productivity) due to illness or death. These include those due to absence from work, lost wages, decreased earnings, and need to change jobs, etc. Indirect cost or productivity losses caused by an intervention should be contrasted with the indirect costs of illness. Indirect costs of an illness are usually measured by an extension of the human capital approach. Reduction in the indirect costs of illness is often estimated as a monetary benefit, especially for cost-benefit studies.

Intangible costs represent nonmonetary costs of illness, such as pain, suffering, and grief expressed in monetary terms. These costs form a part of the denominator in cost-benefit analysis that uses the willingness-to-pay method. In cost-utility analysis, such items are not given a dollar value but are included in the determination of health outcomes, i.e., in the calculation of quality-adjusted life years (QALY). Therefore, even in the cost-utility analysis, intangible costs become a part of the denominator.

An important aspect of cost determination is *cost finding*, a term used to describe the highly complex procedure for cost delineation. This involves classification of costs as *fixed costs* and *variable costs*. Fixed costs are the ongoing costs of providing service, which are unrelated to volume. Salaries of operating room (OR) managers, costs of OR and recovery room monitors, etc. come under the category of fixed costs. Variable costs vary as a function of the volume provided. Examples of variable costs in the OR and recovery room include supplies, drugs, and supplemental nursing services. Most analyses assume only fixed costs and therefore are limited in their utility. Local anesthesia with or without sedation was found in some studies to be cost-effective and patient-appreciated when compared to both regional and general anesthesia.[41,42] In a recent paper, Lennox et al. found that small-dose spinal anesthesia was an effective alternative to a desflurane general anesthetic in terms of cost-and-recovery profiles in ambulatory gynecologic laparoscopy.[43] When comparing inhalation with total intravenous anesthesia (TIVA), Joshi reported that inhalation anesthesia may have an economical advantage over TIVA.[44] However, induction of anesthesia with sevoflurane followed by maintenance with sevoflurane is both costly and offers no advantage over induction with propofol.[45]

Multifactorial Nature of Outcome Assessment

It is imperative to realize that "perioperative" risk is multifactorial, and depends on the interaction of anesthesia-, patient-, and surgery-specific factors (Fig. 9-1). With respect to anesthesia, both the effects of the agents and the skills of the practitioner are important. Similarly, both the surgical procedure itself and the surgeon's skills impact on perioperative risk. From the patient's perspective, the question remains whether the coexisting disease raises the probability of complications to a level such that the benefit of the surgery is outweighed by the risk. As the specialty focuses on its role in the twenty-first century, it is important to acknowledge the patient's perspective and desire to undergo life-prolonging or quality-of-life improving procedures. The ability of the anesthesiologist to impact on the decision process and overall risk is the challenge.

Anesthesia-Related Factors Affecting Outcome

With the introduction of newer inhalation anesthetics, it can be questioned whether there is an improved outcome for patients since the costs incurred to the caregiver as a result of newer anesthetics and drugs have increased substantially. One study looked at outcome measured in terms of recovery and discharge as also postoperative complications following anesthesia with inhalational agents and propofol.[46] Postoperative recovery and complications can be considered as important outcomes for patients following ambulatory surgery. Minor differences were found, specifically in terms of PONV, by the authors. However, their main conclusion was that local practice and techniques rather than outcome should guide the choice of anesthetics. The hypothesis that there would be tremendous savings in terms of reduced personnel due to quicker and earlier recovery has never been shown in practice, despite increasing costs from newer drugs.

Surgery-Related Factors Affecting Outcome

Perhaps the single most important surgical factor that affects outcome is successfully performed surgery. In fact, this factor limits the ability to assess "anesthetic" satisfaction. Surgery-related factors that may result in delayed discharge or longer period of recovery and even reoperation include bleeding, unwanted injury to tissues and organs,

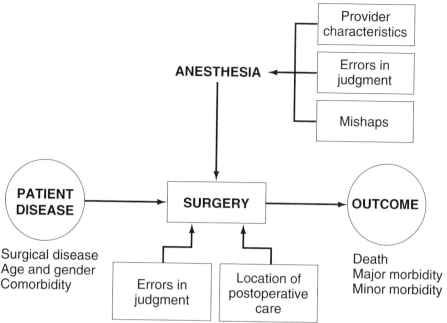

Figure 9-1   Multifactorial nature of outcome assessment. (Reproduced with permission from Miller RD [ed.], *Anesthesia*, Vol. I, 5th ed. New York: Churchill Livingstone, 2000. Copyright © 2000, with permission from Elsevier.)

nerve or tissue injury resulting in chronic pain syndromes, and postdischarge complications, including infection requiring readmission or reoperation. All of these factors affect outcome for the patient and the hospital.

Patient-Specific Factors Affecting Outcome

There has been a great deal of research into identifying those patients at greatest risk for perioperative complications, although virtually all of the work has been for inpatient procedures. In an assessment of Medicare beneficiaries for the years 1994–1999, comorbidity was assessed by the presence of an inpatient hospitalization during the 6 months prior to the 3-month period during which the patient had outpatient surgery. In multivariate models, variables like very old patients, prior admission within 6 months, performance in an office or hospital setting, and invasiveness of surgery identify those patients who are at increased risk of admission or death within 7 days. In an analysis of data from New York State on outpatient surgery from 1997, which has been submitted to the Hospital Cost and Utilization Project (HCUP) and is available through the Agency for Healthcare Research and Quality, outcomes of interest were identified including age > 85, OR duration 60–119 min, OR duration > 120 min, cardiac disease, peripheral vascular disease, cerebrovascular disease, malignancy, HIV-positive, and general anesthesia.

Insurance-Related Factors Affecting Outcome

Most patients in the Western world undergoing surgery are likely to have some form of insurance cover that reimburses, to a varying degree, the costs incurred by the health care provider. Insurance can be of varying degrees that cover the basic costs as a consequence of surgery to full costs including loss of income during the rehabilitation phase. Depending on the type of insurance cover, the health care provider is interested in the cost of drugs, the duration of hospital stay as well as the time to return to work. Most countries in Europe would cover the costs including the loss of income to a major extent, but the system in the United States varies considerably depending on the state, the employer, the insurance company as well as the patient and his/her family status. Thus, outcome becomes increasingly important depending on the type of insurance-cover for the individual. Broadly speaking, most health care providers would prefer the shortest duration of stay in the hospital using the cheapest drugs, operated and anesthetized by the best doctors, resulting in the least risk of complications at the lowest possible costs, and providing the most satisfied patient. Unfortunately, this equation is not easy, and although there is a lot of competition to reach this utopia, costs continue to increase. Fortunately, better techniques and minimally invasive methods with more cost-conscious attitudes among personnel has led to some constraints in expenditure without affecting quality.

SUMMARY

Outcomes of interest in anesthesia and surgery are discussed from different perspectives. The issues covered are complex and no single outcome can be considered to be of paramount interest to all parties except *mortality*. This, although objective, is extremely rare following ambulatory surgery. Many outcomes that are of interest to the patient could be considered to be in conflict with the interests of the care provider since cost containment is an issue. In other words, a management technique may increase costs for the care provider but improve outcome for the patient. Although not the standard of care today, the future will hopefully bring greater attention and rewards for better outcomes. It is important to identify outcomes of significance to the patient and better means of tracking these outcomes given their rare occurrence.

REFERENCES

1. Fleisher LA, Corbett W, Berry C, Poldermans D. Cost-effectiveness of differing perioperative beta-blockade strategies in vascular surgery patients. J Cardiothor Vasc Anesth 2004;18(1):7–13.

2. Gan T, Sloan F, Dear Gde L, et al. How much are patients willing to pay to avoid postoperative nausea and vomiting? Anesth Analg 2001;92:393–400.

3. Buck N, Devlin HB, Lunn JL. Report of a Confidential Enquiry into Perioperative Deaths. London: King's Fund Publishing House, 1987.

4. Beecher HK, Todd DP: A study of deaths associated with anesthesia and surgery. Ann Surg 1954;140:2–34.

5. Newland MC, Ellis SJ, Lydiatt CA, Peters KR, Tinker JH, Romberger DJ, Ullrich FA, Anderson JR. Anesthetic-related cardiac arrest and its mortality: a report covering 72,959 anesthetics over 10 years from a US teaching hospital. Anesthesiology 2002;97:108–15.

6. Cheney FW, Posner K, Caplan RA, Ward RJ. Standard of care and anesthesia liability. JAMA 1989;261:1599–603.

7. Mathew JP, Parks R, Savino JS, Friedman AS, Koch C, Mangano DT, Browner WS. Atrial fibrillation following coronary artery bypass graft surgery: predictors, outcomes, and resource utilization. Multicenter Study of Perioperative Ischemia Research Group. JAMA 1996;276:300–6.

8. Mangano DT. Aspirin and mortality from coronary bypass surgery. N Engl J Med 2002;347:1309–17.

9. Nugent WC. Clinical applications of risk-assessment protocols in the management of individual patients. Ann Thorac Surg 1997;64:S68–72.

10. Grover FL, Shroyer AL, Edwards FH, Pae WE Jr, Ferguson TB Jr, Gay WA Jr, Clark RE. Data quality review program: the Society of Thoracic Surgeons Adult Cardiac National Database. Ann Thorac Surg 1996;62:1229–31.

11. Grover FL, Shroyer AL, Hammermeister KE. Calculating risk and outcome: the Veterans Affairs database. Ann Thorac Surg 1996;62:S6–11.

12. Clark RE. The development of the Society of Thoracic Surgeons voluntary national database system: genesis, issues, growth, and status. Best Pract Benchmarking Healthc 1996;1:62–69.

13. Clark RE. The STS Cardiac Surgery National Database: an update. Ann Thorac Surg 1995;59:1376–80.

14. Ghali WA, Ash AS, Hall RE, Moskowitz MA. Statewide quality improvement initiatives and mortality after cardiac surgery. JAMA 1997;277:379–82.

15. Mukamel DB, Mushlin AI. Quality of care information makes a difference: an analysis of market share and price changes after publication of the New York State Cardiac Surgery Mortality Reports. Med Care 1998;36:945–54.

16. Hannan EL, Racz MJ, Jollis JG, Peterson ED. Using Medicare claims data to assess provider quality for CABG surgery: does it work well enough? Health Serv Res 1997;31:659–78.

17. Guida RA, Mattucci KF. Tonsillectomy and adenoidectomy: an inpatient or outpatient procedure? Laryngoscope 1990;100:491–93.

18. Ruboyianes JM, Cruz RM. Pediatric adenotonsillectomy for obstructive sleep apnea. Ear Nose Throat J 1996;75:430–33.

19. Warner MA, Shields SE, Chute CG. Major morbidity and mortality within 1 month of ambulatory surgery and anesthesia. JAMA 1993;270:1437–41.

20. Pedersen T, Eliasen K, Henriksen E. A prospective study of mortality associated with anaesthesia and surgery: risk indicators of mortality in hospital. Acta Anaesthesiol Scand 1990;34:176.

21. Grazer FM, de Jong RH. Fatal outcomes from liposuction: census survey of cosmetic surgeons. Plast Reconstr Surg 2000;105: 436–46.

22. Vila H Jr, Soto R, Cantor AB, Mackey D. Comparative outcomes analysis of procedures performed in physician offices and ambulatory surgery centers. Arch Surg 2003;138:991–95.

23. Fleisher LA, Pasternak LR, Herbert R, Anderson GF. Safety of outpatient surgery in the elderly: the importance of the patient, system, and location of care. Arch Surg 2004;139:67–72.

24. Warren JL, Riley GF, Potosky AL, Klabunde CN, Richter E, Ballard-Barbash R. Trends and outcomes of outpatient mastectomy in elderly women. J Natl Cancer Inst 1998;90:833–40.

25. Twersky R, Fishman D, Homel P. What happens after discharge? Return hospital visits after ambulatory surgery. Anesth Analg 1997; 84:319–24.

26. Mezei G, Chung F. Return hospital visits and hospital readmissions after ambulatory surgery. Ann Surg 1999;230:721–27.

27. Morello DC, Colon GA, Fredricks S, Iverson RE, Singer R. Patient safety in accredited office surgical facilities. Plast Reconstr Surg 1997;99:1496–500.

28. Wu CL, Berenholtz SM, Pronovost PJ, Fleisher LA. Systematic review and analysis of postdischarge symptoms after outpatient surgery. Anesthesiology 2002;96:994–1003.

29. Myles PS, Weitkamp B, Jones K, Melick J, Hensen S. Validity and reliability of a postoperative quality of recovery score: the QoR-40. Br J Anaesth. 2000;84:11–15.

30. Hogue SL, Reese PR, Colopy M, Fleisher LA, Tuman KJ, Twersky RS, Warner DS, Jamerson B. Assessing a tool to measure patient functional ability after outpatient surgery. Anesth Analg 2000;91:97–106.

31. Myles PS, Reeves MD, Anderson H, Weeks AM. Measurement of quality of recovery in 5672 patients after anaesthesia and surgery. Anaesth Intens Care 2000;28:276–80.

32. Myles PS. Quality in anesthesia. Minerva Anesthesiol 2001;67: 279–83.

33. Fleisher LA, Hogue S, Colopy M, Twersky RS, Warner DS, Jamerson BD, Tuman KJ, Glass PS, Roizen MF. Does functional ability in the postoperative period differ between remifentanil- and fentanyl-based anesthesia? J Clin Anesth 2001;13:401–6.

34. Deutsch N, Wu CL. Patient outcomes following ambulatory anesthesia. Anesthesiol Clin North Am 2003;21:403–15.

35. Yellen E, Davis GC, Ricard R. The measurement of patient satisfaction. J Nurs Care Qual 2002;16:23–29.

36. Pernoud N, Colavolpe JC, Auquier P, Eon B, Auffray JP, Francois G, Blache JL. A scale of perioperative satisfaction for anesthesia. II. Preliminary results. Ann Fr Anesth Reanim 1999;18:858–65.

37. Apfelbaum JL, Chen C, Mehta SS, Gan TJ. Postoperative pain experience: results from a national survey suggest postoperative pain continues to be undermanaged. Anesth Analg 2003;97:534–40.

38. Moore RA, McQuay HJ. An Evidence-Based Resource for Pain Relief. New York: Oxford University Press, 1998, pp. 54–57.

39. Gupta A, Wu CL, Elkassabany N, Krug CE, Parker SD, Fleisher LA. Does the routine prophylactic use of antiemetics affect the incidence of postdischarge nausea and vomiting following ambulatory surgery? A systematic review of randomized controlled trials. Anesthesiology 2003;99:488–95.

40. Johnstone RE, Martinec CL. Costs of anesthesia. Anesth Analg 1993;76:840–48.

41. Callesen T, Bech K, Kehlet H. One-thousand consecutive inguinal hernia repairs under unmonitored local anesthesia. Anesth Analg 2001;93:1373–76.

42. Sungurtekin H, Sungurtekin U, Erdem E. Local anesthesia and midazolam versus spinal anesthesia in ambulatory pilonidal surgery. J Clin Anesth 2003;15:201–5.

43. Lennox PH, Chilvers C, Vaghadia H. Selective spinal anesthesia ver-

sus desflurane anesthesia in short duration outpatient gynecological laparoscopy: a pharmacoeconomic comparison. Anesth Analg 2002;94:565–68.

44. Joshi GP. Inhalational techniques in ambulatory anesthesia. Anesthesiol Clin North Am 2003;21:263–72.

45. Elliott RA, Payne K, Moore JK, Harper NJ, St Leger AS, Moore EW, Thoms GM, Pollard BJ, McHugh GA, Bennett J, Lawrence G, Kerr J, Davies LM. Clinical and economic choices in anaesthesia for day surgery: a prospective randomised controlled trial. Anaesthesia 2003;58:412–21.

46. Gupta A, Stierer T, Zuckerman R, Sakima N, Parker SD, Fleisher LA. Comparison of recovery profile after ambulatory anesthesia with propofol, isoflurane, sevoflurane and desflurane: a systematic review. Anesth Analg 2004;98:632–41.

GENERAL ADMINISTRATIVE PRINCIPLES

Office-Based Anesthesia: Regulatory and Administrative Issues

HECTOR VILA, JR.   •   REBECCA S. TWERSKY

INTRODUCTION

Office Surgery Overview

During the last 10 years the growth in the number of surgical procedures being performed in physicians' offices has been dramatic. It is similar to the shift that occurred in the 1980s, when many surgical procedures moved from hospitals to ambulatory surgery centers (ASCs). It was estimated that more than 10 million patients would receive anesthesia for surgical procedures in physicians' offices in the year 2003.[1] By the year 2005, one-quarter of all ambulatory procedures will be performed in a doctor's office.[2] Surgeon and patient preferences are touted as the main driving forces, according to a survey conducted by the Medical Society of New York.[3] Surgeons prefer this venue because they have increased control over their schedule and they are able to generate facility revenue and minimize the associated procedural cost. New anesthesia techniques and medications have provided for increased safety, faster recovery, and higher patient satisfaction.

Although office surgery is growing in popularity, it is not without problems. There have been numerous reports of injuries and deaths after office surgery in Florida, California, North Carolina, and New York as well as other states.[4] In spite of these reports of adverse outcomes, surgery in the physician's office has been unwatched and unregulated. One article went so far as to describe surgery in the physician's office as the "wild, wild, west of health care."[5] In September 2003, a report of outcomes from Florida offices compared to ASCs showed a greater than 10-fold risk of death and injury in the physician's office. The higher office death and injury rate occurred even though Florida office regulations were stricter than those of most other states.[6] This was the first comprehensive report of office outcomes data based on mandatory reporting. It reported an office mortality of about 1 in 10,000 patients, which was similar to previous reports by Grazer and de Jong in 2000, with a death rate approximating 1 in 5000 cases.[7] In contrast, a report by Morello et al from aggregated self-reporting through the facility's accrediting body showed a lower death rate; however, their data relied on voluntary reporting.[8] Hoefflin et al. in 2001 reported no deaths on 23,000 consecutive office cosmetic procedures under general anesthesia.[9] However, this facility was fully accredited by the American Association for Accreditation of Ambulatory Surgery Facilities (AAAASF), the surgeons were all board-certified, and all the anesthetics were administered by board-certified anesthesiologists. This level of care is similar to that provided in freestanding licensed ASCs, where the death rate was found to be less than 1 in 100,000.[6]

These reports of office mishaps illustrate the many challenges for the physician whose previous practice experience may have been in an established hospital-based operating room (OR). The challenge required is to bring the same standard of care existing in ASCs and hospitals into the office surgical suite. Compared to these other settings, the office-based setting has little or no regulation, oversight, or control under federal, state, or local laws. Therefore, the physician must often assume oversight and responsibility for areas that would be taken for granted in the hospital or ambulatory surgical facility. This includes facility construction, medications, supplies, and equipment. In addition, the physician must ensure that established policies and procedures regarding fire, safety, drug, emergencies, staffing, and emergency patient transfers are in place. This chapter will provide an overview of regulatory requirements in these areas as well as relevant references and contact information.

RULES, REGULATIONS, STANDARDS, AND GUIDELINES

Oversight Mechanisms

There are several different methodologies for office surgery oversight, including legislation, statutes, regulations, rules, standards, and guidelines. Some states even have a combination of these methodologies. Legislation includes bills that have been introduced in the legislature but have yet to become law. Statutes are bills that have been signed into law. Regulations or rules are language that has been adopted by a regulatory body that also has the force of law. Guidelines and standards are language that does not have the force of law that has been adopted by or endorsed by a regulatory or advisory body. When guidelines or standards are adopted by the state medical boards, they often form the basis of disciplinary action against physicians who fail to follow them.

State Activities

Approximately half of the states have proposed or enacted regulations specific to office surgery. Table 10-1 summarizes the activities in the states through the latter part of

Table 10-1 Office-Based Surgery Oversight Activities by State

State	Year	Agency	Action	Facility Accred.	Incident Reporting	Surgeon Credentials	Anesthesia Requirement	ACLS/BLS	Licensing/ Registration	Surgery Time Limit
Alabama	2003	BOM	Rules		+	+		+	+	
Arkansas	2003	BOM	Proposed guidelines	+						
California	1996; 2000	Legislature	Regulations	+	+	+		+		
Colorado	2001	BOM	Policy			+	+			
Connecticut	2001	Legislature	Regulations	+						
District of Columbia	2000	BOM	ASA guidelines						+	
Florida	2000	BOM	Rules and regulations	+	+	+	+	+	+	+
Illinois	2001	DPR	Admin. code	+		+	+	+		
Louisiana	2004	BOM	Regulation	+	+	+		+		
Massachusetts	2002	Legislature	Regulations	+	+	+	+	+		
Mississippi	2003	BOM	Regulations			+		+	+	
New Jersey	1998	BOM	Regulations		+	+	+	+		
New York	2001	DOH	Proposed guidelines		+	+	+			
North Carolina	2002	BOM	Position statement	+	+	+	+			
Ohio	2002; 2004	BOM	Proposed rules/regs	+	+	+	+	+		
Oklahoma	2000	BOM	ASA guidelines							
Oregon	1998; 2003	Med. assoc.	Standards	+		+		+		
Pennsylvania	2000	DOH	Regulations	+	+				+	+
Rhode Island	2000	DOH	Rules	+	+	+	+	+	+	+
South Carolina	2001	BOM	Guidelines	+	+	+	+			
Texas	2000	BOM	Regulations	+	+	+	+		+	
Virginia	2003	BOM	Regulations		+				+	
Washington	2003	SMA/MQAC	Proposed guidelines/regs	+	+	+	+			

Abbreviations: ACLS—Advanced Cardiac Life Support; BLS—Basic Life Support; BOM—Board of Medicine; DOH—Department of Health; DPR—Department of Public Regulator; SMA—State Medical Association.

2003. Because of rapid changes in state-by-state regulations, the authors strongly advise that practitioners in each state consult the respective state board of medicine to determine current requirements. As shown in Table 10-1, 23 states have proposed or enacted some form of oversight. Several other states have begun efforts through entities such as task forces or discussion groups. Fewer than half of the states listed have used active legislation to regulate offices. Most have guidelines or standards by a state medical board or medical association. More states focus on requirements for facility accreditation, mandatory incident reporting, and minimum provider qualifications. Other components considered by fewer states include emergency transfer plans, advanced cardiac life support (ACLS) training, and facility and provider licensure. Regulation of offices in the United States is a new process, demonstrated by the fact that most regulations are less than 3 years old.

Specialty and National Societies

Many of the specialty societies have also promulgated guidelines or standards regarding the conduct of office surgery. These societies include the American College of Surgeons (ACS), the American Society of Plastic Surgeons (ASPS), the American Society for Aesthetic Plastic Surgery (ASAPS), the American Academy of Dermatology Association (AAD), and the American Association of Oral and Maxillofacial Surgeons (AAOMS). These national societies have enacted their own guidelines and set the standard for their professional practice. The ACS was the first surgical society to create guidelines for office surgery in 1994, *Guidelines for Optimal Ambulatory Surgery and Office-Based Care*, now in its third edition. The ASPS has taken the stance of requiring their members to practice only in accredited facilities in order to maintain membership.[10] The ASPS Task Force on Patient Safety and Office-Based Surgery Facilities published several practice advisories for the office-based setting.[11]

The American Medical Association (AMA) convened a work group in 2003 of subspecialty societies and state medical associations with the input of accrediting bodies, to identify specific requirements for office-based surgery that could be used to develop guidelines and model state legislation for use by state regulatory authorities to assure quality of office-based surgery. This resulted in 10 core principles that represent a wide consensus within the medical profession and are intended to promote consistency in the safety and quality of office surgery and anesthesia (Appendix 10-1). These activities followed the report issued in 2002 by the Federation of State Medical Boards, "Special Committee on Office-Based Surgery," which contained recommendations on administration, personnel, patient evaluation, anesthesia, accident reporting, facilities accreditation, and liposuction procedures.[12]

The American Society of Anesthesiologists (ASA) developed guidelines for office anesthesia considered to be the most comprehensive document for office-based anesthesia care and has been adopted by numerous states as part of their requirements[13] (Appendix 10-2). In addition,

the ASA published a comprehensive compendium, *Office-Based Anesthesia: Considerations for Anesthesiologists in Setting Up and Maintaining a Safe Office Anesthesia Environment*,[1] addressing clinical and administrative issues in more detail.

Anesthesia

At this time, it appears that the guidelines and requirements set forth by the ASA exceed the expectations of many states and would well serve the office practitioners. There are special problems that the office practitioner must recognize when administering anesthesia in the office setting. Unlike most acute-care hospitals or licensed ambulatory surgery facilities, offices usually have little or no regulation or control under federal, state, or local law. There is little of the nursing or administrative infrastructure that exists in hospitals and ASCs. Consequently, anesthesiologists must often assume responsibility for areas that would be taken for granted at the other locations. The office anesthesiologist must, for example, ensure that established policies and procedures regarding fire, safety, drug, emergencies, staffing, training, and unanticipated patient transfers are in place and that all regulations regarding reporting of adverse incidents occur. Furthermore, because there are usually no active peer review procedures, it is important to ensure that "near misses" and adverse outcomes are reviewed and that quality improvement steps are performed.

The classification of the surgical facilities used by the accrediting organizations focuses on the level of anesthesia provided. However, the classifications are not standardized. The ASA has provided comments for clarification to these organizations and has suggested the following:

Level I/Class A: Minor surgical procedures performed under topical, local, or infiltration block anesthesia without preoperative or intraoperative sedation.
Level II/Class B: Minor or major surgical procedures performed in conjunction with oral, rectal, parenteral, or intravenous sedation or under analgesic or dissociative drugs.
Level III/Class C: Surgical procedures that require general anesthesia or major conduction blocks and support of vital bodily functions.

Some states have regulations or guidelines containing specific anesthesia requirements (Table 10-1). Many regulations contain language such as the following: "A physician who administers or supervises the administration of anesthesia services in an office shall have credentials reviewed by the medical director or governing body of the office surgical facility. The physicians should: perform a preanesthetic examination and evaluation; prescribe the anesthesia; assure that qualified practitioners participate; remain physically present and immediately available for diagnosis; treat and manage anesthesia-related complications or emergencies; assure the provision of indicated postanesthesia care. The supervising licensed physician or operating practitioner should be specifically trained in the office-based surgery being performed as well as sedation, anesthesia, and rescue techniques appropriate to the type of sedation being provided."

Florida, Mississippi, and South Carolina recommend or require surgeons to obtain Continuing Medical Education (CME) regarding local anesthetic drug dosages and management of toxicity for Level I procedures. Illinois, Mississippi, New Jersey, Ohio, and Virginia have CME requirements for non-anesthesiologists who supervise the administration of anesthesia. Massachusetts, South Carolina, and North Carolina specifically require the physician supervising Certified Registered Nurse Anesthetists (CRNAs) in the office to be competent in the tasks he/she supervises and Florida requires that an anesthesiologist administer or supervise the administration of Level III anesthesia in the office.

OFFICE-ACCREDITING ORGANIZATIONS

Accreditation of office-based practices is currently provided by the four major accrediting bodies (see Table 10-2): JCAHO—Joint Commission on Accreditation of Healthcare Organizations, AAAHC—Accreditation Association for Ambulatory Healthcare, AAAASF—American Association for Accreditation of Ambulatory Surgery Facilities, and the American Osteopathic Association (AOA). Contact information for these organizations is given in Table 10-2. The major accrediting bodies were developed to assure verifiable quality care with definable standards. All these organizations address similar aspects of an office-based practice. These include: the facility's physical layout, patient and personnel records, peer-review/quality assurance, OR personnel, equipment, operations and manage-

Table 10-2   Accrediting Organizations for Office-Based Surgery

Accreditation Association for Ambulatory Health Care (AAAHC), 3201 Old Glenview Road, Suite 300, Wilmette, IL 60091-2992. Telephone: (847)853-6060. (Source for Accreditation Handbook of Ambulatory Health Care). Internet: <www.aaahc.org>.

American Association for Accreditation of Ambulatory Surgery Facilities, Inc. (AAAASF), Manual for Accreditation of Ambulatory Surgery Facilities, 1998, 1202 Allanson Road, Mundelein, IL 60060. Telephone: (888)545-5222. Internet: <www.aaaasf.org>.

American Osteopathic Association—Healthcare Facilities Accreditation Program (AOA-HFAP), 142 E. Ontario Street, Chicago, IL 60611. Telephone: (800)621-1773, ext.8258. Internet: <www.aoa-net.org/Accreditation/HFAP/hfapcontact.htm>.

Joint Commission on Accreditation of Healthcare Organizations (JCAHO), One Renaissance Boulevard, Terrace, IL 60181. Telephone: (630)792-5000. Internet: <www.jcaho.org>.

ment, and environmental safety. The anesthesia requirements for accreditation have all been substantially revised and now reflect many of the ASA standards and guidelines. Alternatives for these accrediting bodies may include a state-recognized entity, or be state-licensed and/or Medicare-certified.

The AAAASF is primarily an office-practice-accrediting body and is made up of over 600 plastic surgery practices. Through a liaison with the ASA, the AAAASF created a special anesthesia standards section that reflects the ASA standards. This includes qualifications of practitioners delivering the pre- and postanesthetic care, postanesthesia care unit (PACU) evaluation, discharge evaluation, anesthesia equipment and supplies, and transfer and emergency plans. The accreditation cycle is 3 years and the facility must maintain the standards of the association in the interim years.

The AAAHC accredits only ambulatory facilities. There are currently over 1200 facilities accredited by the AAAHC nationally, including nearly 200 office-based practices. The AAAHC, using the general core standards, may award accreditation for 6 months, 1 year, or 3 years. The AAAHC has also used ASA input significantly as a part of its anesthesia services requirements.

JCAHO, the largest of the three accrediting bodies, having realized that the obstacles in applying existing hospital standards to an office practice, approved in January 2001 the *Office-Based Surgery Accreditation Handbook*. The handbook includes 146 specific standards that address key patient safety and quality performance expectation. Attention is given to those issues that directly affect patients and their care, and the handbook covers essential areas such as medication and anesthesia, patient safety, practitioner credentials, staff competency, and customer service. The standards were established specifically for single sites of care for up to four physicians, dentists, or podiatrists. Practices eligible for accreditation include oral surgeons, endoscopy suites, plastic surgery practices, podiatry practices, and laser surgery centers. JCAHO accreditation surveys are performed on a 3-year cycle.

The AOA Healthcare Facilities Accreditation Program (HFAP) has been providing medical facilities with an objective review of their services since 1945. The program is recognized nationally by the federal government, state governments, insurance carriers, and managed-care organizations.

ADMINISTRATIVE ISSUES

Practitioner Credentials and Qualifications

All health care practitioners (defined herein as physicians, dentists, podiatrists) and nurses should hold a valid license or certificate to perform their assigned duties. All OR personnel who provide clinical care in the office should be qualified to perform services commensurate with their level of education, training, and experience.

Anesthesiologists and surgeons practicing in an office-based setting should maintain current ACLS training. All other medical personnel, at a minimum, must maintain training in basic cardiopulmonary resuscitation.

Anesthesia services must comply with state requirements and should also meet the perioperative practitioner qualifications and services as summarized in the previous section on anesthesia.

Facility Governance

The facility should have a medical director or formal governing body that establishes policy and is responsible for the activities of the facility and its staff and responsible for ensuring that facilities and personnel are adequate and appropriate for the type of procedures performed. Policies and procedures should be written for the orderly conduct of the facility and reviewed on a regular basis. All applicable state and federal regulations, local laws, codes, and regulations pertaining to fire prevention, building construction and occupancy, accommodations for the disabled, occupational safety and health, and disposal of medical waste and hazardous waste should be observed.

Records and Documentation

All patient records, including anesthesia records, must be available for review and kept on file by both the office-based practice and the anesthesia care provider (anesthesia records). They should be maintained from the time the facility is opened and for the number of years thereafter as mandated by state regulations. The individual anesthesia care provider should also maintain the anesthesia records in a similar manner. Evidence of preoperative and postoperative evaluations must be documented in the patient record. Any necessary laboratory reports, including electrocardiograms or radiographs, medical consultation, and telephone contact with the patient, should be documented and available on the patient record.

Any forms signed by the patient (including consent, "living wills," release of medical records permission, or others) should be kept in the file.

Quality Improvement Activities

An outcomes surveillance reporting system for the office is important to promote high-quality patient care. States should be encouraged to develop a legally privileged adverse-incident reporting system.

The anesthesiologist should participate in ongoing continuous quality improvement and risk management activities of each particular office practice.

1. The quality improvement plan should specify the individual who is responsible for performing each element of the plan.
2. An anesthesiologist or an anesthesiology group that provides anesthesia care at multiple facilities may form its own quality improvement unit to evaluate the total anesthesia care it provides.
3. The written plan should be in place to continually assess, document, and improve the outcome of the anesthesia care provided.

4. There should be a review of quality indicators, including measures of patient satisfaction.
5. There should be an annual review and check of anesthesia equipment to ensure compliance with current safety standards and the standards for the release of waste anesthetic gases.
6. The quality improvement plan should include routine review of anesthesia and surgical morbidity and "adverse" or "sentinel" or outcome events such as recommended by the ASA Committee on Ambulatory Surgical Care and the Task Force on Office-Based Anesthesia (see Table 10-3). The recommendations are designed to encourage quality patient care, but cannot guarantee a specific outcome.

Continuing Education

Anesthesiologists participating in an office-based practice and nonphysicians medically direct should engage in regular and current courses of study of medical, ethical, and safety issues relevant to that office practice.

Professional Liability

The individual practitioner must not take liability coverage for granted and should also carefully examine the policy and all its declarations, amendments, attachments, and qualifications. It is common for insurers to require specific performance criteria, often citing ASA standards or guidelines and making adherence to these as a condition of coverage. Such issues as mandatory oxygen saturation measurement, end-tidal carbon dioxide ($ETCO_2$) monitoring, constant presence in the OR, and, increasingly, temperature measurement may well be part of policy requirements. It is vitally important that these provisions be understood and followed.

There are potential differences between hospital and office-based liability coverage. A few specific areas of difference are:

1. Insurers may lack an established peer review structure to examine the quality of the exclusively office-based practitioner.
2. Insurers may lack a facility accreditation system to assess risk related to adequacy of the equipment, supplies, and protocols and procedures in place for patient protection.
3. Office-based providers will frequently work only 1 or 2 days a week at a given office, so multiple sites complicate underwriting calculations.
4. Practices may cross state lines, giving rise to how multistate coverage is written.
5. Vicarious liability—the legal liability that may exist for others involved in the same incident—takes on a different perspective when considered in an office setting where the surgeon is the determinant of both the surgical risk and the risk associated with ownership and management of the facility and equipment. In some cases the surgeon may have limited or minimal coverage, exposing the anesthesiologist.

Table 10-3   Office-Based Anesthesia Outcome Indicators (Recommended by the ASA Committee on Ambulatory Surgical Care and Task Force on Office-Based Anesthesia, 2003)

Follow-up on postoperative day 1 and day 14

Cancellation rates and reasons

Central nervous system or peripheral nervous system new deficit

Need for reversal agents (e.g., naloxone, flumazenil)

Reintubation

Unplanned transfusion

Aspiration pneumonitis

Pulmonary embolus

Local anesthetic toxicity

Anaphylaxis

Possible malignant hyperthermia

Infection

Return to operating room

Unplanned postprocedural treatment in physician's office or emergency department within 30 days after discharge

Unplanned admission to hospital or acute-care facility within 30 days

Cardiopulmonary arrest or death within 30 days

Continuous quality indicators

Cardiovascular complications in recovery requiring treatment (including: arrhythmias, hypotension, hypertension)

Respiratory complications in recovery requiring treatment (including asthma)

Nausea not controlled within 2 hr in recovery

Pain not controlled within 2 hr in recovery

Postoperative vomiting rate

Prolonged postanesthesia care unit stay (> 2 hr)

Medication error

Injuries, e.g., to eye, teeth

Time to return to light activities of daily living (ADL)

Common postoperative sequelae, e.g., sore throat, muscle pain, headache

Postdural puncture headache or transient radicular irritation

Discharge without escort or against medical advice (AMA)

Patient satisfaction

Equipment maintenance

Facility quality improvement reviews should be conducted annually. A group that includes, at a minimum, the medical director, a representative of the anesthesiologists currently providing patient care, and a representative of the operating room or recovery nursing staff should perform the reviews.

Insurers may or may not consider entity coverage of the office-based site, covering surgeon, anesthesiologist, and facility in a single policy.

FACILITY SAFETY

While state regulatory control is increasing, in the majority of office-based practices there will be no specific state regulatory authority; only general health, fire, and safety provisions will therefore apply. Ultimately, enforcement of any safety codes is up to the local, state, or federal authorities having jurisdiction.

Fire Safety

Both patient and anesthesiologist assume greater challenges with office-based anesthesia in a facility that does not meet the standards described in the National Fire Protection Association (NFPA) 99 Health Care Facilities document. The guidelines of some surgical organizations speak to the use of ether and other flammable compounds for skin preparation; however, these are best avoided to eliminate noxious fumes and the risk of fires and explosions. Office-based anesthesia often involves plastic surgery of the head and neck with the use of electrocautery. The use of supplemental oxygen during these procedures increases the risk of fire.

Medical Gases

The NFPA has described gas supplies at health care facilities as Level 1, 2, or 3. Level 1 is where patients are dependent on mechanical ventilation; Level 2 signifies that the medical, surgical, or diagnostic intervention is dependent on the piped system; and Level 3 is where patients are not on critical life support equipment. NFPA standards are not required in the office setting unless accrediting organizations indicate this. The Level 1 standard is the most comprehensive and one that most anesthesiologists are familiar with from the hospital setting. If one seeks accreditation conforming to NFPA 99 regulations, then facilities conducting procedures on intubated patients on a ventilator will need to meet Level 1 requirements, whereas monitored anesthesia care procedures may only require a Level 2. In an office-based anesthesia practice, the anesthesiologist should evaluate the gas system to see if it is adequate for clinical needs and patient safety in that office.

Options for anesthesia waste gas disposal are limited. Halogenated hydrocarbons or ethers and nitrous oxide are the primary anesthetic concerns for operating-suite air pollution. Hospital or ambulatory surgery facilities make use of either "active" waste gas scavenging (with a piped vacuum system) or a "passive" system (with waste gases directed into the facility ventilation exhaust system). An office may utilize these standard methods or could opt for other methods to use. An exhaust hose may be run to an outside window; however, due care should be taken to ensure that the flow of waste gas does not reenter that, or any other, living space. Another option is adsorption of hydrocarbons or ethers by activated charcoal. If this method is used, the manufacturer's instructions concerning system capacity and replacement should be followed. This method is not effective for nitrous oxide. Obviously, a total intravenous technique eliminates the need for such systems. For an in-depth description of the Occupational Safety and Health Administration's (OSHA) advisory guidelines for anesthetic gas exposure, see http://www.osha-slc.gov/dts/osta/anestheticgases/index.htmlanestheticgases/index.html.

Information and regulations that address the transportation of compressed or liquefied gases come primarily from the Compressed Gas Association (CGA) and the Department of Transportation (DOT), although local and state regulations may also apply. When gas cylinders are transported by motor vehicle, requirements of Title 49 of the Code of Federal Regulations (49 CFR: 171, 177) apply. In addition, the DOT regulates the driver and vehicle carrying the compressed gases (49 CFR: 390–397). Further information may be obtained from http://www.cganet.com/.

Electrical Power Failure

If the anesthetic is conducted in a typical medical arts or commercial building, there may be no source of backup electrical power. In such buildings, emergency lighting is only required to allow a safe and orderly exit from the building.

In a JCAHO-approved acute-care hospital, the essential electrical distribution system must be a Type 1 electrical system that has both an emergency component (lighting and communications, etc.) and a critical component (bedside power to ORs and intensive-care units, etc.). Electrical service is assured through the use of an emergency generator or alternate source of power. In the simplest essential electrical system installation allowed by NFPA (Type 3), the system is capable of supplying only a limited amount of power necessary for life safety and the orderly termination of a procedure during a time that normal electrical service is interrupted. The emergency system must have an alternate source of power separate and independent from the normal source that failed. The alternate source must be effective for a minimum of 1.5 hr.

All equipment needs to be maintained, tested, and inspected according to the manufacturer's specifications. Electrical shock hazard is a concern. The office-based site will not likely be provided with isolated power supplies and therefore will not have line isolation monitors. At best, one may find ground fault circuit interrupters (GFCIs). If the GFCI is triggered by an errant current, all current flow will cease until the fault is corrected and the device is reset.

Infection Control

Poor infection control poses a risk of wound infection to patients and possible cross-contamination between patients. The infection rate should be reviewed on a regular basis. The facility must have an area for cleaning, high-level disinfection or sterilization of surgical equipment and supplies, with appropriate quality control procedures/indicators. A procedure for cleaning and disinfecting procedure rooms must be in place as well as procedures to document training or qualifications of personnel in aseptic technique. Protective clothing, appropriate to the procedure, must be worn by health professionals when surgery is in progress.

Occupational Safety

Office surgical procedures pose risk to personnel (and patients) due to exposure to hazardous/infectious body fluids and/or hazardous materials.

Suggested Practices or Options

- The facility must comply with OSHA Standard 1910.1450 to protect patients and personnel from toxic exposure.
- Policies and procedures must exist to address chemical spills when hazardous chemicals are in use (e.g., formaldehyde, mercury).
- The facility must comply with OSHA Standard 1910.1030 to protect patients and personnel from exposure to biohazardous waste.
- Universal precautions shall be instituted and observed.
- Policies and procedures must exist for handling biohazardous waste (sharp and nonsharp, including containers, labels, transport, and disposal).
- Policies and procedures must exist for management of employee exposure to biohazardous fluids (e.g., needle stick).
- Hepatitis B vaccination must be offered to personnel at employer's expense.

CONTROLLED MEDICATIONS

States may have varying rules and requirements regarding controlled medication. Schedule II, III, IV, and V medications are commonly used in the course of providing sedation, analgesia, and anesthesia. Policies and procedures are required to comply with laws and regulations pertaining to controlled drug supply, storage, and administration. In addition, all medications used in anesthesia care need to be controlled, and regular inspection of the medication supply ensures safe and effective administration to patients. There are separate Federal Drug Enforcement Administration (DEA) registration certificates for manufacturing, distributing, dispensing, and administering controlled medications. A separate state-controlled drug registration may be required.

Suggested Practices or Options

The use of any medication in the office setting must be under the direction of state-licensed medical providers. These individuals should assume professional, organizational, and administrative responsibility for the use of prescriptive medications. It should be clear in the office policies and procedures who is responsible for various medications and how issues such as drug outdating or recall are handled.

Drug Supply

An individual working in the office setting may supply the controlled drugs used for anesthesia care or may use the supply provided by the surgeon's office. If there are multiple office locations where controlled medications may be administered/dispensed, a separate registration number is needed for each one.

These "dispensing entities" must obtain controlled drugs from a medication supplier using DEA form 222 (the DEA Schedule I and II Drug order form). Occasionally, a pharmacy may dispense controlled medications to individual physicians to administer, using a 222 order form.

Drug Inventory

For a physician or office acting as a "dispenser" of controlled drugs, an inventory must be taken on the date of DEA registration and every 2 years thereafter.

Records that account for the use and wastage of all controlled medications on each patient for each date must be maintained. DEA regulations should always be followed. Records must be kept for at least 2 years (some states require longer time periods) and are subject to DEA inspection. The recording method and any backup media should be specified.

Drug Security

Controlled drugs must be kept in a locked cabinet or safe. Any loss or theft of drugs or of a DEA order form must be reported to the regional DEA office. If controlled drugs are transported to the office site, security is essential to protect the drug supply, protect the public from lost or stolen medications, and protect the anesthesiologist from physical harm during attempted theft. For this reason, it may be easier to have the office location order and stock controlled drugs. Other noncontrolled medications should be kept in designated locations and, when patients are not being anesthetized, maintained in a secure or locked place, away from potential tampering or theft. Other medications, although not on the DEA schedule list, can be abused. These include sympathomimetic stimulants and any of the potent anesthesia vapors or nitrous oxide. Sufficient safety precautions must be taken to prevent accidental or intentional misuse.

SUMMARY

An increasing number of surgical procedures are being performed in the physician's office and it is estimated that by the year 2005, one-quarter of all ambulatory procedures will be performed in a doctor's office. The challenge for the medical profession is to bring the same standard of care existing in ASCs and hospitals into the office surgical suite. The physician must often assume oversight and responsibility for areas that would be taken for granted in the hospital or ambulatory surgical facility. This includes ensuring compliance with federal and state regulations. It also includes oversight of facility construction, medications, supplies, equipment, personnel, and policies and procedures. Obtaining accreditation by one of the nationally recognized accrediting bodies can assist in many of these areas. The practitioner must have a thorough understanding to ensure compliance with the requirements of the accrediting and regulatory bodies.

REFERENCES

1. American Society of Anesthesiologists. *Office-Based Anesthesia—Considerations for Anesthesiologists in Setting Up and Maintaining a Safe Office-Anesthesia Environment.* May 10, 2002: http://asaha.org .publicationsAndServices/office.pdf.

2. Rohrich RJ, White PF. Safety of outpatient surgery: is mandatory accreditation of outpatient surgery centers enough? Plast Reconstr Surg 2001;107(1):189–92.

3. MSSNY Survey on Office-Based Surgery and Invasive Procedures. New York State Public Health Council Committee on Quality Assurance in Office-Based Surgery, October 1998.

4. Cosmetic surgery: the hidden dangers. Fort Lauderdale Sun-Sentinel, November 26, 2000.

5. Quattrone MS. Is the physician office the wild, wild west of health care? J Ambul Care Manag 2000;23:64–73.

6. Vila H, Soto R, Cantor AB, Mackey D. Comparative outcomes analysis of procedures performed in physician offices and ambulatory surgery centers. Arch Surg 2003;138:991–95.

7. Grazer FM, de Jong RH. Fatal outcomes from liposuction: census survey of cosmetic surgeons. Plast Reconstr Surg 2000;44:193–98.

8. Morello DC, Colon GA, Fredricks S, Iverson RE, Singer R. Patient safety in accredited office surgical facilities. Plast Reconstr Surg 1997;99:1496–99.

9. Hoefflin SM, Bornstein JB, Gordon M. General anesthesia in an office-based plastic surgical facility: a report on more than 23,000 consecutive office-based procedures under general anesthesia with no significant anesthetic complications. Plast Reconstr Surg 2001;107(1):243–57.

10. American Society of Plastic Surgeons and American Society for Aesthetic Plastic Surgery. Policy statement on accreditation of office facilites. American Society of Plastic Surgeons Web site, http://www .plasticsurgery.org/psf/psfhome/govern/officepol.cfm.

11. Iverson RE. ASPS Task Force on Patient Safety in Office-Based Surgery Facilities: I. Procedures in the office-based surgery setting. Plast Reconstr Surg 2002;110(5):1337–42.

12. Report of the Special Committee on Outpatient (Office-based) Surgery. Federation of State Medical Boards of the United States, Inc. Med. Licensure Discipline 2002;88:160–74.

13. Guidelines for Office-Based Anesthesia. *American Society of Anesthesiologists—Standards, Guidelines and Statements*, October 27, 2003.

APPENDIX 10-1. AMA OFFICE-BASED SURGERY CORE PRINCIPLES 2003 BOARD OF TRUSTEES REPORT 23-A-03 (WWW.AMA-ASSA.ORG)

Principles apply to office-based facilities where moderate or deep sedation/analgesia and/or general anesthesia are administered.

1. States should develop guidelines or regulations based on levels of anesthesia as defined by the ASA.
2. Patient selection should be made using the ASA Physical Status Classification system.
3. Facilities should be accredited, state licensed or Medicare certified.
4. Physicians must have:

   • Admitting privileges at nearby hospital, *or*
   • Transfer agreement with another physician who has admitting privileges, *or*
   • An emergency transfer agreement with a nearby hospital

5. States should follow the Federation of State Medical Board recommendations regarding informed consent.
6. States should consider legally privileged adverse incident reporting, and peer-review and continuous quality improvement programs.
7. Physicians must be:

   • Board certified by a board recognized by the ABMS or AOS
   • Procedures performed must generally be recognized by the certifying board as falling within its scope of training and practice.

8. Physicians may show competency by maintaining core privileges at an accredited or licensed hospital or ASC for the procedures they perform in the office-based surgery facility.

   The governing body is responsible for the peer review process and for a privileging process that is based on nationally recognized credentialing standards.
9. At least one physician present in the office-based surgery facility must be currently trained in advanced resuscitative techniques (advanced trauma life support [ATLS], ACLS, pediatric advanced life support [PALS]).

   Other staff with direct patient contact must be trained in BLS.

   Age appropriate resuscitative equipment must be available.
10. Physicians administering or supervising anesthesia should have appropriate education and training.

APPENDIX 10-2. ASA GUIDELINES FOR OFFICE-BASED ANESTHESIA APPROVED BY THE HOUSE OF DELEGATES, OCTOBER 13, 1999 (WWW.ASAHQ.ORG)

These guidelines are intended to assist ASA members who are considering the practice of ambulatory anesthesia in the office setting: office-based anesthesia (OBA). These recommendations focus on quality anesthesia care and patient safety in the office. These are minimal guidelines and may be exceeded at any time based on the judgment of the involved anesthesia personnel. Compliance with these guidelines cannot guarantee any specific outcome. These guidelines are subject to periodic revision as warranted by the evolution of federal, state and local laws as well as technology and practice.

ASA recognizes the unique needs of this growing practice and the increased requests for ASA members to provide OBA for health care practitioners* who have developed their own office operatories. Since OBA is a subset of ambulatory anesthesia, the ASA "Guidelines for Ambulatory Anesthesia and Surgery" should be followed in the office setting as well as all other ASA standards and guidelines that are applicable.

There are special problems that ASA members must recognize when administering anesthesia in the office setting. Compared with acute care hospitals and licensed ambulatory surgical facilities, office operatories currently have little or no regulation, oversight or control by federal, state or local laws. Therefore, ASA members must satisfactorily investigate areas taken for granted in the hospital or ambulatory surgical facility such as governance, organization, construction and equipment, as well as policies and procedures, including fire, safety, drugs, emergencies, staffing, training and unanticipated patient transfers.

ASA members should be confident that the following issues are addressed in an office setting to provide patient safety and to reduce risk and liability to the anesthesiologist.

Administration and Facility

Quality of Care

• The facility should have a medical director or governing body that establishes policy and is responsible for the activities of the facility and its staff. The medical director or governing body is responsible for ensuring that facilities and personnel are adequate and appropriate for the type of procedures performed.
• Policies and procedures should be written for the orderly conduct of the facility and reviewed on an annual basis.
• The medical director or governing body should ensure that all applicable local, state and federal regulations are observed.
• All health care practitioners and nurses should hold a valid license or certificate to perform their assigned duties.

*Defined herein as physicians, dentists and podiatrists.

- All OR personnel who provide clinical care in the office should be qualified to perform services commensurate with appropriate levels of education, training and experience.
- The anesthesiologist should participate in ongoing continuous quality improvement and risk management activities.
- The medical director or governing body should recognize the basic human rights of its patients, and a written document that describes this policy should be available for patients to review.

Facility and Safety

- Facilities should comply with all applicable federal, state and local laws, codes and regulations pertaining to fire prevention, building construction and occupancy, accommodations for the disabled, occupational safety and health, and disposal of medical waste and hazardous waste.
- Policies and procedures should comply with laws and regulations pertaining to controlled drug supply, storage and administration.

Clinical Care

Patient and Procedure Selection

- The anesthesiologist should be satisfied that the procedure to be undertaken is within the scope of practice of the health care practitioners and the capabilities of the facility.
- The procedure should be of a duration and degree of complexity that will permit the patient to recover and be discharged from the facility.
- Patients who by reason of pre-existing medical or other conditions may be at undue risk for complications should be referred to an appropriate facility for performance of the procedure and the administration of anesthesia.

Perioperative Care

- The anesthesiologist should adhere to the "Basic Standards for Preanesthesia Care," "Standards for Basic Anesthetic Monitoring," "Standards for Postanesthesia Care" and "Guidelines for Ambulatory Anesthesia and Surgery" as currently promulgated by the ASA.
- The anesthesiologist should be physically present during the intraoperative period and immediately available

until the patient has been discharged from anesthesia care.
- Discharge of the patient is a physician responsibility. This decision should be documented in the medical record.
- Personnel with training in advanced resuscitative techniques (e.g., ACLS, PALS) should be immediately available until all patients are discharged home.

Monitoring and Equipment

- At a minimum, all facilities should have a reliable source of oxygen, suction, resuscitation equipment and emergency drugs. Specific reference is made to the ASA "Guidelines for Nonoperating Room Anesthetizing Locations."
- There should be sufficient space to accommodate all necessary equipment and personnel and to allow for expeditious access to the patient, anesthesia machine (when present) and all monitoring equipment.
- All equipment should be maintained, tested and inspected according to the manufacturer's specifications.
- Back-up power sufficient to ensure patient protection in the event of an emergency should be available.
- In any location in which anesthesia is administered, there should be appropriate anesthesia apparatus and equipment which allow monitoring consistent with ASA "Standards for Basic Anesthetic Monitoring" and documentation of regular preventive maintenance as recommended by the manufacturer.
- In an office where anesthesia services are to be provided to infants and children, the required equipment, medication and resuscitative capabilities should be appropriately sized for a pediatric population.

Emergencies and Transfers

- All facility personnel should be appropriately trained in and regularly review the facility's written emergency protocols.
- There should be written protocols for cardiopulmonary emergencies and other internal and external disasters such as fire.
- The facility should have medications, equipment and written protocols available to treat malignant hyperthermia when triggering agents are used.
- The facility should have a written protocol in place for the safe and timely transfer of patients to a prespecified alternate care facility when extended or emergency services are needed to protect the health or well-being of the patient.

Quality Improvement in Ambulatory Anesthesia

TERRANCE W. BREEN

INTRODUCTION

Health care delivery is undergoing a revolution. Patients and purchasers are better informed and want better value, leading health care organizations to reevaluate how they provide and evaluate services. These demands will only increase with time, leading to a need for continuous quality improvement. This chapter will give a brief review of quality and quality improvement and will then focus on new methods and the new agenda for the twenty-first century.

The American National Standards Institute (ANSI) and the American Society for Quality (ASQ) define quality as "the totality of features and characteristics of a product or service that bears on its ability to satisfy given needs." This definition is comprehensive but lacks easy interpretation and application to health care. A modern, more easily understood and applied definition of quality is "meeting or exceeding customer expectations." An important property of quality is that it can be measured and compared; that is, quality is a *relative* term. Quality of anesthesia care can be examined from many points of view, including those of patients, surgeons, nurses, administrators, and financial concerns.[1] This chapter will focus primarily on the point of view of patients where quality anesthesia care provides or exceeds patient's expressed and implied requirements.

Companies have long recognized the importance of both perceived and real quality. Quality assurance (QA) developed as a method to ensure quality and hence improve market share, reputation, or profit. The fundamental concept behind QA was, and still is, to identify variability in the quality of work or product produced and to "improve" quality to a uniformly excellent level. While this idea sounds logical and reasonable, it does not take into account human nature. The practical application of QA to the workplace has often been to identify and eliminate "poor quality" (workers or products) assuming that overall quality would then be improved. Frontline workers have long understood this agenda and recognized the advantage of maintaining uniform (perhaps low) standards with quality that is easily met by all. Consequently, signif-icant peer pressure and inertia retard innovation or raising quality, and the QA approach to optimizing and improving quality is often unsuccessful.[2]

THE MODEL OF IMPROVEMENT

W. Edwards Deming was one of the first to study and try to improve quality.[3] His deliberations led him to develop a method of quality improvement termed the "system of profound knowledge." This system is divided into four parts: (1) appreciation of a system, (2) understanding variation, (3) theory of knowledge, and (4) psychology. Deming recognized that services or products (e.g., health care delivery) involve complex interactions between people, processes, and equipment. Understanding each of these and their interactions is critical to improving products or services. The path to improved quality involves change, but not all change will result in improved quality. Thus, quality must be measured to determine whether change represents improvement. Variation is an inherent property in all processes and measurements. Outcomes of interest must be tracked over time to see whether changes introduced alter quality and whether or not changes are sustained (or if apparent changes simply represent random variation). Individuals or organizations trying to make system or outcome improvements need knowledge of problems, solutions, barriers to implementation, and measurement tools. Improvement is gained by making changes, studying their effect, learning from the result, and making more changes. Knowledge of psychology, including individual motivations and learning styles, and how to change behavior, is also critical to successful change.

The work of Deming and many others has led to development of a technique termed the "model of improvement."[4] This approach involves asking:

- What are we trying to accomplish?
- How will we know that a change is an improvement?
- What changes can we make that will result in improvement?

Organizations need to address the first question in order to answer the myriad of questions that follow. In particular, quality aims must be differentiated from mission statements. An outpatient surgery center might have a mission statement to "be the best outpatient surgery center in the state." However, what does "be the best" mean? Is the aim to be the safest, most profitable, provide the highest patient satisfaction, or some other metric? It is useful to involve many members of the organization in determining which questions to ask; however, health care is becoming increasingly patient-centered. Therefore, the focus of quality should be based on *patient issues* and *patient data*. With the rapid changes in society and health care delivery, organizational aims should be reassessed on a regular basis, probably at least once every 18–24 months.

Once an organization has clear aims, it must develop metrics to assess how well the aims are being met. Good organizations will identify areas for improvement. Leadership must consider the possible positive and negative consequences of change and ensure that metrics assess both. More than one metric is needed to assess the impact of many changes. However, the number of metrics must not be excessive or the measurement will become the central theme, not the change. Metrics of interest should be determined on a regular, but intermittent, basis. If a change is to be introduced, more frequent measurement should be applied. If a change leads to a quality improvement, periodic measurement should continue to ensure that the improvement is sustained. If quality does not change or worsens, then a different change is needed and more measurement is required.

Identification of opportunities to improve process or outcomes should be a collaborative process. Organizational leadership and frontline staff should work together ("brainstorm") to identify possible improvements. Visionary organizations involve customers (patients) in the "brainstorming" sessions and try to look at system redesign to improve processes (i.e., thinking "outside the box").[5] It is normal human tendency to try to fix a problem by throwing more resources (time, money, or people) at the problem. However, most organizations need to make improvements within the framework of existing or even fewer resources. After identification of ideas for possible change, leadership must choose one or more strategies to implement. Ideas with consensus support may be more easily implemented but are not always the best ideas. Regardless of the level of support, change must be implemented, the effects measured, and the results shared so that all can learn and continue to improve.

This process is summarized as the plan-do-study-act or PDSA cycle (Fig. 11-1).

- *Plan* a change. A change may be modifying the current practice or redesigning it completely.
- *Do* the change in a trial or on a small group. It is almost always better to initially implement changes in small groups rather than throughout an organization. If data from a small group show the benefit of a change, that information is a powerful tool to support the change on

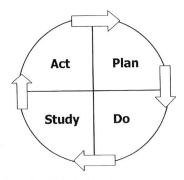

Figure 11-1   The plan-do-study-act cycle.

a larger scale. Conversely, changes that do not work should not be spread throughout the organization.

- *Study* the results of the change. Does the new process result in improvement or less random variation than the previous process?
- *Act* on the finding. Implement the change more widely in the organization, modify it, or discard it. Repeat the PDSA cycle and implement more change.

The combination of the three framing questions and the PDSA cycle are the basis of the *model for improvement* (Fig. 11-2).

STATISTICAL PROCESS CONTROL

The statistical techniques to assess the effect of outcome change over time are different from those used in most basic science or clinical anesthesia research. In general, research studies compare one or more aspect(s) of different groups to determine whether or not there are differences between the groups. In contrast, quality measures seek to show if an intervention has produced a change, if the change is in the desired direction, and if the change is sustained. The approach to analyzing this kind of problem and data is called statistical process control (SPC) and includes

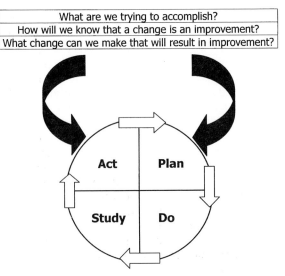

Figure 11-2   Model for improvement.

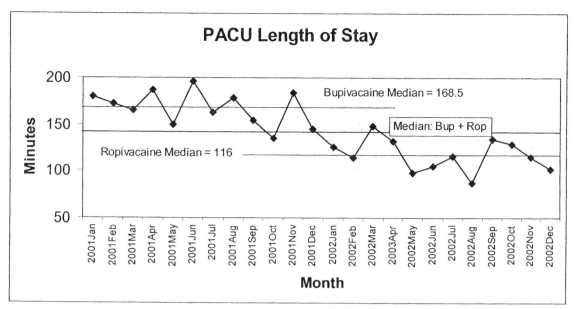

Figure 11-3   PACU length of stay after spinal anesthesia: Bupivacaine in 2001 and ropivacaine in 2002.

control charts (Shewhart charts), run charts, frequency plots, histograms, Pareto analysis, scatter diagrams, and flow diagrams. Refer to Raymond Carey's *Improving Healthcare with Control Charts* (or similar texts) for more information about SPC methods and their analysis, including how to determine when a change is significant.[6] The following example will illustrate a basic SPC technique.

Anesthesia providers in an outpatient surgery facility used bupivacaine for spinal anesthesia. They constructed a *run chart* plotting average postanesthesia care unit (PACU) length of stay (LOS) by month for 2001 (Fig. 11-3). The *median* PACU LOS was 168.5 min and appeared stable, with some values above the median and some below (range 135–196 min). This variation around the median is termed *common cause variation*. The anesthesia providers wanted to decrease the PACU LOS and replaced spinal bupivacaine with spinal ropivacaine. They plotted the 2002 PACU LOS on the same run chart and found that PACU LOS after spinal ropivacaine also exhibited common cause variation and had a median value of 116 min (range 87–148 min).

Further study revealed that the overall median PACU LOS was 140 min with almost all the spinal bupivacaine values greater than 140 min and almost all the spinal ropivacaine values less than 140 min. The change from spinal bupivacaine to ropivacaine represented *special-cause variation* and was a significant change. You might be asking yourself, "Couldn't the anesthesia group have used standard parametric statistics and reached the same conclusion?" In this example, standard parametric statistics would have reached the same conclusion, although the run chart approach would have more rapidly demonstrated a statistically significant change. Another example will illustrate how control charts can be helpful where standard statistical techniques fail.

The same anesthesia group looked at their regional block failure rate in 2001 and found an *average* (not median) failure rate of 5%. At the beginning of 2002 they took a weekend regional anesthesia course to improve their block techniques. By the end of 2002 their block failure rate was down to an average of 4% as shown in the histogram (Fig. 11-4). Did an improvement really occur that reduced the block failure rate by 20%? When the data were plotted as a run chart over 24 months, the *median* value was a block failure rate of 4.5% (Fig. 11-5). Neither the 2001 nor 2002 data exhibited common-cause variation; in fact, the data show *special-cause* variation. The regional block failure rate improved from 8% to 2% in 2001 and worsened from 2% to 6% in 2002! Examination of the histogram and parametric statistics might have erroneously led the practitioners to believe they had improved their care when in fact they had not. The anesthesia group needs to explain the data. Did the weekend regional anesthesia course lead the group to the use of an inferior block technique? Are group members still learning the block technique? Can the data be explained by new group members who joined in March and July? Did the surgeons change their surgical techniques such that the blocks were no longer effective and different block techniques are required? Were their any other changes in the system? After considering these questions, more "drilling down" into the data might be needed. Then, another PDSA cycle will be needed to return to the 2% block failure rate (or even lower).

Where Can a PDSA Cycle Be Applied?

Options for quality improvement may be found in the elements of structure, process, and outcome.[7] Structure refers to the physical plant, equipment used, personnel, administration, and organization. Process involves the interaction of the patient with the system, including what the patient does to affect his/her health and what the system does to affect the patient's health. Process refers to what is done and how it is done. Flowcharts can be help-

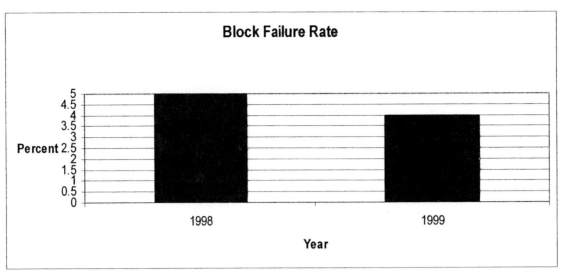

Figure 11-4   Regional anesthesia block failure rate: By year.

ful in understanding process elements and their linkage. Outcome refers to the effect of the treatment(s) on the patient and population(s). Each of these steps can, and should, be examined to look for ways to improve quality. Many changes occur only when a local champion takes charge and acts as a *change agent*. Change agents must be continuously aware of the quality measurement trap— *there is no inherent direct relationship between improved structure and process and improved outcomes*. In addition to measuring elements of process after a change, organizations must measure their real and important outcome(s) to see if they have, or have not, achieved their aim. Analogous to clinical research, quality improvement efforts are shifting to measurement of "meaningful" outcomes.[8–10] Future health care delivery should be based on this kind of information.

What Is Quality in Health Care?

In 2000, the Institute of Medicine (IOM) released a report titled *To Err Is Human: Building a Safer Health System*.[11]

This widely reported dramatic publication estimated that medical errors in hospitals were the cause of up to 98,000 deaths per year, more than motor vehicle accidents, breast cancer, or AIDS. The IOM proclaimed that medical error constituted a crisis in health care requiring urgent attention. Importantly, the IOM recognized that problems occur not because of bad people providing care, but rather good people providing care in systems that need to be improved. The IOM report brought patient safety to the forefront of quality initiatives. A follow-up report, *Crossing the Quality Chasm: A New Health System for the 21st Century*, listed aims to direct future quality care measures and initiatives of importance to the health of the population (Table 11-1).[12] Health care should be patient-centered, safe, effective, timely, efficient, and equitable.

The Institute for Healthcare Improvement (IHI), founded and led by Dr. Donald Berwick, is a driving force for health care improvement in the United States and throughout the world (www.ihi.org). At the fifteenth Annual National Forum, Dr. Berwick made an eloquent, yet readily identifiable plea for improvement on a personal level, entitled "My Right Knee." Dr. Berwick outlined his

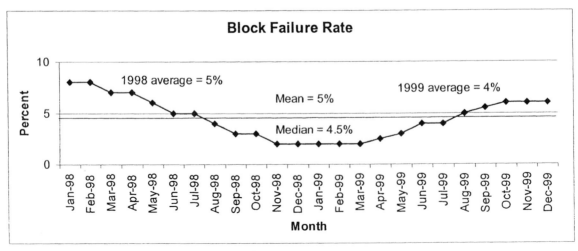

Figure 11-5   Regional anesthesia block failure rate: By month.

Table 11-1 Crossing the Quality Chasm: Aims for the Twenty-First Century

Health care that is	
Patient-centered:	providing care that is respectful of, and responsive to, individual patient preferences, needs, and values and ensuring that patient values guide all clinical decisions
Safe:	avoids injuries to patients from care that is intended to help them
Effective:	provides services based on scientific knowledge to all who could benefit and refrains from providing services to those not likely to benefit
Timely:	reducing waits and sometimes harmful delays for both those who receive and those who give care
Efficient:	avoiding waste, including waste of equipment, supplies, ideas, and energy
Equitable:	providing care that does not vary in quality because of personal characteristics such as gender, ethnicity, geographic location, and socioeconomic status

requirements for a pending total knee replacement and he challenged the audience to deliver the care he will need to meet his (patient-centered) specifications. Dr. Berwick framed his issues as a request for proposals (RFP) as outlined below:

1. Don't kill me
2. Don't hurt me
   a. Don't do things that cannot help me
   b. Reliably do things that can help me
   c. Relieve my pain
      i. Physical pain
      ii. Emotional pain
3. Don't make me feel helpless
   a. Share information
   b. Give me choices
   c. Follow my orders
   d. Remember me
4. Don't make me wait
   a. Manage access
   b. Manage flow
   c. Keep track of things
5. Don't waste money

The IOM and IHI goals apply to anesthesia as well as to other parts of the health care system. The practice of anesthesia needs to become more patient-focused. We need to know what patients want and expect, and we need to better deliver those services. Macario and colleagues identified patient concerns (from most important to least important) as postoperative vomiting, gagging on the endotracheal tube, pain, nausea, and intraoperative recall.[13] Royston and Cox reviewed the literature and presented a similar, but slightly different view.[14] They noted that patients often consider anesthesia as the intervention with the highest risk (not the operation or procedure itself). Many patients worry they will die or suffer neurologic injury during anesthesia (persistent vegetative state, paralysis, nerve injury, or postoperative cognitive dysfunction). Other concerns include awareness during anesthesia, postoperative pain, and postoperative nausea and vomiting (PONV). Each health care organization should develop a patient-centered approach to address these concerns, to provide state-of-the-art care to minimize adverse effects, and to implement strategies to improve care.

Anesthesia allows surgery to be performed without pain, suffering, or awareness; women to deliver babies without experiencing long painful labor; and acute and chronic painful conditions to be treated. Anesthesia exposes patients to risk generally without intrinsic health benefit. Therefore, minimizing risk and maximizing safety are important priorities of anesthesiologists.

Improving safety in anesthesia has long focused on identifying errors and decreasing their frequency. Cooper et al. interviewed volunteer faculty and residents to identify critical incidents that could have led (if not discovered and corrected) or did lead to undesirable outcomes (increased length of hospital stay, permanent disability, death).[15–17] Most of the preventable incidents (82%) involved human error and only 14% involved equipment failure. Suboptimal equipment design, inadequate anesthesia experience, and insufficient familiarity with anesthesia equipment or surgical procedure also contributed to errors. The most common human errors involved the ventilation/breathing circuit, drug administration and labeling errors, anesthesia machine use, and airway management. Equipment failures most commonly involved monitors, the breathing circuit, and airway components. Although many anesthesiologists believe that the highest risk of anesthesia complications is at induction and emergence, errors were most likely during the middle of the surgical procedure. Vigilance throughout anesthesia is essential. Numerous other studies from throughout the world have demonstrated similar findings.[18]

Interest in patient safety led to the formation of the Anesthesia Patient Safety Foundation in the United States (www.apsf.org). This organization promotes anesthesia patient safety and funds research related to patient safety. Similar organizations exist in other countries, including the Australian Patient Safety Foundation. The Australian Incident Monitoring Study was founded to look at anesthesia critical events and errors, to create a database, and to learn how to potentially improve care.[19,20] The American Society of Anesthesiologists (ASA) began a process looking at closed malpractice claims, extracting data from the files, and entering it into a database.[21] Information from these databases has proved useful in alerting practitioners of potentially troublesome or dangerous situations and has helped drive a research agenda through hypothesis generation. Indeed, anesthesiology is a leading field in improving patient safety.[22]

A crude, but commonly used index of patient safety is mortality. Two studies published in 2002 challenge the notion that modern anesthesia is safer than in past decades.[23,24] Certainly, data collection and availability are better today, but has anesthesia-related mortality decreased? Anesthesia mortality may be a low as 1:200,000 in healthy ASA I patients, but may be much higher in patients with higher ASA physical status scores. Indeed, overall anesthesia mortality may not be dramatically different now from decades ago, at least in part because patients once considered unfit for surgery now routinely undergo procedures. Many changes to equipment have occurred since Cooper et al. began their research, but data showing improved patient safety from equipment and monitoring advances have been hard to obtain. A large (20,802 patients) randomized study looked at the effect of pulse oximetry to detect and manage perioperative hypoxemia.[25] The investigators found that when patients were monitored with pulse oximeters, oxygen desaturation was detected much more commonly. However, even with this large sample size, pulse oximetry did not affect the overall rate of postoperative complications. Consistent with Cooper's original findings, improved anesthesia care will involve decreasing human error through equipment and process design changes.

The subject of human error and approaches to decreasing error was well reviewed in the *British Medical Journal*.[26–34] There are two general approaches to human error, the person approach and the system approach. The person approach—identifying individuals and blaming them for error—is prominent in medicine and this culture continues to impede real improvements. The system approach involves acceptance that humans are fallible and that errors will occur—*indeed errors are learning opportunities!* A system interpretation to error is that structure and process produce exactly whatever they were designed to produce—including error and bad outcomes. The way to improve outcomes is to change the system! Human error is termed *active failure* or error occurring at the *"sharp end"* of the system. *Latent conditions* or *"blunt end"* problems are part of systems or processes that can lead to error, particularly when safety mechanisms fail. System factors both contribute to and mitigate against the effects of error. The combination of variability, latent conditions, and human error converge to produce adverse consequences. We must apply ourselves to improve system design in order to reduce harm.[35,36] Several industries have implemented systems changes and have very low error rates. Examples of these high-reliability organizations (HROs) are the commercial airline and nuclear power industries. In addition to identifying latent conditions, HROs embrace crisis resource management techniques and teamwork to identify and solve problems. The systems approach to improving safety is advocated by the IOM and IHI and is the method most likely to reduce error and improve care. Organizations must make identification of latent conditions a priority, preferably before errors occur. In addition, leadership must invest in people and techniques for health care to become an HRO.[26]

The Agency for Healthcare Research and Quality (AHRQ) (www.ahcpr.gov) is an excellent resource for information about quality practice. They recently released an extensive review of practices and used an evidence-based weighting scheme to identify targets for improvement best supported by evidence.[37,38] A number of issues identified are applicable to patients undergoing surgery. One item directly related to anesthesia care is morbidity from central line insertion. The majority of areas for improvement involve personnel from anesthesia, surgery, nursing, and medicine, and include prevention of venous thromboembolism, perioperative cardiac events,[39–41] and infections. Teamwork throughout the organization will be required to obtain and document meaningful improvement.

Accreditation and regulatory agencies are increasingly involved in patient safety and improving health care. The Joint Commission of Accreditation of Healthcare Organizations (JCAHO) began requiring quality improvement data as part of the recredentialing process in 2001. Unfortunately, the JCAHO requires reporting of individual-specific data compared to an appropriate peer group. This is widely perceived as analogous to the person approach to error and in the opinion of this author, is a misguided approach to improving patient outcomes. The JCAHO publishes national safety goals each year (www.jcaho.org) and the 2004 goals are listed in Table 11-2. All of these goals are relevant to operating room (OR) settings and need to be addressed by anesthesia departments as well as organizations.

Patient-Centered Application of the PDSA Cycle

Evidence-based medicine is one example of the PDSA cycle. How might evidence-based medicine be applied to day-to-day anesthesia practice?[42] Understanding how to treat a problem begins with understanding the mechanism of the disease or process, development of therapeutic options, and clinical trials to demonstrate effectiveness. Often clinical trials lack necessary statistical power and are combined into meta-analyses or systematic reviews. Large studies (database studies or meta-analyses) may show (small) statistically significant differences, but they may not be clinically relevant or cost-effective. *The key missing element tends to be assessment of new or different therapies in everyday practice.* Most "advances" or new therapies come with increased cost. It is incumbent on practitioners and organizations to carefully evaluate new drugs and techniques, asking the following questions:

- Is the change a real improvement in day-to-day clinical practice?
- How significant is the improvement?
- What does the improvement cost?
- Can/should the change be adopted throughout the organization?
- What will be the cost of implementing the change across the organization?
- What will be the benefit to the overall organization?

Table 11-2   2004 JCAHO National Patient Safety Goals

1.	Improve the accuracy of patient identification	a) Use at least two patient identifiers whenever taking blood, administering medications or blood products
		b) Prior to the start of any surgical or invasive procedure, conduct a verification process, such as a "time-out," to confirm the correct patient, procedure, and site, using active— not passive—communication techniques
2.	Improve the effectiveness of communication among caregivers	a) Implement a process for taking verbal or telephone orders or critical test results that require a verification "read-back" of the complete order or test result by the person receiving the order or test result
		b) Standardize the abbreviations, acronyms, and symbols used throughout the organization, including a list of abbreviations, acronyms, and symbols *not* to use
3.	Improve the safety of high-alert medications	a) Remove concentrated electrolytes (including, but not limited to, potassium chloride, potassium phosphate, sodium chloride > 0.9%) from patient units
		b) Standardize and limit the number of drug concentrations available in the organization
4.	Eliminate wrong-site, wrong-patient, wrong-procedure surgery	a) Create and use a preoperative verification process, such as a checklist, to confirm that appropriate documents are available
		b) Implement a process to mark the surgical site and involve the patient in the marking process
5.	Improve the safety of using infusion pumps	a) Ensure free-flow protection on all general-use and patient-controlled analgesia (PCA) intravenous infusion pumps used in the organization
6.	Improve the effectiveness of clinical alarm systems	a) Implement regular preventative maintenance and testing of alarm systems
		b) Assure that alarms are activated with appropriate settings and are sufficiently audible with respect to distances and competing noise within the unit
7.	Reduce the risk of health care–acquired infections	a) Comply with current Centers for Disease Control and Prevention (CDC) hand hygiene guidelines
		b) Manage as sentinel events all identified cases of unanticipated death or major permanent loss of function associated with a health care–acquired infection

• Can unforeseen effects be anticipated and how will they be sought?

Recall the patient-centered problem of PONV. A vast amount of literature and study is devoted to PONV and will not be presented here in detail. The pathophysiology of PONV is at least partly understood.[14] Many reviews have been presented and suggestions made about how to prevent or treat PONV.[43,44] Strategies range from no prophylactic therapy to prevent PONV but rapid treatment of PONV in the PACU, to using risk stratification to guide treatment with no agent, one agent, or multiple PONV prevention agents.[45] The question of the ideal agent or agents to treat PONV remains under study as does whether the ideal treatment involves a "PONV" drug[46] or some other therapy such as oxygen.[47] In addition, the problems and treatment for postoperative nausea may be different from those of vomiting.[48] Each practitioner, group, department, or organization should address the questions, determine current practice, measure PONV, and implement a strategy to improve treatment.

The same approach can be used to evaluate treatment of postoperative pain, new technologies such as the bis-

pectral index (BIS) monitor, and numerous other questions in anesthesia. Are nonsteroidal anti-inflammatory agents being used appropriately?[49,50] Are regional anesthesia and analgesia being used to their fullest extent?[51–53] Are opioids given appropriately in the OR and in the PACU? Should the BIS monitor be used in everyday practice? Initial studies with the BIS monitor showed faster emergence from anesthesia and improved recovery,[54–56] including decreased postoperative vomiting.[57] Subsequent studies question whether or not BIS monitoring affects PACU recovery and LOS.[58,59] The challenge for readers of this chapter is to evaluate their practice, implement change, assess the impact of the change, and reevaluate, that is, to make the PDSA cycle part of everyday practice.

SUMMARY

Health care is not as safe or effective as many would like it to be. The challenge for all working in the health care field is to meet the goals of the IOM and IHI and to strive for continuous improvement.[60,61] Look for new ideas from research, other organizations, or other sources, and implement change. Use the PDSA model and implement change in small, clearly identified areas. Monitor the effect of the change over time.[62] If an improvement occurs, make the change more widespread.[63] If no improvement occurs or the outcome worsens, reverse the change or make another change. Organizations that adopt and apply quality improvement and that have buy-in at the highest levels are the organizations most likely to succeed in the twenty-first century.

REFERENCES

1. Eagle CJ, Davies JM. Current models of "quality"—an introduction for anaesthetists. Can J Anaesth 1993;40:851–62.

2. Berwick DM. Continuous improvement as an ideal in health care. N Engl J Med 1989;320:53–56.

3. Deming WE. *Out of the Crisis.* Cambridge, MA: Massachusetts Institute of Technology, 1986.

4. Langley GJ, Nolan KM, Nolan TW, Norman CL, Provost LP. *The Improvement Guide: A Practical Approach to Enhancing Organizational Performance.* San Francisco: Jossey-Bass, 1996.

5. Using patient input in a cycle for performance improvement. J Qual Improv 1995;21:87–96.

6. Carey RG. *Improving Healthcare with Control Charts: Basic and Advanced SPC Methods and Case Studies.* Milwaukee, WI: ASQ Quality Press, 2003.

7. Donabedian A. The quality of care: how can it be assessed? JAMA 1988;260:1743–48.

8. Orkin FK, Cohen MM, Duncan PG. The quest for meaningful outcomes. Anesthesiology 1993;78:417–22.

9. Fisher DM. Surrogate outcomes: meaningful not! Anesthesiology 1999;90:355–56.

10. Mangano DT. Adverse outcomes after surgery in the year 2001—a continuing odyssey. Anesthesiology 1998;88:561–64.

11. Kohn LT, Corrigan JM, Donaldson MS (eds.). *To Err Is Human: Building a Safer Health System.* Washington, DC: The National Academies Press, 2000.

12. Institute of Medicine. *Crossing the Quality Chasm: A New Health System for the 21st Century.* Washington, DC: The National Academies Press, 2001.

13. Macario A, Weinger M, Carney S, Kim A. Which clinical anesthesia outcomes are important to avoid? The perspective of patients. Anesth Analg 1999;89:652–58.

14. Royston D, Cox F. Anaesthesia: the patient's point of view. Lancet 2003;362:1648–58.

15. Cooper JB, Newbower RS, Long CD, McPeek B. Preventable anesthesia mishaps: a study of human factors. Anesthesiology 1978;49:399–406.

16. Cooper JB, Long CD, Newbower RS, Philip JH. Critical incidents associated with intraoperative exchanges of anesthesia personnel. Anesthesiology 1982;56:456–61.

17. Cooper JB, Newbower RS, Kitz RJ. An analysis of major errors and equipment failures in anesthesia management: considerations for prevention and detection. Anesthesiology 1984;60:34–42.

18. James RH. 1000 anaesthetic incidents: experience to date. Anaesthesia 2003;58:856–63.

19. Runciman WB, Sellen A, Webb RK, Williamson JA, Currie M, Morgan C, Russell WJ. Error, incidents and accidents in anaesthetic practice. Anaesth Intens Care 1993;21:506–19.

20. Webb RK, Currie M, Morgan CA, Williamson JA, MacKay P, Russell WJ, Runciman WB. The Australian incident monitoring study: an analysis of 2000 incident reports. Anaesth Intens Care 1993;21:520–28.

21. Cheney FW. The American Society of Anesthesiologists closed claims project: what have we learned, how has it affected practice, and how will it affect practice in the future? Anesthesiology 1999;91:552–56.

22. Cooper JB, Gaba D. No myth: anesthesia is a model for addressing patient safety. Anesthesiology 2002;97(6):1335–37.

23. Newland MC, Ellis SJ, Lydiatt CA, Peters KR, Tinker JH, Romberger DJ, et al. Anesthetic-related cardiac arrest and its mortality: a report covering 72,959 anesthetics over 10 years from a US teaching hospital. Anesthesiology 2002;97:108–15.

24. Lagasse RS. Anesthesia safety: model or myth? Anesthesiology 2002;97:1609–17.

25. Moller JT, Johannessen NW, Espersen K, Pedersen BD, Jensen PF, Rasmussen NH, et al. Randomized evaluation of pulse oximetry in 20,802 patients: II. Perioperative events and postoperative complications. Anesthesiology 1993;78:445–53.

26. Reason J. Human error: models and management. Br Med J 2000;320:768–70.

27. Nolan TW. System changes to improve patient safety. Br Med J 2000;320:771–73.

28. Weingart SN, Wilson RM, Gibberd RW, Harrison B. Epidemiology of medical error. Br Med J 2000;320:774–77.

29. Vincent C, Taylor-Admas S, Chapman EJ, Hewett D, Prior S, Strange P, Tizzard A. How to investigate and analyse clinical incidents: clinical risk unit and association of litigation and risk management protocol. Br Med J 2000;320:777–81.

30. Helmreich R. On error management: lessons from aviation. Br Med J 2000;320:781–85.

31. Gaba D. Anaesthesiology as a model for patient safety in health care. Br Med J 2000;320:785–88.

32. Bates DW. Using information technology to reduce rates of medication errors in hospitals. Br Med J 2000;320:788–91.

33. Cook RI, Render M, Woods DD. Gaps in the continuity of care and progress on patient safety. Br Med J 2000;320:791–94.

34. Pietro DA, Shyavitz LJ, Smith RA, Auerbach BS. Detecting and reporting errors: why the dilemma? Br Med J 2000;320:794–96.

35. Runciman WB, Webb RK, Lee R, Holland R. System failure: an analysis of 2000 incident reports. Anaesth Intens Care 1993;21:684–95.

36. Sentinel events: approaches to error reduction and prevention. J Qual Improv 1998;24:175–86.

37. Shojania KG, Duncan BW, McDonald KM, Wachter RM. Safe but sound: patient safety meets evidence-based medicine. JAMA 2002;288:508–13.

38. Leape LL, Berwick DM, Bates DW. What practices will most improve safety? Evidence-based medicine meets patient safety. JAMA 2002;288:501–7.

39. Fleisher LA, Eagle KA. Lowering cardiac risk in noncardiac surgery. N Engl J Med 2001;345:1677–82.

40. Eagle KA, Berger PB, Calkins H, Chaitman BR, Ewy GA, Fleischmann KE, et al. American College of Cardiology/American Heart Association Task Force on Practice Guidelines. ACC/AHA guideline update for perioperative cardiovascular evaluation for noncardiac surgery—executive summary. Anesth Analg 2002;94:1052–64.

41. Auerbach AD, Goldman L. β-blockers and reduction of cardiac events in non-cardiac surgery: clinical applications. JAMA 2002;287:1445–47.

42. Pedersen T, Moller AM. How to use evidence-based medicine in anaesthesiology. Acta Anaesthesiol Scand 2001;45:267–74.

43. Tramer MR. A rational approach to the control of postoperative nausea and vomiting: evidence from systematic reviews. Part I. Efficacy and harm of antiemetic interventions, and methodological issues. Acta Anaesthesiol Scand 2001;45:4–13.

44. Tramer MR. A rational approach to the control of postoperative nausea and vomiting: evidence from systematic reviews. Part II. Recommendations for prevention and treatment, and research agenda. Acta Anaesthesiol Scand 2001;45:14–19.

45. Gan TJ. Postoperative nausea and vomiting—can it be eliminated? JAMA 2002;287:1233–36.

46. Hill RP, Lubarsky DA, Phillips-Bute B, Fortney JT, Creed MR, Glass PSA, et al. Cost-effectivness of prophylactic antiemetic therapy with

ondansetron, droperidol, or placebo. Anesthesiology 2000;92:958–67.

47. Goll V, Akca O, Grief R, Freitag H, Arkilic CF, Scheck T, et al. Ondansetron is no more effective than supplemental intraoperative oxygen for prevention of postoperative nausea and vomiting. Anesth Analg 2001;92:112–17.

48. Stadler M, Bardiau F, Seidel L, Albert A, Boogaerts JG. Difference in risk factors for postoperative nausea and vomiting. Anesthesiology 2003;98:46–62.

49. Hyllested M, Jones S, Pedersen JL, Kehlet H. Comparative effect of paracetamol, NSAIDs, or their combination in postoperative pain management: a qualitative review. Br J Anaesth 2002;88:199–214.

50. Romsing J, Muiniche S, Dahl JB. Rectal and parenteral paracetamol, and paracetamol in combination with NSAIDs, for postoperative analgesia. Br J Anaesth 2002;88:215–26.

51. Klein SM, Nielsen KC, Greengrass RA, Warner DS, Martin A, Steele S. Ambulatory discharge after long-acting peripheral nerve blockade: 2382 blocks with ropivacaine. Anesth Analg 2002;94:65–70.

52. Rawal N, Allvin R, Axelsson K, Hallen J, Ekback G, Ohlsson T, Amilon A. Patient-controlled regional analgesia (PCRA) at home: controlled comparison between bupivacaine and ropivacaine brachial plexus analgesia. Anesthesiology 2002;96:1290–96.

53. Ilfeld BM, Morey TE, Wright TW, Chidgey LK, Kayser Enneking F. Continuous interscalene brachial plexus block for pain control at home: a randomized, double-blinded, placebo-controlled study. Anesth Analg 2003;96:1089–95.

54. Gan TJ, Glass PS, Windsor A, Payne F, Rosow C, Sebel P, et al. Bispectral index monitoring allows faster emergence and improved recovery from propofol, alfentanil, and nitrous oxide anesthesia. BIS Utility Study Group. Anesthesiology 1997;87:808–15.

55. Song D, vanVlymen J, White PF. Is the bispectral index useful in predicting fast-track eligibility after ambulatory anesthesia with propofol and desflurane? Anesth Analg 1998;87:1245–48.

56. Burrow B, McKenzie B, Case C. Do anesthetized patients recover better after bispectral index monitoring? Anaesth Intens Care 2001;29:239–45.

57. Nelskyla KA, Yli-Hankala AM, Puro H, Korttila KT. Sevoflurane titration using bispectral index decreases postoperative vomiting in phase II recovery after ambulatory surgery. Anesth Analg 2001;93:1165–69.

58. Pavlin DJ, Hong JY, Freund PR, Koerschgen ME, Bower JO, Bowdle TA. The effect of bispectral index monitoring on end-tidal gas concentration and recovery duration after outpatient anesthesia. Anesth Analg 2001;93:613–19.

59. Ahmad S, Yilmaz M, Marcus RJ, Glisson S, Kinsella A. Impact of bispectral monitoring on fast tracking gynecologic patients undergoing laparoscopic surgery. Anesthesiology 2003;98:849–52.

60. Larson EB. Measuring, monitoring, and reducing medical harm from a systems perspective: a medical director's personal reflections. Acad Med 2002;77:993–1000.

61. Berwick DM. Crossing the boundary: changing mental models in the service of improvement. Int J Qual Health Care 1998;10:435–41.

62. Lagasse RL, Steinberg ES, Katz RI, Saubermann AJ. Defining quality of perioperative care by statistical process control of adverse outcomes. Anesthesiology 1995;82:1181–88.

63. Posner KL, Kendall-Gallagher D, Wright IH, Glosten B, Gild W, Cheney FW. Linking process and outcome of care in a continuous quality improvement program for anesthesia services. Am Coll Med Qual 1994;9:129–37.

Billing for Anesthesia and Pain Management in the Ambulatory Setting

JODY LOCKE • DAVID A. LUBARSKY

INTRODUCTION

Perhaps the most significant management challenge facing anesthesiologists today is the migration of more types of surgical cases from inpatient venues to outpatient venues. Aside from the clinical issues associated with the anesthetic management of patients in a variety of new settings, this evolution raises numerous billing and practice management questions as anesthesia providers attempt to determine whether traditional billing guidelines still apply in these nontraditional settings. Except as specifically noted, the following discussion of ambulatory anesthesia billing considerations refers to the whole spectrum of ambulatory venues including ambulatory surgical centers (ASCs) and doctors' offices.

Technically, the site of service does not impact the mechanics of anesthesia billing, although in many cases the decision to pursue clinical opportunities in the ambulatory setting is the result of a strategic decision that may have been inspired by expectations of new revenue opportunities. Even though the same billing guidelines apply to all anesthesia claims, the impact of venue can be significant. New modalities of care inevitably raise questions about appropriate billing policies. While it is logical that reimbursement should stay abreast of new clinical modalities, there is an inevitable lag. The specter of compliance looms large, especially when it comes to sudden and significant changes in billing and practice patterns.

AMBULATORY REIMBURSEMENT CONVENTIONS

Current professional reimbursement for most medical specialties varies based on the place of service. Payer fee schedules are intended to minimize the global cost of a given service by means of financial incentives to the surgeon to perform the procedure in an ambulatory setting. An epidural steroid injection (Current Procedural Terminology—CPT code 62311) performed on a Blue Shield of Michigan patient is worth $89.14 if performed in a hospital or outpatient facility where the facility will be separately reimbursed for $243.26 if the physician performs the service in the physician's office. It is not uncommon for the office or nonfacility rate (so called because the facility is not separately reimbursed) to be 200% of the facility rate (the amount paid to the physician for the professional component alone). Some institutions do not bill the facility fee for pain management blocks performed by anesthesia staff. While it would be unethical for the anesthesiologist to bill the nonfacility fee as that presumes the anesthesiologist is incurring overhead, working with the institution to maximize their billing could lead to either subsidies, or other perks that make such an effort extremely worthwhile.

For purposes solely of understanding Medicare reimbursement options one must consider the additional category that has been created for ASCs. Historically, the Health Care Financing Administration (HCFA) policy allowed for reimbursement to physicians under Part B of the Medicare program based on a fee schedule. Hospitals, by contrast, have been reimbursed for expenses associated with surgical procedures under Part A of the Medicare program based on diagnosis-related groups (DRGs). Consistent with this distinction, physicians have submitted claims on a HCFA 1500 form while hospitals have used a UB 92 claim form. A state-licensed and Medicare-approved ASC is reimbursed for eligible services under Part B. Reimbursement rates (see Table 12-1) are based on levels of service. These payments include all nonprofessional expenses such as drugs and disposable expenses required for the administration of anesthesia. ASC rates are adjusted periodically by the Centers for Medicare and Medicaid Services (CMS). Most chronic pain procedures, for example, fall under ASC reimbursement level 1.[1]

---

[1]There is a particularly useful summary of ASC billing requirements on the HGSAdministrators (HGSA) webpage at www.hgsa.com/professionals/bguides/asc-m.html.

Table 12-1   Reimbursement Rates for State-Licensed or Medicare-Approved Ambulatory Surgery Centers (Part B of Medicare Program Based on Diagnosis-Related Groups)

ASC Payment Group	Effective 10/1/2001	Effective 10/1/2002
Group 1 procedures	$323.00	$333.00
Group 2 procedures	$433.00	$446.00
Group 3 procedures	$495.00	$510.00
Group 4 procedures	$612.00	$630.00
Group 5 procedures	$696.00	$717.00
Group 6 procedures	$806.00	$826.00
Group 7 procedures	$966.00	$995.00
Group 8 procedures	$949.00	$973.00
Group 9 procedures	not applicable	$1339.00

The only specialty for which rates do not vary by site of service is anesthesia. Because of the unique nature of anesthesia services and the exception status established in 1992 when the Medicare program reform known as the Resource-Based Relative Value System (RBRVS) was implemented, anesthesia charges are calculated based on a conversion factor that is adjusted for locality and base and time units that are consistent across the country.[2] This does not preclude the anesthesiologist's realizing additional revenues for work performed in an ambulatory setting, but it does mean that the additional income will not derive specifically from professional fee income.

CHARGE CALCULATIONS AND FEE SCHEDULES

It is a tribute to the persistence of the American Society of Anesthesiologists (ASA) that all payers now recognize the validity of the base-plus-time-unit reimbursement methodology long-promoted by the society and very clearly outlined in the ASA Relative Value Guide.[3] Because anesthesiologists provide a service at the request of surgeons they have little control over key determinants in the risk and time associated with providing care. The ASA Relative Value Guide recognizes this reality. While surgeons get paid flat fees, the anesthesia reimbursement will vary based on the time spent managing the case and a variety of notable or unusual operative conditions, such as the age and ASA physical status of the patient, and operative factors such as emergency care. Some anesthesiologists may bemoan the limitations of this approach to reimbursement especially when dealing with payers that do not reimburse all the

codes and modifiers included in the ASA Relative Value Guide, but given their overall reimbursement is often higher than that of other physicians, anesthesia providers should be grateful for their exception status.

As with any complex calculation, maximizing anesthesia reimbursement in an ambulatory setting is a matter of understanding the subtle relationships between the variables and determining ways of structuring them to optimum advantage. The ambulatory environment is ripe with both challenges and opportunities. New treatment modalities invariably inspire an age-old question: do different treatment protocols mean that the old rules no longer apply? For a while there was a popular belief that the preoperative assessment of a patient in an anesthesia clinic some days prior to surgery was somehow different from the preoperative assessment performed as part of the logical preparation for a general anesthetic for an inpatient candidate. It did not take the payers long to figure out that the sudden increase in evaluation and management codes correlated directly to an abusive billing practice.

Knowing when to take a risk or experiment with new billing protocols is rarely easy to determine, especially when payer policies are still being developed. The good and the bad news about Local Medical Review Policies (LMRPs) is that we tend not to worry until a specific policy is published. Many are waiting for the final verdict on the mad rush to provide monitored anesthesia care (MAC) in endoscopy suites. The current environment and economic realities tend to encourage considerable experimentation. There is a tendency to view the ambulatory environment as a new frontier and to assume that the unique clinical aspects of care allow one to redefine the old rules. Unfortunately, in most cases we will not know until someone pushes a payer too far.

THE IMPACT OF PAYER MIX

There is no more obvious example of the advantage of the ambulatory setting than payer mix. As surgical cases have migrated from traditional inpatient venues to ambulatory venues, a disproportionate percentage of Medicare and Medicaid patients have remained in the hospital. The result is a generally more favorable payer mix for the outpatient cases. In addition, the lower levels of acuity associated with ambulatory patient conditions make for a more predictable workload. Anesthesiologists who are actively considering the expansion of their ambulatory practices would be well advised to calculate the effective net yield per anesthesia unit billed. One method involves dividing actual net collections (gross collections minus refunds) by the number of units billed. Be sure to limit the number of units to those that are generally reimbursable. This will preclude modifier units for Medicare and Medicaid cases.

The financial impact of payer mix cannot be overstated. The revenue potential of an anesthesia practice can be defined as the product of multiplying anesthesia units by the net yield per unit billed. It is a simple mathematical proposition that one can achieve the same result by producing

[2]*Federal Register*, Volume 56, No. 227, November 25, 1991, p. 59521.
[3]*2003 Relative Value Guide*, American Society of Anesthesiologists.

more units in an environment with a lower net yield or fewer units with a higher net yield. For many, this is all part of the attraction of ambulatory venues: shorter cases, lower risk, no call; in short, a place to work smarter rather than harder.

Underlying values and assumptions need to be constantly validated, however, because all too often the advantages of a more favorable payer mix are not commensurate with lower average daily levels of unit production. One of the most significant management challenges associated with ambulatory anesthesia is the lack of consistent levels of productivity. This is especially true in the office setting.

The effective net yield per unit billed can also be calculated on a prospective basis, as indicated in Table 12-2, if reliable payer mix information is available. Valid payer mix data require that all charges are determined using the same conversion factor. This method does not work if charges are determined based on allowable payment amounts. The payment rates represent either the group's usual and customary rate or the contract rate. Typically such calculations also assume that payment is made based on a 15-min time unit. If this is not the case, adjustments may need to be made. Bad-debt percentages are set based on historical experience. The national average effective yield per unit for 2003 is about $33.00 per unit.

In Table 12-2, the weighted average net yield per unit is calculated in the following manner: the gross charges determine each category's percentage of the total practice. This percentage multiplied by the contract or expected payment rate per unit yields a gross expected yield per unit. In the real world, though, an allowance must be made for bad debt, which is factored in as a confidence factor. Thus, Blue Shield represents 16% of practice charges, which are supposed to be reimbursed at $42 per unit. Not all patients pay their copayments and deductibles, so we set the confidence factor at 97% because there is an average bad debt of 3%.

Table 12-2   Surgical Anesthesia Cases

	%	Rate	Confidence (%)	Net Yield/ Unit*
BS of FL	16.0	$42.00	97	6.52
Medicare	12.0	$19.00	96	2.19
Commercial	12.0	$60.00	85	6.12
HMO	50.0	$45.00	95	21.38
Worker's comp	3.0	$27.34	99	0.81
Champus	1.0	$35.00	98	0.34
Self-pay	1.0	$55.00	20	0.11
Medicaid	5.0	$14.00	90	0.63
	100.0			38.10

* = % × Rate × Confidence.

THE MEDICAL DIRECTION OF NONPHYSICIAN PROVIDERS

Anesthesiologists are the only physicians who can be reimbursed specifically for the medical direction of nonphysician providers. This concept was first introduced in 1984 as part of the implementation of the Tax Equity and Fiscal Reduction Act of 1984 (TEFRA) guidelines and has since been integrated into the reimbursement policies of a number of public and private payers. From a purely economic perspective, medical direction is a little more than the leveraging of expensive physician resources by means of less expensive nurse resources.

In Figure 12-1, the revenue impact of the second provider involved in each case is close to neutral, but the overall cost savings can be significant at consistently higher levels of medical direction. The example in Figure 12-1 is a simplified version of a calculation with numerous variables: if a physician grosses $375,000 per year and takes an average of 6 weeks of vacation, and a Certified Registered Nurse Anesthetist (CRNA) makes $150,000, then their respective hourly rates are $232.92 and $116.46, assuming that each spends 70% of the time administering anesthesia and producing billable units. As Figure 12-1 indicates, there is no cost savings for 2:1 coverage but a significant cost savings for 3:1 coverage. This creates a distinct financial opportunity for anesthesia practices that cover surgery centers with three or more rooms and that can be conveniently covered by one physician medically directing three CRNAs.

What entity employs the CRNAs can also impact the overall profitability of medical direction. Clearly, the most profitable practice situations are those in which anesthesiologists medically direct hospital CRNAs because most private payers do not reduce payment for medical direction versus personally performed anesthesia in contrast to the payment reductions defined in the Medicare guidelines. Depending on the state, there is also some opportunity for both the hospital and the anesthesiologist to bill certain payers for the same case. In other words, if an anesthesia group employs the nurses there is only one charge per case, while the group that works with hospital CRNAs will generate one bill and the hospital will also bill for the same case. It should be noted that most commercial payers are following the lead of Aetna and UnitedHealthcare to actively close this loophole.

BILLING COMPLIANCE

Even anesthesia practices that do not rely heavily on the anesthesia care team (ACT) in the main operating room (OR) will probably realize a significant savings by introducing them in the ambulatory setting, especially if overtime is not an issue. It is exactly this type of economic reality, however, that has led CMS to be highly suspicious of the motives of anesthesiologists whose billing patterns suddenly change as they migrate into the ambulatory environment. There is little doubt in many observers' minds

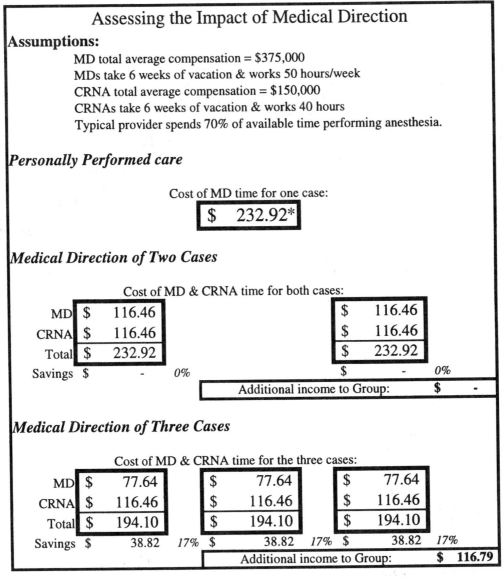

Figure 12-1   Assessing the impact of medical direction.

*$375,000/yr × yr/40 wk × $\frac{50\ hr}{wk}$ × $\frac{0.7\ billable\ hr}{hr\ worked}$ = $232.92

that the additional documentation required for the medical direction of CRNAs is more likely an intentional trap for the unsuspecting physician than a means of ensuring consistency of care. The seven requirements for reimbursement for medical direction, which are listed below, were obviously written by and for the auditors. Anesthesiologists who are contemplating the introduction of nurses into their practice should take note of the fact that the number one compliance risk for anesthesiologists and the greatest source of fine revenue for the government has been inappropriate documentation of the medical direction of CRNAs.

In order to be paid for medical direction an anesthesiologist must:

- Perform a preanesthetic exam and evaluation
- Prescribe the anesthesia plan

- Personally participate in the most demanding aspects of the anesthesia plan, including, if applicable, induction and emergence
- Ensure that any procedures in the anesthetic that he or she does not perform are performed by a qualified individual as defined in operating instructions
- Monitor the course of anesthesia administration at frequent intervals
- Remain physically present and available for immediate diagnosis and treatment of emergencies
- Provide indicated postanesthesia care

Other potential triggers for compliance concern are no less common in the ambulatory setting. Medicare intermediaries and CMS monitor code and modifier usage closely. Significant changes often inspire new policies. Of special note to anesthesiologists working in the ambulatory environment is the increase in the submission of ASA code 00810 for lower-intestinal endoscopy. Use of this code increased by 50% from 2001 to 2002. Because these patients undergo procedure usually under MAC, this increase has resulted in over 25 LMRPs intended to specifically define the conditions for payment for MAC.[4] The common element to all these policies is the need to define the medical necessity of the anesthesia provider's presence, and reimbursement. Some consider specified lists of diagnoses as evidence of medical necessity, while others, such at the Empire Blue Shield policy, require the administration of propofol. This is one area where computer-assisted decision support can be crucial, automatically cross-checking the patient's International Classification of Diseases, Ninth Revision (ICD-9) codes to the list of codes allowing for reimbursement. For example, when last checked in 2001, North Carolina had about 700 different ICD-9 codes that allowed for MAC for certain procedures to be reimbursed, and on multiple occasions, diagnoses for which there was medical evidence and that could have supported payment had not been entered into the patient's record by the surgeon.

Another trap of the requirements for medical direction is the fact that preoperative evaluation and placement of regional blocks in preparation for the next case may not be something allowable while concurrently billing for anesthesia during a procedure. While seemingly absurd, and contrary to the efficiencies expected in an ASC, this is the letter of the law. Yet another trap is the process of running four rooms, extubating the patient who is left safely in the care of the CRNA, and then turning one's attention to the next retrobulbar block or the next preoperative sedation, providing a temporary but financially devastating 5:1 ratio as cases overlap, precluding billing a full fee not only to CMS, but any insurer in whose contract there is a clause "by CMS rules and regulations." This is quite common for many insurance contracts, and should be noted.

DISTINGUISHING FEATURES OF THE AMBULATORY SETTING

To the extent that the ambulatory setting is intended to make life easier for the surgeon and the patient, it may complicate life for the anesthesia provider. The traditional model of anesthetic management, which was developed for general anesthetics provided in the main OR to patients who would recover in their rooms, does not always fit today's ambulatory setting. An increased focus on turnover, prompt emergence, a desire to perform procedures in a wide variety of less-well-outfitted venues, and the logistics of coordinating care in geographically disparate sites all contribute to the need for a different approach to anesthesia management in the ambulatory setting. Sometimes the appeal of such work is the prospect of immediate payment, but more often than not, the anesthesia provider finds him or herself saddled with a unique set of billing and demographic data capture requirements.

Preoperative Assessment

The first and most obvious challenge is the evaluation of the patient preoperatively. The traditional bedside chat the day before surgery is no longer an option. Different facilities have developed different methods for dealing with this critical aspect of the anesthetic experience. Anesthesia clinics have much to commend themselves from a clinical management perspective and can greatly reduce the number of last-minute cancellations. The problem is they must be manned by qualified personnel who usually cannot bill separately for what amounts to a separate service a number of days prior to the surgery. The reasoning for this is that the preoperative assessment is considered part of the base fee for anesthesia. This has led to more creative alternatives, all of which put increasing pressure on the anesthesia providers to assess and manage patients in a single episode of care.

Coding and Documentation

The traditional anesthesia record, which is completed by the anesthesia provider during the case, is a relic of times past when cases were longer and documentation requirements less demanding. Not only is it one of the curious ironies of modern anesthesia that practitioners still complete handwritten records despite all the high-technology monitoring used as part of even a routine anesthetic, but the anesthesia record itself has undergone significant transformation over the years. This medicolegal document must clearly reflect not only what agents were given, how the patient responded, and any particular events of note during the case, but also the comings and goings of each member of the team. Increasingly, payers are requesting copies of anesthesia records to confirm anesthesia start and stop time, the providers of record, and levels of concurrency.

Time constraints associated with ambulatory care make sparer records and more delegation of documentation to nurse anesthetists inevitable. This is one of the obvious trade-offs associated with medical direction. A physician who is responsible for two or three rooms, the intake of new patients, and the oversight of patients in the recovery room will find it fairly difficult to document all care completely. Even when this responsibility is delegated to the CRNAs, the attending anesthesiologist is still responsible for the completeness and accuracy of all records. The only exception would be those situations where the physician has decided to let the nurses' bill go out as "unsupervised care," which is reported to Medicare with a QZ modifier. The use of such a modifier on the claim form implies no physician oversight, a fact that may not exactly describe the intent of the physician practice group or the expectation of the facility. One potential pitfall is that anesthesiologists, who may be involved in the induction and preoperative evaluation, see that they can bill 3 units for medical supervision, even when they do not meet all other billing requirements. In some instances, they have mistakenly combined this with a QZ modifier to bill 3 units for them, and a full fee for the CRNAs. That amounts to

[4]Alex Hahnenberg, MD, Chairman of the ASA Committee on Economics, Presentation to the 2003 SAMBA meeting.

fraud, circumventing the CMS policy of only paying a maximum of 100% of the full fee for each procedure, no matter who is employed. In that case, a QK modifier with 50% reimbursement is more appropriate.

Physicians can be creatures of habit, especially with regard to the completion of anesthesia records, but the world of reimbursement is changing. Historically, payers expected to see a description of the surgical procedure and a surgical, postoperative diagnosis on the physician's documentation. This will still satisfy most payers when the patient receives a general or regional anesthetic, but it may not be adequate if the patient was given a MAC. A growing number of Medicare intermediaries now want a diagnosis that specifically justifies the medical necessity of the anesthesia provider's presence. Many also require evidence of a request by the surgeon for professional anesthesia care.

There is a popular myth that payers routinely compare the codes submitted by surgeons with those submitted by anesthesiologists. There is no reliable evidence to support such a view with regard to either procedure or diagnosis codes. Despite this fact, anesthesia coding is still a potential compliance risk area for many practices. The reason for this relates directly to the possibility of upcoding and unbundling.

Upcoding is defined as the submission of a code with a higher basic value than is supported by the clinical documentation, in this case the anesthesia record. There are two codes for a laparoscopy, for example. Code 00840 has a basic value of 6 units and is intended to be used when there is no upper-abdominal involvement, while code 00790 has a base value of 7, but specifically requires upper-abdominal involvement. Practices that default to the higher code have a higher risk of an audit than those with a reasonable mix of the two.

Unbundling refers to the use of multiple codes when only one is indicated. The ASA Relative Value Guide clearly delineates what services are included in the base value for a code. This includes the preoperative assessment, noninvasive monitoring, and the administration of fluids and blood products. Any attempt to charge separately for these items constitutes unbundling.

CONCURRENT SERVICES

The discussion of medical direction above represented one aspect of concurrent care that is closely monitored by Medicare. Concurrent services or overlapping case times can exist even when there are no nurses involved. Not only can an anesthesiologist not be performing two services at the same time, as defined by an overlap in anesthesia times, but legally he or she cannot be medically directing a nurse and performing a procedure, such as a nerve block, outside the OR. (There is a specific CMS exception to the medical direction rules for the placement and management of epidurals in obstetric patients and the treatment of medical emergencies in the immediate area.) This billing requirement can be a definite restraint in a high-turnover environment, such as an eye clinic, where the anesthesiologist is always trying to get the next patient ready. One would

hope that our component societies, such as the Society for Ambulatory Anesthesia (SAMBA), should be addressing this at a national level for clarification. Currently practices have to rely on individual practices, seeking explanation from local CMS carriers whose ruling on this may or may not be retrospectively held up as acceptable to CMS.

ACUTE PAIN MANAGEMENT

Many patients undergoing orthopedic procedures in the ambulatory setting receive single-injection or continuous peripheral nerve blocks to assist postoperative pain management. These valuable services can greatly enhance patient outcomes. The good news is that the regional procedure (e.g., a brachial plexus, a sciatic, or a femoral nerve block) is separately reimbursable if performed in conjunction with a general anesthetic. However, if a continuous peripheral nerve block is used as the primary technique, there is no separate reimbursement for additional daily management.

Technically, the anesthesiologist is expected to follow up with these patients, which creates a postoperative billing opportunity. For procedures involving the epidural space and the spine, CPT code 01996 is used for subsequent daily management, while an evaluation and management code (99211–99215) must be used for follow-ups for nonneuraxial procedures such as continuous interscalene blocks. While these codes are used quite commonly for inpatient services, their use could raise a red flag if billed in connection with ambulatory care since they cannot be billed on the same day as the anesthetic. This is definitely true if you have billed for the nerve block. Some local CMS carriers may accept a daily management fee if the block placement was the primary anesthetic and use of that block was continuously followed through the day. Because this would represent an exception to the general rule, the provider should always confirm the policy with the payer before making it a standard policy.

CHRONIC PAIN MANAGEMENT

Another logical form of product line extension for anesthesiologists working in an ASC is chronic pain management. The treatment of patients with chronic pain syndromes has nothing to do with ambulatory anesthesia except that those who work in an ambulatory setting may find it convenient to take advantage of the facility to perform nerve blocks at the end of the regular schedule. The integration of such services into a typical workday can dramatically increase the revenue potential of the arrangement. The key to success lies in remembering that the documentation and billing conventions for chronic pain are quite different from those of anesthesia. It should also be noted that there is no riskier proposition, as was evidenced in the prison sentence of Dr. Jeffrey Askenazi, than trying to manage CRNAs while simultaneously performing chronic pain procedures. There is no gray area here. The same person cannot do pain management while supervising CRNAs.

UNIQUE REVENUE OPPORTUNITIES

Anesthesiologists often ask if there are unique revenue opportunities associated with working in an ambulatory environment. The answer is yes. The problem is that most are more trouble than they are worth.

Facility Fees

Few anesthesiologists will ever have an opportunity to participate in the facility fee income received by a hospital. Their only real opportunity to participate in this revenue stream is through ownership in the ASC. Federal guidelines limit the number of facilities a physician can partly own such that at least 33% of the ambulatory services performed by the physician must be at the center in which he has ownership. This is usually not an unreasonable threshold since most anesthesiologists are rarely owners in more than one facility.

The possibility of participating in the revenue stream generated by the facility raises the obvious question whether such business opportunities make sense. The best answer is it depends. A busy surgery center can generate a considerable amount of revenue from a variety of sources. The potential of this passive income can be very enticing. Unfortunately, for all the upside potential, there is also downside. Potential investors should examine the business plan very carefully and consider the risks. More often than not, it does not make sense to pay for a franchise that you would get anyway.

As is true of many aspects of anesthesia practice management, there are the guidelines and then there are the practical considerations associated with the guidelines. Although many anesthesiologists may desire to participate in the ownership of an ASC, although their involvement may not be perceived as in the best interests of the other investors. Typically, when groups of physicians decide to open their own surgery center, they will look to sell shares only to those who can refer business to the facility, which is obviously not the case with most anesthesiologists. The notable exception would be the chronic pain physician, who definitely has the potential to refer significant business to the facility.

OTHER POTENTIAL INCOME

Certain anesthesia groups have discovered other creative means of generating revenue as a result of their participation in ambulatory venues. Some groups have experimented with an equipment charge, but the financial impact of this appears to be negligible since most payers do not consider it a valid expense. Others have been able to negotiate medical director stipends. Even if such arrangements do not represent significant amounts of money, they

may provide the anesthesiologists a critical means of managing the schedule to the advantage of the anesthesia providers.

DISTINCT CHALLENGES ASSOCIATED WITH AMBULATORY ANESTHESIA

Just as most anesthesia practices had to learn to accommodate the unique requirements of obstetric anesthesia, so, too, most will have to deal with the specific requirements of the ambulatory surgical environment. As was true of the evolution of obstetric anesthesia, a significant part of the challenge lies in the variability of clinical and management options. While most ASCs are outfitted with the same types of monitoring as their main OR counterparts, others are not. Some doctors' offices even require the anesthesiologist to bring in an anesthesia machine.

Demographic Verification

The anesthesia provider is always somewhat challenged by the flow of information necessary to bill for professional services. Even under the best of circumstances, anesthesia practices must rely on admitting clerks employed by the hospital or the facility for the details of a patient's address and insurance coverage, all of which is known in the industry as "the demographics." The fundamental problem in a traditional hospital setting is that the admitting clerk has no specific motivation to verify physician coverage, as distinct from that which will reimburse the hospital. To some extent the CMS ASC guidelines help the anesthesia provider, since ASC reimbursement is made from Part B, and not Part A. Even so, and given the large numbers of patients who may be seen in the ambulatory setting, verification of this information can be problematic. As a general rule, unless the anesthesia provider is going to be paid upfront by check or credit card, he or she will need to establish a specific mechanism for obtaining this critical demographic information. For the anesthesiologist working in a doctor's office, an agreement should be made with the office staff to get a copy of the patient's insurance card.

SCHEDULING AND HUMAN RESOURCE MANAGEMENT

Many anesthesiologists have been intrigued by the potential profitability of providing care to a surgeon in his or her office. Invariably the payer mix is very favorable. Because of the lower volume and greater variability of surgical cases in the doctor's office, however, such situations are not always as profitable as they might appear. Professional services must typically be scheduled in blocks of a day. Financial viability of such arrangements should be evaluated in the same terms. The best situations are those with high predictability of case volume. Many anesthesia groups have entered into agreements with surgeons to cover their offices only to find out over time that by the time they factor in downtime and the opportunity costs of the providers, they are actually losing money.

The ambulatory environment lends itself to economies of scale. The larger the pool of anesthetizing locations, the greater the overall predictability of surgical volume. Groups that only have one or two offices to cover often find them problematic, while those that have a larger scale and are more effective at managing around the volume issue tend to do better. Dealing with these issues, however, requires the creation of the necessary infrastructure. It is this reality that has given rise to a growing number of groups that cover only ambulatory settings. These practices function much like the surgical-request practices in the Southwest. They are primarily scheduling offices, dedicated to the coordination of anesthesia manpower and resources across a broad geography. A typical example is Resource Anesthesiology Associates, P.C., a New York–area anesthesia practice that describes itself in its homepage as "the largest accredited office-based anesthesiology practice in the United States. Our large team of board-certified anesthesiologists provides anesthesia care in offices and surgery centers throughout New York, New Jersey and Connecticut."[5]

MAINTAINING STANDARDS OF CARE

Today's consistently safe anesthesia care is the result of significant advances in anesthesia provider training, modern pharmacology, and the extensive use of physiologic monitoring. Patients who have surgery in traditional hospital ORs also benefit from all the other resources available to the anesthesia provider should there be a complication with the case. Ensuring that these same standards and resources are available in the ambulatory setting is a necessary prerequisite for maintaining similar levels of safety outside the hospital OR. While a hospital-based group can assume that certain minimum standards will be met by virtue of the hospital's accreditation by the Joint Commission and Accreditation of Healthcare Organizations, such an assumption cannot always be made in the ambulatory setting. This introduces another dimension into the ambulatory anesthesia management equation and a potential opportunity for the entrepreneurial anesthesiologist who is willing to serve as anesthesia safety consultant to facility owners.

[5]www.officeanesthesia.com.

SUMMARY

Business consultants often refer to a strategic planning tool known as a SWOT analysis. SWOT refers to strengths, weaknesses, opportunities, and threats. The tool can provide an effective means of assessing changes in the business environment. What it often reveals is that the same aspect of a development can be both opportunity and threat. Such is clearly the case with ambulatory anesthesia. There is an inevitability to the migration of many types of low-risk surgical procedures to the ambulatory setting. The loss of the revenue from these cases poses a distinct threat to the practice that is too tightly bound to a specific hospital. Groups that can restructure themselves in such a way as to permit their members to follow the cases will maintain the loyalty of the surgeons and continue to realize this important revenue stream. The problem is that this transformation is ripe with unique billing and management challenges and will require new tools and techniques. As is true of the anesthesiologist who starts focusing on chronic pain management in a clinic or office, the anesthesia group that migrates into the ambulatory setting must focus more closely on the management issues and cost accounting. The group must be more careful in its assessment of risk and profitability. The ambulatory environment is quite different from the traditional inpatient workplace: the very factors that make it financially attractive also make it perilous for those who are not prepared to devote themselves to mastering a new set of practice management skills.

REFERENCES

American Medical Association (AMA). www.amapress.com. The AMA publishes an extensive array of coding references, which can be reviewed at their website.

American Society of Anesthesiologists (ASA). *2003 Relative Value Guide.* Park Ridge, IL: ASA, 2003. This excellent summary of ASA billing guidelines should be considered the de facto standard for all anesthesia billing policy decisions.

Centers for Medicare and Medicaid Services (CMS). http://cms.hhs.gov. The CMS website is an invaluable source of information concerning Medicare policies. It also includes links to individual intermediary websites.

Society for Ambulatory Anesthesia (SAMBA). www.sambahq.org.

United Communications Group. http://www.decisionhealth.com. United Communications Group conducts seminars on anesthesia billing and publishes various billing and compliance newsletters specifically targeting anesthesia providers. All of the details about their services can be obtained at their website.

Profit Maximization for Ambulatory Surgery Centers

TOM ARCHER • STEVE MANNIS • ALEX MACARIO

A STORY AND A CONVERSATION

We begin this chapter on ambulatory surgery center (ASC) profitability by telling a story and by listening in on an imagined conversation:

Drs. Smith, Garcia, Chang, and Gupta are four busy orthopedists practicing at Mountainview Community Hospital (MCH), located in Sunnyslope, a medium-sized city in a rapidly growing Western state. They are excellent, well-respected surgeons and their group has contractual access to patients from all of the major health plans in the area. Nevertheless, they are frustrated and unhappy with their surgical practices.

Their incomes have been declining over the last two decades as insurance companies and Medicare have reduced their professional fees. But their complaints are not limited to the money they earn. When they perform outpatient surgery at MCH, many of their cases get delayed or canceled. Sometimes the anesthesiologists are called away for emergencies and sometimes the anesthesiologist delays or cancels a case because he/she says the preoperative workup is inadequate. Sometimes other more complicated cases performed by other surgeons run over and delay their own cases. What is more, the documentation requirements in the outpatient department are time-consuming and unrealistic.

To add insult to injury, when they ask the hospital administrator for a new piece of equipment, they get quizzed about how many cases they are going to do with the new device, and even if they get the expenditure approved, the whole process takes months. They feel like they have to beg for something that they know will enhance patient care.

The group also knows that other orthopedists in the nearby city of Charlesburg have started their own ASC and have been crowing about how much money they are making. Listen in on a conversation between Dr. Gupta and Dr. Jack Rich, a member of Charlesburg Orthopedic Associates:

"Now that we have our own ASC," boasts Dr. Rich, "we get the whole ball of wax: Not only do we earn our professional fees for performing the surgery, but—as co-owners of the ASC—we also get our share of the facility fees! That means that every time we do surgery we earn twice: once as the operating surgeon and once again as an owner of the facility. We've streamlined our admissions and documentation procedures so we only have to do what's really necessary—either from a patient care standpoint or to satisfy the bean counters. We're not saddled with all that complicated hospital paperwork we used to have to do."

"What do you do if you want a new piece of equipment?" asks Dr. Gupta.

"We just hold a partner's meeting, and if the votes are there, we buy it. Simple as pie."

"Have you been able to do anything about delays and cancellations?"

"We sure have! We got rid of the anesthesiologists from the hospital who always show up late and are always complaining. We just didn't give them privileges. Now we have a team of anesthesiologists who are committed to the success of the facility. They show up on time, they're nice to the patients, they stay late if we need them to and they don't complain too much when we ask them to use cheaper drugs and to help discharge the patients more rapidly. Our patients have less nausea and the anesthesiologists are helping us out with postoperative pain control, so we get the patients out faster. One of the anesthesiologists even came up with a suggestion for scheduling patients more evenly in order to smooth out our need for postanesthesia care unit (PACU) nursing staff. That's helped us to reduce our PACU payroll." He stopped for a moment, chuckled, and then went on. "We're thinking about letting *that* guy buy a share in the ASC. He might be of use to us later on."

"So you mean that all of your anesthesiologists aren't partners in the ASC?"

"Are you kidding? Who brings in the money anyway? *They* certainly don't! *We* negotiated our facility fees with the health plans in our area. Anesthesia didn't have anything to do with it. As far as I'm concerned, anesthesia should just show up on time, turn over the cases promptly, and use the drugs we tell them to use. And be nice to patients, of course. And not kill patients, of course!" He paused. "Believe me, our anesthesiologists are very happy to have the privilege of working in our ASC. They make better money than in the hospital and they have better hours. But they know that if they don't do a good job we can just get rid of them."

"Hey, that sounds great. I sure wish we could get rid of some of the anesthesiologists at our hospital. But hey, couldn't they sue you for loss of privileges?"

"Our lawyers tell us that we don't have to have an open staff. They say that we have the right to use whoever we want as long as there's a legitimate business reason for limiting the privileges to a certain group. And believe me, the whole operation works a lot better when everybody's on the same team! Now that we control the ASC environment we have 5–10 min turnaround times and we have a really caring, friendly atmosphere for the patients. Plus, the patients wind up paying less than if they had gone to the hospital. As for the anesthesiologists, they are just better motivated than that group we had to deal with before. They're more like team players."

IN A PROFITABLE ASC, REVENUE RULES AND COST CONTROL FOLLOWS

The key to a profitable ASC is high revenue. Without a lot of revenue coming in the door, no amount of cost control or cost minimization will make for a profitable ASC.

High ASC revenue depends on high case volume and high facility fees per procedure. The anesthesiologist can only marginally influence the number of cases performed in a given workday (through punctuality and rapid case turnovers) and has no control over facility fee. Hence the anesthesiologist's influence over ASC revenue generation is limited.

A High Volume of Profitable Patients

The key factor in ensuring a high surgical volume at an ASC is that the surgeons who operate there have an ownership stake in the facility.[1] Of the more than 3000 ASCs in the United States, 60–70% are wholly or partly owned by the surgeons who work there. Surgeons, like other physicians, have seen their professional fees eroded over the last couple of decades. One strategy to maintain their incomes is to obtain two income streams—once when they receive their professional fee and again when they receive their stake in the profits of their ASC. Income from ownership of an ASC can represent 10–20% of a successful practitioner's total practice income, so many doctors will take profitable patients to an ASC that they own.

Hospitals Fight Back

This loss of profitable cases represents a threat to full-service hospitals, who often try to prevent "cherry-picking" of profitable cases by insisting that contracting health plans give the hospital the exclusive right to perform *all* surgery for plan beneficiaries—and not just what is left behind after the profitable cases have been skimmed off by the surgeon-owned ASCs.

Fighting back in another way, some hospitals have canceled the privileges of surgeons whose ASCs try to compete with them for profitable cases.

In the future we may see a more coordinated assault (e.g., via changes in laws) on the very idea of physician ownership of medical facilities. The argument—whether justified or not—will be that physicians should not profit from their referrals to medical facilities. ASCs function in a political environment in which victory goes not necessarily to whoever gives the best care, but rather to the group with the best political skills.

Facility Fees

Facility fees are paid by Medicare, by the insurance companies, or even directly by the patient (for example, in cosmetic surgery, where there is no financial intermediary between patient and surgeon). In the case of Medicare, the setting of facility fees is a political process—that is why organized medicine has lobbyists in Washington, D.C.

Historically, ASC facility fees have been generous at first, to encourage the performance of surgery outside of the expensive hospital environment, but once a certain type of case has left the hospital—cataract and intraocular lens operations, for example—the payers begin to ratchet down facility fees. Falling ASC facility fees imply the survival of the low-cost producer in the competitive health care jungle.

COSTS: VARIABLE, FIXED, AND MIXED

ASC costs are a more complicated issue. Here we need to consider three different types of costs—variable costs, fixed costs, and, finally, the cost of labor, which is neither fully variable nor fully fixed.

Definitions of Variable and Fixed Costs

The definitions of variable and fixed costs come from management accounting and—applied to the ASC environment—are as follows:

1. Variable costs vary directly with the number of cases performed.
2. Fixed costs *do not* vary with the number of cases performed (Table 13-1).

We want to emphasize that the term "fixed costs" does not mean or imply "costs that cannot be changed." The terms "fixed" and "variable" simply refer to whether a cost

Table 13-1   Variable Costs and Fixed Costs

Variable Costs	Fixed Costs
Hourly payroll	Salaried payroll
Preoperative clinical evaluation	Real estate debt amortization
Preoperative laboratory tests	Equipment debt amortization
Surgical and anesthesia disposables	Insurance, utilities, permits
Anesthesia and surgical drugs	Consulting fees
Medical waste disposal	

is *directly proportional to case volume or not.* All costs, both variable and fixed, can potentially be reduced if we are creative enough or if we intervene early enough in the decision-making process.

Whether or not costs can be reduced frequently depends on the time frame in which we are working. For example, within any given day our scheduled labor costs (not counting overtime) are fixed, but over time—via productivity-enhancing measures—labor costs per case can be reduced. Figure 13-1 shows how current costs are the result of decisions made at many different times in the past.

Variable Cost Examples

Certain types of variable costs are easy to understand: surgical drapes, sutures, anesthetic circuits, and medications are used once on a case and are then discarded. For each case, a certain quantity of these "variable cost" resources must be consumed and paid for. If no cases are performed, no costs are incurred. One role of management is to attempt to reduce variable costs in surgery, so managers are perpetually seeking out better deals on disposable items.

Fixed Cost Examples

Likewise, certain fixed costs are easy to understand. For example, no matter whether the ASC performs 3000 cases per year or none, the debt service on the land, building, and equipment has to be paid. Similarly, costs for insurance, utilities, and permits will have little or no relation to case volume. Even fixed costs can be managed. Debt service costs can be eliminated or reduced if the owners pay off the mortgage or refinance it at a lower interest rate, and management can shop around for new insurance quotes, or install energy-savings devices to save on utility costs. So—in management accounting—the word "fixed" does not mean "unchangeable."

Labor Costs—Neither Fully Variable Nor Fully Fixed

Unfortunately, there are large gray areas when we talk about variable and fixed costs. The largest gray area—and 70% of the cost of health care—is labor. Labor costs are neither fully variable nor fully fixed.

Labor costs are fixed to the extent that they do not vary with case load. Examples of fixed labor costs in the ASC would be the *salaried employees*: the facility administrator, the director of nursing, and the business office manager. Salaried employees generally earn the same whether the ASC case volume is low or high, whether they work 8 or 14 hr/day.

In contrast, variable labor costs, by definition, will have at least a rough correlation with the number of cases performed in the ASC. We treat hourly employees as variable cost labor. Certainly, as an ASC expands, running longer days or opening new operating rooms (ORs) in order to accommodate more patients, labor costs will rise.

Productivity

But the correlation between case volume and variable labor costs is only rough, and at any given level of labor costs there is a range of possible production, depending on the ASC's *productivity*, or number of cases performed divided by the variable labor cost of performing those cases. The inverse of productivity is variable labor cost per case, so *the higher the productivity, the lower the variable labor cost per case.*

At any given case volume, we may have a productive workforce (which most definitely includes the surgeons and the anesthesiologists) that needs relatively few hours of labor to perform a certain number of cases, or a relatively inefficient or nonproductive workforce. If we have frequent gaps in the ASC schedule, or if we have particularly slow surgeons or employees, then the productivity will be low and the variable labor costs per case will be high.

Some surgeons are faster than others and some employees work with more enthusiasm and are more proactive than others. Labor-savings devices (e.g., staplers or fluoroscopes) enable us to accomplish more in less time and hence with less labor cost. Therefore, we need to be aware that labor productivity—the number of cases performed divided by the variable labor cost of performing those cases—can vary for many reasons, some within management's control and some not.

To summarize: ASC labor costs have a variable and a fixed component and *it is the role of management to minimize total labor costs at any given level of case volume. In other words, it is management's role to maximize labor productivity* (Table 13-2).

Next we present a mathematical model of ASC profitability.

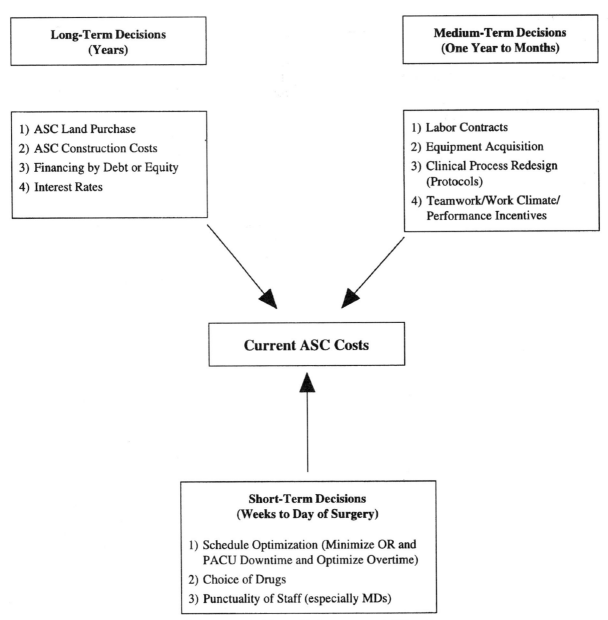

Figure 13-1 Long-term, medium-term, and short-term decisions all influence current ASC costs.

A MATHEMATICAL MODEL OF ASC PROFITABILITY

Our model is based on a hypothetical ASC that performs only one type of procedure and receives the same facility fee (F) for each case.

Revenue

Revenue (R) = Case Volume (V) × Facility Fee (F)

Costs

Total Costs (Ct) = Variable Costs (Cv) + Fixed Costs (Cf)

We assume that the ASC has only two types of variable costs, supplies (S) and labor (L), so:

$$Ct = S + L + Cf$$

Profit Equations

We define profit as the difference between revenue and total costs:

Profit (P) = Revenue (R) − Total Costs (Ct)

Since Revenue (R) = Volume (V) × Facility Fee (F), we can write:

Profit (P) = VF − (S + L) − Cf

We can state this result in words as follows: "ASC profit equals the ASC case volume times the facility fee minus the

Table 13-2   Techniques and Investments to Increase Labor Productivity (Decrease Variable Labor Cost per Case)

Get faster surgeons.

Clinical process redesign (working smarter).

Motivated workforce (working harder and smarter).

Purchase labor-saving technology.

Optimize preoperative evaluation.

Fill gaps in OR schedule (requires schedule control by ASC).

Minimize cancellations (call patient night before).

Optimize use of overtime to avoid excessive staffing costs.

Run fewer rooms longer (accept fewer 07:30 starts).

Cross-train employees (e.g., OR and PACU nurses).

Purchase information technology.

sum of variable supply and labor costs, minus the fixed costs."

Next we can derive profit on a per case basis by dividing each side by V:

$$P/V = F - (S/V + L/V) - Cf/V$$

This result, in words, says that: "ASC profit per case equals the facility fee per case minus the variable costs per case minus the fixed costs per case." In a real ASC we would have to worry about how to "allocate" or attribute our fixed costs to a wide array of different cases that vary in duration and in their utilization of other resources, but in this simplified model (in which all cases are the same), we ignore the cost-accounting nemesis of "fixed-cost allocation" between dissimilar cases.

Contribution Margin

The quantity $F - (S/V + L/V)$—the facility fee per case minus the variable costs per case—is known as the "contribution margin" per case (CM). If the ASC is to be profitable, the CM has to be positive and greater than Cf/V, the fixed costs per case.

Productivity

Productivity is V/L, volume of cases performed divided by the variable labor cost. The reciprocal of this (L/V) is variable labor cost per case.

ASC Profitability Factors

To maximize profit, the business person can work on any of five factors:

Facility fee
Case volume
Productivity (variable labor costs per case)
Variable supply costs per case
Fixed costs (labor and nonlabor)

Since the anesthesiologist normally has influence neither over revenue generation nor over fixed costs, he or she is usually just asked to help reduce variable supply and variable labor costs per case.

In the following fictional example, we put some flesh on these mathematical bones.

LAKEVIEW AMBULATORY SURGERY CENTER: COMPLACENCY AND UNTAPPED PROFIT POTENTIAL

Lakeview Ambulatory Surgery Center (LASC) has been successful over the years. The current owners are several orthopedic surgeons who founded the ASC some 25 years ago. They are now nearing retirement and have done very well for themselves financially. At this point, case volume at the ASC has fallen off a bit and gaps are appearing in the schedule, as some of the surgeon-owners decrease their case volume in order to follow up on other interests. The owners have not cut back on hourly labor costs, either by running fewer rooms or by shortening the workday.

The ASC employees are like family and many of them have been with the ASC for 15 or 20 years. The senior surgeon-owner has been overheard saying, "Oh, I suppose we could be more efficient, but this way we have room to work in an urgent case when we need to. Besides, I've made enough money from this place! We don't have to count every penny!"

In terms of facility fees, the owners are still in good shape. Orthopedics gets relatively high facility fees for the resources required, so the partners have done well over the years.

With respect to variable supply costs, the manager knows that she might be able to get better prices on disposables from some of the new suppliers, but she knows her current vendors well and they take good care of her. She has thought about trying to buy over the Internet, for example, but she is afraid of rocking the boat and the owner-surgeons are comfortable with the products they have been using for years.

Fixed, nonlabor costs are high too. Interest rates have come down a lot since the ASC was last refinanced, so debt service costs could be cut, particularly if the outstanding balance on the loan were reduced. The senior partner of the orthopedic group has been meaning to bring up the topic, but has not gotten around to it yet.

Fixed labor costs are also high. The spouse of one of the partners has been the business manager of the ASC since its inauguration, but she currently does not put in more than 2 or 3 hr a day, if that. By now, the place pretty much runs itself. A few years ago when government regulations got more onerous, the ASC board hired another partner's spouse as "compliance officer" for the ASC. He worked pretty hard for a few years getting the ASC up to speed with the new regulatory environment (and the government still does throw him a new challenge from time to time), but the truth is that the "compliance officer" has a pretty easy job.

One day, the senior partner is approached by one of the younger orthopedists in town, who asks him, "Would you like to sell your ASC to my group?"

The senior partner is intrigued by the idea and promises to take it up with the ASC board.

The ASC board decides that the time may be right to sell. But at what price?

The board realizes that to answer that question they need to critically analyze the ASC's books. The board hires an outside consultant, and asks her two fundamental questions: The first is "What could new management do to increase LASC profits?" The second is "Based on the increased income stream, what would the LASC be worth to an acquirer?"

The consultant (who uses our profitability model) gathers the data in Table 13-3 and makes the following presentation to the ASC's owners.

Recommendation 1: Increase Case Volume

The existing ASC could easily accommodate 200 more cases per OR per year, especially if the ASC had more control over the scheduling process.

By encouraging more surgeons to work at LASC, or by increasing the types of cases that can be performed in the

Table 13-3   Lakeview Ambulatory Surgery Center–Before Management Intervention

Number of ORs: 3
Cases per OR/year: 1000
Facility fee/case: $1300
ASC revenue/year: $3,900,000
Variable labor cost/case: $197
Supply cost/case: $260
Fixed labor cost/year: $265,000
ASC debt: $2,921,700
Interest rate: 14%
Debt service/year: $409,038
Other fixed, non labor costs/year: $100,000
Yearly profit: $1,755,962

ASC, we can increase case volume. Figure 13-2 shows ASC profit as a function of case volume, *with all of the other profitability factors held constant.*

A 20% increase in case volume from 1000 to 1200 cases/OR/year causes a 28.8% increase in profit from $1,755,962 to $2,261,962, despite our need to increase our variable labor and supply costs by 20%. Despite the fact that the facility fee and per case labor and supply costs remain constant, profit increases for two reasons: first, there

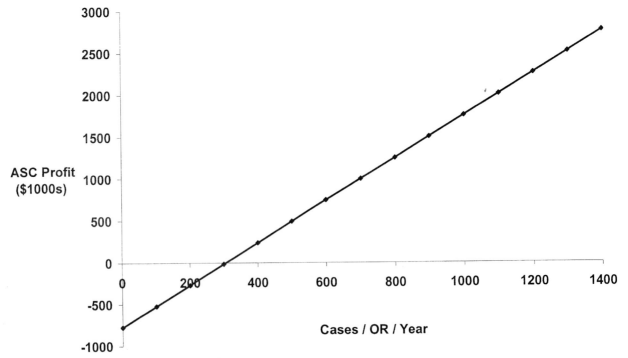

Figure 13-2   ASC profit as a function of case volume.

are more cases (each with its unchanged contribution margin), and second, the fixed costs per case are decreased. In cost-accounting parlance, we can "allocate" our total fixed costs across more cases, diminishing their effect on the profitability of each case. For these two reasons, profit increases greatly with increased volume and managers should work hard to attract new surgeons and new types of cases to their ASC, even if they have to hire more labor and use more supplies.

Recommendation 2: Perform More Cases with High Facility Fees

Changes in facility fees impact contribution margin, and hence have an extremely powerful effect both on the profitability of the ASC and on its *break-even point* (case volume at which profit is zero).

Figure 13-3 shows profit as a function of facility fee, at three different levels of case volume.

At 1000 cases/OR/year, a 20% increase in facility fee per case from $1300 to $1560 results in a 44.4% increase in profit from $1,755,962 to $2,535,962!

As facility fees *decrease*, the profit lines for different case volumes converge. This illustrates that, *as facility fees fall, it is harder and harder to maintain profit by increasing case volume.* As facility fees fall, the contribution margin approaches zero and we are just spinning our wheels when we increase case volume. When facility fees are low we produce lots of activity but no profit! In that situation, the only remedy is to restore contribution margin by decreasing variable costs—or to go out of business.

Figure 13-4 shows the effect of a 20% decrease in facility fee from $1300 to $1040 per case. At 1000 cases/OR/year, ASC profit falls 44.4%, from $1,755,962 to $975,962. Reduction

in facility fees decrease contribution margin dollar for dollar, with no countervailing decreases in labor or supply costs. In other words, for ASC profits, increases in facility fee are an undiluted benefit and decreases are an undiluted detriment.

No wonder that facility fees are the object of intense political lobbying activity and that potential cuts in facility fees strike fear in the hearts of ASC owners!

LASC should take measures to increase not only volume, but average facility fee as well. Perhaps LASC should try to recruit a new cardiologist or chronic-pain specialist because pacemakers and pain pumps are currently commanding high facility fees. By adding these high-value cases, the average facility fee for the ASC could be increased from $1300 to $1400 per case.

Recommendation 3: Increase Labor Productivity

Additional cases and higher average facility fees will boost revenue, of course, but *labor productivity* will also be increased by filling gaps in the OR schedule. Productivity can also be boosted by using new software to schedule patients more cost-effectively and by cross-training some employees—for example, OR and PACU nurses. Productivity could be enhanced as well by adopting new anesthetic techniques and new protocols to speed up discharge from the PACU.

If all these measures were instituted, variable labor costs could be cut by $33 per case, to $164 per case. Stated another way, *productivity will increase 20%,* meaning that for an unchanged $590,000 yearly variable labor cost, the ASC will be able to perform 1200 cases per OR per year, rather than 1000—or conversely, that 1000 cases could be performed for a variable labor cost of only $491,667.

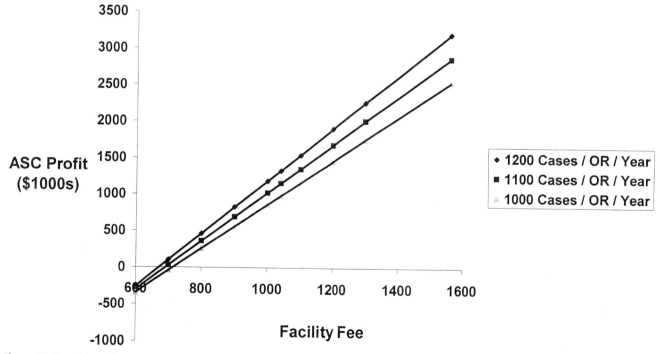

Figure 13-3   ASC profit as a function of facility fee, at three different levels of case volume.

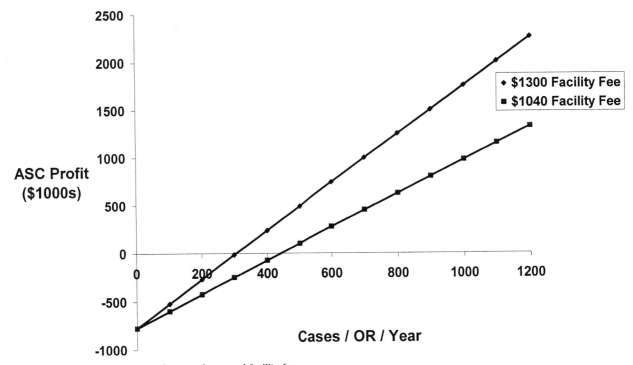

Figure 13-4   Profit as a function of case volume and facility fee.

Figure 13-5 shows the effect of increased productivity on ASC profits.

At 1000 cases/OR/year, a 20% increase in the productivity of the hourly labor force leads to a 5.6% increase in profit, from $1,755,962 to $1,854,295. We may note in passing that this "productivity increase" may have nothing to do with the nonsurgeon workers at the ASC. If we simply recruit faster surgeons, or fill gaps in the OR schedule, we may accomplish the goal of increased productivity. In other words, an ASC that is not very "productive" may be the result of slow surgeons, and not the result of poor employees. Assuming reasonable management, surgeon productivity (facility fee and number of cases performed per day) is by far the most important factor in ASC productivity and profitability.

Note that an isolated 20% productivity increase—at constant case volume—leads to a relatively modest profit increase. Remember that a productivity increase at fixed case volume implies a shorter workday—not a desirable attribute if we want to maximize profits.

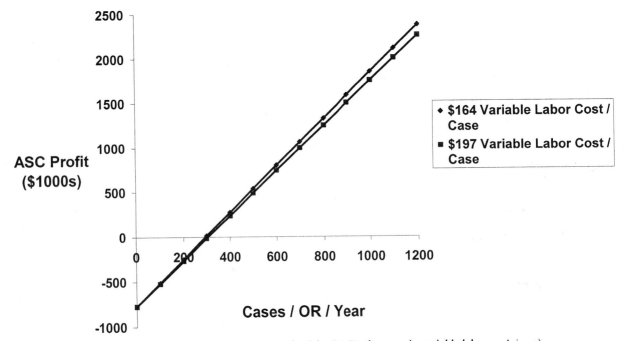

Figure 13-5   ASC profit before and after a 20% increase in productivity (16.7% decrease in variable labor costs/case).

It is only when we combine a productivity increase with increased case volume (fitting more cases into a normal workday) that we see outstanding profit performance. Hence, we can see that the "mantra" of the financially successful ASC needs to be "volume, volume, volume."

Volume trumps productivity, but certainly it is best to maximize both. If we *combine* a 20% increase in case volume with a 20% increase in the productivity of variable-cost labor—in other words, if we can do 20% more cases without increasing variable labor costs—we will enjoy a 35.5% profit increase, from $1,755,962 to $2,379,962.

As of the summer of 2003, a nursing shortage in many parts of the United States severely limits case production and adds urgency to the need to optimize the productivity (and work satisfaction) of nursing labor. Large gaps in the elective schedule combined with compulsory overtime leads to worker dissatisfaction. If nurses feel they are being abused, or if they have to work in an unfriendly and poorly managed ASC, they often will just quit and take their skills to a more nurse-friendly environment. Sometimes compulsory overtime leads to staff resignations, despite generous overtime payments. "We have lives outside the OR," these nurses say, "even if the surgeons don't."

Recommendation 4: Cut Variable Supply Costs

Figure 13-6 shows that at 1000 cases/OR/year, a 20% decrease in variable supply costs (from $260 to $208 per

case) causes an 8.9% increase in profit from $1,755,962 to $1,911,962.

When we save money on the variable supply costs (e.g., drugs or disposables), we directly increase contribution margin and savings go "straight to the bottom line." For every $5 we save on variable supply costs we increase the ASC profit by $5 times the ASC case volume. In an environment of decreasing facility fees, we can expect intense pressure on variable costs, in an attempt to maintain contribution margins.

By using less expensive medications, by cutting down on drug wastage, and by changing suppliers for other disposables, LASC could cut supply costs from $260 to $242 per case.

Recommendation 5: Cut Fixed Costs

In Figure 13-7 we see the effect on ASC profit of a 20% cut in fixed costs.

By cutting fixed costs 20% we boost profit at 1000 cases/OR/year by 8.8%, from $1,755,962 to $1,910,770, and our break-even point is a lower number of cases. Fixed costs act as a drag on profitability at any level of cases per year, and if the ASC were to close its doors temporarily owing to licensing or code problems (and do no cases at all), the yearly loss would be cut from $774,038 to $619,230, as shown by the intercepts on the y-axis.

With respect to fixed nonlabor costs, LASC was built and its basic equipment was acquired years ago, when interest rates were much higher than they are today. A local

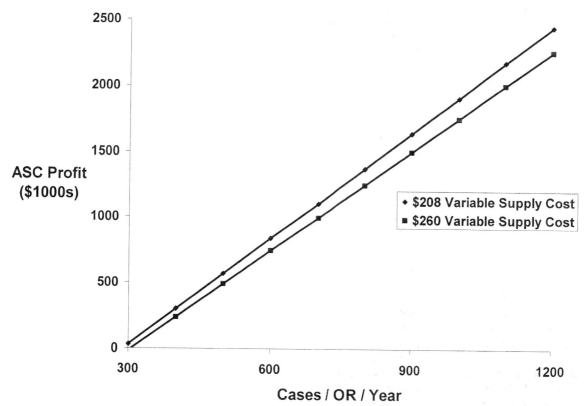

Figure 13-6   ASC profit before and after a 20% decrease in variable supply costs.

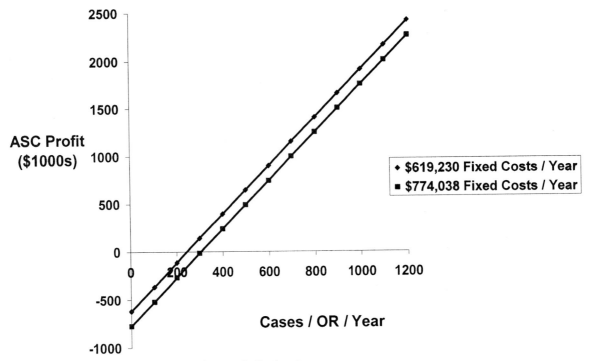

Figure 13-7 ASC profit before and after a 20% decrease in fixed costs.

banker has expressed a willingness to refinance the ASC's debt at a lower interest rate if the principal amount could be reduced. Specifically, if the debt can be reduced by $1,000,000, the interest rate could fall from 14% to 7%.

Insurance and utility bills—other fixed, nonlabor costs—are much too high as well. Getting new insurance quotes (in light of an excellent safety record and a quality improvement program) and installing energy-efficient lighting, could reduce other fixed, nonlabor costs from $100,000 to $50,000 per year.

Fixed, nonlabor costs (debt service and other fixed, nonlabor costs) could be cut from $509,038 to $184,519.

The business manager and the compliance officer have done great work over the years, but they really are not needed anymore, so fixed labor costs could be cut from $265,000 to $160,000.

Profit Potential Realized

After all of these management interventions, the financial picture of the ASC would be much improved (Table 13-4).

The Bottom Line: Increased Profit and Increased ASC Value

By taking in new surgeon-owners and thereby increasing the average facility fee from $1300 to $1400 and the case-load per OR per year from 1000 to 1200, by increasing productivity, and by decreasing variable supply costs and fixed costs, management could increase yearly ASC profit from $1,755,962 to $3,234,281, an increase of 84.1%.

Under these new conditions, what would be the increase in value of the ASC?

ASCs are sold at a multiple of cash flow, anywhere from 3 to 9× yearly cash flow, based on the degree of perceived risk.[2]

For purposes of illustration, we choose a multiple of 6× cash flow (what we have been calling "profit"). Assuming that our valuation multiple remains the same (and a better-managed ASC with less debt and more owners might well be able to command a higher multiple), we can see that the value of the ASC might increase as follows:

Table 13-4 Lakeview Ambulatory Surgery Center–After Management Intervention

Number of ORs: 3
Cases per OR/year: 1200
Facility fee/case: $1400
ASC revenue/year: $4,680,000
Variable labor cost/case: $164
Supply cost/case: $242
Fixed labor cost/year: $160,000
ASC debt: $1,921,700
Interest rate: 7%
Debt service/year: $134,519
Other fixed, nonlabor costs/year: $50,000
Yearly ASC profit: $3,234,281

Old Value = 6 × $1,755,962 = $10,535,772
New Value = 6 × $3,234,281 = $19,405,606

Hence, proper ASC management not only increases yearly profit, but also increases the capitalized value of the ASC's yearly income stream.

WHAT ARE WE DOING EVERY DAY?

Rearranging Deck Chairs or Avoiding Icebergs?

Control of variable supply costs and fixed costs is fairly straightforward and easy to understand and to implement. We know what our supplies cost currently and we can easily get competing bids from other suppliers. We know what the ASC mortgage is, and what interest rate we are paying on it. Besides the fact that these two types of costs are easily quantified and understood, they have another advantage for the manager—the involvement of ASC employees is minimal!

When we come to labor costs, people are involved and for that reason management of these costs gets sticky. We can minimize labor costs per case by preventing gaps in the OR schedule, but in order to do this the ASC needs control of the schedule. But what do we do when a surgeon-owner asks to do his/her cases exactly when it suits him/her and not when it would minimize labor costs for the ASC? Clearly, there exist potential conflicts between the desires of individual surgeon-owners to control the schedule in "their" ASC and the desires of the very same owner-surgeons to keep labor costs per case as low as possible.

The owners of the ASC need to set policies that establish a compromise between maximizing surgeon convenience and maximizing ASC profit. One common problem is that of inappropriate block times—time that is set aside for a surgeon but is routinely underutilized. The owners of such an ASC have to decide which is more important to them—profit or soothing the ego of a big producer.

Another specific obstacle is the fact that many surgeons would always like to start at 07:30, as the first case of the day. If ASC management can resist this preference to some extent, then profit can be increased by running fewer rooms for a longer period of time during the day. Also, ASC management that wants to maximize profit should be willing to run different numbers of ORs on different days, depending on variation in demand between the various days of the week.

Another important approach to reducing labor costs per case is the "redesign" of patient care processes by discarding the irrelevant and redundant aspects of care. This redesign can occur in the ordering of preoperative laboratory tests, in the preoperative evaluation, in ASC patient documentation requirements, or in the PACU through fast tracking techniques and through the prevention or control of postoperative pain and nausea. Attempts to redesign patient care processes are aided by employees who are happy and proactive and who take pride in their work. Teamwork and attitude are somewhat fuzzy concepts, but nevertheless very real in determining the success of an ASC.

Is physician ownership all good? At its best, physician ownership facilitates efficient, sympathetic, and high-quality surgical care with a minimum of bureaucracy. At its worst, physician ownership leads to tyrannical management and compulsory overtime to the point where employees rebel and quit.

How does one affect physician behavior once the ASC partners are in place? Be careful whom you pick as partners. Being a co-owner of an ASC—or of any other business—is like being in marriage.

Financial arguments for efficient management may not carry much weight if the ASC generates only a tiny percentage of a physician's income. Faced with the choice between efficient management and personal service, the doctor-owner may opt for personal service. He/she may be willing to lose a little on his/her ASC profits in order to be able to take his/her kids to soccer practice.

Similarly, it may be that the financial heyday of ASCs is over. Over the next 20 years, American society will face an aging population and burgeoning health care and Social Security costs. We expect pressures on facility fees will be severe and unremitting, since there will always be more voters than there are health care providers. Politicians will serve their constituents' interests.

SUMMARY

Today's costs are the result of thousands of decisions, some made years, months, or weeks ago and some made this morning. The potential for cost minimization on any given surgical day has already been achieved owing steady prior planning—refining scheduling techniques and OR and PACU procedures, cutting supply costs and usage, and promoting a sense of ownership and teamwork in the staff.

Routine care should represent the best we can do at the present state of our knowledge.

Frantic, superhuman effort on the day of surgery is frequently disruptive and counterproductive. Irritable, impatient, and chronically overscheduled surgeons may want to rush in order to make it back to the office or to their tennis games, but their impatience has no financial justification. On the day of surgery the best way to proceed is by simply taking care of each patient in a relaxed, cheerful, and supportive way. Rushing to save a few minutes here or there can be dangerous, stressful, and is financially trivial.

So, we should finally ask ourselves what we are doing each day we come to work. Are we rearranging the deck chairs on the *Titanic*—that is, are we struggling to "optimize" an obsolete and unworkable reality—or are we critically and creatively examining our environment in order to avoid the looming icebergs and arrive safely in port?

REFERENCES

1. Lynk WJ, Longley CS. The effect of physician-owned surgicenters on hospital outpatient surgery. Health Aff 2002; 21(4):215–21.
2. Becker's ASC, http://www.beckersasc.com/Review/review2.htm, June 4, 2003.

Cost–Benefit and Cost–Utility Analyses: Outpatient Implications

BRIAN A. WILLIAMS • MICHAEL L. KENTOR • JACQUES E. CHELLY

INTRODUCTION

In the United States, the annual number of outpatient surgery procedures for all musculoskeletal conditions (4.3 million) is predominated by patients under the age of 65 (3.7 million, or 86%).[1] Thus, this is a patient population with significant numbers of patients in both privately insured and government-assisted (e.g., Medicare) sectors. With diminishing payments from both private insurers and Medicare, physicians and administrators are now forced to focus energies toward cost containment in order to maintain an operating margin free from deficits. Cost analysis is an emerging tool in health care economics that can help physicians and administrators meet these new challenges presented by health care market forces.

Cost analysis examines health care expenditures, but many subtypes of cost analysis also examine factors that are inserted into a denominator of a cost equation. Such factors include monetary benefits (e.g., cost-benefit analysis), incremental changes of health status variables (e.g., cost-effectiveness analysis), and patient-reported quality of life (e.g., cost-utility analysis).[2] If outcomes are determined to be equivalent regardless of the treatment program implemented, then a basic cost-minimization analysis is all that is required, because the denominators are equal and the only relevant comparison is between the cost numerators of the compared programs.

With respect to complex outpatient orthopedic surgery, it is highly unlikely that comparing exclusively administered regional anesthesia (RA) techniques with exclusively administered general anesthesia (GA) techniques would show equal benefits or equal effectiveness (i.e., life-years gained, days of disability avoided). RA significantly differs from GA with volatile agents, and the relevant side-effect profiles and risks are quite different as well. In fact, in the past few years, it has become very clear in ambulatory procedures that the choices of the anesthetic and postopera-tive analgesic techniques have significant consequences on both the length of hospital stay and the frequency of unplanned hospitalization,[3,4] and consequently the overall cost of the surgery. As a result, comparisons between RA and GA would require a cost-benefit, cost-utility, and/or cost-effectiveness analysis. On the other hand, comparison of two medications delivered in an otherwise standardized continuous-catheter RA technique, for example, may lend itself to a cost-minimization analysis, if outcomes are otherwise essentially equal.

As physicians caring for individual patients, it is important to note that basing one's entire practice strictly on cost analysis is not well advised, as individual patients have individual needs. However, there is no substitute for proper education of patients regarding the benefits of RA techniques, such that patients agreeing to and receiving such techniques may then benefit while the hospital and health care system enjoys any cost benefits achieved.

TYPES OF COST ANALYSES

Textbooks on the topic[2,5] consider cost-effectiveness analysis (CEA) the standard cost analysis technique, while categorizing cost-minimization, cost-benefit, and cost-utility analyses as subtypes of CEA. For this discussion, we will assume that there is thematic overlap among all subtypes of CEA, but we will try to distinguish the subtypes as best as possible, and perform illustrations of each subtype later in the chapter.

An important assumption in any cost analysis is to determine the perspective of the analyst (hospital administrator, health care provider, third-party payer, patient, family). The perspective of the analyst may yield very different results for a given subtype of cost analysis.

Cost-Minimization Analysis

Cost-minimization analysis (CMA) can be used to provide an economic basis of comparing various anesthesia techniques and antiemetic interventions, for example, but assumes that the outcomes achieved between compared techniques are equal. CMA differs from cost-benefit analysis, the latter of which ascribes a monetary value to both costs and benefits,[2] and from CEA, which measures benefits in terms of a clinical outcome such as "life-years gained" or "days of disability avoided."[2,5] CMA is also distinguished from cost-utility analysis in that the latter ascribes a patient-specific value to the denominator regarding the utility of a given outcome (more details will be described below).

CMA can be performed from any perspective (patient, family, health care provider, administrator). For example, a hospital administrator can compute CMA values to correspond with the hospital costs of nursing interventions (for postoperative pain and postoperative nausea and vomiting [PONV]) and unplanned hospital admission (for refractory pain and PONV). From an administrative viewpoint, the incremental costs of anesthesia techniques can be addressed by evaluating recovery nurse staffing requirements, and unplanned admissions for each anesthesia technique being compared. Since there is no denominator in CMA, there is no basis for demonstrating "trade-offs" of a given outcome versus a given cost.

Even though CMA appears relatively simple, it is not. If one were to accurately compare GA versus RA, for example, one would need to consider all costs involved with the techniques in question. For example, GA involving use of an anesthesia machine and breathing circuit requires tabulation of not only costs of disposable supplies (the cost of a disposable anesthesia circuit is about $3) but also costs related to capital equipment (maintenance contracts, depreciation, etc.). New anesthesia machines are not inexpensive; each new machine can cost $40,000–$50,000. In a large hospital with 50 anesthesia machines (a capital cost that may approach $2.5 million if all machines were new), an annual maintenance contract can exceed $80,000, with newer machines requiring at least one preventive maintenance service per year, and older machines requiring three such services per year, assuming each machine is used 8–12 hr/day, 5 days/week. Our institution's biomedical engineers believe that the maintenance contract would be less (for older machines) if utilization was only 3–4 hr/day (e.g., with high-volume RA practice), leading to only one preventive maintenance service per year. In our institution, anesthesia machines are budgeted to last 10–12 years, so annual depreciation costs would be one-eighth to one-tenth of the purchase price per machine (assuming "straight-line" depreciation). Other depreciation methods can be used, however, to help gain immediate taxation advantages. "Half-life" depreciation for a $50,000 machine would involve sequential annual depreciation costs of $25,000, $12,500, $6250, etc. The higher up-front depreciation costs help to buttress the immediate tax burden of high purchasing costs of new capital equipment, and may better match resale values of such equipment.

Meanwhile, total intravenous anesthesia (TIVA) techniques would need to incorporate the expenditures related to disposables such as syringes and tubing, as well as capital equipment such as electronic infusion pumps. Such pumps cost from $1000 to $1500, and also are assumed to last 10–12 years. In our institution, biomedical engineers perform preventive maintenance on infusion pumps, making outsourced maintenance costs difficult to quantify. Finally, RA techniques featuring peripheral nerve blocks would need to include cost data for disposables (needles, sterile prep supplies) and capital equipment (nerve stimulators with or without automated current-control features, automated injection devices, and the like). Nerve stimulators typically cost from $500 to $1000, with disposable single-injection needles costing from $10 to $15.

For a facility with 20 anesthetizing locations, the cost savings in capital equipment and maintenance is readily apparent if new anesthesia machines were earmarked for critical-care operating rooms (ORs), while older machines were reserved for rooms in which regional and/or intravenous anesthesia techniques were used.

Given the complexities of costing capital equipment, depreciation, and maintenance, the costing of personnel is even more complex. Seventy percent of all costs in a service organization are attributed to personnel. Individual centers use different strategies to "right-size" personnel deployment, such as flexible shifts with different start and stop times, "call" from home, "paid time off," elective overtime, forced overtime, etc. A useful but detailed personnel-costing technique is a time-motion study; another, more straightforward approach is tabulating the counts of the most labor-intensive activities (such as postoperative nursing interventions for any symptoms).[6–10]

To summarize, in any cost analysis involving RA versus GA techniques, one must not ignore the costs of capital equipment, depreciation, and maintenance, in order to account for potentially "hidden" costs. Accounting for all such costs generated by any health care program (drugs, disposables, capital equipment, and personnel involved with all perioperative care) is applicable to all categories of cost analysis, and all need to be considered together if the compared techniques potentially differ in any of these cost categories.

Cost-Effectiveness Analysis

Unlike CMA, CEA, and the cost analyses that follow, incorporate a denominator into the calculation. After computing the costs of a health care program, exemplified in the discussion above, the analyst would then determine parameters of "effectiveness." For this discussion, the authors will use "days of disability avoided" (or relevant proxy measures) as an ideal denominator comparing RA and GA techniques using CEA.

After costs are calculated using the approach described in "Cost-Minimization Analysis," the effectiveness is calculated by gathering data relating to the variable of interest. For patients undergoing total joint replacement, the variable may be something like "length of stay in the hospital before the patient is eligible for outpatient rehabilitation." For an adolescent undergoing arthroscopic reconstruction of the anterior cruciate ligament (ACL), the variable may be "days before returning to school." Obviously, these indicators can be highly patient-dependent. Unmotivated students may not be eager to return to school, and depressed elderly patients may meet inpatient rehabilitation objectives more slowly than nondepressed cohorts. It is important, therefore, to try to gather as much relevant demographic information as possible when performing such analyses, in order to adjust for patient motivation, in this example, or other variables that may influence return to work.

Cost-Benefit Analysis

Cost-benefit analysis (CBA) is useful for incorporating multiple variables into the calculation of effectiveness.[2] However, CBA is complex in that the denominator (benefits) assumes a monetary value, and translating nonmonetary benefits into a monetary value can be difficult. For administrators focused on revenues only, hospital collections when comparing different treatment programs would be well-suited for use in the denominator as "benefits." However, monetary values that are patient-specific are much more difficult to ascertain. One emerging economic analysis, called "willingness to pay" (WTP), does have applications in anesthesia care. WTP is defined as a sum of money a patient would be willing to spend to avoid a given side effect, or to achieve a given outcome. Details about WTP will follow.

The availability of WTP values, which could be easily inserted into the denominator of a cost-benefit equation, renders CBA a viable analysis to perform from the patient's perspective. Analysts who wish to present institutional data to potential managed-care contractors could use these values to demonstrate the patient-oriented outcomes of one's institutional treatment programs, especially if the contractor is lobbying on behalf of companies wary of reduced health care quality per insurance dollar spent. Unfortunately, there have been no published manuscripts on CBA in the anesthesia literature using WTP values.

Cost-Utility Analysis

Cost-utility analysis (CUA) is especially useful to incorporate patient-reported benefits into the denominator of a cost analysis. Unlike CBA from the patient's perspective, CUA does not use monetary values, rather using outcomes that relate to the quality of life. Generally accepted denominators used in CUA are "quality-adjusted life-years" (QALY) or "healthy-years equivalent" (HYE).[2] QALY values conveniently capture changes in both quantity (i.e., reduced mortality) and quality (i.e., reduced morbidity). However, comparisons of GA and RA in outpatient orthopedics are unlikely to show differences in mortality, whereas morbidity changes may be significantly favorable with successful RA techniques, or potentially catastrophic with RA techniques with rare but severe complications (such as permanent nerve damage). When determining a proxy measure for quality of life, especially since mortality is not a likely factor, it is important to use validated out-

come measures, such as the Medical Outcomes Study Short Form 36 (SF-36).[11] Other useful validated patient-reported outcome measures for this purpose include the Quality of Recovery (after anesthesia)—40-Item Scale, as reported by Myles et al.[12] Such patient-reported outcome measures allow the individual patient to determine which health factors are most relevant to him/her, by using Likert-scale responses that provide meaningful interval changes when compared with the patient's baseline assessment. Details about these survey instruments will be presented later in the chapter.

ANESTHESIOLOGISTS' INTERVENTIONS APPLICABLE TO COST ANALYSES

Selection of Techniques, Drugs, and Agents

In our clinical practice, we have found for invasive outpatient orthopedic surgery that the routine use of general endotracheal anesthesia without peripheral nerve blocks (as the centerpiece of a multimodal analgesic plan) leads to the following expensive outcomes: (i) postanesthesia care unit (PACU) admission; (ii) multiple nursing interventions for pain and PONV; (iii) PACU and same-day surgery discharge delays; and (iv) unplanned hospital admission.[6–10] Although the least expensive GA technique using thiopental, succinylcholine, opioids, and volatile agents is certainly favorable for the budgets of the anesthesia department and the hospital pharmacy, the technique is fraught with "downstream" expenses for the hospital, and is a likely basis for extreme patient dissatisfaction. We should understand that most hospital pharmacy and therapeutics committees are primarily focused on the pharmacy budget. Six percent or less of all hospital costs related to surgical care are attributed to pharmacy drug costs,[13] and examining drug costs in isolation without regard for patient outcomes is ill-advised.

Within emerging RA practices, pharmacy committees may be loath to incorporate drugs such as levobupivacaine and ropivacaine to replace the less-expensive but potentially hazardous bupivacaine in the hospital formulary. This common-sense barrier is likely defended by the number of cardiac arrests (unresponsive to resuscitation) encountered with bupivacaine before one is encountered with levobupivacaine or ropivacaine. The legal costs of defending the use of bupivacaine in such a complication will well exceed the savings achieved by pharmacy's mandating the cheaper drug.

Minimizing Anesthesia-Controlled Time in the Operating Room

The value of the regional anesthesia induction room should not be underestimated. Peripheral nerve block techniques performed before OR entry have been shown to be associated with a time savings of approximately 9 min of OR time per case, when compared with using GA without blocks.[8] When the patient enters the OR ready for surgical preparation, and has a faster emergence (and exit) due to the use of sedation versus GA, an OR with five cases can save 45 min/day. If the cost of a minute of OR time is estimated to be $30, then 1 day of this amount of time savings for five cases carries a potential cost reduction of $1350. A portion of this theoretical savings is likely "real" in centers operating at or above 80% capacity, in which forced overtime (of preoperative, intraoperative, and postoperative nursing/ancillary staff) is a major budgetary expenditure. The cost savings becomes even more significant when cases later in the day (e.g., after 3 P.M. or 5 P.M.) are commonly "stacked" into fewer available staffed ORs, further lengthening already-long clinical days. Dexter et al. estimated that emergence which is 6 min faster than baseline likely translates to a per-case overtime reduction ranging from 1.3 to 2.6 min.[14] In a 50-case surgical pavilion, this translates to 65–130 min of overtime saved.

Bypass of the Postanesthesia Care Unit

We have shown that PACU bypass can be achieved in nearly 90% of patients receiving exclusively RA techniques (including neuraxial techniques if hemodynamic criteria are met).[9] Dexter et al. have shown that in surgical pavilions with large caseloads (e.g., 50 cases per day), an 80% PACU bypass rate (when compared with no PACU bypass) can lead to a PACU nurse full-time equivalent (FTE) staffing reduction of up to 4 FTE if the PACU nurses are full-time employees, or by 20 nursing hours if the PACU nurses are part-time employees.[14] When combined with forced overtime of OR staff and step-down recovery staff, OR time savings and PACU bypass, documented to be achievable with exclusive use of RA, can present important cost-saving opportunities for the hospital.

In our patient population of ACL reconstruction, we found that patients who bypassed PACU had an associated cost reduction of $420.[15] Some of this reduction is likely attributable to PACU staffing reductions highlighted by Dexter et al. above, since we bypassed many outpatient orthopedic surgery patients, not just those undergoing ACL reconstruction. The cost-savings component from the initial of $420 per PACU bypass patient excluding nurse staffing reductions were likely attributable to RA patients having fewer symptoms compared with GA patients. Interestingly, in our main campus university hospital, during peak use of PACU bypass (3000 outpatient orthopedics per year), PACU nurse staffing requirements for 25,000 patients per year consisted of 28 FTE, or one PACU nurse per 890 patients. When the main campus relocated outpatient orthopedics to another hospital in the health system, and PACU bypass was used for monitored anesthesia care (MAC) cases only, PACU nurse staffing requirements increased to 33 FTE for an annual caseload of 22,500, or one FTE per 680 patients).[15]

Successful Same-Day Discharge

Woolhandler and Himmelstein have estimated that the cost of hospital admission (for all types of diagnoses and procedures) is $1050.[16] We found that the hospital cost of an overnight admission after ACL reconstruction was $385.[15] The likely cost difference in our findings versus those of Woolhandler and Himmelstein is likely related to the generally healthy status of outpatients presenting for ACL reconstruction. The key point is that it will always be less expensive for a patient to go home immediately after outpatient surgery than to be admitted overnight for observation.[17] That said, precautions are required to ensure that costs are not incurred later in the form of requiring hospital readmission for complications improperly managed during the initial admission, especially since these readmissions are often ineligible for third-party reimbursement.

PATIENT-BASED INDICATORS OF THE UTILITY OF CARE

Hospital-Based Satisfaction Surveys

It should be noted that the vast majority of hospital-based patient satisfaction surveys are not designed with due attention to psychometric theory. The psychometric properties required when developing a patient satisfaction survey instrument are based on extensive theoretical principles[18] and require high levels of expertise to ensure that items are presented in an unbiased fashion, with minimized repetition or confounding among individual items. In the landmark textbook *Measuring Health,*[19] the theoretical detail involved with properly developing a health measurement is provided, and a large number of existing survey instruments are evaluated critically. Surveys created *de novo* should not randomly "pick and choose" a few questions from each of several validated survey instruments, trying to assemble a "suitable package" for a specific patient population. *The psychometric properties of a validated survey— validity, reliability, and responsiveness to change—are based on the individual survey from start to finish.* Merely sampling a few questions from several surveys and combining them all into one survey eliminates the rigorousness of the method. A most simplistic recommendation is to use an existing, validated instrument that most closely matches the needs of an individual institution, such as those described below in "Validated Outcome Survey Instruments."

Patient Willingness-to-Pay

Three important studies in the anesthesia literature address WTP. Most recently, Leslie et al. asked 200 patients if they would be willing to pay for monitoring to prevent awareness during anesthesia, and determined that only 34% would pay if they were at low risk for awareness. However, 50% of patients surveyed would be WTP if they were considered to be at high risk for awareness.[20] Thus, WTP studies such as this can address the straightforward question of whether patients are WTP at all (such as the study by Leslie et al. above), and if so, how much patients would be WTP for a given outcome (with examples described below).

Two approaches may be taken in determining specific WTP values. The first allows patients to spend for various utilities from a finite sum of money.[21] The second approach asks patients to estimate the absolute value of a specific utility or health care resource (e.g., medical hotel stay vs. hospital admission,[22] or avoiding PONV symptoms).[23] Monetary value is ascribed to both positive and negative benefits.

Three WTP values are cited in the literature. In the first study, Gan et al. showed that patients were WTP $100 to avoid PONV.[23] In the second study, Lehmann et al., in their study of "pilot" outpatients, demonstrated that this population was WTP $400 for symptom-free same-day discharge after laparoscopic cholecystectomy, rather than have an unplanned hospital admission.[22] The third study cited in the literature is by Macario et al., who reviewed general surgery patients undergoing general anesthesia.[13] In this study, patients were theoretically allocated $100 to spend for the avoidance of various symptoms. For example, from the $100 available, patients were WTP $30 to avoid PONV and $17 to avoid pain.[13]

To summarize the last paragraph, in one study, patients were WTP $400 to avoid an unplanned hospital admission and have a symptom-free same-day discharge.[22] In two other studies, symptom-specific WTP values are given and/or can be calculated. Given an absolute value of $100 that patients would be WTP to avoid PONV,[23] one can calculate that patients would be WTP $57 to avoid pain.[21] Thus, it is important as a specialist in outpatient RA to pay even more attention to the prevention and/or treatment of PONV than pain. Certainly, the avoidance of opioids will assist in this effort, but the use of volatile agents versus propofol for maintenance has been associated with a 300% increase in PONV.[24] Thus, recent data indicate that patients are WTP finite sums to avoid the common complications of pain, PONV, and unplanned hospital admission.

The major disadvantage of WTP studies to date is that they do not distinguish methods used for pain management. As such, future studies that evaluate WTP sums for RA and GA should include questions such as "How much would you be willing to pay for effective pain relief that carries a risk of side effects such as somnolence, PONV, and itching?" versus "How much would you be willing to pay for pain relief in which your extremity is rendered insensate and involves procedures with long needles and involuntary twitches?" Granted, these last two paragraphs represent the extremes of opinions regarding GA (many nuisance side effects) versus RA (additional complex procedures with the rare potential for nerve damage). However, further work is needed to incorporate patient WTP perspectives on both procedural complexity and analgesic benefits of RA.

Validated Outcome Survey Instruments

Quality of Recovery (QoR) Scales

The QoR-40, described by Myles et al., is one of the first instruments designed to address patients' early postoperative health status in detail.[12] Most previous postanesthesia assessments focused on time to awakening, pain, nausea,

Table 14-1   Patient Outcome Dimensions Queried by the Quality of Recovery Score–9-Item Scale

- Feeling of general well-being
- Feeling that others are supportive
- Ability to understand instructions and advice
- Ability to attend to personal hygiene needs
- Bowel and bladder control
- Ease in respiratory effort
- Freedom from headache, backache, and myalgia
- Freedom from nausea, retching, and emesis
- Freedom from moderate to severe pain

SOURCE: Adapted from Myles PS, Hunt JO, Nightingale CE, et al. Development and psychometric testing of a Quality of Recovery score after general anesthesia and surgery in adults. Anesth Analg 1999;88:83.

vomiting, confusion, or length of hospital stay. The QoR-40 has incorporated measures deemed important by focus groups of patients and families. The five dimensions measured by the QoR-40 are emotional state, physical comfort, psychologic support, physical independence, and pain. The QoR-40 has demonstrated the best construct validity, test-retest reliability, internal consistency, and responsiveness of the few instruments available.[12,25,26] and is recommended for use in evaluating hospital surgical practice. This 40-item instrument consists of five-point Likert Scale items, with responses ranging from "none of the time" to "all of the time." The highest possible score is 200. The QoR-40 instrument has demonstrated good internal consistency and high test-retest reliability.[12]

The QoR-40 was preceded by a shorter version, which we will call the QoR-9.[25] This version has nine items with three responses available per item ("not at all," "some of the time," and "most of the time"). The total score achievable is 18 points, and patients are able to complete it in less than 2 min. Overall, these features render the QoR-9 an ideal quality-of-care auditing tool, and we strongly recommend its use to replace any existing hospital-based satisfaction surveys. The current disadvantage of the QoR-9 is that it has not been tested for RA; however, using the instrument to compare patients receiving GA and RA for similar surgical procedures should produce meaningful results. The items comprising the QoR-9 are listed in Table 14-1.

Medical Outcome and Health Status Surveys: SF-36, SF-8

The SF-36 is a 36-item survey that measures eight general health concepts, which are summarized in Table 14-2.[11] Each of the eight subscales is scored from 0 to 100 after a linear transformation that renders 0 as the least desirable health state and 100 the most desirable. The SF-36 also includes a single item measuring health transition, which is not used in the calculation of the other eight general health scores.

From these eight scale scores, two summary scores are computed: the physical component summary (PCS) and the mental component summary (MCS). These scores are normalized so that the population means equal 50 and the

Table 14-2   Patient Outcome Dimensions Queried by the Medical Outcomes Study SF-36, and Its Derivative SF-8 Scale

- Physical functioning
- Able to accomplish work and daily roles based on physical functioning
- Effects of bodily pain
- Personal evaluation of general health
- Vitality, or energy level
- Social functioning related to physical or emotional health
- Able to accomplish work and daily roles based on social functioning
- Personal evaluation of mental health

SOURCE: Adapted from Ware JE, Snow KK, Kosinski M, et al. *SF-36 Health Survey: Manual and Interpretation Guide.* Boston: Health Institute, 1997.

standard deviation equals 20. For the SF-36, data analysis and interpretation follows the protocols described by Ware et al.[11] These protocols include detailed guidelines for the timing of data collection, administration and completion, data entry, item recoding and calibration, treatment of missing data, computing raw scale scores, and transformation of scale scores.

The SF-36 has been commonly used as a generic patient-reported outcome measure after knee and hip replacement surgery.[27–29] These studies recommend that the SF-36 be used (more so than condition-specific knee outcome surveys) to assess patients with multiple comorbidities. The SF-36 has also been used for generic health assessment of patients with deficiency of the ACL, for example, and has reflected improved physical function with both surgical and nonsurgical treatment.[30]

The only published study that has used the SF-36 to compare patient outcomes after outpatient orthopedic surgery based on anesthesia and pain management technique was described by Wurm et al.[31] In this study, patients undergoing shoulder surgery were randomized to receive single-injection nerve blocks of the brachial plexus either before or after shoulder surgery with general anesthesia. The SF-36 was administered 7 days postoperatively and showed no differences between study groups on any SF-36 parameter. Patients receiving nerve blocks before surgery required less opioid during surgery and for 8 hr after surgery when compared with patients receiving the postoperative nerve block.

Daily postoperative assessments with the SF-36 are not recommended.[11,32] This is because the shortest recall period for the SF-36 (acute form) is 1 week. A new generation of single-item health measures, called the SF-8, is available for use in monitoring population health status and outcomes.[33] The SF-8 consists of eight items, one for each of the eight dimensions of health measured by the widely used SF-36 (summarized in Table 14-2). The SF-8 is designed for daily assessments. Scoring options include an eight-dimension health profile, as well as summary measures of the physical and mental components of health. A noteworthy feature of the SF-8 is that its health profile

and summary measures are scored on the same standard metrics as the SF-36 using norm-based scoring. Thus, the scores for all three instruments have the same means and standard deviations in the general U.S. population. Scores differ only in precision between SF-36 and SF-8 forms; and means can be compared directly.

It is likely that the SF-8 will fill a noteworthy gap in the field since it appears to be practical, psychometrically sound, and has a known relationship to widely used full-length measures that are the accepted standards in the field (e.g., SF-36). The SF-8 will likely make it possible to greatly increase the comprehensiveness of very acute monitoring efforts while keeping respondent burden to a minimum. For the same reasons as listed above for choosing the QoR-9 versus the QoR-40, using the SF-8 as a measure of general health status during the first week after surgery is likely to provide a meaningful assessment of patient outcomes that can be traced back to the anesthesia techniques used. We recommend the use of both the QoR-9 and the SF-8 in routine auditing of patient outcomes, replacing any nonvalidated hospital-based survey instruments.

Condition-Specific Patient-Reported Survey Instruments

For advanced clinical research involving comparisons of RA and GA, researchers should include a condition-specific outcome survey instrument. In orthopedic surgery, two such instruments include the Knee Outcome Survey,[34] and the Disabilities of the Arm, Shoulder, and Hand (DASH).[35] Condition-specific instruments are able to focus greater specificity on the rehabilitation process, more so than instruments simply querying general health status.

EXAMPLES OF COST ANALYSIS CALCULATIONS RELEVANT TO REGIONAL ANESTHESIA IN OUTPATIENT SURGERY

Cost-Minimization Analysis

For this analysis, we shall assume that the outcomes are equal for patients undergoing continuous peripheral nerve block for analgesia comparing ropivacaine 0.2% and levobupivacaine 0.125%, in conjunction with a standardized anesthetic technique. The cost analysis is then simplified: the product cost of the two local anesthetic agents is tabulated, and the results are achieved. If a cost analysis were performed on the recent study by Casati et al. comparing these two interscalene infusion drugs where pain and physical function outcomes were considered equal,[36] the only difference would be in the costs of the two drugs used.

Cost-Effectiveness Analysis

For the CEA, we shall assume that patients are undergoing unicompartmental knee arthroplasty using a standardized anesthetic technique, and continuous peripheral nerve block techniques comparing the use of ropivacaine 0.2%

with clonidine versus levobupivacaine 0.125% with clonidine. The surgical objective is to achieve full ambulation by the morning after surgery. Let us assume that analgesia is equal, but motor block is greater in the levobupivacaine-clonidine combination (strictly speculation for this example), and patients in this group are unable to ambulate until postoperative day 2, whereas the ropivacaine-clonidine patients are fully able to ambulate on the first postoperative day. When the costs are calculated, the result is reported as follows: The cost for the levobupivacaine-clonidine combination was $X, but the incremental cost of the ropivacaine-clonidine combination was $X+Y, with the effectiveness variable of 1 day of disability avoided with the ropivacaine-clonidine combination.

Cost–Benefit Analysis

Using the same study design for the CEA example above, the effectiveness variable for CBA now takes on a monetary value. Assume the primary inclusion criterion for males undergoing unicompartmental knee arthroplasty was being a factory foreman paid an hourly wage, who is not paid for time off for medical leave. The "return to work" outcome takes the form of "achieved wages." Patients who are able to return to work 1 day sooner are then concluded to have required a cost increment of $Y to achieve $200 (for example) in daily wages. This concludes the example of unicompartmental knee replacement.

In a more complex example of different anesthetic techniques, assume patients are willing to pay $400 for a successful surgery and to avoid an unplanned hospital admission,[22] whereas they are only willing to pay $1 for an otherwise successful surgery complicated by symptomatic pain and PONV requiring an unplanned hospital admission. In the comparison of two patients with anesthetic techniques and outcomes as follows: (1) thiopental-succinylcholine-endotracheal tube-isoflurane anesthesia associated with a $50 drug/supplies cost,[6] a $420 cost associated with a PACU admission and symptom management, and a $380 cost associated with an unplanned admission and symptom management,[15] and (2) exclusive RA technique including prolonged single-injection peripheral nerve block analgesia (and propofol sedation) costing $90 (with PACU bypass and a symptom-free same-day hospital discharge). The first (GA) scenario's cost-benefit ratio would be 850:1, whereas the cost-benefit ratio for the second scenario would be 90:400 (or 0.225:1). The magnitude of monetary benefit-to-cost, using patient WTP values would be 850:0.225, or 3556. Obviously, these differences in outcomes of the two patients in question are quite dramatic; the necessary inclusion of the outcomes of the entire sample size would mandate the use of weighted-average decision-tree techniques to determine a cost-benefit value that is closer to "reality."

Cost–Utility Analysis

Cost-utility analysis involves the insertion of a patient-reported effectiveness variable into the denominator of the cost analysis. We will use the QoR-9 of Myles et al.[25] as a measure of utility from the patient's perspective, and compare the GA patient ($850 cost) with the RA/peripheral nerve block patient ($90 cost) in the previous paragraph. Let us assume that in the first day after surgery, the GA patient has a QoR-9 score of 10 (out of a possible 18), whereas the RA patient has a QoR-9 score of 17 (of 18). The cost-utility ratios would be 850:10 versus 90:17. When the denominator is corrected to the value of 1, the cost-utility magnitude of difference between the 2 outcomes described is 16.

Obviously, the preceding examples are quite simplistic and do not account for the significant variability in the care of many patients. However, the core structure of the analyses, including multiple variables that are important contributors to costs and outcomes, can be analyzed using decision analysis trees and weighted-average techniques, to provide meaningful comparisons of health care programs.

SUMMARY

Cost analysis techniques are valuable tools to help physicians and administrators meet these new challenges presented by health care market forces. Health care expenditures and various forms of outcomes such as monetary benefits in CBA, health status changes in CEA, and patient-reported quality of life in CUA can be studied in reasonable detail. Meaningful equations and comparisons among techniques can be derived. If outcomes are determined to be equivalent regardless of the treatment program implemented, then a fundamental CMA is all that is required.

Comparisons between RA and GA require a cost-benefit, cost-utility, and/or cost-effectiveness analysis, as it is unlikely that outcomes will be similar. On the other hand, comparison of two medications delivered in an otherwise standardized continuous catheter RA technique, for example, may lend itself to a CMA, if outcomes are otherwise essentially equal.

As physicians caring for individual patients, it is important to not base one's practice strictly on cost analysis; instead, one should use cost analysis as a tool to justify RA programs in the institution, while providing ample time for individual patient education to justify the use of RA techniques for the upcoming surgical procedure.

REFERENCES

1. Praemer A, Furner S, Rice DP. *Musculoskeletal Conditions in the United States.* Rosemont, IL: American Academy of Orthopaedic Surgeons, 1999.
2. Drummond MF, O'Brien B, Stoddart GL, et al. (eds.). *Methods for the Economic Evaluation of Health Care Programmes,* 2nd ed. Oxford: Oxford University Press, 1997.
3. Pavlin DJ, Rapp SE, Polissar NL, et al. Factors affecting discharge time in adult outpatients. Anesth Analg 1998;87:816–26.
4. Pavlin DJ, Chen C, Penaloza DA, et al. Pain as a factor complicating recovery and discharge after ambulatory surgery. Anesth Analg 2002;95:627–34.
5. Gold MR, Siegel JE, Russell LB, et al (eds.). *Cost-Effectiveness in Health and Medicine.* New York: Oxford University Press, 1996.

6. Williams BA, DeRiso BM, Engel LB, et al. Benchmarking the perioperative process. II. Introducing anesthesia clinical pathways to improve processes and outcomes, and reduce nursing labor intensity in ambulatory orthopedic surgery. J Clin Anesth 1998;10:561–69.

7. Williams BA, DeRiso BM, Figallo CM, et al. Benchmarking the perioperative process. III. Effects of regional anesthesia clinical pathway techniques on process efficiency and recovery profiles in ambulatory orthopedic surgery. J Clin Anesth 1998;10:570–78.

8. Williams BA, Kentor ML, Williams JP, et al. Process analysis in outpatient knee surgery: effects of regional and general anesthesia on anesthesia-controlled time. Anesthesiology 2000;93:529–38.

9. Williams BA, Kentor ML, Williams JP, et al. PACU bypass after outpatient knee surgery is associated with fewer unplanned hospital admissions but more phase II nursing interventions. Anesthesiology 2002;97:981–88.

10. Williams BA, Kentor ML, Vogt MT, et al. Femoral-sciatic nerve blocks for complex outpatient knee surgery are associated with less postoperative pain before same-day discharge: a review of 1200 consecutive cases from the period 1996–1999. Anesthesiology 2003;98:1206–13.

11. Ware JE, Kosinski M, Kemoun G. SF-36 Physical and Mental Health Summary Scales: A User's Manual, 5th printing. Boston: Health Assessment Lab, 1994.

12. Myles PS, Weitkamp B, Jones K, et al. Validity and reliability of a postoperative quality of recovery score: the QoR-40. Br J Anaesth 2000;84:11–15.

13. Macario A, Vitez TS, Dunn B, et al. Where are the costs in perioperative care? Analysis of hospital costs and charges for inpatient surgical care. Anesthesiology 1995;83:1138–44.

14. Dexter F, Macario A, Manberg PJ, et al. Computer simulation to determine how rapid anesthetic recovery protocols to decrease the time for emergence or increase the phase I postanesthesia care unit bypass rate affect staffing of an ambulatory surgery center. Anesth Analg 1999;88:1053–63.

15. Williams BA, Kentor ML, Vogt MT, et al. The economics of nerve block pain management after anterior cruciate ligament reconstruction: significant hospital cost savings via associated PACU bypass and same-day discharge. Anesthesiology 2004;100(3):697–706.

16. Woolhandler S, Himmelstein DU. Costs of care and administration at for-profit and other hospitals in the United States. N Engl J Medi 1997;336:769–74.

17. Kitz DS, Slusary-Ladden C, Lecky JH. Hospital resources used for inpatients and ambulatory surgery. Anesthesiology 1988;69:383–86.

18. DeVellis RF. Scale Development: Theory and Applications. Newbury Park: Sage Publications, 1991.

19. McDowell I, Newell C. Measuring Health, 2d ed. New York: Oxford University Press, 1996.

20. Leslie K, Lee L, Myles PS, et al. Patients' knowledge of and attitudes towards awareness and depth of anaesthesia monitoring. Anaesth Intens Care 2003;31:63–68.

21. Macario A, Weinger M, Carney S, et al. Which clinical anesthesia outcomes are important to avoid? The perspective of patients. Anesth Analg 1999;89:652–58.

22. Lehmann HP, Fleisher LA, Lam J, et al. Patient preferences for early discharge after laparoscopic cholecystectomy. Anesth Analg 1999;88:1280–85.

23. Gan T, Sloan F, Dear G, et al. How much are patients willing to pay to avoid postoperative nausea and vomiting? Anesth Analg 2001;92:393–400.

24. Sneyd JR, Carr A, Byrom WD, et al. A meta-analysis of nausea and vomiting following maintenance of anaesthesia with propofol or inhalational agents. Eur J Anaesthesiol 1998;15:433–45.

25. Myles PS, Hunt JO, Nightingale CE, et al. Development and psychometric testing of a Quality of Recovery score after general anesthesia and surgery in adults. Anesth Analg 1999;88:83–90.

26. Dexter F, Aker J, Wright WA. Development of a measure of patient satisfaction with monitored anesthesia care: the Iowa Satisfaction with Anesthesia Scale. Anesthesiology 1997;87:865–73.

27. Kantz ME, Harris WJ, Levitsky K, et al. Methods for assessing condition-specific and generic functional status outcomes after total knee replacement. Med Care 1992;30:MS240–52.

28. Hawker G, Melfi C, Paul J, et al. Comparison of a generic (SF-36) and a disease specific (WOMAC) instrument in the measurement of outcomes after knee replacement surgery. J Rheumatol 1995;22:1193–96.

29. Bombardier C, Melfi CA, Paul J, et al. Comparison of a generic and a disease-specific measure of pain and physical function after knee replacement surgery. Med Care 1995;33:AS131–44.

30. Shapiro ET. The use of a generic, patient-based health assessment (SF-36) for evaluation of patients with anterior cruciate ligament injuries. Am J Sports Med 1996;24:196–200.

31. Wurm WH, Concepcion M, Sternlicht A, Carabuena JM, Robelen G, Goudas LC, et al. Preoperative interscalene block for elective shoulder surgery: loss of benefit over early postoperative block after patient discharge to home. Anesth Analg 2003;97(6):1620–26.

32. Ware JE, Snow KK, Kosinski M, et al. SF-36 Health Survey: Manual and Interpretation Guide. Boston: Health Institute, 1997.

33. Ware JE, Kosinski M, Dewey JE, et al. How to Score and Interpret Single-Item Health Status Measures: A Manual for Users of the SF-8(TM) Health Survey. Lincoln, RI: QualityMetric, 2001.

34. Irrgang JJ, Snyder-Mackler L, Wainner RS, et al. Development of a patient-reported measure of function of the knee. J Bone Joint Surg 1998;80-A:1132–45.

35. Beaton DE, Katz JN, Fossel AH, et al. Measuring the whole or the parts? Validity, reliability, and responsiveness of the Disabilities of the Arm, Shoulder and Hand outcome measure in different regions of the upper extremity. J Hand Ther 2001;14:128–46.

36. Casati A, Borghi B, Fanelli G, et al. Interscalene brachial plexus anesthesia and analgesia for open shoulder surgery: a randomized, double-blinded comparison between levobupivacaine and ropivacaine. Anesth Analg 2003;96:253–59.

PART III

GENERAL SEDATION AND ANALGESIA PRINCIPLES

Inhalation Agents for Ambulatory Anesthesia

KAREN J. SOUTER   •   D. JANET PAVLIN

INTRODUCTION

At the beginning of the twenty-first century, four inhalational anesthetics are in routine use in ambulatory anesthesia: the halogenated ethers isoflurane, sevoflurane, and desflurane, and the anesthetic gas nitrous oxide. The aims of this chapter are to consider how closely each approaches the ideal for ambulatory anesthesia. Characteristics proposed by a number of authors for an ideal outpatient anesthetic are shown in Table 15-1.[1–3]

INDUCTION OF ANESTHESIA

Induction of general anesthesia should be rapid, smooth, and pleasant for the patient. In adults, the vast majority of inductions are performed using intravenous anesthetic agents, particularly propofol. None of the volatile anesthetics are comparable to propofol with respect to attaining a rapid, smooth induction, although certain characteristics of propofol induction such as pain on injection, apnea, or hypotension may be considered relatively undesirable. However, there are circumstances where an inhalational induction is desirable or specifically indicated (Table 15-2) and where induction characteristics become particularly relevant.

Induction of anesthesia with a volatile anesthetic requires the development of a drug concentration in the brain sufficient to cause loss of consciousness. The concentration and partial pressure of anesthetic in the brain are directly proportional to partial pressure in alveoli. The rate of rise of partial pressure and concentration in the alveolus determines the rate of rise of concentration in the brain and the speed of induction. All other factors being equal, the rate of rise of alveolar anesthetic concentration (F_A) is inversely proportional to the blood solubility of the anesthetic agent,[4,5] commonly expressed as the blood/gas partition coefficient (relative affinity of an anesthetic for the gaseous phase in the alveolus vs. the liquid phase in blood) (Table 15-3). Of the agents in common use, desflurane would be expected to produce the most rapid anesthetic induction based on its very low solubility in blood, and thus, rapid equilibration between partial pressures of gas in alveoli and blood (Fig. 15-1).

Table 15-1   Properties of the Ideal Volatile Agent for Ambulatory Anesthesia

Rapid, smooth onset of anesthesia
Produces sedation, hypnosis, amnesia, analgesia, and muscle relaxation
Lacks undesirable intraoperative side effects
Provides rapid recovery profile without postoperative side effects
Provides residual analgesia during the early postoperative period
Cost-effective relative to other available drugs

SOURCE: Adapted from Smith J, Nathanson MH, White PF. The role of sevoflurane in outpatient anesthesia. Anesth Analg 1995;81:567–72.

Table 15-2   Indications for Inhalational Induction

The technique of choice in many pediatric patients
A technique for adults who are needle-phobic
Occasional patient preference
A rapid recovery free from the hangover effects of intravenous induction agents
To maintain spontaneous ventilation

Table 15-3   Blood/Gas Partition Coefficients at 37° C

Anesthetic	Blood/Gas Partition Coefficient
Desflurane	0.42
Cyclopropane	0.46
Nitrous oxide	0.47
Sevoflurane	0.69
Isoflurane	1.4
Enflurane	1.92
Halothane	2.54
Diethyl ether	12
Methoxyflurane	15

However, an additional important factor to be considered when describing the induction characteristics of an anesthetic is its effect on the airway. Airway irritation can provoke breath holding, coughing, laryngospasm, and excessive salivation, all of which may reduce ventilation, potentially impeding anesthetic uptake, or causing hypoxia. Such effects may not only be unpleasant for the patient, but also potentially harmful. In fact, desflurane has a propensity to cause airway irritation, particularly in

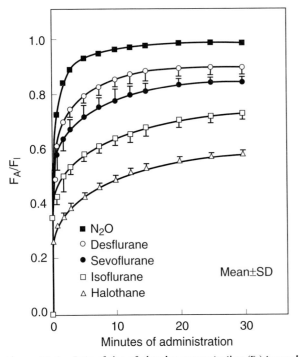

Figure 15-1   Rate of rise of alveolar concentration (F_A) toward inspired concentration (F_I) with volatile anesthetic agents. (Reproduced with permission from Yasuda N, Lockhart SH, Eger EI, Weiskopf RB, Liu J, Laster MJ, et al. Comparison of kinetics of sevoflurane and isoflurane in humans. Anesth Analg 1991;72:316–24.)

children,[6] making it less desirable for gas induction than is sevoflurane.

Inhalational Induction Techniques

Tidal Breathing Inhalational Induction[7]

The classic slow method of inhalational induction is to administer an anesthetic in low concentration in a carrier gas mixture of oxygen and nitrous oxide and to slowly increase the inspired concentration of the volatile anesthetic in a stepwise manner to avoid causing airway irritation.[8]

Vital Capacity Rapid Inhalation Induction

The first description of a rapid single breath induction was reported for cyclopropane in 1954.[9] The low blood gas solubility of cyclopropane (0.46) and its lack of airway irritability allowed induction by a single breath of anesthetic. In 1985 Ruffle et al. described a *vital capacity rapid inhalation induction* (VCRII) technique for halothane.[10] The technique involved priming a circle system with high concentrations of volatile anesthetic using high flows (10 L/min) for 2 min. Volunteers were instructed to exhale to residual volume, then take a slow vital capacity breath (VCB) from the primed circuit and hold their breath for 30–90 sec. After this, they continued breathing from the circuit for 2 min. With 4% halothane in oxygen, induction was achieved in less than 3.5 min. When 67% nitrous oxide was incorporated in the gas mixture, speed of induction was further reduced to 83 sec.[11]

Isoflurane

This VCRII technique has since been applied to newer volatile anesthetics. Isoflurane has a lower blood gas solubility than halothane, and theoretically, should produce a more rapid inhalational induction. In children, however, isoflurane induction caused significantly more airway irritation, breath holding, and laryngospasm, actually prolonging induction.[12,13] In adults, 2% isoflurane administered as a single VCB in 66% nitrous oxide produced rapid induction with fewer airway-related side effects than a conventional stepwise induction with isoflurane.[14] Subsequent studies demonstrated that premedication with fentanyl (5 μg/kg) and glycopyrrolate[15] or humidification of inspired gases[16,17] further reduced the incidence of side effects. However, gas induction with isoflurane has never really become popular and the introduction of sevoflurane into clinical practice has made further attempts to improve induction with isoflurane redundant.

Sevoflurane

The blood gas solubility of sevoflurane is half that of isoflurane (0.65), and perhaps more significantly, sevoflurane is much less irritating to the airways.

There are numerous studies examining the induction time in adults with sevoflurane. These are summarized in Table 15-4. When these studies are scrutinized, two factors appear

Table 15-4   Comparison of Induction Agents and Inhalational Induction Techniques in Adults

Author (Date)	Induction Method[a]	Drugs Compared	O₂/N₂O	Definition of Induction	Induction Time (sec)[b]	Premedication	Acceptable
Fredman[27] (1995)	TBII	3–4% Sevoflurane	40/60	Loss of response to verbal commands	153	Fentanyl	Yes
		Propofol			92 (S)		
Yurino[128] (1993)	VCB	4.5 % sevoflurane	100/0	Failure to respond to commands	81 (S)	None	Yes
		2% halothane			153		
Yurino[20] (1993)	VCB	4.5% sevoflurane	33/66	Failure to respond to commands	54 (S)	None	Yes
	TBII	Sevoflurane increased 0.5% every 3 breaths			108		Yes
Sloan[129] (1996)	VCB	5% sevoflurane	50/50	Loss of eyelash reflex	75	Midazolam	Yes
		5% isoflurane			67 (NS)		
Smith[22] (1992)	TBII	5% sevoflurane	40/60	Failure to respond to commands	109	Fentanyl	Not determined
		Propofol			<60 (S)		
Shah[30] (2001)	VCB	6% sevoflurane Propofol	33/66	BIS value below 70	95 70 (S)	None	Yes
Muzi[25] (1996)	VCB ×3	6–7% sevoflurane	28/66	Loss of eyelid reflex	66 (NS)	None	Not determined
		6–7% sevoflurane	100/0		66		
Yurino[21] (1995)	VCB	7.5% sevoflurane	33/66	Failure to respond to commands	41 (S)	None	Yes
	TBII				52		Yes
Ti[24] (1998)	VCB	7.5% sevoflurane	33/67	Loss of response to verbal commands	45	Midazolam	Yes
		3.5% isoflurane			71		
Muzi[23] (1997)	VCB	8% sevoflurane	33/66	Loss of eyelash reflex	80 (S)	Fentanyl	Not determined
					93	Midazolam	
					89	Fentanyl + Midazolam	
Siau[7] (2002)	TBII	8% sevoflurane	33/66	Cessation of finger tapping/loss eyelid reflex	62 (NS)	None	Yes
			100/0		60		
Dashfield[18] (1998)	VCB	8% sevoflurane	33/66	Loss eye-lash reflex	54 (S)	Fentanyl	Not determined
		Propofol			92		
		8% sevoflurane		Time to drop a weight[c]	75 (S)		
		Propofol			93		

(Continued)

Table 15–4   Comparison of Induction Agents and Inhalational Induction Techniques in Adults (*Continued*)

Author (Date)	Induction Method[a]	Drugs Compared	O₂/N₂O	Definition of Induction	Induction Time (sec)[b]	Premedication	Acceptable
Thwaites[29] (1997)	TBII	8% sevoflurane	33/66	Time to drop a weight	84	None	"Mask induction unpleasant"
		Propofol			57 (S)		
Kirkbride[19] (2001)	TBII	8% sevoflurane	50/50	Time to drop a weight	97	None	Yes
		Sevoflurane increased by 1% every 3 breaths to 8%			130 (S)		
		Propofol			107		
Hall[26] (1997)	VCB	8% sevoflurane	33/66	Cessation of finger tapping	53	None	Yes
		8% sevoflurane	100/0		57		
		Propofol			40 (S)		

[a]Induction methods: VCB = vital capacity breath; TBII = tidal breathing inhalational induction.

[b]S = significant difference; NS = not significantly different.

[c]Held between the thumb and index finger of the dominant hand.

to be important in determining induction time with sevoflurane: the inspired concentration and the induction technique.

The higher the initial inspired concentration the more rapid the induction. In one study induction was found to be faster with 8% sevoflurane than with propofol[18] and in another, induction with 8% sevoflurane was comparable to propofol.[19] The remaining studies all show that propofol is the faster-onset induction agent (Table 15-4).

Use of the VCB technique speeds up inhalational induction with sevoflurane compared to tidal breathing inhalational induction (TBII) techniques.[20,21] The incidence of complications during induction, including laryngeal spasm, coughing, salivation, breath holding, and involuntary movements, varies considerably between studies; overall sevoflurane produces fewer complications during induction than propofol.[19,22] These complications appear to be less with the VCB technique.[21]

The Effects of Premedication

Most studies report very little benefit from premedication with either fentanyl or midazolam.[22–24] In one example, fentanyl increased the incidence of airway complications such as apnea and breath holding, making airway management more difficult during induction.[23]

The Effects of Nitrous Oxide

Nitrous oxide is traditionally used as a carrier gas for inhalational induction. However, when higher concentrations of sevoflurane are used[7,25] there is no improvement in speed of induction with nitrous oxide as the carrier gas.

Cardiovascular Stability

Generally the cardiovascular effects of sevoflurane induction are similar to those of other agents including propofol.[18,26–28] Some studies, however, report greater degrees of hypotension with intravenous induction with propofol than with sevoflurane inhalational induction techniques;[29,30] this was also noted in a group of elderly patients.[19]

Laryngeal Mask Airway Insertion and Tracheal Intubation

Several investigations examine the time taken to achieve satisfactory conditions for laryngeal mask airway (LMA) insertion and tracheal intubation after gaseous induction with sevoflurane. Using 6–7% sevoflurane LMA insertion was possible after 1.7 min[25] and 2.2 min.[31] LMA insertion was achieved in 3.5 min with 8% sevoflurane in 100% oxygen and in 2.8 min with 8% sevoflurane in 66% nitrous oxide.[26]

Tracheal intubation (without the use of muscle relaxants) was possible in 4.7 min (6–7% sevoflurane in 66% nitrous oxide) and 6.4 min (6–7% sevoflurane in 100% oxygen). The minimal alveolar concentration (MAC) value of sevoflurane for tracheal intubation has variously been estimated as 4.52%[32] and 3.55%.[33]

Desflurane

As the least soluble of available anesthetic agents, desflurane would be expected to provide the most rapid inhalational induction. However, using a stepwise technique, induction times have been reported as approximately 2 min with or without nitrous oxide,[34,35] with a high incidence of coughing, breath holding, and excitatory movements. Loss of consciousness occurred at end tidal desflurane concentrations of 5.9% with nitrous oxide and 6.5% without nitrous oxide. When compared to propofol, induction times with desflurane were significantly longer owing to airway irritability precipitated by desflurane.[35,36] Nitrous oxide decreased induction time but this was still not equivalent to propofol.[37] In children, who have a relatively low functional residual capacity (FRC), use of nitrous oxide was sometimes associated with bothersome desaturation and has generally resulted in abandonment of this technique. Airway irritation appears to be maximal when inspired concentrations of desflurane approach 1 MAC (7%). It has been suggested[38] that irritation may be overcome by rapidly increasing the anesthetic concentration above 1 MAC, theoretically shortening the duration of the excitement phase. However, this hypothesis has not been tested or proven to be true. Other studies have demonstrated that rapid escalation of inspired desflurane concentrations is associated with "autonomic activation" (hypertension and tachycardia).[39] Airway irritability with desflurane may be overcome to some extent by premedication with fentanyl and midazolam,[38] although induction still takes approximately 100 sec. Desflurane, however, is still considered by many, as being too pungent for routine inhalational induction, particularly in children.

MAINTENANCE OF ANESTHESIA

Minimal Alveolar Concentration

Minimal alveolar concentration was originally defined by Merkel and Eger in 1963 as the minimal alveolar concentration of an anesthetic required to prevent movement in 50% of subjects in response to a surgical incision.[40] The values of MAC for sevoflurane and desflurane are shown in Table 15-5.

Physiologic Side Effects and Toxicity of Inhaled Anesthetics

Cardiovascular System

Hemodynamic effects of the various inhalational anesthetics are similar.[41–44] All three volatile anesthetics decrease myocardial contractility, cardiac output, blood pressure, and peripheral resistance in a dose-dependent fashion.

Isoflurane, and desflurane to a lesser extent, typically produce a dose-related increase in heart rate. This tends to compensate for any reduction in contractility such that cardiac output tends to be well maintained up to 1 MAC. Sevoflurane produces less increase in heart rate than occurs with isoflurane.[45] Myocardial blood flow is better maintained with desflurane than with isoflurane or halothane. "Coronary steal" (whereby dilation of coronary blood vessels in areas of normal perfusion diverts blood flow away from areas of compromised perfusion) has not been proven to occur with desflurane,[46] nor with sevoflurane.[47]

In human volunteers, sudden increases of inspired desflurane concentration have been associated with significant but transient increases in heart rate and mean arterial blood pressure (autonomic activation).[39,48] These effects were less apparent when studied in patients.[42,49] Sympathetic stimulation caused by desflurane is thought to be due to either direct stimulation of medullary centers in the brain, or the effects on irritant receptors in the airway, and is accompanied by increases in circulating levels of catecholamines.[39]

All three potent inhalants tend to preserve regional blood flow to viscera and kidneys up to concentrations exceeding 1 MAC, above which hepatic and splanchnic blood flow are reduced. As is typical of ethers, none of the three commonly used inhalants predispose to epinephrine-induced cardiac arrhythmias.

Respiratory System[44,46]

Desflurane and sevoflurane decrease the ventilatory response to carbon dioxide (CO_2), causing ventilatory depression and mild hypercarbia in spontaneously breathing subjects, and may cause apnea at between 1.5 and 2 MAC. Increasing concentrations cause a progressive decline in tidal volume with a compensatory increase in respiratory rate that in part offsets the decreased tidal volume. Sevoflurane is not irritating to the airway and is effective at reversing bronchospasm. Isoflurane and desflurane (as described above) are both irritating to the airways[46] at the inception of anesthesia, making inhalational induction potentially difficult. However, desflurane and sevoflurane, as well as isoflurane, are bronchodilators and are safe for maintenance of anesthesia in asthmatic patients.

Central Nervous System[50]

The effects of sevoflurane, desflurane, and isoflurane on the central nervous system (CNS) are comparable. Up to 1 MAC cerebral blood flow does not increase and cerebral autoregulation remains intact. The effects on intracranial pressure

Table 15-5 MAC (%) of Sevoflurane and Desflurane at Various Ages with and without Nitrous Oxide

Agent	Neonates	With N₂O	Adults	With N₂O	Elderly (age in years)	With N₂O
Sevoflurane	3.3	2.5	2.05	1.6	1.3 (87)	0.65 (87)
Desflurane	9.96	7.15	6.0	2.83	5.17 (70)	1.67 (70)

SOURCE: Adapted from Young CJ, Apfelbaum JL. Inhalational anesthetics: desflurane and sevoflurane. J Clin Anesth 1995;7:564–77.

are also similar although may be more marked with desflurane. Desflurane, sevoflurane, and isoflurane all produce dose-dependent depression of the electroencefalogram (EEG) and neither agent provokes epileptiform activity.

Musculoskeletal System

Sevoflurane and isoflurane produce dose-dependent muscle relaxation comparable to that seen with isoflurane and potentiate the effects of nondepolarizing neuromuscular blocking agents. Studies comparing desflurane and sevoflurane to propofol infusions for maintenance of anesthesia in spontaneously breathing patients have found that the volatile agents are less likely to cause spontaneous movements during surgery.[51,52] All three volatile agents have the potential to trigger malignant hyperpyrexia.

Hepatorenal Effects and Drug Toxicity

None of the three inhalational anesthetics appear to have toxic effects on the liver or kidney when used in clinical concentrations. With halothane, it has been speculated that drug metabolites may be causally related to cases of "halothane hepatitis." Approximately 15–20% of halothane is metabolized, in comparison to only 2–5% of sevoflurane[53] and 0.2% for isoflurane. Desflurane is relatively inert; only 0.02% is metabolized,[54] theoretically making it least likely to be associated with toxicity to the liver or other organs assuming toxicity is truly related to drug metabolites.

Compound A toxicity.   Compound A is a degradation product of sevoflurane that is nephrotoxic in rats, although Eger has recently suggested[55] that compound A is not a cause of any great concern in humans. The package label in the United States warns that sevoflurane should not be administered with a flow rate less than 1 L/min. The production of compound A can be minimized by using smaller canisters of absorbent[56] and also by using absorbents that contain little or no sodium and potassium hydroxide.[57]

Carbon monoxide formation.   Of greater concern than compound A, is the degradation of desflurane and isoflurane to carbon monoxide (CO) by desiccated or partly desiccated absorbents. Of all agents deflurane produces the greatest and sevoflurane the least amount of CO.[58] Carbon monoxide formation occurs in situations where the absorbent has been allowed to dry out, particularly in anesthesia machines that have been unused for prolonged periods. With the rapid turnover of cases in an ambulatory surgery department, desiccation of absorbent is unlikely to be a problem and frequent changes of the absorbent reduce CO production. Absorbents that contain sodium and particularly potassium hydroxide produce more CO than those that are free of these strong bases.[57]

RECOVERY CHARACTERISTICS

In rats, the speed of recovery has been related directly to the blood gas partition coefficient of volatile anesthetics, and to the depth and duration of anesthesia (MAC hr)[59]

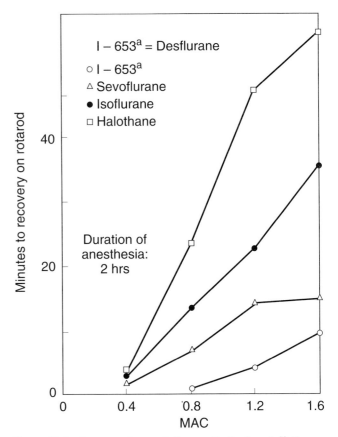

Figure 15-2   Recovery from volatile anesthetics in rats.[59] (Reproduced with permission from Eger EI, Johnson BH. Rates of awakening from anesthesia with I-653, halothane, isoflurane, and sevoflurane: a test of the effect of anesthetic concentration and duration in rats. Anesth Analg 1987;66(10):977–82.)

(Fig. 15-2). In humans however, although the same pharmacokinetic factors are operant, the pharmacodynamic characteristics of anesthetics appear to be of near-equal or greater importance in determining the speed or quality of recovery in ambulatory surgery.

When comparing recovery characteristics of different anesthetics, it is important to consider which factors correlate with speed of recovery and discharge after ambulatory surgery. In one prospective analysis of patients undergoing ambulatory surgery,[60] the most important predictor of speed of recovery was the identity of the recovery room nurse caring for the patient. The anesthetic drugs utilized for induction and maintenance of general anesthesia were of some significance in women (accounting for approximately 4% of variability in recovery times), but less so in men. In individual patients, factors that most commonly delayed discharge from Phase 1 or Phase 2 recovery included pain, drowsiness, postoperative nausea and vomiting (PONV), unresolved local anesthetic block, inability to void, and shivering. PONV and postoperative pain[61] are also two of the most important factors accounting for unexpected hospital admissions in day surgery patients. These observations are important to understanding and interpreting studies that have compared recovery rates and discharge times after various anesthetics.

End points that are commonly used to characterize recovery after ambulatory surgery are shown in Table 15-6. Generally, they include initial emergence parameters, intermediate milestones of recovery, and, last, actual time of discharge (or time to achieve "discharge readiness"). In humans, the initial recovery period, referred to as "emergence," is probably most directly related to the blood gas solubility of the volatile anesthetics. Theoretically, a less soluble drug will be more rapidly eliminated and will be associated with more rapid awakening. In animals, speed of recovery was strongly influenced by the duration and depth of anesthesia (MAC hr) for more soluble anesthetics (halothane), but less so for relatively insoluble anesthetics such as desflurane.[59] Consistent with this prediction, Tsai et al.[62] reported there was no significant difference in patient recovery times after desflurane/nitrous oxide anesthesia when comparing anesthetics that lasted less than 100 min, 100–140 min, or over 150 min. Because of its low solubility in blood and brain tissue, partial pressures of desflurane equilibrate rapidly between body compartments. As a result, increasing duration of anesthesia causes a relatively small increment in the amount of anesthetic stored in the body that must be eliminated.

Sevoflurane

Recovery from Sevoflurane Compared to Isoflurane and Propofol

In an analysis of eight studies comparing recovery after sevoflurane to recovery after isoflurane,[63] times to achieving early end points of recovery (emergence) were significantly shorter with sevoflurane (on average 3.3 min), except in cases lasting less than 1 hr, when there was no difference. Although another study has demonstrated significantly faster emergence from sevoflurane compared to isoflurane in cases lasting less than 1 hr,[43] the actual difference was small (2 min). Other outpatient studies[64–66] have confirmed that early emergence is more rapid with sevoflurane, but the time to home readiness or discharge is typically not different to isoflurane.

A number of studies have demonstrated that patients receiving sevoflurane for maintenance emerge more rapidly than those maintained with propofol infusion, irrespective of whether induction was with sevoflurane or propofol.[66–68] In these studies, although the time for emergence was statistically faster with sevoflurane, the actual differences were only a matter of minutes. Furthermore, comparisons of later recovery parameters (psychomotor tests, recovery scores, and time to discharge) show no significant differences. A few studies[27,63] have reported finding no difference in emergence times between patients anesthetized with sevoflurane compared to propofol.

Desflurane

Recovery from Desflurane Compared to Isoflurane and Propofol

In outpatient studies,[69] including a meta-anylsis,[70] patients emerged from desflurane anesthesia on average 4.4 min earlier than from isoflurane. A few studies have also demonstrated more rapid discharge with desflurane when compared to isoflurane.[49] Other studies have reported more rapid recovery of psychomotor function with desflurane, but with no effect on time to discharge.[62,71]

When comparing recovery from desflurane to recovery from propofol infusion, the results are mixed. Some studies reported more rapid emergence, by an average of 3 min, and improved recovery of psychomotor tests after desflurane compared to propofol.[34,35,72,73] Recovery was particularly fast when desflurane was used for induction and maintenance.[34] Other investigators, however, have not been able to demonstrate any differences in emergence times between propofol and desflurane anesthetics.[51,74] A meta-anylsis of studies where propofol was used for induction and either desflurane or propofol was the maintenance agent[70] reported that patients receiving propofol tended to be able to sit up earlier. These patients were also

Table 15-6   End Points of Recovery from General Anesthesia

Phase of Recovery	Assessment Modality	Time (min) from Discontinuing Anesthesia
Emergence	Opens eyes	0–15
	Obeys commands	
	Extubation	
	Orientation	
Intermediate recovery		
Clinical assessment	Aldrete scores[130]	15–60
	Modified Aldrete scores	
Cognitive and psychomotor function	Trieger test	30–120
	Digital Symbol Substitution test	
	Deletion test	
	Critical Flicker Fusion Threshold test	
	Critical reaction time	
Discharge (Home) readiness	Able to sit up	60–180
	Able to stand	
	Minimal PONV	
	Minimal pain	
	Able to eat and drink	
	Able to void	

discharged home 17 min earlier, probably as a result of experiencing less nausea and vomiting.

Desflurane Compared to Sevoflurane

Desflurane has a lower blood gas solubility than sevoflurane and recovery from anesthesia should be faster with desflurane. In studies comparing recovery from these two inhalational anesthetics in outpatients,[42,75] early emergence was faster by approximately 3 min with desflurane. Recovery of psychomotor function was marginally, but not significantly, better. When sevoflurane and desflurane were compared using the bispectral index (BIS) to titrate to a particular anesthetic depth,[76] emergence was significantly shorter in BIS-titrated desflurane patients than in a BIS-titrated sevoflurane group. In all studies, however, there were no differences in the length of postanesthesia care unit (PACU) stay and time to home readiness.

Fast-Tracking and Volatile Anesthetics

"Fast-tracking" in ambulatory surgery refers to bypassing the PACU by transferring patients directly from the operating room (OR) to a step-down (phase II) recovery area.[77,78] When fast-tracking is used for appropriate patients, overall recovery times have been reduced and significant cost savings reported.[79] In theory, use of anesthetic agents with a rapid recovery spectrum should allow more patients to be fast-tracked although other factors may determine whether fast-tracking of patients actually occurs.[79] Coloma et al.[80] compared propofol infusion with sevoflurane and desflurane for maintenance of anesthesia using the BIS to titrate anesthetic depth to a value of 60. Significantly more patients maintained with volatile agents were judged to be eligible for fast-tracking at the end of an anesthetic than those who received propofol, although only between 35% and 53% of these patients were actually fast-tracked. The time to home readiness was the same in all patients. Another study[81] also shows that desflurane and sevoflurane perform better than propofol in achieving fast-tracking criteria in ambulatory patients.

Postoperative Side Effects

Pain

There are obvious advantages to rapid emergence from anesthesia in ambulatory surgery, but it is not beneficial if the patient awakens in severe pain. Halothane in subanesthetic concentrations has been shown to antagonize the effects of opioid analgesics.[82] If this is true for currently used inhalational anesthetics, rapid elimination might have a beneficial effect on postoperative pain. On the other hand, if an anesthetic has analgesic properties at subanesthetic concentrations, slower elimination might be beneficial. When desflurane was compared to isoflurane and propofol, there were no differences in the amounts of analgesics required postoperatively[37,74,83] or pain scores.[34] In one study patients receiving desflurane required more postoperative opioids than those who had

propofol infusions.[84] However, extra fentanyl was administered intraperatively to the group receiving propofol. Similarly, patients receiving sevoflurane did not have increased analgesic requirements compared to a group anesthetized with isoflurane.[43]

Postoperative Nausea and Vomiting

PONV frequently delays discharge and is the most likely nonsurgical reason for unexpected hospitalization after ambulatory surgery[85] in both adults and children. It is important to remember that the causes of PONV are multifactorial. The use of opioids for pain relief, and the type of surgery in particular, have a major influence on the incidence of PONV.

Desflurane, sevoflurane, and isoflurane compared. Studies investigating PONV during recovery from volatile anesthetics are summarized in Table 15-7. Results of comparisons of the incidence of PONV after desflurane, sevoflurane, and isoflurane have been variable and inconsistent, or sometimes contradictory. Most studies show no significant differences in the incidence of PONV after the volatile agents (Table 15-7). In one study on women undergoing breast surgery,[86] there was a lower incidence of PONV with isoflurane compared to both desflurane and sevoflurane in the early postoperative period, possibly explained by the fact that patients were more drowsy after isoflurane anesthesia. In this study desflurane contributed most significantly to overall PONV. Sevoflurane was associated with a significantly lower incidence of PONV compared to isoflurane in another study in ambulatory patients.[43] However, several other investigations failed to confirm any significant differences in emetogenic sequelae with sevoflurane compared to isoflurane.[63,64,87] In a study investigating the effects of subhypnotic doses of propofol at the end of an anesthetic,[88] patients receiving desflurane had significantly more emetogenic sequelae than those who had received sevoflurane.

It has been suggested that there is a dose-related effect of sevoflurane on postoperative vomiting.[89] Sevoflurane anesthesia was titrated to a BIS value of 50–60 and compared with anesthetic titration using standard clinical signs. Patients in the BIS-monitored group received less sevoflurane and had a significantly lower incidence of vomiting (16% compared to 40% in phase II recovery).

Desflurane and sevoflurane compared to propofol. Studies comparing PONV after the volatile agents with propofol anesthesia are shown in Table 15-8. In all studies that compared desflurane to propofol (Table 15-8), there was significantly less PONV with propofol.[35,74,84] One study[90] found that the incidence of postoperative emesis in patients undergoing gynecologic laparoscopy after desflurane anesthesia could be reduced to levels comparable to propofol by giving ondansetron, 4 mg intravenously.

A triple antiemetic therapy regimen (ondansetron, metoclopramide, and droperidol) has been effective in eliminating PONV that followed desflurane administered for dental surgery.[52] The use of prophylactic antiemetics has

Table 15-7   The Incidence of PONV with Volatile Agents

Study (Date)	Type of Surgery	N₂O	Agents Compared	Incidence of PONV (%)		Significant (S) Not Significant (NS)	Comments
				Early	Late		
Frink[87] (1992)	Elective general	Yes	Isoflurane Sevoflurane	12 10	52 36	NS	
Karlsen[86] (2000)	Breast	Yes	Isoflurane Sevoflurane Desflurane	4 (together) = 28	22 36 67	S (Desflurane)	
Jakobsson[131] (1997)	Gynecologic laparoscopy		Isoflurane Desflurane	34 51		NS	PONV more frequent after leaving PACU. PONV delayed PACU discharge by 15 min.
Eriksson[64] (1995)	Gynecologic laparoscopy	Yes	Isoflurane Sevoflurane	32 63	56 46	NS	
Ghouri[83] (1991)	Surgical procedures	Yes	Isoflurane Desflurane	43 35		NS	
Philip[43] (1996)	Ambulatory surgery	Yes	Isoflurane Sevoflurane	51 36	24 9	(S) (Nausea only)	
Ebert[63] (1998)	Meta-analysis		Isoflurane Sevoflurane		50 51	NS	

permitted taking advantage of the rapid recovery that is characteristic of desflurane without incurring the unpleasant emetic side effects that may otherwise follow its use.

In most studies comparing sevoflurane and propofol, there is a greater incidence of PONV after sevoflurane anesthesia.[18,27,68] One study did report a higher incidence of nausea[67] (two patients compared to none) after propofol infusion; however, these patients received more fentanyl intraoperatively than the sevoflurane group.

COST OF THE VOLATILE ANESTHETICS

When the costs of the various inhalational techniques are compared, several factors need to be considered: the cost of the anesthetic itself, drugs used to treat the anesthetic side effects, and cost savings incurred if patients are fast-tracked or go home earlier. In addition, one should discriminate between costs to the institution and charges to the patient.

Determining the actual cost of a volatile anesthetic utilized is dependent on[91] the cost per milliliter of anesthetic liquid, the volume of vapor that results from each milliliter of liquid, the concentration of anesthetic that must be delivered from the vaporizer to provide clinical anesthesia (potency), and the background flow of anesthetic gas.

A low flow or closed circuit will help to offset the cost of the volatile agent as less volatile anesthetic will be vaporized and once equilibrium is approached, only minimal amounts of anesthetic need to be added to the circuit

(Table 15-9). The potency and the solubility of the vapor are also important factors to consider. At the time of writing (June 2003), the prices in the authors' hospital pharmacy for volatile anesthetics were as follows:

Desflurane (240-mL bottle): $97.45 ($0.41/mL)
Sevoflurane (250-mL bottle): $195.75 ($0.78/mL)
Isoflurane (100-mL bottle): $9.95 ($0.10/mL)

A cost analysis study[92] published in 1998 compared the cost of desflurane, sevoflurane, and isoflurane to that of propofol and found that the three volatile agents had similar costs and these were significantly lower than the cost of propofol. Patients receiving propofol, however, required significantly fewer drugs in the PACU and had lower PACU costs compared to the volatile agents. The calculated cost of propofol was $30.73 per patient compared to $16.68, $15.74, and $15.78 for desflurane, sevoflurane, and isoflurane, respectively. Other cost analysis studies have also found desflurane and sevoflurane to be cheaper than propofol.[93–97] It is interesting to note, however, that the wasted propofol remaining in the syringe at the end of an intravenous anesthetic contributes significantly to the cost of the anesthetic. On the other hand, only the actual volume of volatile agent used is calculated and the rest remains in the vaporizer to be administered to the next patient.[96,97]

Other economic factors are also important to consider. An anesthetic that allows more rapid awakening in theory may improve OR turnover times allowing a greater case

Table 15-8   Incidence of PONV after Volatile Anesthesia Compared to Propofol

Study	Type of Surgery	N$_2$O	Agents Compared	Incidence of PONV (%) Early	Incidence of PONV (%) Late	Significant (S) Not Significant (NS)	Comments
Rapp[74] (1992)	Peripheral and orthopedic	Yes	Induction/maintenance Propofol/propofol Propofol/desflurane Desflurane/desflurane		13 41 68	S Nausea only	
Raeder[84] (1998)	Outpatient laparoscopic cholecystectomy	No	Propofol Desflurane		17 40	S	
Eriksson[90] (1996)	Gynecologic laparoscopy		Propofol Desflurane Desflurane and Ondansetron		20 80 40	S	PONV with desflurane reduced using ondansetron (S)
Dashfield[18] (1998)	Minor arthroscopy	Yes	Propofol Sevoflurane	NS S	NS NS		Nausea score rather than percentages
Fredman[27] (1995)	Outpatient gynecology and ENT	Yes	Induction/maintenance Propofol/propofol Propofol/sevoflurane Sevoflurane/sevoflurane	10 18 33		S (vomiting only)	
Peduto[67] (2000)	Outpatient lower abdominal and ENT	Yes	Propofol Sevoflurane		7 0	S	Propofol group given more fentanyl intraperatively
Raeder[68] 1997	Knee arthroscopy	Yes	Propofol Sevoflurane		18 32	S	
Ebert[63] (1998)	Meta-analysis		Propofol Sevoflurane		40 48	NS	

throughput. An anesthetic that permits a higher incidence of fast-tracking may also reduce the cost of PACU care. In practice, however, these cost savings may be difficult to demonstrate, or to realize.

Ghouri et al.[83] demonstrated more rapid recovery from desflurane anesthesia compared to isoflurane. The cost savings from this was calculated to be $145 but was only realized if the vacant OR was used again more quickly.

In a study performed in patients undergoing ambulatory knee arthroscopy,[94] emergence times with the volatile anesthetics were 3 min shorter than when target-controlled infusions of propofol were used. When these times were added up over eight procedures, the time saved was 24 min. The cost saving of this amount of time must be assessed in terms of staffing costs, etc., which will vary with the institution. In a comparison of the effects of adding nitrous oxide to sevoflurane anesthesia in patients undergoing outpatient knee arthroscopy,[98] nitrous oxide reduced the cost of sevoflurane by 59% and hourly anesthetic costs by 41%, with no differences in postoperative course.

Use of the BIS monitor to accurately titrate the anesthetic concentration has been shown to decrease the amount of volatile anesthetic used.[89,99,100] In short ambulatory procedures, use of the BIS monitor reduced the cost of anesthetic agents, but the initial outlay for the BIS monitor itself actually increased the overall cost of the anesthetic.[100]

NITROUS OXIDE IN AMBULATORY SURGERY

Nitrous oxide is a widely used anesthetic agent. Its low solubility in oil (oil/gas partition coefficient) means that it has a high MAC (105), and is not effective by itself as an anesthetic agent. It has a low blood gas solubility (0.47) comparable to that of desflurane and therefore is associated with rapid onset and offset of effect. Nitrous oxide may be delivered in high concentrations and by increasing the inspired concentration, the alveolar concentration

Table 15-9   Cost of Inhalation Anesthesia per Hour Maintenance with and without Nitrous Oxide with Different Fresh Gas Flows (FGF),[107] 1995 Study (modified to reflect 2003 costs of volatile agents)

Agent	Price ($)/ bottle	Cost ($)/mL liquid (2003 cost)	Cost ($)/ L vapor	FGF L/min	Cost ($) per hr (2003)	Cost ($) per hr with N$_2$O (2003)
Isoflurane	77.99	0.78 (0.10)	4.00	1	8.14 (1.04)	
				3	15.81 (2.03)	6.65 (0.85)
Sevoflurane	180.00	0.72 (0.78)	3.96	1	9.52 (10.3)	
				3	20.92 (22.7)	8.60 (9.32)
Desflurane	73.05	0.30 (0.41)	1.46	1	8.59 (11.74)	
				3	20.45 (27.95)	8.79 (12.0)

SOURCE: Reproduced and modified with permission from Philip BK. Practical cost-effective choices: ambulatory general anesthesia. J Clin Anesth 1995;7: 606–13.

increases more rapidly (the so-called "concentration effect").[101] The uptake of large volumes of nitrous oxide during induction concentrates both the nitrous oxide and any other gas delivered concurrently in the alveoli; this is the second gas effect.[102] Based on these two principles, nitrous oxide should increase the rate of induction with other volatile anesthetic agents. Early confirmatory studies were performed in animals and the relevance of these effects to humans has been questioned.[103] Recently, however, the concentration and second gas effects have been shown to exist in studies with desflurane and 65% nitrous oxide,[104] although the clinical significance of these effects is minimal. Inhalational induction with desflurane can be difficult owing to airway irritation and the addition of nitrous oxide hastens but does not improve the quality of induction.[35] There was no improvement in induction time when nitrous oxide was added to 8% sevoflurane,[7,26] probably owing to the low blood gas solubility of sevoflurane (0.60), which approaches that of nitrous oxide (0.47).

Nitrous oxide is an inexpensive anesthetic and has been shown to significantly reduce the use of propofol with no increase in side effects or delay in discharge.[105,106] It will also significantly reduce the cost of coadministered volatile anesthetics[98,107] and propofol[108] (Table 15-9).

Nitrous Oxide and Postoperative Nausea and Vomiting

There is debate as to whether nitrous oxide increases the rate of postoperative emesis. Investigations into the effects of nitrous oxide when used concurrently with propofol have not demonstrated an emetogenic effect of nitrous oxide. However, this may be due to the antiemetic effects of propofol masking the effects of nitrous oxide. A meta-analysis[109] concluded that omitting nitrous oxide had no

effect on the incidence of nausea after anesthesia with either propofol or volatile anesthetics, but was associated with a statistically significant reduction in early and late vomiting.

Another analysis of 27 studies that investigated the incidence of emesis after volatile anesthetic agents with and without nitrous oxide[110] found that in 24 of these investigations there was increased nausea and vomiting with nitrous oxide, but only in 12 investigations was the effect statistically significant.

In summary, the use of nitrous oxide in ambulatory surgery will significantly reduce the use of other anesthetic agents, helping to keep drug costs down. It may contribute to PONV in patients who are at high risk of developing emetogenic sequelae and it would be prudent to avoid nitrous oxide in these cases.

VOLATILE AGENTS IN PEDIATRIC AMBULATORY ANESTHESIA

Pediatric patients represent a group in whom inhalational induction of anesthesia is very common and in many cases advantageous.

Halothane was the mainstay of inhalational induction in pediatric patients for all types of surgery for many years. It had a pleasant odour and smooth inhalation induction, although induction and emergence could be prolonged.

Isoflurane has been tried as a replacement for halothane, postulating that its relative insolubility compared to halothane and minimal cardiac depressant effects would make it superior. However,[13,111] when isoflurane was compared to halothane in unpremedicated pediatric patients, inhalational induction was significantly shorter and had a lower incidence of airway complication using halothane. In short cases lasting approximately 20 min, the patients who received halothane had a more pleasant recovery. The children who were maintained with isoflurane had a more irritable, violent recovery and had a higher incidence of airway complications than those who had been maintained with halothane. The children who received isoflurane did wake up a few minutes earlier, but these time differences were regarded as being clinically insignificant.

Sevoflurane has been shown to produce a smooth inhalational induction in children,[112] and in some studies produces a statistically, but not clinically significant, faster induction than halothane.[113–115] In other studies, however,[116–118] induction times with sevoflurane and halothane in children were very similar. Emergence has been shown to be significantly more rapid after sevoflurane when compared to halothane in pediatric patients.[114,117–121] The times to discharge, however, were the same. Only in one study[117] have recovery times been significantly delayed with halothane. In that study patients received 1–1.5 MAC of sevoflurane or halothane for procedures lasting an average of 40 min. In another study, however, in children undergoing myringotomy,[116] recovery times after sevoflurane and halothane were the same. In this particular study the surgical times were all less than 10 min, which implies a lower exposure to the anesthetic agent in the latter patients.

Postoperative Complications

A trend toward a greater incidence of restlessness and agitation has been demonstrated in children who have received sevoflurane when compared with halothane.[117] When halothane and sevoflurane were compared in children undergoing ear, nose, and throat procedures with mild upper-respiratory-tract infections,[119] sevoflurane produced significantly faster induction and recovery. There was no increase in the incidence of intra- and postoperative complications. The children who received sevoflurane, however, were noted to be increasingly restless and agitated after surgery. Postoperative restlessness and agitation have been noted by others following sevoflurane.[113,114,120] In one study specifically designed to investigate recovery characteristics of children aged 1–3 years anesthetized with sevoflurane or halothane[121] for adenoidectomy, recovery was faster in the sevoflurane group. Children who had received sevoflurane complained of more postoperative pain and required analgesics at an earlier stage. The only factor in the recovery profile that was significantly different was an increased incidence of vomiting in the halothane group. There was a trend toward postanesthetic excitement in the sevoflurane group, but this was not significant.

Although no studies have shown significant differences, an increased number of children may be restless and agitated in the early postoperative period and will require analgesics at an earlier time. The reasons for restlessness after sevoflurane have been attributed to more rapid emergence, and awareness of postoperative pain.[122] Sevoflurane has been shown to produce epileptogenic activity in children.[123,124] Agitation associated with rapid emergence is also seen following desflurane anesthesia in children,[125,126] and in most instances can be relieved by treating postop-

erative pain with acetominophen.[113] Midazolam premedication also reduces the incidence of postoperative restlessness.[116]

Desflurane, as in adult patients, is associated with a high incidence of airway complications to be considered as an induction agent in pediatric patients.[6] Emergence from desflurane is more rapid than after isoflurane.[127] When sevoflurane, desflurane, and halothane were compared in children undergoing adenoidectomy and myringotomy,[125] emergence after similar MAC concentrations of anesthetic was significantly more rapid after desflurane than sevoflurane or halothane. There were no significant differences between sevoflurane and halothane in this study. There was a greater incidence of postoperative agitation after desflurane (55%) related to rapid emergence. However, times to discharge were no different in the three groups.

REFERENCES

1. Heijke S, Smith G. Quest for the ideal inhalation anaesthetic agent. Br J Anaesth 1990;64(1):3–6.
2. Smith I, Nathanson MH, White PF. The role of sevoflurane in outpatient anesthesia. Anesth Analg 1995;81:S67–S72.
3. White PF. Studies of desflurane in outpatient anesthesia. Anesth Analg 1992;75:S47–S54.
4. Yasuda N, Lockhart SH, Eger EI, Weiskopf RB, Liu J, Laster MJ, et al. Comparison of kinetics of sevoflurane and isoflurane in humans. Anesth Analg 1991;72:316–24.
5. Yasuda N, Lockhart SH, Eger EI, Weiskopf MD, Johnson BH, Freire BA, et al. Kinetics of desflurane, isoflurane, and halothane in humans. Anesthesiology 1991;74:489–98.
6. Zwass MS, Fisher DM, Welborn LG, Cote CJ, Davis PJ, Dinner M, et al. Induction and maintenance characteristics of anesthesia with desflurane and nitrous oxide in infants and children. Anesthesiology 1992;76(3):373–78.
7. Siau C, Liu EH. Nitrous oxide does not improve sevoflurane induction of anesthesia in adults. J Clin Anesth 2002;14(3):218–22.
8. Drummond GB. Rapid inhalation induction of anaesthesia. Br J Anaesth 1988;61(4):373–75.
9. Bourne JG. General anaesthesia for out-patients, with special reference to dental extraction. Proc Roy Soc Med 1954;47:416–22.
10. Ruffle JM, Snider MT, Rosenberger JL, Latta WB. Rapid induction of halothane anaesthesia in man. Br J Anaesth 1985;57(6):607–11.
11. Wilton NC, Thomas VL. Single breath induction of anaesthesia, using a vital capacity breath of halothane, nitrous oxide and oxygen. Anaesthesia 1986;41(5):472–76.
12. Phillips AJ, Brimacombe JR, Simpson DL. Anaesthetic induction with isoflurane or halothane: oxygen saturation during induction with isoflurane or halothane in unpremedicated children. Anaesthesia 1988;43(11):927–29.
13. Pandit UA, Steude GM, Leach AB. Induction and recovery characteristics of isoflurane and halothane anaesthesia for short outpatient operations in children. Anaesthesia 1985;40(12):1226–30.
14. Lamberty JM, Wilson IH. Single breath induction of anaesthesia with isoflurane. Br J Anaesth 1987;59(10):1214–18.
15. Loper K, Reitan J, Bennett H, Benthuysen J, Snook L Jr. Comparison of halothane and isoflurane for rapid anesthetic induction. Anesth Analg 1987;66(8):766–68.
16. van Heerden PV, Bukofzer M, Edge KR, Morrell DF. Rapid inhalational induction of anaesthesia with isoflurane or halothane in humidified oxygen. Can J Anaesth 1992;39(3):242–46.
17. van Heerden PV, Wilson IH, Marshall FP, Cormack JR. Effect of hu-

midification on inhalation induction with isoflurane. Br J Anaesth 1990;64(2):235–37.

18.   Dashfield AK, Birt DJ, Thurlow J, Kestin IG, Langton JA. Recovery characteristics using single-breath 8% sevoflurane or propofol for induction of anaesthesia in day-case arthroscopy patients. Anaesthesia 1998;53(11):1062–66.

19.   Kirkbride DA, Parker JL, Williams GD, Buggy DJ. Induction of anesthesia in the elderly ambulatory patient: a double-blinded comparison of propofol and sevoflurane. Anesth Analg 2001;93(5):1185–87.

20.   Yurino M, Kimura H. Induction of anesthesia with sevoflurane, nitrous oxide and oxygen: a comparison of spontaneous ventilation and vital capacity rapid inhalation induction (VCRII) techniques. Anesth Analg 1993;76:598–601.

21.   Yurino M, Kimura H. A comparison of vital capacity breath and tidal breathing techniques for induction of anaesthesia with high sevoflurane concentration in nitrous oxide and oxygen. Anaesthesia 1995;50:308–11.

22.   Smith I, Ding Y, White PF. Comparison of induction, maintenance and recovery characteristics of sevoflurane-N_2O and propofol-sevoflurane-N_2O with propofol-isoflurane-N_2O. Anesth Analg 1992;74:253–59.

23.   Muzi M, Colinco MD, Robinson BJ, Ebert TJ. The effects of premedication on inhaled induction of anesthesia with sevoflurane. Anesth Analg 1997;85:1143–48.

24.   Ti LK, Pua HL, Lee TL. Single vital capacity inhalational anaesthetic induction in adults—isoflurane vs sevoflurane. Can J Anaesth 1998;45:949–53.

25.   Muzi M, Robinson BJ, Ebert TJ, O'Brien TJ. Induction of anesthesia and tracheal intubation with sevoflurane in adults. Anesthesiology 1996;85(3):536–43.

26.   Hall JE, Stewart JI, Harmer M. Single-breath inhalation induction of sevoflurane anaesthesia with and without nitrous oxide: a feasibility study in adults and comparison with an intravenous bolus of propofol. Anaesthesia 1997;52(5):410–15.

27.   Fredman B, Nathanson MH, Smith I, Wang J, Klein K, White PF. Sevoflurane for outpatient anesthesia: a comparison with propofol. Anesth Analg 1995;81(4):823–28.

28.   Ebert TJ, Muzi M, Lopatka CW. Neurocirculatory responses to sevoflurane in humans: a comparison to desflurane. Anesthesiology 1995;83(1):88–95.

29.   Thwaites A, Edmends S, Smith I. Inhalation induction with sevoflurane: a double-blind comparison with propofol. Br J Anaesth 1997;78(4):356–61.

30.   Shah MK, Tan HM, Wong K. Comparison of sevoflurane-nitrous oxide anaesthesia with the conventional intravenous-inhalational technique using bispectral index monitoring. Anaesthesia 2001;56(4):302–8.

31.   Molloy ME, Buggy DJ, Scanlon P. Propofol or sevoflurane for laryngeal mask airway insertion. Can J Anaesth 1999;46(4):322–26.

32.   Kimura T, Watanabe S, Asakura N, Inomata S, Okada M, Taguchi M. Determination of end-tidal sevoflurane concentration for tracheal intubation and minimum alveolar anesthetic concentration in adults. Anesth Analg 1994;79(2):378–81.

33.   Katoh T, Nakajima Y, Moriwaki G, Kobayashi S, Suzuki A, Iwamoto T, et al. Sevoflurane requirements for tracheal intubation with and without fentanyl. Br J Anaesth 1999;82(4):561–65.

34.   Wrigley SR, Fairfield JE, Jones RM, Black AE. Induction and recovery characteristics of desflurane in day case patients: a comparison with propofol. Anaesthesia 1991;46(8):615–22.

35.   Van Hemelrijck J, Smith I, White PF. Use of desflurane for outpatient anesthesia: a comparison with propofol and nitrous oxide. Anesthesiology 1991;75:197–203.

36.   Rampil IJ, Lockhart SH, Zwass MS, Peterson NA, Yasuda N, Eger EI, et al. Clinical characteristics of desflurane in surgical patients: minimal alveolar concentration. Anesthesiology 1991;74:429–33.

37.   Lebenbom-Mansour MH, Pandit SK, Kothary SP, Randel GI, Levy

L. Desflurane versus propofol anesthesia: a comparative analysis in outpatients. Anesth Analg 1993;76:936–41.

38.   Kelly RE, Hartmann GS, Embree PB, Sharp G, Artusio JF Jr. Inhaled induction and emergence from desflurane anesthesia in the ambulatory surgical patient: the effect of premedication. Anesth Analg 1993;77:540–43.

39.   Weiskopf RB, Moore MA, Eger EI, Noorani M, McKay L, Chortkoff B, et al. Rapid increase in desflurane concentration is associated with greater transient cardiovascular stimulation than with rapid increase in isoflurane concentration in humans. Anesthesiology 1994;80(5):1035–45.

40.   Merkel G, Eger EI. A comparative study of halothane and halopropane anesthesia: including a method for determining equipotency. Anesthesiology 1963;24:346–57.

41.   Young CJ, Apfelbaum JL. Inhalational anesthetics: desflurane and sevoflurane. J Clin Anesth 1995;7:564–77.

42.   Nathanson MH, Fredman B, Smith I, White PF. Sevoflurane versus desflurane for outpatient anesthesia: a comparison of maintenance and recovery profiles. Anesth Analg 1995;81(6):1186–90.

43.   Philip BK, Kallar SK, Bogetz MS, Scheller MS, Wetchler BV. A multicenter comparison of maintenance and recovery with sevoflurane or isoflurane for adult ambulatory anesthesia: the Sevoflurane Multicenter Ambulatory Group. Anesth Analg 1996;83(2):314–19.

44.   Eger EI. New inhaled anesthetics. Anesthesiology 1994;80:906–22.

45.   Ebert TJ. Cardiovascular and autonomic effects of sevoflurane. Acta Anaesthesiol Belg 1996;47(1):15–21.

46.   Warltier DC, Pagel PS. Cardiovascular and respiratory actions of desflurane: is desflurane different from isoflurane? Anesth Analg 1992;75(4 Suppl):S17–S29.

47.   Kersten JR, Brayer AP, Pagel PS, Tessmer JP, Warltier DC. Perfusion of ischemic myocardium during anesthesia with sevoflurane. Anesthesiology 1994;81(4):995–1004.

48.   Ebert TJ, Muzi M. Sympathetic hyperactivity during desflurane anesthesia in healthy volunteers: a comparison with isoflurane. Anesthesiology 1993;79(3):444–53.

49.   Loan PB, Mirakhur RK, Paxton LD, Gaston JH. Comparison of desflurane and isoflurane in anaesthesia for dental surgery. Br J Anaesth 1995;75: 289–92.

50.   Koenig HM. What's up with the new volatile anesthetics, desflurane and sevoflurane, for neurosurgical patients? J Neurosurg Anesthesiol 1994;6(4):229–32.

51.   Ashworth J, Smith I. Comparison of desflurane with isoflurane or propofol in spontaneously breathing ambulatory patients. Anesth Analg 1998;87(2):312–18.

52.   Tang J, White PF, Wender RH, Naruse R, Kariger R, Sloninsky A, et al. Fast-track office-based anesthesia: a comparison of propofol versus desflurane with antiemetic prophylaxis in spontaneously breathing patients. Anesth Analg 2001;92(1):95–99.

53.   Kharasch ED. Biotransformation of sevoflurane. Anesth Analg 1995;81(6 Suppl):S27–S38.

54.   Sutton TS, Koblin DD, Gruenke LD, Weiskopf RB, Rampil IJ, Waskell L, et al. Fluoride metabolites after prolonged exposure of volunteers and patients to desflurane. Anesth Analg 1991;73(2):180–85.

55.   Eger EI. Compound A: does it matter? Can J Anaesth 2001;48(5): 427–30.

56.   Yamakage M, Kimura A, Chen X, Tsujiguchi N, Kamada Y, Namiki A. Production of compound A under low-flow anesthesia is affected by type of anesthetic machine. Can J Anaesth 2001;48(5):435–38.

57.   Kharasch ED, Powers KM, Artru AA. Comparison of Amsorb, sodalime, and Baralyme degradation of volatile anesthetics and formation of carbon monoxide and compound A in swine in vivo. Anesthesiology 2002;96(1):173–82.

58.   Fang ZX, Eger EI, Laster MJ, Chortkoff BS, Kandel L, Ionescu P. Carbon monoxide production from degradation of desflurane, enflurane, isoflurane, halothane, and sevoflurane by soda lime and Baralyme. Anesth Analg 1995;80(6):1187–93.

59.   Eger EI, Johnson BH. Rates of awakening from anesthesia with I-

653, halothane, isoflurane, and sevoflurane: a test of the effect of anesthetic concentration and duration in rats. Anesth Analg 1987;66(10):977–82.

60. Pavlin DJ, Rapp SE, Polissar NL, Malmgren JA, Koerschgen M, Keyes H. Factors affecting discharge time in adult outpatients. Anesth Analg 1998;87(4):816–26.

61. Gold BS, Kitz DS, Lecky JH, Neuhaus JM. Unanticipated admission to the hospital following ambulatory surgery. JAMA 1989;262(21): 3008–10.

62. Tsai SK, Lee C, Kwan WF, Chen BJ. Recovery of cognitive functions after anaesthesia with desflurane or isoflurane and nitrous oxide. Br J Anaesth 1992;69(3):255–58.

63. Ebert TJ, Robinson BJ, Uhrich TD, Mackenthun A, Pichotta PJ. Recovery from sevoflurane anesthesia: a comparison to isoflurane and propofol anesthesia. Anesthesiology 1998;89(6):1524–31.

64. Eriksson H, Haasio J, Korttila K. Recovery from sevoflurane and isoflurane anaesthesia after outpatient gynaecological laparoscopy. Acta Anaesthesiol Scand 1995;39(3):377–80.

65. O'Hara DA, DeAngelis V, Lee H, Zedie N, Seuffert PA, Amory DW. The effects of sevoflurane and isoflurane on recovery from outpatient surgery. Pharmacotherapy 1996;16(3):446–52.

66. Robinson BJ, Uhrich TD, Ebert TJ. A review of recovery from sevoflurane anaesthesia: comparisons with isoflurane and propofol including meta-analysis. Acta Anaesthesiol Scand 1999;43(2):185–90.

67. Peduto VA, Mezzetti D, Properzi M, Giorgini C. Sevoflurane provides better recovery than propofol plus fentanyl in anaesthesia for day-case surgery. Eur J Anaesthesiol 2000;17:138–43.

68. Raeder J, Gupta A, Pedersen FM. Recovery characteristics of sevoflurane- or propofol-based anaesthesia for day-care surgery. Acta Anaesthesiol Scand 1997;41(8):988–94.

69. Gupta A, Kullander M, Ekberg K, Lennmarken C. Anaesthesia for day-care arthroscopy: a comparison between desflurane and isoflurane. Anaesthesia 1996;51(1):56–62.

70. Dexter F, Tinker JH. Comparisons between desflurane and isoflurane or propofol on time to following commands and time to discharge: a metaanalysis. Anesthesiology 1995;83(1):77–82.

71. Fletcher JE, Sebel PS, Murphy MR, Smith CA, Mick SA, Flister MP. Psychomotor performance after desflurane anesthesia: a comparison with isoflurane. Anesth Analg 1991;73(3):260–65.

72. Apfelbaum JL, Lichtor JL, Lane BS, Coalson DW, Korttila KT. Awakening, clinical recovery, and psychomotor effects after desflurane and propofol anesthesia. Anesth Analg 1996;83(4):7215–25.

73. Song D, Chung F, Wong J, Yogendran S. The assessment of postural stability after ambulatory anesthesia: a comparison of desflurane with propofol. Anesth Analg 2002;94:60–64.

74. Rapp SE, Conahan TJ, Pavlin DJ, Levy WJ, Hautman B, Lecky J, et al. Comparison of desflurane with propofol in outpatients undergoing peripheral orthopedic surgery. Anesth Analg 1992;75: 572–79.

75. Tarazi EM, Philip BK. A comparison of recovery after sevoflurane or desflurane in ambulatory anesthesia. J Clin Anesth 1998;10(4): 272–77.

76. Song D, Joshi GP, White PF. Titration of volatile anesthetics using bispectral index facilitates recovery after ambulatory anesthesia. Anesthesiology 1997;87(4):842–48.

77. White PF. Criteria for fast-tracking outpatients after ambulatory surgery. J Clin Anesth 1998;11:78–79.

78. Lubarsky DA. Fast track in the postanesthesia care unit: unlimited possibilities? J Clin Anesth 1996;8(3 Suppl):70S–72S.

79. Apfelbaum JL. Bypassing PACU: a cost effective measure. Can J Anaesth 1998;45(5 Pt 2):R915–R94.

80. Coloma M, Zhou T, White PF, Markowitz SD, Forestner JE. Fast-tracking after outpatient laparoscopy: reasons for failure after propofol, sevoflurane, and desflurane anesthesia. Anesth Analg 2001;93:112–15.

81. Song D, Joshi GP, White PF. Fast-track eligibility after ambulatory

anesthesia: a comparison of desflurane, sevoflurane, and propofol. Anesth Analg 1998;86(2):267–73.

82. Kissin I, Jebeles JA. Halothane antagonizes effect of morphine on the motor reaction threshold in rats. Anesthesiology 1984;61(6): 671–76.

83. Ghouri AF, Bodner M, White PF. Recovery profile after desflurane-nitrous oxide versus isoflurane nitrous oxide in outpatients. Anesthesiology 1991;74:419–24.

84. Raeder JC, Mjaland O, Aasbo V, Grogaard B, Buanes T. Desflurane versus propofol maintenance for outpatient laparoscopic cholecystectomy. Acta Anaesthesiol Scand 1998;42(1):106–10.

85. White PF, Shafer A. Nausea and vomiting: causes and prophylaxis. Semin Anesth 1987;6:300–308.

86. Karlsen KL, Persson E, Wennberg E, Stenqvist O. Anaesthesia, recovery and postoperative nausea and vomiting after breast surgery: a comparison between desflurane, sevoflurane and isoflurane anaesthesia. Acta Anaesthesiol Scand 2000;44(4):489–93.

87. Frink EJ Jr, Malan TP, Atlas M, Dominguez LM, DiNardo JA, Brown BR Jr. Clinical comparison of sevoflurane and isoflurane in healthy patients. Anesth Analg 1992;74(2):241–45.

88. Song D, Whitten CW, White PF, Yu SY, Zarate E. Antiemetic activity of propofol after sevoflurane and desflurane anesthesia for outpatient laparoscopic cholecystectomy. Anesthesiology 1998;89:838–43.

89. Nelskyla KA, Yli-Hankala AM, Puro PH, Korttila KT. Sevoflurane titration using bispectral index decreases postoperative vomiting in phase II recovery after ambulatory surgery. Anesth Analg 2001; 93:1165–69.

90. Eriksson H, Korttila K. Recovery profile after desflurane with or without ondansetron compared with propofol in patients undergoing outpatient gynecological laparoscopy. Anesth Analg 1996; 82(3):533–38.

91. Weiskopf RB, Eger EI. Comparing the costs of inhaled anesthetics. Anesthesiology 1993;79(6):1413–18.

92. Boldt J, Jaun N, Kumle B, Heck M, Mund K. Economic considerations of the use of new anesthetics: a comparison of propofol, sevoflurane, desflurane, and isoflurane. Anesth Analg 1998;86(3): 504–9.

93. Philip BK, Mushlin PS, Manzi D, Freiberger D, Roaf E. Isoflurane versus propofol for maintenance of anesthesia for ambulatory surgery: a comparison of costs and recovery profiles. Anesthesiology 1992;77:A44.

94. Dolk A, Cannerfelt R, Anderson RE, Jakobsson J. Inhalation anaesthesia is cost-effective for ambulatory surgery: a clinical comparison with propofol during elective knee arthroscopy. Eur J Anaesthesiol 2002;19:88–92.

95. Suttner S, Boldt J, Schmidt C, Piper S, Kumle B. Cost analysis of target-controlled infusion-based anesthesia compared with standard anesthesia regimens. Anesth Analg 1999;88(1):77–82.

96. Rosenberg MK, Bridge P, Brown M. Cost comparison: a desflurane-versus a propofol-based general anesthetic technique. Anesth Analg 1994;79(5):852–55.

97. Smith I, Terhoeve PA, Hennart D, Feiss P, Harmer M, Pourriat JL, et al. A multicentre comparison of the costs of anaesthesia with sevoflurane or propofol. Br J Anaesth 1999;83(4):564–70.

98. Jakobsson J, Heidvall M, Davidson S. The sevoflurane-sparing effect of nitrous oxide: a clinical study. Acta Anaesthesiol Scand 1999;43(4):411–14.

99. Pavlin DJ, Hong JY, Freund PR, Koerschgen ME, Bower JO, Bowdle TA. The effect of bispectral index monitoring on end-tidal gas concentration and recovery duration after outpatient anesthesia. Anesth Analg 2001;93(3):613–19.

100. Yli-Hankala A, Vakkuri A, Annila P, Korttila K. EEG bispectral index monitoring in sevoflurane or propofol anaesthesia: analysis of direct costs and immediate recovery. Acta Anaesthesiol Scand 1999;43(5):545–49.

101. Eger EI. Effect of inspired anesthetic concentration on the rate of rise of alveolar concentration. Anesthesiology 1963;24:153–57.

102. Epstein RM, Rackow H, Salanitre E, Wolf GL. Influence of the concentration effect on the uptake of anesthetic mixtures: the second gas effect. Anesthesiology 1964;25:364–71.

103. Sun X-G, Su F, Shi YQ, Lee C. The "second gas effect" is not a valid concept. Anesth Analg 1999;88(1):188–92.

104. Taheri S, Eger EI. A demonstration of the concentration and second gas effects in humans anesthetized with nitrous oxide and desflurane. Anesth Analg 1999;89:774–80.

105. Sengupta P, Plantevin OM. Nitrous oxide and day-case laparoscopy: effects on nausea, vomiting and return to normal activity. Br J Anaesth 1988;60(5):570–73.

106. Arellano RJ, Pole ML, Rafuse SE, Fletcher M, Saad YG, Friedlander M, et al. Omission of nitrous oxide from a propofol-based anesthetic does not affect the recovery of women undergoing outpatient gynecologic surgery. Anesthesiology 2000;93(2):332–39.

107. Philip BK. Practical cost-effective choices: ambulatory general anesthesia. J Clin Anesth 1995;7:606–13.

108. Heath KJ, Sadler P, Winn JH, McFadzean WA. Nitrous oxide reduces the cost of intravenous anaesthesia. Eur J Anaesthesiol 1996;13(4):369–72.

109. Tramer M, Moore A, McQuay H. Omitting nitrous oxide in general anaesthesia: meta-analysis of intraoperative awareness and postoperative emesis in randomized controlled trials. Br J Anaesth 1996;76(2):186–93.

110. Hartung J. Twenty-four of twenty-seven studies show a greater incidence of emesis associated with nitrous oxide than with alternative anesthetics. Anesth Analg 1996;83(1):114–16.

111. Kingston HG. Halothane and isoflurane anesthesia in pediatric outpatients. Anesth Analg 1986;65(2):181–84.

112. Lerman J, Sikich N, Kleinman S, Yentis S. The pharmacology of sevoflurane in infants and children. Anesthesiology 1994;80:814–24.

113. Johannesson GP, Floren M, Lindahl SG. Sevoflurane for ENT-surgery in children: a comparison with halothane. Acta Anaesthesiol Scand 1995;39(4):546–50.

114. Lerman J, Davis PJ, Welborn LG, Orr RJ, Rabb M, Carpenter R, et al. Induction, recovery, and safety characteristics of sevoflurane in children undergoing ambulatory surgery: a comparison with halothane. Anesthesiology 1996;84(6):1332–40.

115. Agnor RC, Sikich N, Lerman J. Single-breath vital capacity rapid inhalation induction in children 8% sevoflurane versus 5% halothane. Anesthesiology 1998;89:379–84.

116. Hallen J, Rawal N, Gupta A. Postoperative recovery following outpatient pediatric myringotomy: a comparison between sevoflurane and halothane. J Clin Anesth 2001;13(3):161–66.

117. Naito Y, Tamai S, Shingu K, Fujimori R, Mori K. Comparison between sevoflurane and halothane for paediatric ambulatory anaesthesia. Br J Anaesth 1991;67(4):387–89.

118. Piat V, Dubois MC, Johanet S, Murat I. Induction and recovery characteristics and hemodynamic responses to sevoflurane and halothane in children. Anesth Analg 1994;79(5):840–44.

119. Rieger A, Schroter G, Philippi W, Hass I, Eyrich K. A comparison of sevoflurane with halothane in outpatient adenotomy in children with mild upper respiratory tract infections. J Clin Anesth 1996; 8(3):188–97.

120. Sury MR, Black A, Hemington L, Howard R, Hatch DJ, Mackersie A. A comparison of the recovery characteristics of sevoflurane and halothane in children. Anaesthesia 1996;51(6):543–46.

121. Viitanen H, Baer G, Annila P. Recovery characteristics of sevoflurane or halothane for day-case anaesthesia in children aged 1–3 years. Acta Anaesthesiol Scand 2000;44(1):101–6.

122. Aono J, Ueda W, Mamiya K, Takimoto E, Manabe M. Greater incidence of delirium during recovery from sevoflurane anesthesia in preschool boys. Anesthesiology 1997;87(6):1298–1300.

123. Vakkuri A, Jantti V, Sarkela M, Lindgren L, Korttila K, Yli-Hankala A. Epileptiform EEG during sevoflurane mask induction: effect of delaying the onset of hyperventilation. Acta Anaesthesiol Scand 2000;44(6):713–19.

124. Komatsu H, Taie S, Endo S, Fukuda K, Ueki M, Nogaya J, et al. Electrical seizures during sevoflurane anesthesia in two pediatric patients with epilepsy. Anesthesiology 1994;81(6):1535–37.

125. Welborn LG, Hannallah RS, Norden JM, Ruttimann UE, Callan CM. Comparison of emergence and recovery characteristics of sevoflurane, desflurane, and halothane in pediatric ambulatory patients. Anesth Analg 1996;83(5):917–20.

126. Grundmann U, Uth M, Eichner A, Wilhelm W, Larsen R. Total intravenous anaesthesia with propofol and remifentanil in paediatric patients: a comparison with a desflurane-nitrous oxide inhalation anaesthesia. Acta Anaesthesiol Scand 1998;42(7):845–50.

127. Wilhelm W, Berner K, Grundmann U, Palz M, Larsen R. Desflurane or isoflurane for paediatric ENT anaesthesia: a comparison of intubating conditions and recovery profile. Anaesthesist 1998; 47(12):975–78.

128. Yurino M, Kimura H. Vital capacity rapid inhalation induction technique: comparison of sevoflurane and halothane. Can J Anaesth 1993;40(5):440–43.

129. Sloan MH, Conard PF, Karsunky PK, Gross JB. Sevoflurane versus isoflurane: induction and recovery characteristics with single-breath inhaled inductions of anesthesia. Anesth Analg 1996; 82(3):528–32.

130. Aldrete JA, Kroulik D. A postanesthetic recovery score. Anesth Analg 1970;49(6):924–34.

131. Jakobsson J, Rane K, Ryberg G. Anaesthesia during laparoscopic gynaecological surgery: a comparison between desflurane and isoflurane. Eur J Anaesthesiol 1997;14(2):148–52.

Sedative–Hypnotic Agents for Ambulatory Anesthesia

DARYN H. MOLLER • PETER S.A. GLASS

INTRODUCTION

Ambulatory surgical procedures have seen phenomenal growth in recent decades. The most common ambulatory procedures remain ophthalmologic, plastic, gastroenterologic, pediatric, and gynecologic. Intravenous sedatives and hypnotics (see Table 16-1) are a component of nearly every anesthetic/sedation. The challenge for the anesthesia provider is not just one of efficiency but primarily of patient safety despite diverse patient characteristics of age and medical condition. The appropriate selection and use of intravenous anesthetic agents can enhance patient tolerance of a procedure as well as facilitating early discharge and high patient satisfaction.

PROPOFOL

Propofol (2,6-diisopropylphenol) was introduced into clinical practice after approval by the Food and Drug Administration (FDA) in October 1989. It is poorly soluble in aqueous solution and is available in an emulsion of 1% propofol (wt/vol), 1.2% egg lecithin, 2.25% glycerol, and 10% soybean oil. Known hypersensitivity to either of these components is a contraindication to the use of propofol. There have been several case reports of allergic-type reactions associated with the administration of propofol.[1,2] A generic propofol is available that uses metabisulfite as a preservative; known hypersensitivity to sulfites is a precaution in the administration of the generic propofol.

Pharmacology

Propofol is a sedative hypnotic agent that is believed to have its primary action in the central nervous system (CNS) through gamma-aminobutyric acid (GABA) channel binding and potentiating chloride conductance. Its sedative effects may also be potentiated through actions on the alpha-2 adrenoreceptor[3] (with alterations in central norepinephrine release)[4] and N-methyl-D-aspartate (NMDA) systems.[5] Propofol has rapid onset of hypnosis after bolus dose with a peak effect seen in 90–100 sec following a 2.5-mg/kg dose with a duration of action of 5–10 min.[6] The induction dose of propofol is age-dependent and greatest at 2 years of age[7] with substantial decline associated with increasing age.[8] In adult volunteers, amnesia requires 33.3 μg/kg/min infusion rates for unstimulated individuals,[9] which corresponds with a plasma concentration of 1 μg/mL. Depth of anesthesia as measured by bispectal index (BIS) monitoring is correlated with plasma propofol concentration, with 50% of volunteers unable to respond to verbal commands (i.e., are unconscious) at a BIS score of 63.[10]

Propofol undergoes rapid metabolism in the body, primarily via the liver to inactive glucuronide metabolites that are excreted via the kidney. A small amount (less than 5%) of propofol is excreted unchanged via the urine and feces.[11] The clearance of propofol exceeds that of hepatic blood flow and one of the principal sites of extrahepatic metabolism appears to be the lungs, which may account for up to 30% of its total metabolism.[12] The dose of propofol may be greater in children owing to a greater volume of the central compartment as well as more rapid clearance.[13]

Propofol, when used as an induction agent, should be administered between 1 and 2.5 mg/kg, with lean body mass, age, and other concurrent medications significantly effecting the dose.[14,15] Titration of propofol in 10–30 mg doses can further reduce the incidence of hypotension. A reduced dose of 1–1.75 mg/kg is recommended for patients over the age of 60.[16] For patients with end-stage renal disease (ESRD), a slightly higher dose of propofol may be needed to obtain adequate hypnosis (1.42 mg/kg vs. 0.89 mg/kg).[17] For the maintenance of general anesthesia, doses of 100–200 μg/kg/min are generally satisfactory.[18] The use of concomitant opioid therapy will reduce the total propofol requirement. Intubating conditions after a 2 mg/kg propofol bolus are found to be superior to thiopental or etomidate when given with an opioid background of 3 μg/kg remifentanil in the absence of muscle relaxant.[19]

Table 16-1 Dosing of Common Intravenous Sedative/Hypnotic Agents

Drug	Dose	Use
Propofol	1–2.5 mg/kg	Induction
	25–100 μg/kg/min	Sedation (IV)
	50–200 μg/kg/min	Maintenance general anesthesia
Midazolam	0.01–0.1 mg/kg	Sedation (IV)
	0.25–0.5 mg/kg (20 mg max)	Sedation (PO)
Flumazenil	0.01 mg/kg (1 mg max)	Benzodiazepine reversal (IV)
Ketamine	0.15 mg/kg	IV analgesic adjuvant
	1–1.5 mg/kg	Primary operative analgesic
Etomidate	0.2–0.3 mg/kg	Sedation/induction
Dexmede-tomidine	0.4–1 μg/kg (slow over 10 min)	Bolus
	0.2–0.7 μg/kg/hr	Sedation (IV)
Droperidol	0.625–1.25 mg (adult)	PONV prophylaxis
Scopolamine	0.3–0.6 mg	Sedation, PONV prophylaxis

Abbreviations: IV = intravenous; PO = oral; PONV = postoperative nausea and vomiting.

Cardiorespiratory Effects

When given for anesthetic induction, propofol causes a 20–30% incidence of apnea. Apnea is prolonged in the presence of other intravenous agents, particularly opioids, and may be longer than with other intravenous induction agents.[20] The decrease in tidal volume exceeds the decrease in respiratory rate during the initial bolus. When a steady-state infusion of propofol is reached at 100 μg/kg/min, there is a 40% decrease in tidal volume with a 20% increase in respiratory rate. There is a flattening of the curve for the ventilatory response to carbon dioxide (CO_2)[21] as well as inhibition of hypoxic ventilatory drive.[22] Propofol is known to have bronchodilating abilities.[23]

When propofol is given at an induction dose (2–2.5 mg/kg), the most prominent cardiovascular side effect is a decrease in systolic blood pressure of 25–40%, which is attributed to reductions in both preload and afterload.[24] Propofol does not seem to have significant negative inotropic effects in animal studies.[25] During induction with propofol, heart rate does not change, perhaps as a result of resetting of the baroreceptors.[26] Propofol at infusions of 167 μg/kg/min have been shown to alter the number of patients who respond with tachycardia to atropine therapy.[27] The potential antiarrhythmic effects of propofol are poorly

understood, but the loss of sympathetic tone associated with propofol administration may be responsible for its observed effects in abolishing supraventricular and ventricular tachycardias and may be of potential use during cardioversion.[28–31] Propofol has been shown to be safe and efficacious for external cardioversion. For unpremedicated patients, there is no difference in hemodynamics when compared to etomidate. At 15 min postprocedure, recovery scores were better for propofol, but by 20 min, no difference could be detected.[32]

Safe Handling

Propofol itself will support growth of microorganisms, particularly at room temperature. There have been many reports of systemic infections and five deaths traced to contamination of propofol.[33–35] In an effort to reduce the potential for bacterial contamination from propofol, the Anesthesia Patient Safety Foundation (APSF) released guidelines recommending the disinfection of vials and ampules with isopropyl alcohol, the use of single-patient syringes within 6 hr, and infusions to be completed within 12 hr of "spiking" of a vial sign.[36] The storage of propofol at reduced temperatures (12–14°C) does not appear to affect bacterial contamination.[37] There have been suggestions that combining propofol with other drugs such as methohexital[38] or lidocaine[39–41] may reduce its ability to support bacterial growth. However, these data remain inconclusive and adherence to previously established guidelines by the APSF is recommended.

Clinical Use

During the administration of propofol for sedation or for the induction of general anesthesia, the unpleasant side effect of burning or pain upon injection is common. Various strategies have been investigated to minimize this. Some include the application of eutetic mixture of local anesthetics (EMLA) cream to the intravenous site,[42] preadministration filtration of propofol,[43] preadministration of metoprolol,[44] ketorolac,[45] remifentanil,[46] inhaled nitrous oxide,[47] magnesium sulfate,[48] granisetron,[49] mixing propofol with thiopental,[50] and adjusting the infusion rate.[51] None appear to be superior to the administration of lidocaine. The method of lidocaine delivery that is associated with the least amount of discomfort is 0.5 mg/kg injected intravenously 30–120 sec prior to propofol with proximal venous occlusion.[52] Variations on the propofol formulation have led to experimental water-soluble prodrugs that are converted to propofol in vivo, which cause less pain upon injection. The time to peak plasma concentration and context-sensitive half-times are slightly prolonged compared to the lipid emulsion.[53]

Recovery times from propofol are obviously affected by the infusion rates used intraoperatively and the total dose given. The use of BIS monitoring can shorten patient recovery times when compared to adjustment of propofol infusion rates based on standard practice aimed at fast emergence times. Infusion rates for the standard practice were

134 μg/kg/min compared to 116 μg/kg/min in the BIS-titrated group.[54] Return to cognitive function after propofol anesthesia also appears delayed in the elderly, despite titration based on BIS monitoring.[55] The addition of propofol to an opioid results in significant decrement in verbal memory skills even at 6 hr postadministration.[56] The use of propofol in conjunction with the ultrashort-acting opioid remifentanil can result in faster emergence times and recovery of cognitive function when compared to the use of inhalational agent alone.[57] Though this combination may hasten actual recovery, it does not appear to significantly shorten postanesthesia care unit (PACU) duration of stay.[58]

Conscious Sedation

Propofol is considered an excellent agent for brief hypnosis during unpleasant and painful procedures both in the operating room and in procedure suites. The combination of propofol (0.5 mg/kg) and remifentanil (0.5 μg/kg) is associated with the least number of adverse events and highest percentage of satisfactory conditions during retrobulbar block.[59] Propofol can also be mixed with remifentanil to form a stable mixture.[60] The combination of these two drugs has been used as patient-controlled sedation during shock wave lithotripsy with some success.[61] The combination of propofol and remifentanil has also been used for colonoscopies but has a higher incidence of apnea and hypotension when compared to a midazolam, fentanyl, and propofol technique.[62] Propofol has also been mixed with alfentanil (400 mg propofol/1 mg alfentanil) and infused simultaneously. An infusion scheme of 166 μg/kg/min for 10 min, followed by 133 μg/kg/min and maintenance at 100 μg/kg/min, was shown to have equal outcomes compared to separate infusions.[63] The separate administration of propofol and fentanyl compared to midazolam and meperidine is associated with higher patient satisfaction.[64] A propofol-based sedation for endoscopy is also being used by non-anesthesia providers with relatively few complications.[65,66]

Propofol is also a commonly used drug for nonoperative procedures such as magnetic resonance imaging (MRI) for children. Infusion rates between 100 and 250 μg/kg/min were calculated via a drop/minute technique in the absence of MRI-compatible equipment for successful hypnosis.[67]

Economic Aspects

With the introduction of rapidly acting inhalational agents, the economics of propofol use for maintenance of general anesthesia has been examined. When used for outpatient knee arthroscopy, propofol infused via target-controlled infusion results in slightly longer emergence times (2–3 min). Cost for maintenance with inhalational agents was 45% lower than when propofol was used for maintenance. In this study, there was no difference between postoperative nausea, emesis, or recovery stay.[68] It has also been hypothesized that the rapid offset action of propofol when used for relatively short surgeries (under

1 hr) may hasten the ability of ambulatory patients to be "fast-tracked" as compared to the inhalational agents sevoflurane and desflurane. When looking at laparoscopic tubal ligations, the use of propofol for maintenance is associated with longer emergence times, longer times to reach Aldrete scores of 10, and fewer patients viewed as able to bypass phase 1 recovery. Of those patients who were not "fast-tracked," excess sedation in the propofol group was the primary reason for admission to the PACU.[69] There was no difference in PACU length of stay or in total time to home readiness for any of the groups.[70] The use of propofol for induction and an inhalational agent for maintenance appears to be the most economical approach to actual costs of anesthetic drugs when compared to propofol induction/propofol maintenance. On the day after surgery, no differences could be detected between the inhalational or propofol groups.[71] While this technique has the lowest direct costs associated with it, there is a trend toward increased risk of nausea and vomiting with the inhalational maintenance group. To further reduce direct costs of anesthetic drugs, titration to BIS monitoring has been proposed. While propofol consumption decreased by 29%, the increased cost of monitoring did not reach the "break-even" point, which was calculated to be an anesthetic of 704 min in duration.[72] The total costs must be weighed, including cost of antiemetics and prolonged PACU stay, among others. After ambulatory surgical procedures, two of the main anesthetic factors affecting length of stay are subjective complaints of dizziness and of postoperative nausea.[73] Patient satisfaction also appears to be reduced with inhalational maintenance when compared to the propofol maintenance group.[74,75] To further cost savings, methohexital has been used for induction with an inhalational agent for maintenance with equal recovery times and side effect profile when compared to propofol induction/inhalational maintenance.[76]

Propofol as an Antiemetic

The antiemetic effects of propofol have been well established in the literature.[77,78] In 2003, a consensus conference for the managing of postoperative nausea and vomiting (PONV) was established. Systematic reviews of the literature led to an evidence-based review of strategies for the reduction in risk of PONV (Fig. 16-1). In these, the use of propofol for both induction and maintenance of anesthesia is the only anesthetic technique that is viewed as having good evidence in the literature for the reduction of PONV.[79]

The precise antiemetic action of propofol remains unclear. It may be related to alterations in serotonin levels in the area postrema.[80] It does not appear to be related to peripheral prokinetic effects on gastric emptying[81] or to dopamine subtype 2 receptor blockade,[82] a common site of action of other antiemetic agents. However, propofol has been shown to increase dopamine concentrations in the nucleus accumbens, an area of the brain associated with reward and substance abuse.[83] Experimentally, there is a threshold plasma concentration of propofol that is seen to have antiemetic activity. When propofol was given in in-

Use of regional anesthesia (IIIA)

Use of propofol for induction and maintenance of anesthesia (IA)

Use of intraoperative supplemental oxygen (IIIB)

Use of hydration (IIIA)

Avoidance of nitrous oxide (IIA)

Avoidance of volatile anesthetics (IA)

Minimization of intraoperative (IIA) and postoperative (IVA) opioids

Minimization of neostigmine (IIA)

Figure 16-1 Evidence-based strategies for the reduction in baseline risk of postoperative nausea and vomiting. (From Gan TJ, Meyer T, Apfel C, et al. Consensus guidelines for managing postoperative nausea and vomiting. Anesth Analg 2003;97:62–71.)

creasing amounts to patients experiencing nausea and vomiting postoperatively, a 93% success rate was noted in the reduction of subjective symptoms of nausea. From this study, a plasma concentration of propofol associated with a 50% reduction in PONV was determined to be 343 ng/mL.[84] For most adults, this corresponds to a 10-mg bolus followed by an infusion of 10 μg/kg/min. Empirical clinical treatment with propofol in the PACU for nausea shows a 25–29% reduction in nausea scores for 20- and 40-mg doses respectively. Several patients receiving the higher dose (40 mg) experienced oversedation, leading to the recommendation of 20 mg as a standard antiemetic dose.[85]

The antiemetic effect of these small doses of propofol is most likely short-lived. A continuous postoperative infusion of propofol (16 μg/kg/min) has been shown to significantly reduce the incidence of nausea during the study period (24 hr).[86] Currently this is a non-FDA-approved indication for propofol use.

The antiemetic effects of propofol have impacted anesthesia drug selection by anesthesiologists. Of 150 anesthesiologists surveyed, 84% use propofol specifically for its antiemetic effects. For cases expected to last under 1 hr, the majority of anesthesiologists are using propofol solely for induction. Another one-third are using propofol as part of a "sandwich" technique, with propofol being used as an induction agent followed by maintenance with an inhalational agent. An additional bolus of propofol is given within the final minutes of surgery. Using pharmacokinetic modeling, the plasma concentration of propofol falls below that known to have an antiemetic effect in 32 min after a 2-mg/kg induction dose. When a 20-mg "sandwich" dose is supplied 60 min later, the plasma concentration of propofol is in the therapeutic antiemetic range for only 7 min (Fig. 16-2).[87] This fairly common clinical practice has been shown to not function well as an antiemetic. The propofol "sandwich" functioned no better as an antiemetic than a propofol induction alone when studied in breast surgery. Only when propofol was used as an maintenance agent, significant antiemetic activity occur, which was equal in magnitude to ondansetron, 4 mg.[88]

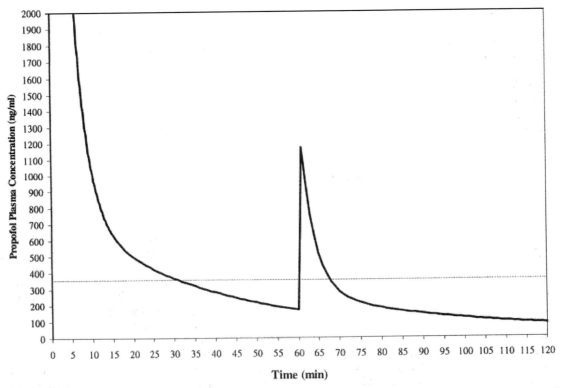

Figure 16-2 Pharmacokinetic modeling of plasma propofol concentration during antiemetic "sandwich" technique. (From Soppitt AJ, Glass PS, Howell S, et al. The use of propofol for its antiemetic effect: a survey of clinical practice in the United States. J Clin Anesth 2000;12:265–69.)

BENZODIAZEPINES

Three main benzodiazepines are used in anesthesia: diazepam, lorazepam, and midazolam. All benzodiazepines are thought to work via the GABA receptor, though the interaction with the receptor may be different than that of barbiturates. All are lipid-soluble agents with rapid onset of action when administered intravenously, though slower than other routinely used intravenous induction agents. Common uses for benzodiazepines include anxiolysis, sedation/amnesia for procedures or during regional anesthesia, as a premedication to general anesthesia, or as an induction agent. Diazepam, lorazepam, and midazolam are all principally metabolized in the liver. The half-life of these agents vary: diazepam, 20–50 hr; lorazepam, 11–22 hr; and midazolam, 1.7–2.6 hr.[89] The liver metabolism of midazolam may be inhibited by the presence of other medications or foods such as grapefruit juice[90] or ethanol.[91] Midazolam has found itself in common clinical use owing to a relative lack of active metabolites and to its shorter half-life than lorazepam and diazepam.

Pharmacology

All benzodiazepines have rapid onset of action when administered intravenously because of their relatively high lipid solubility. Of the three agents, midazolam is the most lipid-soluble, but is available in a water-soluble formula containing 0.8% sodium chloride, 0.01% disodium edetate, and 1% benzyl alcohol as a preservative at pH 3.5.[92] At physiologic pH, closure of an imidazole ring accounts for its increased lipid solubility. Parenteral midazolam received FDA approval in December 1985 and an oral version received approval in October 1998. An oral version of midazolam can also be "created" on site by combining parenteral midazolam with a palatable liquid such as Syrpalta (Humco Labs, Texarkana, TX) syrup to a final concentration of 2 mg/mL, similar to the commercially available form. Plasma concentrations of midazolam may be higher when using this combination compared to the commercially available one.[93] Other potential routes of midazolam administration include nasal and rectal.[94,95] These alternative routes of administration of intravenous midazolam, though common, are considered non-FDA-approved uses.

Cardiorespiratory Effects

Benzodiazepines produce respiratory depression in a dose-dependent manner, with 0.15 mg/kg midazolam being equivalent to 0.3 mg/kg of diazepam.[96] The speed of administration is a determinant of the rapidity of respiratory depression[97] with a flattening of the response curve to CO_2.[98] The hemodynamic effects of induction doses of midazolam are principally a mild reduction in systemic vascular resistance.[99] As with many lipid-soluble agents, repeat dosing may lead to a prolonged duration of clinical action.

Clinical Use

The use of benzodiazepines for preoperative sedation in ambulatory surgery is believed to be an effective means to reduce anxiety perioperatively. In addition to patient comfort, this can result in lower blood pressures and heart rates preinduction.[100] Urinary catecholamine levels are reduced after benzodiazepine premedication.[101] The clinical significance of this is unclear, but patients receiving preprocedural sedation with midazolam report improved recovery and reduced analgesic use,[102] though this is an inconsistent finding.[103] The use of preprocedural sedation may also lessen intraoperative anesthetic requirements.[104,105] For children undergoing surgical procedures, midazolam has been compared to parental presence during the induction of anesthesia, and for repeat surgical procedures parents prefer their presence compared to preoperative sedation with oral midazolam.[106] When used as an oral premedication for children, doses 0.25 mg/kg, 0.5 mg/kg, and 1 mg/kg have been investigated, with an increase in adverse events such as respiratory depression and nausea in the higher dose group. The smaller dose of 0.25 mg/kg appears to be as effective as 0.5 mg/kg.[107] The use of 0.5 mg/kg oral midazolam can be associated with prolonged emergence times from general anesthesia, but is not associated with delayed discharge in the ambulatory setting.[108,109] Other studies suggest that delayed emergence from general anesthesia correlates with the presence of excess preoperative sedation from the midazolam.[110] Intravenous midazolam (0.04 mg/kg) is shown to reduce performance on motor tests in the PACU, but not to delay emergence or discharge readiness in adults.[111] Administration of oral midazolam (0.2 mg/kg) has also been shown to reduce emergence agitation associated with sevoflurane anesthesia.[112]

Midazolam is frequently used as a component of sedation/analgesia by both anesthesia and non-anesthesia providers. The combination of midazolam and opioid produces greater patient tolerance than midazolam alone when used for outpatient colonoscopy.[113] For ambulatory surgical procedures, the use of midazolam as a hypnotic is associated with prolonged return to baseline functional status. Sleep latency is decreased for up to 4 hr after 0.07 mg/kg midazolam with 2 μg/kg fentanyl when compared to a propofol/fentanyl technique.[114] Performance on psychomotor tests and short-term memory were measured after 2 mg midazolam and 50 μg fentanyl and found to be of equal impairment to a blood alcohol level of 0.11 for 90–120 min postinjection.[115] When compared to alprazolam, premedication with midazolam provides better amnesia and more rapid return to baseline on motor function tests.[116] Age correlates with reduced dose to achieve the same effect as well as delayed return to functional status.[117]

Flumazenil

Flumazenil is structurally related to the benzodiazepines, but functions as an antagonist. It was approved for clinical use in December 1991. It has high receptor affinity and low intrinsic activity.[118] It is a competitive antagonist and will occupy the receptor in place of the agonist as it undergoes normal association/dissociation kinetics. Flumazenil undergoes rapid liver metabolism and has a half-life of about 1 hr. This is even shorter than midazolam and may allow for resedation of a patient as the antagonist is metabolized.[119] Flumazenil is typically given incrementally in doses of 0.2–0.5 mg up to 3 mg. It will not reverse the respiratory depressant effects of drugs from other classes such as opioids. Reversal of benzodiazepines has been used to shorten postprocedure times after endoscopy with improved sedation scores 30 min postinjection.[120] In an attempt to prolong the duration of action of flumazenil, it has been given orally (3 mg). Antagonist effects are seen within 20 min, but performance on alertness testing remained poor.[121]

KETAMINE

Pharmacology

Ketamine is a schedule III controlled substance that received FDA approval in 1970. It is structurally related to phencyclidines (PCP) and has been attributed to have many of the same adverse effects, including psychosis with hallucinations (primarily visual). Its primary method of action is believed to be blockade of the NMDA receptor. The incidence of psychosis has been reported to be greater than 30% at 1–3 mg/kg. This can be reduced by pretreatment with benzodiazepines (e.g., midazolam). Ketamine is classically described as a neurostimulant resulting in increases in cerebral metabolic rate and cerebral blood flow.[122] Subanesthetic doses of ketamine appear to have no effect on cerebral metabolic rate, and cause only slight increases in cerebral blood volume in the frontal region.[123] Ketamine has minimal respiratory depression, is a bronchodilator, and can increase myocardial oxygen consumption.

Ketamine is a highly lipid-soluble drug and when administered intravenously has a rapid onset of action. A single dose of 0.5 mg/kg has rapid metabolism with a decline to undetectable concentrations by 180 min.[124] Clinical action is terminated by both redistribution and metabolism with hepatic metabolites about one-third as active and excreted primarily renally. Upon administration, typical patient findings would include papillary dilation, nystagmus, increased lacrimation and salivation as well as increased skeletal muscle tone. Certain reflexes may be intact, but airway reflexes should not be assumed to be protected. The pharmacodynamics of ketamine has been assessed using BIS as a monitor. Ketamine is known to increase theta waves on the electroencephalogram (EEG). In propofol-sedated individuals, ketamine administered as a bolus (0.4 mg/kg) followed by an infusion rate of 1 mg/kg/hr resulted in a statistically significant rise in BIS score from 3 to 8 min after bolus.[125] The rise in BIS scores is paralleled by a rise in the spectral edge (95%).[126] After a 1.5-mg/kg intubating dose of ketamine, BIS scores remained greater than 90 in the absence of other anesthetic agents, despite the clinical appearance of an anesthetized patient.[127] Alternative routes of administration of ketamine include oral, intramuscular, nasal, rectal, and epidural with a preservative-free solution.

Clinical Use

Low-dose ketamine (0.15 mg/kg) has been shown to decrease postoperative pain scores, decrease analgesic requirements, and improve mobility after knee arthroscopy,[128] as well as anterior cruciate ligament repair.[129] A similar dose of ketamine was found to decrease analgesic requirements after outpatient surgery.[130] major abdominal surgery,[131] and renal surgery.[132] The addition of ketamine to an intraoperative analgesic regimen has been shown to reduce the hypertension associated with tourniquet pain.[133] Low-dose ketamine (0.5 mg/kg) has also been associated with mood elevation in the first 24 hr in depressed patients who underwent orthopedic procedures,[134] but can cause deficits in information processing.[135]

The analgesic effects of ketamine have made it an alternative to opioids as analgesics for procedural sedation/analgesia. With increasing dose, there is noted to be an increased incidence of nausea and vomiting[136] as well as delayed emergence and discharge times.[137,138] For cases where general anesthesia is associated with a high risk of PONV, ketamine has been examined as an alternative to traditional opioid-based analgesics. During outpatient tubal ligation surgery, ketamine (1–1.5 mg/kg) was used as a replacement for fentanyl (3–5 μg/kg). There appeared to be no difference in the incidence of nausea or in PACU discharge times. However, there was an increased incidence of PACU analgesic administration and dreaming in the ketamine group.[138] The incidence of postoperative psychologic effects appears to be greater in this study (17%) compared to other reports of propofol/ketamine-based anesthesia. When used for tumescent liposuction, propofol/ketamine anesthesia results in dreaming in 1% of patients.[139] The difference has been attributed to the duration of the surgical procedure, 30–40 min versus 151–160 min,[138] and the continued administration of an hypnotic agent (propofol) in the period after ketamine administration.

Ketamine has also been investigated as an adjunct to sedation during central neuraxial anesthesia. When it was given at a low dose (100 μg/kg) and followed by a 300-μg/kg/hr infusion, no detectable difference was observed in sedation score or amount of propofol used to achieve a set level of sedation. Those administered ketamine had significantly higher blood pressures however.[140] When used in combination with propofol for brief painful procedures such as retrobulbar block, ketamine results in better tolerance with less respiratory depression.[141] For preoperative sedation, ketamine appears to be an effective sedative when given orally in the 4–8-mg/kg dose, though higher doses are associated with longer recovery times.[142,143] Intranasal administration at 3 mg/kg appears an effective premedication.[144]

Though currently not approved for clinical use in the United States, the S+ isomer of ketamine is associated with less decline in cognitive function when compared to the R–.[145,146] It is unclear whether the perioperative analgesia of the S+ isomer will be equal to that of the racemic mixture.[147]

BARBITURATES

Historically, barbiturates have been the primary intravenous induction agents. They can be categorized based on structure into thio- and oxybarbiturates. The common thiobarbiturates used in anesthesia include thiopental and thiamylal, with methohexital being the only commonly used oxybarbiturate. For barbiturates, a decrease in the pH of the solution can result in decreased solubility of the drug; combining thiopental and vecuronium or rocuronium may result in precipitation and blocking of an intravenous line.

Pharmacology

Barbiturates are primarily metabolized in the liver, with methohexital having a shorter metabolic half-life than thiopental (4 hr vs. 12 hr).[148] These actions occur primarily via GABA both by enhancing and by mimicking the action of the neurotransmitter.[149] Barbiturates have respiratory depressant effects with apnea after rapid intravenous administration as well as causing decrease in systolic blood pressure related to venous pooling of blood upon administration. A well-known side effect of barbiturates at low doses is "antianalgesia" where the patient has a heightened awareness to pain.[150]

Clinical Use

In the ambulatory setting, propofol has surpassed the barbiturates as intravenous induction agents, mostly related to propofol short half-life, rapid metabolism, decreased accumulation with repetitive dosing, antiemetic effect, and sense of well-being. For patients with allergy to components of propofol such as egg or soybean, the barbiturates represent a functional alternative.

The barbiturates have also been examined as a cost-effective alternative to propofol. When used for sedation for ambulatory breast biopsy, the actual cost of drug used was slightly less for methohexital compared to propofol. However, when drug wastage was accounted for, there was no difference.[151] When used for outpatient gynecologic procedures, the cost of methohexital was less than one-half that of propofol.[152] The potential complications and success rate of short, painful procedures such as joint and fracture reductions seem no different between propofol and methohexital.[153] Patient satisfaction with either propofol or thiopental as induction agent appears equal, though there may be slightly faster awakening with propofol.[154] Other studies have found that the total costs (including PACU stay) associated with a propofol induction may be less than an equivalent thiopental induction.[155] Recent difficulties in obtaining methohexital commercially have made its usage less common.

ETOMIDATE

Etomidate is a short-acting intravenous hypnotic that is believed to have its actions via GABA transmission in the CNS. Etomidate is rapidly hydrolyzed in the liver and undergoes renal excretion of metabolites. It gained FDA approval in September 1982 and is formulated in a 35% propylene glycol solution. Initial enthusiasm for the drug was tainted by reports of inhibition of steroid hormone synthesis. Evidence suggests that the inhibition of steroid hormone synthesis is brief and of questionable clinical significance when etomidate is used as an induction agent.[156-158]

Clinical Use

Etomidate has developed a niche as an anesthetic induction agent with hemodynamic stability. Doses of 0.3 mg/kg are well tolerated without significant hemodynamic changes. The respiratory depressant effects of etomidate seem less than those of the barbiturates.[159] For brief sedation during painful procedures, etomidate is frequently used by non-anesthesia providers safely and with high patient satisfaction.[160] However, propofol is suggested to have faster recovery after brief procedures.[161] Etomidate has a high incidence of pain upon injection, which is believed to be related to its solvent preparation[162] that is equal in magnitude to propofol.[161] Etomidate also has a high incidence of thrombophlebitis associated with its use.[163] The incidence of nausea associated with etomidate may vary, but may not exceed that of other intravenous induction agents.[164]

Etomidate has been used successfully for outpatient cardioversion. When compared to propofol, there is a mild increase in blood pressure compared to a decrease with propofol.[165] Recovery times appear equal between the two drugs.[166] Etomidate has been used in the pediatric population for procedural sedation such as MRI in a 0.2-mg/kg dose.[167]

ALPHA-2 ADRENEGIC AGONISTS

Alpha-2 adrenergic agonists were introduced into medicine as antihypertensive agents. Their role as anesthetic adjuvants came about after observations of patients on clonidine therapy undergoing anesthesia. Clonidine is available in an oral, transdermal, and preservative-free preparation. The preservative-free preparation received FDA approval in 1997. Clonidine is known to reduce the minimum alveolar concentration (MAC) of inhalational anesthetics[168-170] as well as decrease the dose of intravenous agents to provide for loss of consciousness.[171,172] Intravenous administration of clonidine (2 μg/kg) has been shown to reduce the incidence of PONV after breast surgery.[173] Intra-articular administration of clonidine (1 μg/kg) has been shown to potentiate the effects of intra-articular morphine as well as have significant analgesic activity of its own.[174,175] Intrathecal administration of clonidine (15 μg) has been used as an adjuvant to prolong the duration of action of ropivacaine spinal anesthesia for ambulatory knee arthroscopy without significant hemodynamic effects.[176] The systemic administration of clonidine in the ambulatory setting is limited by the drug's relatively long duration of action.

Dexmedetomidine is a short-acting alpha-2 agonist that was approved by the FDA in December 1999 as an intravenous sedative for periods less than 24 hr. It has a short redistribution half-life (6 min) and is primarily metabolized in the liver. Renal failure does not appear to significantly alter its pharmacokinetics.[177] The most prominent side effects associated with administration of the drug include bradycardia and hypotension. Dexmedetomidine has a 1600 times affinity for the alpha-2 receptor compared to the alpha-1, but under higher dosing, the alpha-1 effects may be seen with resultant hypertension.[178] It is believed to have similar effects as clonidine both for MAC reduction of inhalational anesthetics and for intravenous agents as well.[179–181] Perioperative dexmedetomidine is associated with reduced heart rate and catecholamine levels upon emergence.[182]

Clinical Use

When used as an intraoperative sedative, the dose range is typically 0.4–0.7 µg/kg/hr maintenance following a 1-µg/kg load dose over 10 min. This is associated with slightly longer recovery times, lower blood pressures, and less analgesic requirements in the PACU when compared to propofol for sedation.[183] Experimentally, dexmedetomidine has been shown to have an amnestic, analgesic, and blood-pressure-lowering effect in humans with doses as small as 0.2 µg/kg/hr. Mild desaturation (not less than 95%) on room air was also noted at this low dose.[184] This is consistent with the known mild respiratory depressant effect of the drug.[185] The sedative effects of dexmedetomidine have also been used to decrease the emergence delirium associated with sevoflurane without significant delay in PACU discharge times,[186] as well as decrease the emergence delirium associated with ketamine anesthesia.[187] Dexmedetomidine has also been used in conjunction with meperidine to synergistically reduce shivering in response to hypothermia.[188]

The use of dexmedetomidine is associated with changes in BIS scores comparable to that of propofol for equal levels of clinical sedation.[189] There is an associated increase in duration of rocuronium blockade associated with the use of dexmedetomidine that may be related to distribution of blood flow. However, it is of questionable clinical significance.[190] Increased familiarity with this sedative/analgesic is leading to its increased use in the ambulatory setting.

OTHER AGENTS

Droperidol

Although not typically thought of as an intravenous sedative, droperidol is chemically a butyrophenone related to haloperidol. Its sedative properties may be based on actions at the GABA receptor when it is used as a component of neuroleptic-anesthesia. Droperidol is most commonly used for its antiemetic activity, which is believed to occur via actions on dopamine, and to a lesser extent serotonin and norepinephrine, and has historically been considered a cost-effective first-line agent for PONV prophylaxis.[191]

Droperidol was first approved by the FDA in 1970, but underwent reevaluation in December 2001 when the FDA announced a "black box warning" to be placed on droperidol based on its potential to cause serious cardiac dysrhythmias, including torsade de pointes and QT interval prolongation. It also restricted its approved indications to the prevention of PONV. A preadministration 12-lead electrocardiogram (ECG) is recommended to evaluate for the presence of prolonged QT syndrome, as well as continuous ECG monitoring for 2–3 hr after administration. The need for such monitoring has been questioned by several recent editorials when droperidol is used at the typical antiemetic doses of 0.625–1.25 mg[192–194] as there have been no reports of dysrhythmias at the antiemetic doses.

As an antiemetic, droperidol is considered as efficacious as ondansetron for the prophylaxis of PONV with number needed to treat between 5 and 6.[195,196] Routine use of droperidol has been shown to be as effective and have as high patient satisfaction as the use of ondansetron for high-risk ambulatory surgeries with significantly less cost.[197] Droperidol (0.625 or 1.25 mg) has also been used as an antiemetic in combination with the 5-Hydroxytryptamine 3 (5-HT$_3$) antagonists or steroids for improved response compared to individual drugs alone.[198,199]

Scopolamine

Scopolamine is considered a muscarinic antagonist by pharmaceutic classification that its tertiary amine structure has penetration into the CNS. Scopolamine had a role in anesthesia both as a sedating premedication and as an antiemetic.[200] It is an effective treatment for motion sickness and has been used effectively for the treatment of PONV. In the ambulatory setting, this is its primary role with the transdermal application requiring application at least 1–2 hr prior to surgery. Its usefulness is limited by the potential side effects, including blurred vision and dry mouth.[201]

REFERENCES

1. Laxenaire, MC, Mata-Bermejo E, Moneret-Vautrin D, Gueant JL. Life-threatening anaphylactoid reactions to propofol (Diprivan). Anesthesiology 1992;77:275–80.

2. Hofer KN, McCarthy MW, Buck ML, Henderick AE. Possible anaphylaxis after propofol in a child with food allergy. Ann Pharmacother 2003;37:398–401.

3. Kushikata T, Hirota K, Yoshida H, et al. Alpha-2 adrenoreceptor activity affects propofol-induced sleep time. Anesth Analg 2002;94:1201–6.

4. Kubota T, Hirota K, Yoshida H, et al. Effects of sedatives on noradrenaline release from the medial prefrontal cortex in rats. Psychopharmacology 1999;146:335–38.

5. Lingamaneni R, Birch ML, Hemmings HC. Widespread inhibition

of sodium channel-dependent glutamate release from isolated nerve terminals by isoflurane and propofol. Anesthesiology 2001;94: 1460–66.

6.   Major E, Verniquet AJ, Wadell TK, et al. A study of three doses of ICI 35868 for induction and maintenance of anesthesia. Br J Anaesth 1981;53:267–72.

7.   Aun CS, Short SM, Leung DH, Oh TE. Induction dose-response of propofol in unpremedicated children. Br J Anaesth 1992;68:64–67.

8.   Vuyk J, Oostwounder CJ, Vletter AA, et al. Gender differences in the pharmacokinetics of propofol in elderly patients during and after continuous infusion. Br J Anaesth 2001;86:183–88.

9.   Zacny JP, Lichtor JL, Coalson DW, et al. Subjective and psychomotor effects of sub-anesthetic doses of propofol in healthy volunteers. Anesthesiology 1992;76:696–702.

10. Glass PS, Bloom K, Kearse L, et al. Bispectral analysis measures sedation and memory effects of propofol, midazolam, isoflurane and alfentanil in healthy volunteers. Anesthesiology 1997;86:836–47.

11. Simons P, Cockshott I, Douglas E. Blood concentrations, metabolism, and elimination after a subanesthetic dose of (14 C) propofol (Diprivan) to male volunteers. Postgrad Med J 1985; 61:64.

12. Dawidowicz AL, Fornal E, Mardarowicz M, Fijalkowska A. The role of human lungs in the biotransformation of propofol. Anesthesiology 2000;93:922–27.

13. Marsh B, White M, Morton N, Kenny GN. Pharmacokinetic model driven infusion of propofol in children. Br J Anaesth 1991;67: 41–48.

14. Kazama T, Morita K, Ikeda T, et al. Comparison of predicted induction dose with predetermined physiologic characteristics of patients and with pharmacokinetic models incorporating those characteristics as covariates. Anesthesiology 2003;98:299–305.

15. Briggs LP, White M. The effects of premedication on anaesthesia with propofol (Diprivan). Postgrad Med J 1985;61(Supp 3):35–37.

16. Steib A, Freys G, Beller JP, et al. Propofol in elderly high risk patients. A comparison of haemodynamic effects with thiopentone during induction of anesthesia. Anaesthesia 1988;43(Supp):111–14.

17. Goyal P, Puri GD, Pandey CK, Srivastva S. Evaluation of induction doses of propofol: comparison between endstage renal disease and normal renal function patients. Anaesth Intens Care 2002;30: 584–87.

18. Turtle MJ, Cullen P, Pyrs-Roberts C, et al. Dose requirements of propofol by infusion during nitrous oxide anaesthesia in man. II: Patients premedicated with lorazepam. Br J Anaesth 1987;59: 283–87.

19. Erhan E, Ugur G, Gunusen I, et al. Propofol-not thiopental or etomidate- with remifentanil provides adequate intubating conditions in the absence of neuromuscular blockade. Can J Anaesth 2003;50:108–15.

20. Taylor MB, Grounds RM, Mulrooney PD, Morgan M. Ventilatory effect of propofol during induction of anaesthesia: comparison with thiopentone. Anaesthesia 1986;41:816–20.

21. Goodman NW, Black AM, Carter JA. Some ventilatory effects of propofol as sole anaesthetic agent. Br J Anaesth 1987;59:1497–503.

22. Blouin R, Seifert H, Conrad P. Propofol significantly decreases hypoxic ventilatory drive during conscious sedation. Anesthesiology 1992;A1215.

23. Conti G, DellUtri D, Vilardi V, et al. Propofol induces bronchodilation in mechanically ventilated chronic obstructive pulmonary disease (COPD) patients. Acta Anaesthesiol Scand 1993;37:105–9.

24. Aun C, Major E. The cardiorespiratory effects of ICI 35868 in patients with valvular heart disease. Anaesthesia 1984;39:1096–100.

25. Graham MR, Thiessen DB, Mutch WA. Left ventricular systolic and diastolic function is unaltered during propofol infusion in newborn swine. Anesth Analg 1998;86:717–23.

26. Cullen PM, Turtle M, Prys-Roberts C, et al. Effect of propofol anesthesia on baroreceptor activity in humans. Anesth Analg 1987;66: 1115–20.

27. Horiguchi T, Nishikawa T. Heart rate response to atropine during propofol anesthesia. Anesth Analg 2002;95:389–92.

28. Miro O, de la Red G, Fontanals J. Cessation of paroxysmal atrial fibrillation during acute intravenous propofol administration. Anesthesiology 2000;92:910.

29. Hermann R, Vettermann J. Change of ectopic supraventicular tachycardia to sinus rhythm during administration of propofol. Anesth Analg 1992;75:1030–32.

30. Burjorjee JE, Milne B. Propofol for electrical storm: a case report of cardioversion and suppression of ventricular tachycardia by propofol. Can J Anaesth 2002;49:473–77.

31. Wu M. Propofol and the supraventricular tachydysrhythmias in children. Anaesth Analg 1998;86:814.

32. Herregods LL, Bossyut GP, De Baerdemaeker LE, et al. Ambulatory external electrical cardioversion with propofol or etomidate. J Clin Anesth 2003;15:91–96.

33. Bennett SM, McNeil MM, Bland LA, et al. Postoperative infections traced to contamination of an intravenous anesthetic, propofol. N Engl J Med 1995;333:147–54.

34. Henry B, Plante-Jenkins C, Ostrsowska K. An outbreak of *Serratia marcescens* associated with the anesthetic agent propofol. Am J Infect Control 2001;29:312–15.

35. McNeil MM, Lasker BA, Lott TJ, Jarvis WR. Post surgical *Candida albicans* infections associated with an extrinsically contaminated intravenous anesthetic. J Clin Microbiol 1999;37:1398–1403.

36. Berry AJ. *Recommendations for Handling Parenteral Medications Used for Anesthesia or Sedation.* Pittsburgh: Anesthesia Patient Safety Foundation, 1995.

37. Aydin N, Aydin N, Gultekin B, et al. Bacterial contamination of propofol, the effects of temperature and lidocaine. Eur J Anaesthesiol 2002;19:455–58.

38. Harvey BR, Ganzberg S. Growth of microorganisms in propofol and methohexital mixtures. J Oral Maxillofac Surg 2003;61:818–23.

39. Wachowski I, Jolly DT, Hrazdil J, et al. The growth of microorganisms in propofol and mixtures of propofol and lidocaine. Anaesth Analg 1999;88:209–12.

40. Vidovich MI, Peterson LR, Wong HY. The effect of lidocaine on bacterial growth in propofol. Anesth Analg 1999;88:936–38.

41. Sakuragi T, Yanagisawa K, Shirari Y, Dan K. Growth of *Escherichia coli* in propofol, and mixtures of propofol and lidocaine. Acta Anaesthesiol Scand 1999;43:476–79.

42. McCluskey A, Currer BA, Sayeed I. The efficacy of 5% lidocaine/prilocaine (EMLA) cream on pain during intravenous injection of propofol. Anesth Analg 2003;97:713–14.

43. Hellier C, Newell S, Barry J, Brimacombe J. A 5-micron filter does not reduce propofol-induced pain. Anaesthesia 2003;58:802–3.

44. Asik I, Yorukoglu D, Gulay I, Tulunay M. Pain on injection of propofol: comparison of metoprolol and lidocaine. Eur J Anaesthesiol 2003;20:487–89.

45. Huang YW, Buerkle H, Lee TH, et al. Effect of pretreatment with ketorolac on propofol injection pain. Acta Anaesthesiol Scand 2002; 46:1021–24.

46. Roehm KD, Piper SN, Maleck WH, Boldt J. Prevention of propofol-induced pain by remifentanil: a placebo controlled comparison with lidocaine. Anaesthesia 2003;58:165–70.

47. Harmon D, Rozario C, Lowe D. Nitrous oxide/oxygen mixture and the prevention of pain during injection of propofol. Eur J Anaesthesiol 2003;20:158–61.

48. Memis D, Turan A, Karamanlioglu B, et al. The use of magnesium sulfate to prevent pain on injection of propofol. Anesth Analg 2002; 95:606–8.

49. Dubey PK, Prasad SS. Pain on injection of propofol: the effect of granisetron pretreatment. Clin J Pain 2003;19:121–24.

50. Jones D, Prankerd R, Lang C, et al. Propofol-thiopentone admixture-hypnotic dose, pain on injection and effect on blood pressure. Anaesth Intensive Care 1999;27:346–56.

51. Grauers A, Liljeuth E, Akeson J. Propofol infusion rate does not af-

fect local pain on injection. Acta Anaesthesiol Scand 2002;46: 361–63.

52. Picard P, Tramer MR. Prevention of pain on injection with propofol: a quantitative systemic review. Anesth Analg 2000;90:963–69.

53. Fechner J, Ihmsen H, Hatterscheid D, et al. Pharmacokinetics and clinical pharmacodynamics of the new propofol prodrug GPI 15715 in volunteers. Anesthesiology 2003;99:303–13.

54. Gan TJ, Glass PS, Winsdor A, et al. Bispectral index monitoring allows faster emergence and improved recovery from propofol, alfentanil, and nitrous oxide anesthesia. Anesthesiology 1997;87: 808–15.

55. Shinozaki M, Usui Y, Yamaguchi S, et al. Recovery of psychomotor function after propofol sedation is prolonged in the elderly. Can J Anaesth 2002;49:927–31.

56. N'Kaoua B, Veron AL, Lespinet VC, et al. Time course of cognitive recovery after propofol anesthesia: a level of processing approach. J Clin Exp Neuropsychol 2002;24:713–19.

57. Larsen B, Seitz A, Larsen R. Recovery of cognitive function after remifentanil-propofol anesthesia: a comparison with desflurane and sevoflurane anesthesia. Anesth Analg 2000;90:168–74.

58. Montes FR, Trillos JE, Rincon IE, et al. Comparison of total intravenous anesthesia and sevoflurane-fentanyl anesthesia for outpatient otorhinolaryngeal surgery. J Clin Anesth 2002;14:324–28.

59. Rewari V, Madan R, Kaul HL, Kumar L. Remifentanil and propofol sedation for retrobulbar nerve block. Anaesth Intens Care 2002;30:433–37.

60. Stewart JT, Warren FW, Maddox FC, et al. The stability of remifentanil hydrochloride and propofol mixtures in polypropylene syringes and polyvinylchloride bags at 22°C–24°C. Anesth Analg 2000;90:1450–51.

61. Joo HS, Perks WJ, Kataoka MT, et al. A comparison of patient-controlled sedation using either remifentanil or remifentanil-propofol for shock wave lithotripsy. Anesth Analg 2001;93: 1227–32.

62. Rudner R, Jalowiecki P, Kawiecki P, et al. Conscious analgesia/sedation with remifentanil and propofol versus total intravenous anesthesia with fentanyl, midazolam, and propofol for outpatient colonoscopy. Gastrointest Endosc 2003;57:657–63.

63. Taylor IN, Kenny GN, Glen JB. Pharmacodynamic stability of a mixture of propofol and alfentanil. Br J Anaesth 1992;69:168–71.

64. Koshy G, Nair S, Norkus EP, et al. Propofol versus midazolam and meperidine for conscious sedation in GI endoscopy. Am J Gastroenterol 2000;95:1476–79.

65. Sipe BW, Rex DK, Latinovich D, et al. Propofol versus midazolam/meperidine for outpatient colonoscopy: administration by nurses supervised by endoscopists. Gastrointest Endosc 2002;55: 815–25.

66. Vargo JJ, Zuccaro G, Dumot JA, et al. Gastroenterologist administered propofol versus meperidine and midazolam for advanced upper endoscopy: a prospective, randomized trial. Gastroenterology 2002;123:8–16.

67. Usher A, Kearney R. Anesthesia for magnetic resonance imaging in children: a survey of Canadian pediatric centres. Can J Anaesth 2000;50:425.

68. Dolk A, Cannerfelt R, Anderson RE, Jakobsonn, J. Inhalational agent is cost-effective for ambulatory surgery: a clinical comparison with propofol during elective knee arthroscopy. Eur J Anaesthesiol 2002;19:88–92.

69. Coloma M, Zhou T, White PF, et al. Fast-tracking after outpatient laparoscopy: reasons for failure after propofol, sevoflurane and desflurane anesthesia. Anesth Analg 2001;93:112–15.

70. Song D, Joshi GP, White PF. Fast-track eligibility after ambulatory anesthesia: a comparison of desflurane, sevoflurane and propofol. Anesth Analg 1998;86:267–73.

71. Struys MM, Somers AA, Van Den Eynde N, et al. Cost-reduction analysis of propofol versus sevoflurane: maintenance of anaesthe-

sia for gynecological surgery using the bispectral index. Eur J Anaesthesiol 2002;19:724–34.

72. Yli-Hankala A, Vakkuri A, Annila P, Korttila K. EEG bispectral index monitoring in sevoflurane or propofol anesthesia: analysis of direct costs and immediate recovery. Acta Anaesthesiol Scand 1999;43:545–49.

73. Chung F, Mezei G. Factors contributing to prolonged stay after ambulatory surgery. Anesth Analg 1999;89:1352–59.

74. Raeder JC, Mjaland O, Asabo V, et al. Desflurane versus propofol maintenance for outpatient laparoscopic cholecystectomy. Acta Anaesthesiol Scand 1998;42:106–10.

75. Smith I, Terhoeve PA, Hennart D, et al. A multicentre comparison of the costs of anaesthesia with sevoflurane or propofol. Br J Anaesth 1999;83:564–70.

76. Sun R, Watcha MF, White PF, et al. A cost comparison of methohexital and propofol for ambulatory surgery. Anesth Analg 1999; 89:311–16.

77. Sneyd JR, Carr A, Byrom WD, Bilaski ZJ. A meta-analysis of nausea and vomiting following maintenance of anesthesia with propofol or inhalational agents. Eur J Anaesthesiol 1998;15:433–45.

78. Tramer M, Moore A, McQuay H. Propofol anaesthesia and postoperative nausea and vomiting: quantitative systemic review of randomized controlled studies. Br J Anaesth 1997;78:247–55.

79. Gan TJ, Meyer T, Apfel C, et al. Consensus guidelines for managing postoperative nausea and vomiting. Anesth Analg 2003;97: 62–71.

80. Cechetto DF, Diab T, Gibson CJ, Gelb AW. The effects of propofol in the area postrema in rats. Anesth Analg 2001;92:934–42.

81. Chassard D, Lansiaux S, Duflo F, et al. Effects of sub-hypnotic doses of propofol on gastric emptying in healthy volunteers. Anesthesiology 2002;97:96–101.

82. Appadu BL, Strange PG, Lambert DG. Does propofol interact with D2 dopamine receptors? Anesth Analg 1994;79:1191–92.

83. Pain L, Gobaille S, Schleef C, et al. In vivo dopamine measurements in the nucleus accumbens after nonanesthetic and anesthetic doses of propofol in rats. Anesth Analg 2002;95:915–19.

84. Gan TJ, Glass PS, Howell ST, et al. Determination of plasma concentrations of propofol associated with a 50% reduction in postoperative nausea. Anesthesiology 1997;87:779–84.

85. Gan TJ, El-Molem H, Ray J, Glass PS. Patient controlled antiemesis: a randomized, double-blind comparison of two doses of propofol versus placebo. Anesthesiology 1999;90(6):1564–70.

86. Ewalenko P, Janny M, DeJonckheere G, et al. Antiemetic effect of subhypnotic doses of propofol after thyroidectomy. Br J Anaesth 1996;77:463–67.

87. Soppitt AJ, Glass PS, Howell S, et al. The use of propofol for its antiemetic effect: a survey of clinical practice in the United States. J Clin Anesth 2000;12:265–69.

88. Gan TJ, Ginsberg B, Grant AP, Glass P. Double blinded, randomized comparison of ondansetron and intraoperative propofol to prevent postoperative nausea and vomiting. Anesthesiology 1996;85:1036–42.

89. Reeves JG. Benzodiazepines. In: Prys-Roberts C, Hugg CC (eds.), Pharmacokinetics of Anesthesia. Boston: Blackwell Scientific Publications, 1984, p. 157.

90. Greenblatt DJ, von Moltke LL, Harmatz JS, et al. Time course of recovery of cytochrome P450 3A after single dose of grapefruit juice. Clin Pharmacol Ther 2003;74:121–29.

91. Kassai A, Toth G, Eichelbaum M, Klotz U. No evidence of genetic polymorphism in the oxidative metabolism of midazolam. Clin Pharmacokinet 1988;15:319–25.

92. Greenblatt DJ, Shader RI, Abernethy DR. Drug therapy: current status of benzodiazepines. N Engl J Med 1983;306:354–58.

93. Brosius KK, Bannister CF. Midazolam premedication in children: a comparison of two oral dosage formulations on sedation score and plasma midazolam levels. Anesth Analg 2003;96:392–95.

94. Knoester PD, Jonker DM, van der Hoeven RT, et al. Pharmaco-

kinetics and pharmacodynamics of midazolam administered as a concentrated intranasal spray: a study in healthy volunteers. Br J Clin Pharmacol 2002;53:501–7.

95. Kogan A, Katz J, Efrat R, Eidelman LA. Premedication with midazolam in young children: a comparison of four routes of administration. Paediatr Anaesth 2002;12:685.

96. Foster A, Gardaz JP, Suter, PM, Gemperle M. Respiratory depression by midazolam and diazepam. Anesthesiology 1980;53:494–97.

97. Brogden RN, Goa KL. Flumazenil: a reappraisal of its pharmacological properties and therapeutic efficacy as a benzodiazepine antagonist. Drugs 1991;42:1061–89.

98. Sunzel M, Paalzow L, Berggren L, Eriksson I. Respiratory and cardiovascular effects in relation to plasma level of midazolam and diazepam. Br J Clin Pharmacol 1988;25:561–69.

99. Reves J, Gelman S. Cardiovascular effects of intravenous anesthetic drugs. In: Covino B, Fozzard H, Rehder K (eds.), *Effects of Anesthesia*. Bethesda, MD: American Physiological Society, 1985, p. 179.

100. Abdul-Latif MS, Putland AJ, McCluskey A, et al. Oral midazolam premedication for day case breast surgery, a randomized prospective double-blind placebo-controlled study. Anaesthesia 2001;56:990–94.

101. Duggan M, Dowd N, O'Mara D, et al. Benzodiazepine premedication may attenuate the stress response in day case anesthesia: a pilot study. Can J Anaesth 2002;49:932–35.

102. Kain ZN, Sevarino F, Pincus S, et al. Attenuation of the preoperative stress response with midazolam: effects on postoperative outcomes. Anesthesiology 2000;93:141–47.

103. Klain ZN, Sevarino FB, Rinder C, et al. Preoperative anxiolysis and postoperative recovery in women undergoing abdominal hysterectomy. Anesthesiology 2001;94:415–22.

104. Maranets I, Kain ZN. Preoperative anxiety and intraoperative anesthetic requirement. Anesth Analg 1999;89:1346–51.

105. Wilder-Smith OH, Ravussin PA, Decosterd LA, et al. Midazolam premedication reduces propofol dose requirements for multiple anesthetic endpoints. Can J Anaesth 2001;49:439–45.

106. Kain ZN, Caldwell-Andrews AA, Wang S, et al. Parental intervention choices for children undergoing repeated surgeries. Anesth Analg 2003;96:970–75.

107. Cote CJ, Cohen IT, Suresh S, et al. A comparison of three doses of commercially prepared oral midazolam syrup in children. Anesth Analg 2002;94:37–43.

108. Viitanen H, Annila P, Viitanen M, Yli-Hankala A. Midazolam delays recovery from propofol induced sevoflurane anesthesia in children 1–3 yr. Can J Anaesth 1999;46:766–71.

109. Viitanen H, Annila P, Viitanen M, Tarkkila P. Premedication with midazolam delays recovery after ambulatory sevoflurane anesthesia in children. Anesth Analg 1999;89:75–79.

110. Brosius KK, Bannister CF. Oral midazolam premedication in preadolescents and adolescents. Anesth Analg 2002;94:31–36.

111. Richardson M, Wu C, Asadullah H. Midazolam premedication increases sedation but does not prolong discharge times after brief outpatient general anesthesia for laparoscopic tubal sterilization. Anesth Analg 1997;85:301–5.

112. Ko YP, Huang CJ, Su NY, et al. Premedication with low dose oral midazolam reduces the incidence and severity of emergence agitation in pediatric patients following sevoflurane anesthesia. Acta Anaesthesiol Scand 2001;39:169–77.

113. Radaelli F, Meucci G, Terruzzi V, et al. Single bolus of midazolam versus both midazolam plus meperidine for colonoscopy: a prospective, randomized, double blind trial. Gastrointest Endosc 2003;57:329–35.

114. Lichtor JL, Alessi R, Lane BL. Sleep tendency as a measure of recovery after drugs used for ambulatory surgery. Anesthesiology 2002;96:878–83.

115. Thapar P, Zacny JP, Choi M, Apfelbaum JL. Objective and subjective impairment from often used sedative/analgesic combinations in ambulatory surgery, using alcohol as a benchmark. Anesth Analg 1995;80:1092–98.

116. De Witte JL, Alegret C, Sessler DI, Cammu G. Preoperative alprazolam reduces anxiety in ambulatory surgical patients: a comparison with oral midazolam. Anesth Analg 2002;95:1601–6.

117. Fujisawa T, Suzuki S, Tanaka K, et al. Recovery of postural stability following conscious sedation with midazolam in the elderly. J Clin Anaesth 2002;16:198–202.

118. Haefely W. The preclinical pharmacology of flumazenil. Eur J Anaesthesiol 1988;(Suppl 2):25–36.

119. Lauven PM, Schwilden H, Stoeckel H, Greenblatt DJ. The effects of a benzodiazepine antagonist Ro 15-1788 in the presence of stable concentrations of midazolam. Anesthesiology 1985;63:61–64.

120. Chang AC, Solinger MA, Yang DT, Chen YK. Impact of flumazenil on recovery after outpatient endoscopy. Gastrointest Endosc 1999;49:573–79.

121. Girdler NM, Lyne JP, Wallace R, et al. A randomized, controlled trial of cognitive and psychomotor recovery from midazolam sedation following reversal with oral flumazenil. Anaesthesia 2002;57:868–76.

122. Takeshita H, Okuda Y, Sari A. The effects of ketamine on cerebral circulation and metabolism in man. Anesthesiology 1972;36:69.

123. Langsjo JW, Kaisti KK, Aalto SM, et al. Effects of sub-anesthetic doses of ketamine on regional cerebral blood flow, oxygen consumption and blood volume in humans. Anesthesiology 2003;99:614–23.

124. Xie H, Wang X, Liu G, et al. Analgesic effects and pharmacokinetics of a low dose of ketamine preoperatively administered epidurally or intravenously. Clin J Pain 2003;19:317–22.

125. Vereecke HE, Struys MM, Mortier EP. A comparison of bispectral index and ARX-derived auditory evoked potential index in measuring the clinical interaction between ketamine and propofol anaesthesia. Anaesthesia 2003;58:957–61.

126. Hirota K, Kubota T, Ishihara H, et al. The effects of nitrous oxide and ketamine on the bispectral index and 95% spectral edge frequency during propofol-fentanyl anaesthesia. Eur J Anaesthesiol 1999;16:779–83.

127. Wu CC, Mok MS, Lin CS, Han SR. EEG-bispectral index changes with ketamine versus thiamylal induction of anesthesia. Acta Anaethesiol Scand 2001;39:11–15.

128. Menigaux C, Guignard B, Fletcher D, et al. Intraoperative small dose ketamine enhances analgesia after outpatient knee arthroscopy. Anaesth Analg 2001;93:606–12.

129. Menigaux C, Fletcher D, Dupont X, et al. The benefits of intraoperative small dose ketamine on postoperative pain after anterior cruciate ligament repair. Anesth Analg 2000;90:129–35.

130. Suzuki M, Tseuda K, Lansing PS, et al. Small-dose ketamine enhances morphine induced analgesia after outpatient surgery. Anesth Analg 1999;89:98–103.

131. Guignard B, Coste C, Costes H, et al. Supplementing desflurane-remifentanil anesthesia with small dose ketamine reduces perioperative opioid analgesic requirements. Anesth Analg 2002;95:103–8.

132. Kararmaz A, Kaya S, Karaman H, et al. Intraoperative intravenous ketamine in combination with epidural analgesia: postoperative analgesia after renal surgery. Anesth Analg 2003;97:1092–96.

133. Satsumae T, Yamaguchi H, Sakaguchi M, et al. Preoperative small dose ketamine prevented tourniquet induced arterial pressure increase in orthopedic patients under general anesthesia. Anesth Analg 2001;92:1286–89.

134. Kudoh A, Takahira Y, Katagai H, et al. Small dose ketamine improves the post-operative state of depressed patients. Anesth Analg 2002;95:114–18.

135. Micallef J, Guillermain Y, Tardieu S, et al. Effects of subanesthes-

tic doses of ketamine on sensimotor information processing in healthy subjects. Clin Neuropharmacol 2002;25:101–6.

136. Deng XM, Xiao WJ, Luo GZ, et al. The use of midazolam and small-dose ketamine for sedation and analgesia during local anesthesia. Anesth Analg 2001;93:1174–77.

137. Badrinath S, Avramov MN, Shadrick M, et al. The use of ketamine-propofol combination during monitored anesthesia care. Anesth Analg 2000;90:858–62.

138. Vallejo MC, Romeo RC, Davis DJ, et al. Propofol-ketamine vs propofol-fentanyl for outpatient laparoscopy: comparison of postoperative nausea, emesis, analgesia and recovery. J Clin Anesth 2002;14:426–31.

139. Friedberg BL. Propofol-ketamine technique: dissociative anesthesia for office-based surgery: a five year review of 1264 cases. Anesth Plast Surg 1999;23:70–75.

140. Frizelle HP, Duranteau J, Samii K. A comparison of propofol with a propofol-ketamine combination during spinal anesthesia. Anesth Analg 1997;84:1318–22.

141. Frey K, Sukhani R, Pawlowski J, et al. Propofol versus propofol-ketamine sedation for retrobulbar nerve block: comparison of sedation quality, intraocular pressure changes and recovery profiles. Anesth Analg 1999;89:317–21.

142. Turhanoglu S, Kararmaz A, Ozylimaz MA, et al. Effects of different doses of oral ketamine for premedication of children. Eur J Anaesthesiol 2003;20:56–60.

143. Gutstein HB, Johnson KL, Heard MB, Gregory GA. Oral ketamine preanesthetic medication in children, Anesthesiology 1992;76:28–33.

144. Diaz JH, Intranasal ketamine preinduction of paediatric outpatients. Paediatr Anaesth 1997;7:273–78.

145. Persson J, Hasselstrom J, Maurset A, et al. Pharmacokinetics and non-analgesic effects of S- and R-ketamines in healthy volunteers with normal and reduced metabolic capacity. Eur J Clin Pharmacol 2002;57:869–75.

146. Pfenninger EG, Durieux ME, Himmelseher S. Cognitive impairment after small-dose ketamine isomers in comparison to equianalgesic racemic ketamine in human volunteers. Anesthesiology 2002;96:357–66.

147. Jaksch W, Lang S, Reichhalter R, et al. Perioperative small dose (S+) ketamine has no incremental beneficial effects on postoperative pain when standard practice opioid infusions are used. Anesth Analg 2002;94:981–86.

148. Bremier D. Pharmacokinetics of methohexitone following intravenous infusions in humans. Br J Anaesth 1976;48:643.

149. Tanelian DL, Kosek P, Mody I, MacIver MB. The role of the GABA receptor/chloride channel complex in anesthesia. Anesthesiology 1993;78:757–76.

150. Dundee J. Alterations in response to somatic pain associated with anesthesia: the effect of thiopentone and pentobarbitone. Br J Anaesth 1960;32:407.

151. Sa Rego MM, Inagaki Y, White PF. The cost-effectiveness of methohexital versus propofol for sedation during monitored anesthesia care. Anesth Analg 1999;88:723–28.

152. Licthenberg ES, Hill LJ, Howe M, et al. A randomized comparison of propofol and methohexital as general anesthetics for vacuum abortion. Contraception 2003;68:211–17.

153. Miner JR, Biros M, Krieg S, et al. Randomized clinical trial of propofol versus methohexital for procedural sedation during fracture and dislocation reduction in the emergency department. Acad Emerg Med 2003;10:931–37.

154. Kern C, Weber A, Aurilio C, Forster A. Patient evaluation and comparison of the recovery profile between propofol and thiopentone as induction agents in day surgery. Anaesth Intens Care 1998;26:156–61.

155. Wagner BK, O'Hara DA. Cost analysis of propofol versus thiopental induction anesthesia in outpatient laparoscopic gynecological surgery. Clin Ther 1995;17:770–76.

156. Absalom A, Pledger D, Kong A. Adrenocortical function in critically ill patients 24 hours after a single dose of etomidate. Anaesthesia 1999;54:861–67.

157. Duthie DJ, Fraser R, Nimmo WS. Effect of induction of anaesthesia with etomidate on corticosteroid synthesis in man. Br J Anaesth 1985;57:156–59.

158. Crozier TA, Beck D, Schlaeger M, et al. Endocrinological changes following etomidate, midazolam or methohexital for minor surgery. Anesthesiology 1987;66:628–35.

159. Stoelting RK. Nonbarbiturate induction drugs. In: *Pharmacology and Physiology in Anesthetic Practice*, 3rd ed. Philadelphia: Lippincott-Raven, 1999, p. 140.

160. Vinson DR, Bradbury DR. Etomidate for procedural sedation in emergency medicine. Ann Emerg Med 2002;39:592–98.

161. Boysen K, Sanchez R, Krintel JJ, et al. Induction and recovery characteristics of propofol, thiopental and etomidate. Acta Anaesthesiol Scand 1989;33:689–92.

162. Doenicke AW, Roizen MF, Hoernecke R, et al. Solvent for etomidate may cause pain and adverse effects. Br J Anaesth 1999;83:464–66.

163. Korttila K, Aromaa U. Venous complications after intravenous injection of diazepam, flunitrazepam, thiopentone, and etomidate. Acta Anaesthesiol Scand 1980;24:227–30.

164. St Pierre M, Dunkel M, Rutherford A, Hering W. Does etomidate increase postoperative nausea? A double blind controlled comparison of etomidate in lipid emulsion with propofol for balanced anesthesia. Eur J Anaesthesiol 2000;17:634–41.

165. Hullander RM, Leivers D, Wingler K. A comparison of propofol and etomidate for cardioversion. Anesth Analg 1993;77:690–94.

166. Herregods LL, Bossuyt GP, Baerdemaeker LE, et al. Ambulatory electrical external cardioversion with propofol or etomidate. J Clin Anesth 2003;15:91–96.

167. Rupprecht T, Kuth R, Bowing B, et al. Sedation and monitoring of paediatric patients undergoing open low field MRI. Acta Paediatr 2000;89:1077–81.

168. Bloor BC, Flacke WE. Reduction in halothane anesthetic requirement by clonidine, an alpha-adrenergic agonist. Anesth Analg 1982;61:741–45.

169. El-Kerdawy HM, Zalingen EE, Bovill JG. The influence of the alpha-2 adrenoreceptor, clonidine, on the EEG and on the MAC of isoflurane. Eur J Anaesthesiol 2000;17:105–10.

170. Inomata S, Kihara S, Miyabe M, et al. The hypnotic and analgesic effects of oral clonidine during sevoflurane anesthesia in children: a dose response study. Anesth Analg 2002;94:1479–83.

171. Higuchi H, Adachi Y, Arimura S, et al. Oral clonidine premedication reduces the EC-50 of propofol concentration for laryngeal mask airway insertion in male patients. Acta Anaesthesiol Scand 2002;46:372–77.

172. Higuchi H, Adachi Y, Dahan A, et al. The interaction between propofol and clonidine for loss of consciousness. Anesth Analg 2002;94:886–91.

173. Oddby-Muhrbeck E, Eksborg S, Bergendahl HT, et al. Effects of clonidine on postoperative nausea and vomiting in breast cancer surgery. Anesthesiology 2002;96:1109–14.

174. Buerkle H, Hugh V, Wolfgart M, et al. Intra-articular clonidine after knee arthroscopy. Eur J Anaesthesiol 2000;17:295–99.

175. Joshi W, Reuben SS, Kilaru PR, et al. Postoperative analgesia for outpatient arthroscopic knee surgery with intra-articular clonidine and/or morphine. Anesth Analg 2000;90:1102–6.

176. De Knock M, Gautier P, Fanard L, et al. Intrathecal ropivacaine and clonidine for ambulatory knee arthroscopy. Anesthesiology 2001;94:574–78.

177. De Wolf AM, Fragen RJ, Avram MJ, et al. The pharmacokinetics of dexmedetomidine in volunteers with severe renal impairment. Anesth Analg 2001;93:1205–9.

178. Bloor BC, Ward DS, Belleville JP, Maze M. Effects of intravenous dexmedetomidine in humans: hemodynamic changes. Anesthesiology 1992;77:1134–42.

179. Khan ZP, Munday IT, Jones RM, et al. Effects of dexmedetomidine on isoflurane requirements in healthy volunteers: pharmacodynamic and pharmacokinetic interactions. Br J Anaesth 1999;83: 372–80.

180. Dutta S, Karol MD, Cohen T, et al. Effect of dexmedetomidine on propofol requirements in healthy subjects. J Pharm Sci 2002;90: 172–81.

181. Peden CJ, Cloote AH, Stratford N, Prys-Roberts C. The effect of intravenous dexmedetomidine premedication on the dose requirement of propofol to induce loss of consciousness in patients receiving alfentanil. Anaesthesia 2001;56:408–13.

182. Talke P, Chen R, Thomas B, et al. The hemodynamic and adrenergic effects of perioperative dexmedetomidine infusion after vascular surgery. Anesth Analg 2000;90:834–39.

183. Arain SR, Egert TJ. The efficacy, side effects, and recovery characteristics of dexmedetomidine versus propofol when used for intraoperative sedation. Anesth Analg 2002;95:461–66.

184. Hall JE, Uhrich TD, Barney JA, et al. Sedative, amnestic and analgesic properties of small-dose dexmedetomidine infusions. Anesth Analg 2000;90:699–705.

185. Nishida T, Nishimura M. Kagawa K, et al. The effects of dexmedetomidine on the ventilatory response to hypercapnia in rabbits. Intens Care Med 2000;28:969–75.

186. Ibacache ME, Munoz HR, Brandes V, Morales AL. Single-dose dexmedetomidine reduces agitation after sevoflurane anesthesia in children. Anesth Analg 2004;98:60–63.

187. Levanen J, Makela ML, Scheinin H. Dexmedetomidine premedication attenuates ketamine-induced cardiostimulatory effects and post-anesthetic delirium. Anesthesiology 1995;82:1117–25.

188. Doufas AG, Lin CM, Suleman MI, et al. Dexmedetomidine and meperidine additively reduce the shivering threshold in humans. Stroke 2003;34:1218–23.

189. Venn RM, Grounds RM. Comparison between dexmedetomidine and propofol for sedation in the intensive care unit: patient and clinical perceptions. Br J Anaesth 2001;87:684–90.

190. Talke PO, Caldwell JE, Richardson CA, et al. The effects of dexmedetomidine on neuromuscular blockade in human volunteers. Anesth Analg 1999;88:633–39.

191. Watch MF, White PF. Postoperative nausea and vomiting: prophylaxis versus treatment. Anesth Analg 1999;89:1337–39.

192. Gan TJ, White PF, Scuderi PE, et al. FDA "black box" warning regarding the use of droperidol for postoperative nausea and vomiting: is it justified? Anesthesiology 2002;97:287.

193. Dershwitz M, Habib AS, Gan TJ. There should be a threshold dose for the FDA black-box warning on droperidol. Anesth Analg 2003;97:1542–43.

194. Bailey P, Norton R, Karan S. The FDA droperidol warning: is it justified? Anesthesiology 2002;97:288–89.

195. Henzi I, Sonderegger J, Tramer MR. Efficacy, dose-response, and adverse effects of droperidol for the prevention of postoperative nausea and vomiting, Can J Anaesth 2000;47:537–51.

196. Tramer MR, Reynold DJ, Moore RA, et al. Efficacy, dose-response, and safety of ondansetron in prevention of postoperative nausea and vomiting: a quantitative systemic review of randomized placebo controlled trials. Anesthesiology 1997;87:1277–89.

197. Hill RP, Lubarsky DA, Phillips-Bute B, et al. Cost-effectiveness of prophylactic antiemetic therapy with ondansetron, droperidol or placebo. Anesthesiology 2000;92:958–67.

198. Pueyo FJ, Lopez-Olaondo L, Sanchez-Ledesma MJ, et al. Cost-effectiveness of three combinations of antiemetics in the prevention of postoperative nausea and vomiting. Br J Anaesth 2003;91:589–92.

199. Sanchez-Ledesma MJ, Lopez-Olaondo L, Pueyo FJ, et al. A comparison of three antiemetic combinations for the prevention of postoperative nausea and vomiting. Anesth Analg 2002;95:1590–95.

200. Kovac AL. Prevention and treatment of postoperative nausea and vomiting. Drugs 2000;59:213–43.

201. Kranke P, Morin AM, Roewer N, et al. The efficacy and safety of transdermal scopolamine for the prevention of postoperative nausea and vomiting: a quantitative systematic review. Anesth Analg 2002;95:133–43.

Opioid Analgesics and Antagonists for Ambulatory Anesthesia

MOEEN K. PANNI   •   BEVERLY K. PHILIP

INTRODUCTION

The ideals for the perioperative use of opioid receptor agents (agonist and antagonist) include the reduction of postoperative pain sensation while minimizing opioid side effects. If these goals are met, early discharge from the ambulatory surgery recovery room is possible. With the increasing complexities of surgery performed in the ambulatory setting, untreated or poorly treated postoperative pain substantially delays "home readiness" after ambulatory surgery.[1] Indeed a recent survey found 82% of patients who were discharged from the day-case surgery facility had some residual pain; 21% of these patients worried about experiencing more severe pain, and 88% of all the patients continued to have residual pain 2–4 days postoperatively.[2] In another study looking at several different types of ambulatory surgical procedures, pain itself was shown to complicate the recovery process.[3]

Opioid analgesics are one of the main classes of therapeutic agents used to prevent and treat moderate to severe pain after ambulatory surgery (Fig. 17-1). Unfortunately the side effect profile of opioid receptor agents can substantially impact their use in these patients. The most notable of these side effects are nausea and vomiting. Postoperative nausea and vomiting (PONV) has been reported to occur in 20–30% of day surgery patients,[4] and some even report a greater range of 20–60%.[5]

Nausea and vomiting can affect patient satisfaction, comfort, and discharge time. Other undesired opioid side effects include excessive sedation, urinary retention, constipation, respiratory depression, delirium, pruritus, and headache. All of these can lead to further delay in the recovery room and increase the cost of care.[6] The route of administration, the choice of agent, and amount given can all contribute to these effects.

In this chapter we will summarize the current literature published on the commonly used agents, typical routes of administration, and the problems that arise with each. Other modalities of perioperative analgesia for ambulatory surgery, such as inhalation agents, intrathecal agents (including opioids), and nonsteroidal anti-inflammatory analgesics, all of which can interact with the effects of systemically administered opioids, are discussed in other chapters of this book.

INTRAVENOUS AGENTS

Fentanyl

In the ambulatory surgery setting, fentanyl is the most commonly used opioid analgesic. It is available in a generic form and is one of the least expensive opioids currently available. Typical doses of fentanyl range between 1 and 2 μg/kg. The onset of analgesia is rapid, with an effect seen within 2 min after intravenous administration, peak effect site time of 3.6 min,[7] and a short duration of action lasting up to 45 min. The duration of respiratory depression with fentanyl is comparable to morphine, and may recur between 30 min to 4 hr in the recovery period.[8] When used in these doses fentanyl has minimal hemodynamic side effects. Bradycardia is the most prominent of these, which is secondary to stimulation of the central vagal nucleus. With the shorter duration of action of fentanyl, its quality of analgesia has been shown to be less good than that of the longer-lasting morphine. One study was done in 58 patients undergoing ambulatory surgery. Patients were randomized to receive either morphine or fentanyl, in equipotent doses titrated to pain scores less than a visual analog score (VAS) of 40 mm. Higher pain scores were seen in the fentanyl group. There was an increased incidence of PONV with morphine compared to fentanyl.[9]

The problem of nausea may be a substantial issue with fentanyl administration, as the duration of nausea may

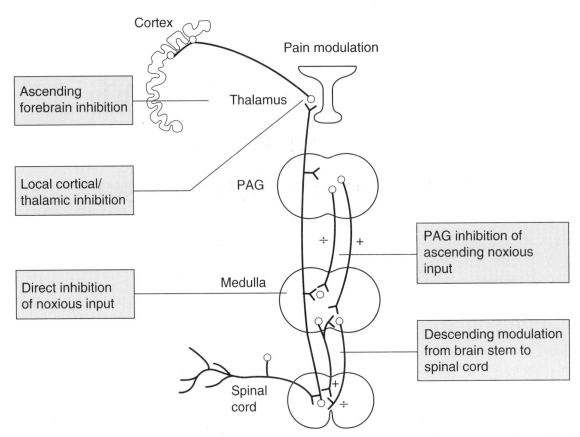

Figure 17-1   Diagram illustrating proposed antinociceptive mechanisms of morphine in the central nervous system. (Reproduced with permission from Miller RD [ed.], *Anesthesia*, Vol. I, 5th ed. New York: Churchill Livingstone, 2000. Copyright © 2000 Churchill Livingstone, Inc. Figure 10-5.)

outlast the duration of analgesia. In one study, 100 μg of fentanyl was compared to 60 mg of ketorolac, given during anesthesia induction, for 1 hr laparoscopic surgery. There was a higher incidence of postoperative emesis requiring treatment in the fentanyl patients, as well as delayed ambulation and discharge in those patients, than with ketorolac.[10] Increased total perioperative fentanyl dose was also shown to be associated with more PONV,[11] and higher doses were more resistant to antiemetic therapy.[12]

A multimodal approach to perioperative analgesia can be effectively used in ambulatory surgery patients, by adding nonsteroidal drugs or inhalational anesthetics intraoperatively. This can reduce the doses of perioperative analgesics needed, such as fentanyl, and in so doing, the associated opioid side effects may also be reduced.

In common with other opioids, fentanyl also causes muscle rigidity of supraspinal origin.[13] Rigidity is seen in the chest wall muscles, extremities, and larynx, which may lead to interference of bag mask ventilation during induction of anesthesia. Rigidity should not be a concern in the postoperative period, because large bolus doses of fentanyl are not used at that stage. Pretreatment with midazolam in the induction period can reduce the amount of muscle rigidity, but not completely prevent it.[14]

Sufentanil

Sufentanil is a structurally related opioid to fentanyl with approximately 10 times the potency. Sufentanil has a similar onset and duration of effect as fentanyl, with similar opioid side effects, even when small doses (0.1–0.25 μg/kg) appropriate for the ambulatory surgery patient are used. There are few studies of sufentanil use in ambulatory surgery. One study showed that maintenance of general anesthesia in ambulatory arthroscopic surgery patients with sufentanil allowed a faster awakening than isoflurane anesthesia. This followed an induction with methohexitone and vecuronium. There was, however, a higher incidence of nausea.[15] Sufentanil was also shown to be a better premedication opioid to reduce anxiety in ambulatory patients. This study showed sufentanil to give a more satisfactory induction, maintenance, and recovery from anesthesia than either morphine, meperidine, or fentanyl, and with a similar incidence of PONV.[16]

The use of sufentanil in ambulatory anesthesia is, however, limited by its relatively high acquisition cost and little kinetic advantage over fentanyl.

Alfentanil

Alfentanil is a short-acting analog of fentanyl. Both onset and offset of this opioid occur via drug elimination rather

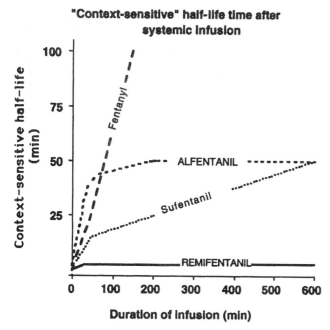

Figure 17-2   Computer simulation of the "context-sensitive" half-life time (CSHT) for remifentanil (3.65 min), alfentanil (58.5 min), sufentanil (240 min), and fentanyl (262.5 min). Note that remifentanil's CSHT is independent of the duration of infusion. (From Burkle H, Dunbar S, Van Aken H. Remifentanil: a novel, short-acting, mu-opioid. *Anesth Analg* 1996 Sep;83(3):646–51. Figure 2.)

than redistribution, which is substantially more rapid than with fentanyl. Single-bolus dosing of alfentanil for placement of regional blocks can be useful. As repeated bolus dosing for maintenance of anesthesia can result in hemodynamic instability, continuous infusion may be the optimal method of administration in this situation (Fig. 17-2). Alfentanil also has typical opioid side effects. Respiratory depression occurs, but is shorter than after fentanyl.[17] Delayed respiratory depression and respiratory arrest have been reported after large doses of alfentanil, related to decreased stimulation in the postanesthesia-care unit (PACU) rather than the reappearance of drug from peripheral storage sites.[18] Alfentanil also exhibits the typical opioid side effects of rigidity and vagal-mediated bradycardia, as well as PONV, which occurs at rates comparable to fentanyl.[19] In one study, however, no difference in PONV was seen in the PACU (immediate recovery), but PONV was significantly lower with alfentanil in later recovery, compared with fentanyl or sufentanil.[20] The use of alfentanil has declined since remifentanil has become available.

Remifentanil

The increase in ambulatory surgical procedures is concurrent with an increase in the number of longer and more complex procedures, which require intense periods of surgical stimulation. This deep anesthetic state may only be necessary for portions of the surgical procedure, and may be required in patients who do not tolerate large shifts in their hemodynamic variables. Hemodynamic stability is achieved by most opioid agonists, but a truly short dura-

tion of action is a difficult goal. Furthermore, residual postoperative opioid sedation and respiratory depression are not ideal, especially in patients with significant respiratory disease.

Remifentanil is another fentanyl class opioid receptor agonist that can be appropriately used for ambulatory anesthesia. In addition to its opioid structure, remifentanil has an ester linkage that can be metabolized by nonspecific blood and tissue esterase, resulting in an ultrashort terminal half-life of 10 min, which is independent of its duration of administration (Fig. 17-2). Metabolism is unrelated to pseudocholinesterase levels or to renal or hepatic dysfunction. The time required for a 50% decrease in effect site concentration after 1-hr infusion has been calculated to be 3.65 min for remifentanil, 33.9 min for sufentanil, and 58.5 min for alfentanil.[21]

Remifentanil also has a rapid onset of action of around 60–90 sec. Typical doses for general endotracheal ambulatory anesthesia begin with a bolus dose of 1 μg/kg, given immediately after the induction hypnotic to minimize rigidity, and continued with an infusion rate of 0.25 (0.05–2) μg/kg/min, given with an inhaled or intravenous (IV) hypnotic. Single-bolus doses of 1 μg/kg are also very effective at the time of placement of a regional or ophthalmic block. Significant duration of respiratory depression is uncommon if simultaneously administered sedatives are avoided and the patient is well oxygenated, but greater than 10 sec of apnea is not uncommon with this technique. Remifentanil infusions of 0.025–0.2 μg/kg/min are also effective supplements to local or regional blocks during surgery, providing substantial IV analgesia, but the clinician must be attentive to avoid hypoventilation or rigidity. Bolus doses added to an ongoing analgesic infusion are particularly likely to cause side effects. Remifentanil does cause nausea and vomiting, and the incidence compared to other opioids appears to be similar but of shorter duration.[22]

When reminfentanil is used, it is important to implement adequate postoperative analgesia, by either local/regional blocks, longer-acting analgesics such as fentanyl, or possibly using a continued remifentanil infusion. With its kinetic and cost advantages, remifentanil has replaced alfentanil as the choice of opioid infusion for maintenance of ambulatory surgery procedures.

Tramadol

Tramadol is a synthetic weak opioid agonist with sympathomimetic activity.[23,24] Tramadol's analgesic effect has been suggested to be similar to that of meperidine, but with fewer side effects. It is not classified as a controlled substance and it may be a good choice in patients undergoing ambulatory surgery.[25] In one randomized trial in ambulatory hand surgery patients, following 6 hr postoperative dosing, tramadol (100 mg) was shown to be superior to acetaminophen (1 g) and metamizol (1 g) (a nonopioid analgesic with antipyretic, antispasmodic, and anti-inflammatory components) for analgesia.[26] Although tramadol was more effective, its use was associated with a high frequency and intensity of adverse effects, with substantial patient dissatisfaction. In a pediatric study using 1.5 mg/kg tramadol drops with midazolam premedication, substantial reduction in postoperative analgesic requirements was seen compared to placebo (rescue with acetaminophen), but again some residual sedation was seen in the tramadol patients.[27] The side effect profile of tramadol may make it unsuitable for use in ambulatory surgery as substantial side effects may outweigh potential benefit.

MIXED AGONISTS AND ANTAGONISTS

Two mixed agonist/antagonist opioids, butorphanol and nalbuphine, have limited use in ambulatory anesthesia. Butorphanol has analgesic and sedative properties, without causing profound respiratory depression. It is an acceptable choice for the opioid component of long-monitored sedation cases. Cook presented 400 cases in which butorphanol was used intravenously for a broad spectrum of ambulatory facial plastic surgery procedures, over a period of 18 months, with good results.[28]

Butorphanol (20 μg/kg) has been compared with fentanyl (1 μg/kg) as the opioid component of general anesthesia for ambulatory gynecologic laparoscopy.[29] Postoperatively there were no differences in analgesic need (no advantage with longer-acting drug) and more early postoperative sedation with butorphanol, but discharge times were not different. More patients reported satisfaction with their anesthesia on the first postoperative day with butorphanol. Similarly a double-blinded study comparing equipotent doses of butorphanol (40 μg/kg) with fentanyl (2 μg/kg) in ambulatory laparoscopic surgery patients showed similar high incidences of PONV, hemodynamic stability, and induction and maintenance characteristics when either was used as a preinduction-dose opioid.[30]

Nalbuphine (0.25 μg/kg) was compared with alfentanil (20 μg/kg) and fentanyl (2 μg/kg) in patients undergoing general anesthesia for ambulatory surgery.[31] Nalbuphine was found to have similar incidence of PONV, discharge time, and need for antiemetics as well as nonsteroidal anti-inflammatory drugs supplementation. Nalbuphine (300–500 μg/kg) has also been compared with fentanyl (1.5 μg/kg) as the opioid component of ambulatory general anesthesia.[32] The use of nalbuphine in this study was associated with dose-related increases in nausea, length of stay, dreaming, and unpleasant dreams.

In a recent study nalbuphine was used as a prophylactic agent for PONV, either with or without the addition of droperidol, in patients having ambulatory knee arthroscopy under lidocaine-fentanyl spinal anesthesia; 4 mg of nalbuphine with 0.625 mg droperidol was shown to be better at reducing PONV and pruritus than nalbuphine alone. This combination reduced the occurrence of prolonged discharge delay, albeit with a slightly increased drowsiness in this group of patients.[33] The duration of both of these mixed agonist/antagonist opioids is long (3–4 hr), and their benefits should be carefully weighed against their side effects.

The use of a pure opioid receptor antagonist such as naloxone or nalmephene may be important in the acute and sustained reversal of troublesome and potentially dangerous opioid agonist side effects; such as respiratory depression and excessive sedation. There has been some suggestion to use these pure antagonists in lower doses, to prevent or attenuate a number of the less dangerous but unpleasant opioid agonist side effects. Nalmephene at doses of both 15 μg and 25 μg was shown to significantly reduce the need for antiemetic and antipruritic treatment in abdominal surgery patients after IV morphine patient-controlled analgesia (PCA).[34] In another study naloxone at an IV infusion of 2 μg/kg/hr and nalbuphine infused at 60 μg/kg/hr were shown to alleviate the frequency of PONV and pruritus after epidural morphine in hysterectomy surgery patients. Immediate postoperative analgesia was adequate with both, but there was an increase in the requirements for late analgesic rescue in the group receiving naloxone (i.e., somewhat attenuating the epidural morphine analgesia given).[35]

INTRANASAL AGENTS

As an alternative to oral and IV dosing, other routes to deliver analgesia have been investigated. Rectal administration has been shown to have low bioavailability and more variability than oral dosing, so may not been an ideal choice for ambulatory surgery patients. Administering medications transcutaneously can avoid the hepatic degradation of the oral route, but leads to a slower onset of action. Sublingual administration can be rapid and also avoids hepatic degradation. Nasal administration also yields rapid onset, with avoidance of hepatic metabolism, as well as ease of patient use and control, with some moderate variation in absorption.

While there are a number of reports of successful intranasal fentanyl use for postoperative PCA,[36–38] there are few studies of intranasal opioids in ambulatory surgery patients. In pediatric ambulatory surgery of less than 2 hr both intranasal midazolam (0.2 mg/kg) and intranasal sufentanil (2 μg/kg) were shown to give rapid, safe, and effective sedation, with sufentanil providing better induction and emergence conditions than midazolam.[39] In another study, good steady-state plasma concentrations were achieved with intranasal fentanyl (2 μg/kg) with reduced postoperative excitement (after sevoflurane), in pediatric patients undergoing bone marrow transplant. This occurred without an increase in vomiting, hypoxemia, or discharge times.[40] Intranasal meperidine (six intranasal puffs of 27 mg/dose) was used to good effect in one study of orthopedic patients.[41]

Intranasal butorphanol was effective in relieving postoperative pain in dental surgery patients (single doses given from 0.25 mg to 2 mg)[42] and pediatric myringotomy patients (25 μg/kg).[43] Butorphanol by the intranasal route may therefore be a valid choice for the ambulatory surgery patient if a longer-acting opioid is required. Further investigation is necessary to establish the effectiveness and side effect profile of this and other opioid analgesics via the intranasal route in ambulatory patients.

TRANSDERMAL THERAPY

There are numerous studies showing the efficacy of delivering transdermal opioid via patches in animals.[44,45] Unfortunately there has been a paucity of transdermal opioid use in the ambulatory surgery literature to date, but there have been studies with major surgeries that may provide insight.

One study in humans showed no significant improvement in analgesia with the use of transdermal fentanyl patch (50 μg/hr and 75 μg/hr) in patients receiving IV morphine PCA after major orthopedic surgery.[46] Another study showed some improvement in moderate to severe postoperative pain when a postoperative fentanyl patch (55–65 μg/hr, or 70–80 μg/hr if weighing over 60 kg) was added to intramuscular (IM) ketorolac (60 mg).[47] After abdominal surgery, patients who were given 0.16 mg/cm^2 fentanyl patches needed a reduced amount of parenteral opioids compared to patients who received 60 mg ketorolac IM.[48] Patches generated plasma fentanyl concentrations at 12 and 24 hr after their application, of 0.98 (±0.14) ng/mL and 1.22 (±0.17) ng/mL, respectively.

When 50 μg/hr and 75 μg/hr fentanyl patches were given to women 2 hr before abdominal hysterectomy under general anesthesia, significantly lower VAS pain scores were found in the 75-μg/hr group of patients, with decreased morphine requirements in both groups. Although good analgesia was provided with this combination therapy, it was associated with a high incidence of respiratory depression requiring intensive monitoring and oxygen supplementation, with removal of the patches in 11% of the patients and opioid reversal with naloxone in 8% of the patients.[49]

In ambulatory patients having hemorrhoidectomy surgery, the fentanyl patch was shown to be successful in reducing meperidine rescue doses compared to placebo patch. The patches also allowed smooth transition to non-invasive pain management options.[50] Overall, however, the slow termination of opioid analgesic administration when the patch is removed, coupled with a high incidence of side effects, indicates that fentanyl by transdermal patch may have a limited role in the ambulatory surgery patient.

ORAL THERAPY

Use of oral analgesic therapy in ambulatory surgery both as a premedication and for its residual postoperative analgesic action is another option that can be considered. Even though there has been a reevaluation of fasting guidelines for elective surgery,[51] the safe timing of oral medication prior to surgery has not yet been clearly outlined. More commonly patients are transitioned onto oral analgesic regimes from intraoperative IV analgesia. Use of oral tramadol in the postoperative period was discussed earlier and shown to be effective but with a high incidence of side effects.[25] Considering other agents, one study showed little difference in either pain or anxiety reduction between placebo and oral lorazepam (2 mg) and hydromorphone (2 mg), given preoperatively, in adult ambulatory bone marrow biopsy/aspiration patients.[52]

Another group studied various formulations of oxycodone in patients undergoing reconstruction of the anterior cruciate knee ligament. After a standard general anesthetic they compared three postoperative analgesic regimens: oxycodone, 10 mg every 4 hr as needed; oxycodone, 10 mg every 4 hr; and continuous-release (CR) oxycodone, 20 mg every 12 hr. The patients in the oxycodone CR group had the least sleep disturbance, least PONV, and were most satisfied with their analgesia.[53]

An interesting modality used to deliver oral opioids is the transmucosal route, which has been developed as oral transmucosal fentanyl citrate (OTFC) or fentanyl oralet. OTFC is a sweetened matrix containing fentanyl with a lollipop-like handle.[54] In the mouth, the matrix dissolves and releases fentanyl that can be absorbed by the transmucosal membranes.

While usually used to treat cancer pain[55] in adults, OTFC has also been shown to successfully reduce postoperative pain after joint replacement surgery (7–10 μg/kg)[56] and lower-abdominal surgery (one dose of either 200 or 800 μg OTFC).[57] A study of preoperative anxiolysis in adult ambulatory surgery patients was done comparing the OTFC (300 μg, or 400 μg if weighing more than 70 kg) versus placebo oralet or placebo (no oralet). Patients receiving the OTFC had more anxiolysis preoperatively with no difference in sedation levels. Gastric volumes measured were similar in all groups. There was an increase in mild dizziness or light-headedness in the OTFC group.[58] OTFC is more commonly used as anxiolytic premedication in children. An upper-dose limit of 15 μg/kg OTFC has been suggested to prevent a high incidence of PONV and occasional respiratory depression.[59] OTFC may be a reasonable option for preoperative anxiolysis and postoperative analgesia, in both adult and pediatric ambulatory surgery patients.

SUMMARY

Ambulatory surgical procedures are being performed increasingly commonly both in the United States and in other parts of the world. Fast tracking patients to bypass the PACU and be discharged home more quickly is possible using the more potent and shorter-acting anesthetic agents. Both postoperative pain and PONV are the major reasons why patients are unable to be discharged in a timely manner, and may even require unplanned overnight hospital admission after ambulatory surgery. Opioid analgesics play a large role in alleviating postoperative pain for ambulatory surgery patients, despite their potential for side effects such as PONV and sedation. There are a number of effective routes of administration of opioid receptor agents. Intranasal, transdermal, and oral routes of administration should be considered, when appropriate, for continued postoperative analgesia, along with the more established perioperative IV routes.

REFERENCES

1. Chung F. Recovery pattern and home-readiness after ambulatory surgery. Anesth Analg 1995 May;80(5):896–902.

2. McHugh GA, Thoms GM. The management of pain following day-case surgery. Anaesthesia 2002 Mar;57(3):270–75.

3. Pavlin DJ, Chen C, Penaloza DA, Polissar NL, Buckley FP. Pain as a factor complicating recovery and discharge after ambulatory surgery. Anesth Analg 2002 Sep;95(3):627–34.

4. Watcha MF, White PF. Postoperative nausea and vomiting: its etiology, treatment, and prevention. Anesthesiology 1992 Jul;77(1):162–84.

5. Gan TJ. Postoperative nausea and vomiting—can it be eliminated? JAMA 2002 Mar 13;287(10):1233–36.

6. Philip BK, Reese PR, Burch SP. The economic impact of opioids on postoperative pain management. J Clin Anesth 2002 Aug;14(5): 354–64.

7. Shafer SL, Varvel JR. Pharmacokinetics, pharmacodynamics, and rational opioid selection. Anesthesiology 1991 Jan;74(1):53–63.

8. Rigg JR, Goldsmith CH. Recovery of ventilatory response to carbon dioxide after thiopentone, morphine and fentanyl in man. Can Anaesth Soc J 1976;23:370–82.

9. Claxton AR, McGuire G, Chung F, Cruise C. Evaluation of morphine versus fentanyl for postoperative analgesia after ambulatory surgical procedures. Anesth Analg 1997 Mar;84(3):509–14.

10. Sukhani R, Vazquez J, Pappas AL, Frey K, Aasen M, Slogoff S. Recovery after propofol with and without intraoperative fentanyl in patients undergoing ambulatory gynecologic laparoscopy. Anesth Analg 1996;83:975–81.

11. Rosenblum M, Weller RS, Conard PL, Falvey EA, Gross JB. Ibuprofen provides longer lasting analgesia than fentanyl after laparoscopic surgery. Anesth Analg 1991;73:255–59.

12. Polati E, Verlato G, Finco G, Mosaner W, Grosso S, Gottin L, Pinaroli AM, Ischia S. Ondansetron versus metoclopramide in the treatment of postoperative nausea and vomiting. Anesth Analg 1997 Aug;85(2):395–99.

13. Fu MJ, Tsen LY, Lee TY, Lui PW, Chan SH. Involvement of cerulospinal glutamatergic neurotransmission in fentanyl-induced muscular rigidity in the rat. Anesthesiology 1997 Dec;87(6):1450–59.

14. Neidhart P, Burgener MC, Schwieger I, Suter PM. Chest wall rigidity during fentanyl- and midazolam-fentanyl induction: ventilatory and haemodynamic effects. Acta Anaesthesiol Scand 1989 Jan;33 (1):1–5.

15. Zuurmond WW, van Leeuwen L. Recovery from sufentanil anaesthesia for outpatient arthroscopy: a comparison with isoflurane. Acta Anaesthesiol Scand 1987 Feb;31(2):154–56.

16. Pandit SK, Kothary SP. Intravenous narcotics for premedication in outpatient anaesthesia. Acta Anaesthesiol Scand 1989 Jul;33(5):353–58.

17. Mildh LH, Scheinin H, Kirvela OA. The concentration-effect relationship of the respiratory depressant effects of alfentanil and fentanyl. Anesth Analg 2001 Oct;93(4):939–46.

18. Persson MP, Nilsson A, Hartvig P. Pharmacokinetics of alfentanil in total i.v. anaesthesia. Br J Anaesth 1988 Jun;60(7):755–61.

19. White PF, Coe V, Shafer A, Sung ML. Comparison of alfentanil with fentanyl for outpatient anesthesia. Anesthesiology 1986 Jan;64(1): 99–106.

20. Langevin S, Lessard MR, Trepanier CA, Baribault JP. Alfentanil causes less postoperative nausea and vomiting than equipotent doses of fentanyl or sufentanil in outpatients. Anesthesiology 1999 Dec;91(6):1666–73.

21. Westmoreland CL, Hoke JF, Sebel PS, Hug CC Jr, Muir KT. Pharmacokinetics of remifentanil (GI 87084B) and its major metabolite (GI 90292) in patients undergoing elective inpatient surgery. Anesthesiology 1993 Nov;79(5):893–903.

22. Philip BK. The use of remifentanil in clinical anesthesia. Acta Anaesthesiol Scand (Suppl) 1996;109:170–73.

23. Mildh LH, Leino KA, Kirvela OA. Effects of tramadol and meperidine on respiration, plasma catecholamine concentrations, and hemodynamics. J Clin Anesth 1999 Jun;11(4):310–16.

24. Lewis KS, Han NH. Tramadol: a new centrally acting analgesic. Am J Health Syst Pharm 1997;54:643–52.

25. Budd K, Langford R. Tramadol revisited. Br J Anaesth 1999 Apr;82(4):493–95.

26. Rawal N, Allvin R, Amilon A, Ohlsson T, Hallen J. Postoperative analgesia at home after ambulatory hand surgery: a controlled comparison of tramadol, metamizol, and paracetamol. Anesth Analg 2001 Feb;92(2):347–51.

27. Roelofse JA, Payne KA. Oral tramadol: analgesic efficacy in children following multiple dental extractions. Eur J Anaesthesiol 1999 Jul; 16(7):441–47.

28. Cook TA. Butorphanol tartrate: an intravenous analgesic for outpatient surgery. Otolaryngol Head Neck Surg 1983 Jun;91(3):251–54.

29. Philip BK, Scott DA, Freiberger D, Gibbs RR, Hunt C, Murray E. Butorphanol compared with fentanyl in general anesthesia for ambulatory laparoscopy. Can J Anaesth 1991;38:183–86.

30. Pandit SK, Kothary SP, Pandit UA, Mathai MK. Comparison of fentanyl and butorphanol for outpatient anaesthesia. Can J Anaesth 1987 Mar;34(2):130–34.

31. Cepeda MS, Gonzalez F, Granados V, Cuervo R, Carr DB. Incidence of nausea and vomiting in outpatients undergoing general anesthesia in relation to selection of intraoperative opioid. J Clin Anesth 1996 Jun;8(4):324–28.

32. Garfield JM, Garfield FB, Philip BK, Earls F, Roaf E. Comparison of clinical and psychologic effects of fentanyl and nalbuphine in ambulatory gynecological patients. Anesth Analg 1987;66:1303–7.

33. Ben-David B, DeMeo PJ, Lucyk C, Solosko D. Minidose lidocaine-fentanyl spinal anesthesia in ambulatory surgery: prophylactic nalbuphine versus nalbuphine plus droperidol. Anesth Analg 2002 Dec;95(6):1596–600.

34. Joshi GP, Duffy L, Chehade J, Wesevich J, Gajraj N, Johnson ER. Effects of prophylactic nalmefene on the incidence of morphine-related side effects in patients receiving intravenous patient-controlled analgesia. Anesthesiology 1999 Apr;90(4):1007–11.

35. Wang JJ, Ho ST, Tzeng JI. Comparison of intravenous nalbuphine infusion versus naloxone in the prevention of epidural morphine-related side effects. Reg Anesth Pain Med 1998 Sep–Oct;23(5):479–84.

36. Striebel HW, Oelmann T, Spies C, Rieger A, Schwagmeier R. Patient-controlled intranasal analgesia: a method for noninvasive postoperative pain management. Anesth Analg 1996 Sep;83(3):548–51.

37. Striebel HW, Olmann T, Spies C, Brummer G. Patient-controlled intranasal analgesia (PCINA) for the management of postoperative pain: a pilot study. J Clin Anesth 1996 Feb;8(1):4–8.

38. Toussaint S, Maidl J, Schwagmeier R, Striebel HW. Patient-controlled intranasal analgesia: effective alternative to intravenous PCA for postoperative pain relief. Can J Anaesth 2000 Apr;47(4): 299–302.

39. Zedie N, Amory DW, Wagner BK, O'Hara DA. Comparison of intranasal midazolam and sufentanil premedication in pediatric outpatients. Clin Pharmacol Ther 1996 Mar;59(3):341–48.

40. Galinkin JL, Fazi LM, Cuy RM, Chiavacci RM, Kurth CD, Shah UK, Jacobs IN, Watcha MF. Use of intranasal fentanyl in children undergoing myringotomy and tube placement during halothane and sevoflurane anesthesia. Anesthesiology 2000 Dec;93(6):1378–83.

41. Striebel HW, Bonillo B, Schwagmeier R, Dopjans D, Spies C. Self-administered intranasal meperidine for postoperative pain management. Can J Anaesth 1995 Apr;42(4):287–91.

42. Desjardins PJ, Norris LH, Cooper SA, Reynolds DC. Analgesic efficacy of intranasal butorphanol (Stadol NS) in the treatment of pain after dental impaction surgery. J Oral Maxillofac Surg 2000 Oct; 58(10 Suppl 2):19–26.

43. Bennie RE, Boehringer LA, Dierdorf SF, Hanna MP, Means LJ. Transnasal butorphanol is effective for postoperative pain relief in children undergoing myringotomy. Anesthesiology 1998 Aug;89(2): 385–90.

44. Glerum LE, Egger CM, Allen SW, Haag M. Analgesic effect of the transdermal fentanyl patch during and after feline ovariohysterectomy. Vet Surg 2001 Jul–Aug;30(4):351–58.

45. Franks JN, Boothe HW, Taylor L, Geller S, Carroll GL, Cracas V, Boothe DM. Evaluation of transdermal fentanyl patches for analgesia in cats undergoing onychectomy. J Am Vet Med Assoc 2000 Oct 1;217(7):1013–20.

46. Sevarino FB, Paige D, Sinatra RS, Silverman DG. Postoperative analgesia with parenteral opioids: does continuous delivery utilizing a transdermal opioid preparation affect analgesic efficacy or patient safety? J Clin Anesth 1997 May;9(3):173–78.

47. Reinhart DJ, Goldberg ME, Roth JV, Dua R, Nevo I, Klein KW, Torjman M, Vekeman D. Transdermal fentanyl system plus im ketorolac for the treatment of postoperative pain. Can J Anaesth 1997 Apr;44(4):377–84.

48. Lehmann LJ, DeSio JM, Radvany T, Bikhazi GB. Transdermal fentanyl in postoperative pain. Reg Anesth 1997 Jan–Feb;22(1):24–28.

49. Sandler AN, Baxter AD, Katz J, Samson B, Friedlander M, Norman P, Koren G, Roger S, Hull K, Klein J. A double-blind, placebo-controlled trial of transdermal fentanyl after abdominal hysterectomy: analgesic, respiratory, and pharmacokinetic effects. Anesthesiology 1994 Nov;81(5):1169–80.

50. Kilbride M, Morse M, Senagore A. Transdermal fentanyl improves management of postoperative hemorrhoidectomy pain. Dis Colon Rectum 1994 Nov;37(11):1070–72.

51. Warner, MA, Caplan RA, Epstein BS, Gibbs CP, Keller CE, Leak, JA, Maltby R, Nickinovich DG, Schreiner, MS, Weinlander CM. Practice guidelines for preoperative fasting and the use of pharmacologic drugs to reduce the risk of pulmonary aspiration: application to healthy patients undergoing elective procedures. Anesthesiology 1999 Mar;90(3):896–905.

52. Wolanskyj AP, Schroeder G, Wilson PR, Habermann TM, Inwards DJ, Witzig TE. A randomized, placebo-controlled study of outpatient premedication for bone marrow biopsy in adults with lymphoma. Clin Lymphoma 2000 Sep;1(2):154–57.

53. Reuben SS, Connelly NR, Maciolek H. Postoperative analgesia with controlled-release oxycodone for outpatient anterior cruciate ligament surgery. Anesth Analg 1999 Jun;88(6):1286–91.

54. Streisand JB, Varvel JR, Stanski DR, Le Maire L, Ashburn MA, Hague BI, Tarver SD, Stanley TH. Absorption and bioavailability of oral transmucosal fentanyl citrate. Anesthesiology 1991 Aug;75(2):223–29.

55. Farrar JT, Cleary J, Rauck R, Busch M, Nordbrock E. Oral transmucosal fentanyl citrate: randomized, double-blinded, placebo-controlled trial for treatment of breakthrough pain in cancer patients. J Natl Cancer Inst 1998;90: 611–16.

56. Ashburn MA, Lind GH, Gillie MH, de Boer AJ, Pace NL, Stanley TH. Oral transmucosal fentanyl citrate (OTFC) for the treatment of postoperative pain. Anesth Analg 1993 Feb;76(2):377–81.

57. Lichtor JL, Sevarino FB, Joshi GP, Busch MA, Nordbrock E, Ginsberg B. The relative potency of oral transmucosal fentanyl citrate compared with intravenous morphine in the treatment of moderate to severe postoperative pain. Anesth Analg 1999 Sep;89(3):732–38.

58. Macaluso AD, Connelly AM, Hayes WB, Holub MC, Ramsay MA, Suit CT, Hein HA, Swygert TH. Oral transmucosal fentanyl citrate for premedication in adults. Anesth Analg 1996 Jan;82(1):158–61.

59. Epstein RH, Mendel HG, Witkowski TA, Waters R, Guarniari KM, Marr AT, Lessin JB. The safety and efficacy of oral transmucosal fentanyl citrate for preoperative sedation in young children. Anesth Analg 1996 Dec;83(6):1200–1205.

Muscle Relaxants and Reversal Agents for Ambulatory Anesthesia

MARCY S. TUCKER

In the outpatient setting, neuromuscular blocking drugs (NMBDs) are primarily used with general anesthetics to facilitate intubation. While most outpatient procedures are brief and do not require muscle relaxation, others such as laryngoscopy or laporoscopy may be variable in length with periods requiring profound relaxation. Without muscle relaxants, larger amounts of inhalation and intravenous amnesiacs, hypnotics, and analgesics are required to provide optimal surgical conditions. Thus, NMBDs not only serve a role at induction, but also can enhance relaxation such that excessive doses of sedating anesthetic agents can be avoided. A balanced approach to general anesthesia in an ambulatory setting can hasten recovery and discharge from the facility.

The choice of a NMBD for an outpatient surgical procedure depends on patient factors, the type of anesthetic planned, and the surgical procedure. An ideal muscle relaxant for day-case surgery has yet to be developed, but clinicians generally agree that characteristics of one for use in outpatient surgical procedures should include the following properties: rapid onset (1–2 min), short duration of action (15–20 min), and predictable clearance. Additional attributes are listed in Table 18-1. Ambulatory patients are presenting with increasingly more complex histories, including renal, cardiac, and neuromuscular disorders which influence the distribution, clearance, and effect of given medications. This chapter will present some of the common available muscle relaxants and reversal agents in order to clarify their uses in ambulatory anesthesia.

AFFERENT NEUROMUSCULAR SIGNALING

Central corticospinal fibers relay information from the somatomotor cortex to the anterior horn cells in the spinal cord. Thus, the corticospinal tract is a relay between the central nervous system (CNS) and the peripheral nervous system (PNS). Central muscle relaxation can be accomplished by interfering with this pathway. Peripheral nerves develop from the axons of anterior horn cells or the alpha motor neurons as they travel to the different skeletal muscles. Peripheral nerve blocks accomplish muscle relaxation by interrupting nerve transmission at this level. The region where the peripheral nerve fibers synapse on or innervate skeletal muscle is called the neuromuscular junction (NMJ). The NMJ is the site of action of our conventional NMBDs. This junction, or the synaptic cleft, is 20–30 nm wide and contains extracellular fluid. Nicotinic cholinergic receptors are located on both the presynaptic and

Table 18-1 Characteristics of an Ideal Muscle Relaxant for Ambulatory Anesthesia

Rapid onset of action

Short duration of action

Predictable redistribution and elimination

Absence of cumulative effects with repetitive dosing

Absence of active metabolites

Minimal to no side effects

Easy reversibility

Easy administration

Low cost

Long shelf life

highly folded postsynaptic membranes. Extrajunctional postsynaptic receptors may proliferate if the muscle is damaged or denervated. These additional receptors are not involved in normal neuromuscular signaling and may exaggerate the response to neuromuscular blocking agents.

Acetylcholine (ACh) is the neurotransmitter synthesized in the presynaptic neuron from the substrates choline and acetate. Upon electrical stimulation of the presynaptic neuron, voltage-dependent calcium channels open, allowing the influx of calcium and fusion of the presynaptic vesicles containing ACh with the cell membrane. Exocytosis results in the release of ACh into the synaptic cleft. If the interstitial fluid is deficient in calcium, the release of ACh may be compromised. Calcium channel blocking agents or an excess of magnesium can decrease calcium entry across cell membranes, compromising neurotransmission as well. In the synaptic cleft, ACh can reversibly bind to the postsynaptic nicotinic receptor and initiate signaling events. At the cholinergic junction, the action of ACh is terminated by its hydrolysis to choline and acetic acid by acetylcholinesterase, also called "true" cholinesterase. This enzyme resides on the motor endplate and in lesser amounts in red blood cells. The rapid degradation of ACh by acetylcholinesterase prevents sustained postsynaptic receptor activation.

Currently, researchers are investigating a protein kinase at the NMJ (Abl kinase) that prepares the postsynaptic receptors to respond to ACh. A prerequisite for the ACh receptors to cluster is the interaction of Abl kinase with muscle-specific receptor tyrosine kinase (MuSK), a muscle cell surface receptor, and agrin, a large protein in the neuromuscular synapse.[2] This interaction of signaling proteins at the NMJ is demonstrated in Figure 18-1.

POSTSYNAPTIC IMPULSE TRANSMISSION

The binding of ACh to its receptor in the muscle cell membrane stimulates the opening of chemically gated channels within the receptor. The postjunctional nicotinic receptor is a 25-kd glycoprotein comprised of five subunits, namely two alpha subunits, and one each of beta, gamma, and delta arranged in a concentric circle around a channel, allowing for the flow of ions. ACh binds to the two alpha subunits, inducing a conformational change in the protein that opens the channel, altering the permeability to potassium and sodium in the postsynaptic membrane. A potential is the difference in "charge" inside and outside of a cell. This potential is created by the relative differences of charged

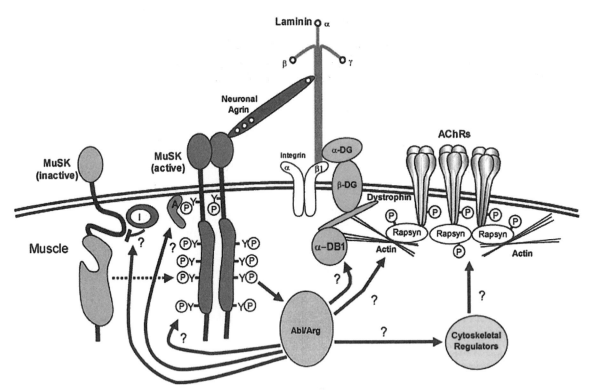

Figure 18-1 Postsynaptic organization of the neuromuscular junction. Critical components are indicated, including the muscle-specific receptor tyrosine kinase (MuSK); neuronal agrin in the synaptic cleft; Abl tyrosine kinases Abl and Arg; the dystrophin–glycoprotein complex (DGC) proteins α-dystrobrevin (α-DB1), dystrophin, and α- and β-dystroglycan (α- and β-DG) linking laminin in the extracellular matrix to cytosolic actin; and acetylcholine receptors (AChRs) tethered to the cytoskeleton by the DGC, the adaptor protein rapsyn, and other cytoskeletal regulatory proteins. Potential points of regulation by Abl kinases comprise (from left to right) binding of inhibitory (I) and activating (A) factors to the MuSK juxtamembrane domain, phosphorylation of the MuSK intracellular domain, phosphorylation of α-DB1, and regulation of the cytoskeleton by direct bundling of actin and phosphorylation of cytoskeletal proteins. (Modified with permission from Finn AJ, Feng G, Pendergast AM. Postsynaptic requirement for Abl kinases in assembly of the neuromuscular junction. Nat Neurosci 2003;6:717–23.)

ions across the cell membrane. ACh increases the conductance of sodium more than potassium through voltage-gated channels, such that the postsynaptic membrane potential, or EPP, moves in a more positive direction, from a transmembrane potential of approximately −90 mV to -45 mV. An action potential is generated when a threshold of depolarization is reached, triggering the muscle to contract. A single action potential in a motor axon evokes a contraction in all the muscle fibers of that unit.[3] After ACh hydrolysis by acetylcholinesterase, normal ion permeability is restored, the end plate membrane is repolarized, and muscle contraction is terminated.

NEUROMUSCULAR BLOCKING DRUGS

NMBDs block the transmission of neural impulses at the NMJ by either mimicking or interfering with the neurotransmitter, ACh. Those that mimic ACh are called depolarizing muscle relaxants, while those that competitively antagonize ACh are called nondepolarizing muscle relaxants. Nondepolarizing NMBDs can further be classified as either benzylisoquinolinium or aminosteroid compounds.[4] These classifications, as well as the chemical structures of some available NMBDs, are shown in Table 18-2 and Figure 18-2, respectively. The positively charged nitrogen ion in these quaternary ammonium compounds causes these agents to be ionized at physiologic pH, making them water-soluble and limited in their ability to cross lipid membranes. Thus, these drugs are generally unable to cross the blood-brain, placental, renal tubular, or gastrointestinal epithelium. This characteristic minimizes CNS effects or effects on a fetus when given to a pregnant female. However, negatively charged cholinergic sites, such as cardiac muscarinic and autonomic ganglia nicotinic receptors are susceptible to NMBD effects. The presence of a tertiary amine increases the likelihood of a histaminergic effect.

Table 18-2   Classification of NMBDs

Class	Duration of Action
Depolarizing NMBDs	
Succinylcholine	Short-acting
Nondepolarizing NMBDs	
Isoquinolines	
Tubocurarine	Long-acting
Atracurium (Tracrium)	Intermediate-acting
Cisatracurium (Nimbex)	Intermediate-acting
Doxacurium (Nuromax)	Long-acting
Mivacurium (Mivacron)	Short-acting
Steroid derivatives	
Pancuronium (Pavulon)	Long-acting
Vecuronium (Norcuron)	Intermediate-acting
Pipecuronium (Arduan)	Long-acting
Rocuronium (Zemuron)	Intermediate-acting

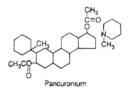

Short-acting

Intermediate-acting

Long-acting

Figure 18-2   Chemical structures and classification of commonly used NMBDs.

The effects of muscle relaxants may be enhanced by hemodynamic perturbations or medications administered in the perioperative period. For example, the action of nondepolarizing NMBDs is augmented by volatile anesthetics,[5-7] aminoglycoside antibiotics, local anesthetics, and cardiac antidysrhythmic drugs. The order of potentiation is as follows: enflurane and isoflurane > halothane > intravenous anesthetic agents.[8] Because the volume of distribution is dependent on the extracellular fluid compartment, increased protein binding, hemorrhage, or dehydration augments the potency of the NMBD.

Depolarizing Neuromuscular Blocking Drugs—Succinylcholine

The only depolarizing NMBD used clinically is succinylcholine (SCh). SCh is able to mimic ACh because its structure is actually two molecules of ACh linked through acetate methyl groups (Fig. 18-2). By binding to the alpha sites on the postsynaptic nicotinic receptor, SCh, like ACh, initiates ion flow through the receptor channel, resulting in depolarization of the postsynaptic membrane. In contrast to ACh, SCh is hydrolyzed at a much slower rate; thus, the receptor ion channel remains open longer, sustaining the ion flow and period of depolarization and muscle cell paralysis, relative to that produced by ACh. This period of sustained depolarization, when the membrane is immune to any further actions of ACh, is referred to as the phase I blockade. Phase II blockade occurs when the postjunctional membrane repolarizes but remains unable to respond normally to ACh. This can occur with excessive doses of SCh (greater than 3–5 mg/kg IV).

SCh produces a rapid onset of profound neuromuscular block in all muscles, including those of the vocal cords, making it the gold standard for intubation of the trachea.[9] SCh may be administered as an IV bolus (0.5–1.5 mg/kg) to facilitate optimal intubating conditions or as an infusion for brief surgeries in which profound muscle relaxation is needed. SCh can also be administered intramuscularly (4–5 mg/kg), making it valuable for treatment of laryngospasm during inhalational induction of anesthesia in the pediatric population. The duration of action of SCh is between 3 and 5 min, with its clinical action attenuated after hydrolysis by plasma cholinesterase. Its rapid onset combined with its short duration of action make it the most commonly used muscle relaxant in day surgical procedures.

A prolonged duration of SCh can be seen in multiple clinical settings such as in the presence of atypical forms of the plasma cholinesterase enzyme and with the administration of adjunct anticholinesterase agents. These agents include those used for treatment of glaucoma and/or myasthenia gravis, as well as chemotherapeutic drugs such as cyclophosphamide. The action of SCh can also be prolonged in patients inadvertently exposed to organophosphate insecticides. In these settings, additional respiratory support must be provided until the neuromuscular block resolves. Small decreases in the synthesis of plasma cholinesterase activity, as can be seen in liver disease, are usually clinically insufficient to alter the duration of SCh.

In the healthy surgical outpatient, particularly young adults undergoing minor surgical procedures, postoperative muscle pain is commonly seen after the use of SCh. The incidence has been reported to be as high as 65% of studied patients.[10–12] The muscles of the neck, back, and abdomen are the most commonly cited areas of pain. Transient generalized skeletal muscle contractions or fasciculations are often seen in a patient within a minute after SCh administration and have been linked to postoperative myalgias. However, postoperative muscle pain can occur in patients without clinical evidence of fasciculations or in patients receiving vecuronium in place of SCh.[13] Pretreatment with small doses of pancuronium or other nondepolarizing NMBDs has been ineffective in abolishing myalgias despite their ability to eliminate fasciculations.[14,15] Thus, the association of depolarizing agents with postoperative myalgias is unclear.

Other associated side effects of SCh administration relate to its structural similarity to ACh. Cardiac arrhythmias after SCh administration are the result of cardiac postganglionic muscarinic receptor stimulation, where SCh mimics the normal actions of ACh at these receptors. A second dose of SCh given 5 min after the first dose can precipitate sinus bradycardia, junctional rhythms, and even sinus arrest. These cardiac responses can be minimized with an IV dose of atropine or subparalyzing doses of nondepolarizing NMBDs (pretreatment) 1–3 min before SCh. SCh can have autonomic effects as well, mimicking the effects of ACh at autonomic ganglia.

Increases in intraocular, intragastric, and intracranial pressures have been an inconsistent finding after SCh treatment. SCh-induced increases in intraocular pressure were shown to be unrelated to contraction of extraocular muscles. SCh has not caused complications in patients with open eye injuries.[16] Increases in intracranial and intragastric pressures following SCh treatment are felt to be dependent on the presence of fasciculations as they are abolished by pretreatment with a nondepolarizing NMBD.

Potential life-threatening side effects of SCh include hyperkalemic cardiac arrest and malignant hyperthermia. The hyperkalemia is believed to be a result of the proliferation of extrajunctional receptors, which allows more potassium to leak outside of the cell during depolarization. This side effect is particularly ominous in children and patients who are in the acute phase of burns or have injuries in which there has been extensive denervation of skeletal muscles. The risk of hyperkalemia in these patients increases with time after injury, peaking 7–10 days after the injury. The duration of susceptibility is unknown. SCh is one of the triggers for malignant hyperthermia in susceptible patients. After exposure to SCh, these patients develop a hypermetabolic state in which there is sustained muscle contraction which, if unrecognized and treated, can lead to death. Another possible adverse effect of SCh is myoglobinuria, especially in pediatric patients.

Nondepolarizing Neuromuscular Blocking Drugs

In contrast to depolarizing NMBDs, which promote ion flow through the muscle cell membrane, nondepolarizing NMBDs occlude the postsynaptic ACh receptor channel, limiting ion flow and subsequent depolarization of the postsynaptic membrane. When bound to one or both of the alpha subunits on the nicotinic receptor, the large and bulky structure of the nondepolarizing NMBDs competitively antagonizes the binding of ACh to its receptor. The duration of this phase II blockade can be classified clinically as either short-, intermediate-, or long-acting (Table 18-2). The dose needed to produce 95% suppression of the single-twitch response (ED95) can be used to differentiate

Table 18-3   Comparative Properties among NMBDs

Drug	ED95 (mg/kg IV)	Time to Intubation (min)[a]	Duration ED95 (min)[b]	Cardiovascular Effects	Elimination
Succinylcholine	0.25	1	3–5	Cardiac arrythmias	Hydrolysis by plasma cholinesterase
Rocuronium	0.30	1–2	30–36	None	Liver > kidney
Mivacurium	0.08	2–3	20–25	Hypotension	Hydrolysis by plasma cholinesterase
Atracurium	0.20	2–3	25–30	Hypotension	Ester hydrolysis, Hofmann elimination
Cisatracurium	0.05	1.5–2	25–30	None	Hofmann elimination
Vecuronium	0.05	1.5–3	25–30	None	Liver > kidney
Pancuronium	0.07	3–5	60–90	Tachycardia	Kidney > liver

[a]Times represent the use of customary doses for intubation after induction of adequate general anesthesia.

[b]The neuromuscular blocking action of all agents is potentiated by volatile anesthetics. There is variability among responses to relaxants at extremes of age and clinical condition.

the potency of the various NMBDs. A comparison of properties among the nondepolarizing NMBDs is provided in Table 18-3.

Short-Acting Nondepolarizing Neuromuscular Blocking Drugs

Short-acting nondepolarizing NMBDs have been introduced as alternatives to SCh. However, one drug of this group, rapacuronium, has been discontinued secondary to the presence of unacceptable intubating conditions after its administration.[17]

Mivacurium

Mivacurium is a short-acting nondepolarizing bisquaternary benzylquinolinium diester with an ED95 of 80 μg/kg. When used at double the ED95 (0.16 mg/kg), its onset time is approximately 2–3 min with spontaneous recovery to 95% control twitch height in approximately 25 min. Thus, its duration is twice that of SCh. Mivacurium is hydrolyzed by plasma cholinesterase into three inactive compounds at a rate that is 88% of SCh.[18] Recovery from mivacurium is predictable and unrelated to whether it is given as a bolus or as an infusion.[19,20] Like SCh, a prolonged neuromuscular block can be demonstrated in patients with atypical plasma cholinesterase.[21]

While the hemodynamic profile is remarkably stable at doses used for intubation, cardiovascular effects become apparent with increasing doses and rapid injection. The major disadvantage of mivacurium is its weak effect on histamine release. The increases in plasma histamine levels are accompanied by decreases in blood pressure and tachyphylaxis, as well as facial erythema.[22] Furthermore, its onset time has been considered a disadvantage by some investigators.[23]

Intermediate-Acting Nondepolarizing Neuromuscular Blocking Drugs

The intermediate-acting NMBDs are advantageous for use in the ambulatory setting because of their predictable clearance and noncumulative effects. The onset of this category of NMBDs is approximately 3–5 min. Excluding rocuronium, their onset is comparable to that of the long-acting NMBDs. Rocuronium has a more rapid onset similar to SCh. This class of NMBDs is more expensive than SCh or pancuronium.

Atracurium

Atracurium is a bisquaternary benzylisoquinolinium diester with an ED95 of 0.2 mg/kg, producing sufficient intubating conditions in 4 min.[24] Increasing the dose to twice the ED95 has been shown to produce excellent intubating conditions in less than 3 min, though increasing the intubating dose increases the duration of action from 44 min to 60–70 min.[24] Atracurium undergoes ester hydrolysis and spontaneous degradation in a process known as Hofmann elimination. Thus, its clearance is independent of hepatic and renal function and not affected by atypical plasma cholinesterase. With noncumulative effects on repeat dosing and a rapid and reliable reversal and recovery, atracurium is a very attractive nondepolarizing NMBD for ambulatory surgery.[25,26] The main disadvantages of atracurium involve histamine release and subsequent hypotension after rapid bolus doses in excess of the ED95. Laudanosine, the inactive metabolite of atracurium, can produce CNS stimulation in high doses in animals.[9]

Cisatracurium

Cisatracurium is the R-cis isomer of atracurium and is a benzylisoquinolinium nondepolarizing NMBD. At doses equal to three times its ED95 of 50 μg/kg (0.15 mg/kg), excellent intubating conditions are observed in 1.5–2 min. The clinical duration ranges from approximately 25 to 55 min. Cisatracurium is also degraded by Hofmann elimination to laudanosine, though much less laudanosine is produced with cisatracurium elimination compared to that produced by atracurium elimination. Unlike atracurium, there is no degradation of cisatracurium by plasma esterases. The longer and less predictable duration of action of cisatracurium relative to atracurium makes it slightly less suitable for day case patients. However, its lack of histamine-releasing effects and associated cardiovascular effects are advantages over atracurium.

Vecuronium

Vecuronium is a monoquaternary aminosteroid derivative of pancuronium with an ED95 of 50 μg/kg. At this dose, the onset time is 4 min with a duration of action of 20–25 min. At doses three to five times the ED95, the onset time decreases to 1–2 min at the expense of a longer duration of action. Stevens and colleagues reported a more rapid onset time of vecuronium compared to cisatracurium when vecuronium was used at doses twice the ED95 for vecuronium.[27] In neonates and infants, vecuronium can be considered a long-acting NMBD.[9]

Vecuronium is eliminated by both hepatic and renal mechanisms, with its increased lipid solubility enhancing biliary excretion. Renal failure has little effect on the duration of action of vecuronium, though repeated or large doses may result in a cumulative effect. Vecuronium can precipitate bradycardia and asystole in the presence of vagotonic, beta-blocking, or calcium-channel-blocking drugs. Other adverse effects include its association with myalgias in the ambulatory setting.[13] Because vecuronium is unstable in solution, it is supplied as a lyophilized powder that must be used within 24 hr of reconstitution.

Rocuronium

Rocuronium is a monoquaternary aminosteroid structurally related to vecuronium. When used at twice the ED95 dose of 0.3 mg/kg, it produces profound neuromuscular blockade at 1–2 min, relaxing the vocal cords at a rate similar to that of SCh.[28] This shorter onset time is its major advantage compared to other currently available NMBDs. Its main disadvantage is its clinical duration of approximately 30–36 min, which is slightly longer than that of the other NMBDs.[29] With a reduced dose of 0.45 mg/kg, the clinical duration decreases to approximately 25 min, but the onset speed is delayed to approximately 3 min. Therefore, rocuronium is better utilized for procedures of more than an hour duration.[30] The role of intramuscular (IM) rocuronium was investigated as a possible alternative to SCh in pediatric patients. The 7–8-min time to peak effect made IM rocuronium an unsatisfactory replacement for SCh when rapid intubation was needed.[31]

Rocuronium is largely unchanged in the bile. Renal failure could increase the duration of action, for as much as 30% of a dose may be renally excreted. No significant his-

tamine release or cardiovascular effects have been reported with rocuronium.

Long-Acting Nondepolarizing Neuromuscular Blocking Drugs

Pancuronium

Long-acting NMBDs are generally inappropriate for ambulatory surgery. However, in unusual circumstances, muscle relaxation is required for a lengthy procedure. Pancuronium is inexpensive and offers advantages over other long-acting NMBDs such as doxacurium and pipecuronium. Pancuronium is a bisquaternary aminosteroid nondepolarizing NMBD with an onset of action of 3–5 min and duration of action of 60–90 min. The ED95 is 70 μg/kg. Pancuronium levels increase with renal failure, resulting in prolonged blockade duration. Cardiovascular effects are due to the ability of pancuronium to selectively block cardiac muscarinic receptors, and thus heart rate is increased. This effect is more pronounced in the setting of atrial fibrillation. Pancuronium has been avoided in patients with coronary artery disease because of these cardiac-stimulating effects and their potential contribution to the development of myocardial ischemia in these patients. Pancuronium does not produce any significant histamine release or autonomic ganglia blockade.

MONITORING OF NEUROMUSCULAR BLOCKADE

Neuromuscular blockade is generally evaluated by observing mechanically evoked responses following the delivery of electrical stimulation from a peripheral nerve stimulator. Common sites of stimulation include the ulnar nerve at the wrist and the facial nerve on the lateral aspect of the face. Evoked muscle tension at the adductor pollicis muscle or the orbicularis oculi muscle is estimated after graded impulses of electrical current are delivered at specified frequencies. A quantitative response to nerve stimulation can be obtained by analysis of an integrated electromyogram (EMG) of the muscle.

Common patterns of nerve stimulation include single-twitch, tetanus, post-tetanic potentiation (PTP), and train-of-four stimulation (TOF). A single-twitch response reflects events at the postjunctional membrane, while responses to continuous stimulation (50–100 Hz) or TOF reflect events at the presynaptic membrane. A TOF stimulation consists of four 2-HZ electrical pulses at 0.5 sec intervals, after which the presence of and relative intensity of resulting muscle twitches is monitored. The type of clinical blockade is correlated with the assessment of muscle tension generated in the fourth twitch relative to the first muscle twitch (TOF ratio). Depolarizing muscle relaxants generate a TOF ratio approximating 1.0 (phase I block), while nondepolarizers elicit a "faded" response, or a TOF ratio less than 1.0 (phase II block, Fig. 18-3). A faded response after repeated SCh administration suggests a tran-

Single twitch response to a NMBD:

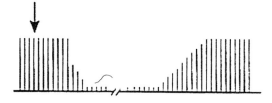

TOF response after:
A. injection of a depolarizing NMBD or

Succinylcholine

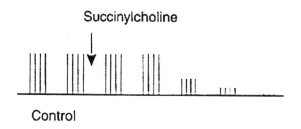

Control

B. injection of a nondepolarizing NMBD.

Nondepolarizing Drug

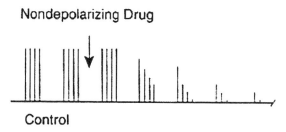

Control

Figure 18-3   Twitch responses to mechanical stimulation.

sition to a phase II blockade. The TOF ratio is also used to assess reversal of neuromuscular blockade, since an increase in the ratio to 0.7 after a nondepolarizing relaxant correlates with adequate clinical recovery.

Tetanus (continuous or tetanic electrical stimulation) for 5 sec at about 50 Hz is an intense stimulus for the release of ACh at the NMJ. An increase in twitch after tetanus indicates increased mobilization and synthesis of ACh, which suggests residual nondepolarizing blockade. PTP is seen after nondepolarizing blockade, but not in normal muscle or depolarizing phase I blockade.

Muscles have differing rates of response to the NMBDs, reflecting their varying ACh receptor densities and blood flow. The peripheral muscles (adductor pollicis) are

blocked before those of the diaphragm but after the laryngeal muscles (vocal cords). Greater than 90% depression of twitch response in the periphery correlates with adequate skeletal muscle relaxation for tracheal intubation. It is important to note at emergence that spontaneous ventilation may precede laryngeal recovery. With nondepolarizing muscle relaxants, the orbicularis oculi muscle has been shown to correlate better with laryngeal muscle blockade, while after SCh, the twitch response at the adductor pollicis is more likely to parallel the intensity of drug effect at the laryngeal adductors. Furthermore, adequate recovery from a general anesthetic when a regional technique is used concurrently must take into consideration any exacerbation of underlying weakness by the regional anesthesia.[32]

REVERSAL OF NEUROMUSCULAR BLOCKING DRUGS

Airway-related complications can result from residual nondepolarizing NMBD-induced weakness. This has prompted the routine use of anticholinesterase agents to ensure adequate recovery of muscle tone prior to tracheal extubation. Diplopia, dysphagia, an increased risk of aspiration, and a decreased ventilatory response to hypoxia are all risks of residual neuromuscular blockade. The function of cholinesterase inhibitors is to inhibit the activity of acetylcholinesterase, increasing ACh at nicotinic (NMJ) and muscarininc sites. This restores neuromuscular transmission. Anticholinergic drugs are used in combination with cholinesterase blockers to prevent the muscarinic side effects of the anticholinesterase treatments.

The anticholinesterases commonly used are neostigmine, pyridostigmine, or edrophonium. These are combined with the anticholinergic agents, atropine or glycopyrrolate. Atropine is often used with edrophonium because its prompt onset of anticholinergic effects parallels the rapid muscarinic effects of edrophonium. Glycopyrrolate is often combined with neostigmine because of the similar rates of their effects.

Stimulation of the muscarinic sites on the gastrointestinal tract by reversal agents has been linked to postoperative nausea and vomiting (PONV). However, the contributions of different combinations of anticholinesterase-anticholinergic treatments to PONV is unclear.[33] Clinical trials have not shown that the omission of pharmacologic reversal decreases the risk of PONV. While PONV is uncomfortable for the patient, it is not as potentially harmful as residual paralysis. For this reason, neuromuscular monitoring should be routine in the ambulatory setting when NMBDs are utilized and residual paralysis prevented by reversing neuromuscular block.[34]

CLINICALLY RELEVANT SITUATIONS

Patients with neuromuscular disorders are more frequently presenting for outpatient surgery. Neuromuscular perturbations can involve ACh directly or its receptor, or be secondary to a traumatic injury or a burn. An example of a disorder in which the ACh receptor is directly altered is myasthenia gravis (MG). In this autoimmune disease, the concentration of nicotinic ACh receptor in end-plate membranes is reduced by the immune reaction. Therefore, even if acetylcholine is released, it cannot effect neuromuscular transmission. This can be treated by blocking acetylcholinesterase, thereby increasing the amount of ACh available to bind to the reduced number of receptors. Patients with MG are generally resistant to depolarizing agents (if not on anticholinesterases) and markedly sensitive to nondepolarizing agents. Shorter-acting nondepolarizing muscle relaxants are the most prudent choices. Treated MG patients can be resistant to nondepolarizing relaxants and sensitive to depolarizers. Neuromuscular monitoring is mandatory.

In myasthenic syndrome, or Eaton Lambert syndrome, the receptors are normal, but a decreased amount of ACh is released. These patients are sensitive to both depolarizing and nondepolarizing agents but demonstrate a poor response to anticholinesterases. Inherited forms of muscular dystrophy or myotonic syndromes may present with an exaggerated response to depolarizers and a normal response to nondepolarizers, but the dose may need to be decreased secondary to innate muscle weakness.

Denervation of skeletal muscle can occur if motor fibers are traumatized or exposed to thermal injury. Within a week of denervation, the ACh receptors multiply, colonizing areas of the muscle fiber outside of the motor end-plate. The proliferation of extrajunctional receptors may occur after periods of prolonged inactivity or sepsis, as well. Thus, the motor fiber becomes exquisitely sensitive to ACh released anywhere in the vicinity of the fiber, causing depolarization at lower-than-usual levels of transmitter. Moreover, the extrajunctional receptors remain open longer when stimulated, allowing increased ion transport through these chemically gated channels. The increased influx of potassium ions in response to SCh administration in patients with denervation or burn injury makes them particularly susceptible to hyperkalemic complications. This supersensitivity later resolves, and after some months, the fibers will not respond to ACh at all.[3]

SUMMARY

While some outpatient surgical procedures may not require muscle relaxation or be accomplished with regional nerve blockade, other procedures may require general anesthesia with neuromuscular blockade. The need for neuromuscular blockade may be brief, only to facilitate endotracheal intubation, or extended, to provide profound muscle relaxation throughout the surgical procedure. While newer nondepolarizing NMBDs have been developed with minimal unwanted side effects, the depolarizing agent SCh remains the most commonly used relaxant in outpatient surgery today. It has a rapid onset and short duration of action, two requirements for an ideal ambulatory muscle relaxant. However, associated side effects, such as myalgias, and contraindications to its use in specific patient populations make it less than ideal for certain cases. For these cases, rocuronium, an intermediate-acting nondepolarizing mus-

cle relaxant with a rapid onset, may serve as an appropriate alternative. Atracurium and cisatracurium are degraded by Hofmann elimination and nonspecific ester hydrolysis and thus would be good relaxants for use in patients with renal or liver disease. The relative lack of histamine and cardiovascular effects with vecuronium and cisatracurium makes them useful in the setting of heart disease where hemodynamic stability is desired.

The risks of nausea and vomiting and prolonged ventilation have been theorized to be disadvantages to general anesthesia techniques with the use of NMBDs in an ambulatory setting. Lubarsky and colleagues did not find any change in the incidence of PONV in patients undergoing general anesthesia nor any significant postoperative ventilatory problems in patients receiving muscle relaxants in an ambulatory center.[35,36] Because the risk of postoperative respiratory muscle weakness is more critical than nausea and vomiting, the use of reversal agents is recommended when recovery from neuromuscular blockade is questioned. General anesthesia techniques with the use of muscle relaxants in an ambulatory setting should be associated with a rapid return to the preanesthetic state without any adverse effects. The careful use of muscle relaxants and appropriate reversal agents can facilitate a more rapid recovery from general anesthesia, hasten discharge from the surgical center, and result in a more satisfied patient.

REFERENCES

1. Apfelbaum JL. Muscle relaxants for outpatient surgery: old and new. J Clin Anesth 1992;4(5 Suppl 1):2S–8S.
2. Finn AJ, Feng G, Pendergast AM. Postsynaptic requirement for Abl kinases in assembly of the neuromuscular junction. Nat Neurosci 2003;6(7):717–23.
3. Somjen GG. Neurophysiology: The Essentials. Baltimore: Williams & Wilkins, 1983.
4. Hunter JM. New neuromuscular blocking drugs. N Engl J Med 1995;332(25):1691–99.
5. Bevan JC, Reimer EJ, Smith MF, Scheepers Ld, Bridge HS, Martin GR, et al. Decreased mivacurium requirements and delayed neuromuscular recovery during sevoflurane anesthesia in children and adults. Anesth Analg 1998;87(4):772–78.
6. Xue FS, Liao X, Tong SY, Liu JH, An G, Luo LK. Dose-response and time-course of the effect of rocuronium bromide during sevoflurane anaesthesia. Anaesthesia 1998;53(1):25–30.
7. Zhou TJ, Coloma M, White PF, Tang J, Webb T, Forestner JE, et al. Spontaneous recovery profile of rapacuronium during desflurane, sevoflurane, or propofol anesthesia for outpatient laparoscopy. Anesth Analg 2000;91(3):596–600.
8. Caldwell JE, Laster MJ, Magorian T, Heier T, Yasuda N, Lynam DP, et al. The neuromuscular effects of desflurane, alone and combined with pancuronium or succinylcholine in humans. Anesthesiology 1991;74(3):412–18.
9. Meakin GH. Muscle relaxants in paediatric day case surgery. Eur J Anaesthesiol Suppl 2001;23:47–52.
10. Collins L, Prentice J, Vaghadia H. Tracheal intubation of outpatients with and without muscle relaxants. Can J Anaesth 2000;47(5):427–32.
11. Churchill-Davidson HC. Suxamethonium (succinylcholine) chloride and muscle pains. Br Med J 1954;4853:718–25.
12. Smith I. Anesthesia for laparoscopy with emphasis on outpatient laparoscopy. Anesthesiol Clin North Am 2001;19(1):21–41.

13. Zahl K, Apfelbaum JL. Muscle pain occurs after outpatient laparoscopy despite the substitution of vecuronium for succinylcholine. Anesthesiology 1989;70(3):408–11.

14. Brodsky JB, Brock-Utne JG, Samuels SI. Pancuronium pretreatment and post-succinylcholine myalgias. Anesthesiology 1979;51(3):259–61.

15. Blitt CD, Carlson GL, Rolling GD, Hameroff SR, Otto CW. A comparative evaluation of pretreatment with nondepolarizing neuromuscular blockers prior to the administration of succinylcholine. Anesthesiology 1981;55(6):687–89.

16. Libonati MM, Leahy JJ, Ellison N. The use of succinylcholine in open eye surgery. Anesthesiology 1985;62(5):637–40.

17. Denman WT, Kaplan RF, Goudsouzian NG, Uejima T, Barcelona SL, Cote CJ, et al. Intramuscular rapacuronium in infants and children: a comparative multicenter study to confirm the efficacy and safety of the age-related tracheal intubating doses of intramuscular rapacuronium (ORG 9487) in two groups of pediatric subjects. Anesthesiology 2001;94(1):3–7.

18. Savarese JJ, Ali HH, Basta SJ, Embree PB, Scott RP, Sunder N, et al. The clinical neuromuscular pharmacology of mivacurium chloride (BW B1090U): a short-acting nondepolarizing ester neuromuscular blocking drug. Anesthesiology 1988;68(5):723–32.

19. Ali HH, Savarese JJ, Embree PB, Basta SJ, Stout RG, Bottros LH, et al. Clinical pharmacology of mivacurium chloride (BW B1090U) infusion: comparison with vecuronium and atracurium. Br J Anaesth 1988;61(5):541–46.

20. Basta SJ. Clinical pharmacology of mivacurium chloride: a review. J Clin Anesth 1992;4(2):153–63.

21. Cook DR, Freeman JA, Lai AA, Kang Y, Stiller RL, Aggarwal S, et al. Pharmacokinetics of mivacurium in normal patients and in those with hepatic or renal failure. Br J Anaesth 1992;69(6):580–85.

22. Savarese JJ, Ali HH, Basta SJ, Scott RP, Embree PB, Wastila WB, et al. The cardiovascular effects of mivacurium chloride (BW B1090U) in patients receiving nitrous oxide-opiate-barbiturate anesthesia. Anesthesiology 1989;70(3):386–94.

23. Geldner G, Wulf H. Muscle relaxants suitable for day case surgery. Eur J Anaesthesiol 2001;18(Suppl. 23):43–46.

24. Basta SJ, Ali HH, Savarese JJ, Sunder N, Gionfriddo M, Cloutier G, et al. Clinical pharmacology of atracurium besylate (BW 33A): a new nondepolarizing muscle relaxant. Anesth Analg 1982;61(9):723–29.

25. Pearce AC, Williams JP, Jones RM. Atracurium for short surgical procedures in day patients. Br J Anaesth 1984;56(9):973–76.

26. Dodgson MS, Heier T, Steen PA. Atracurium compared with suxamethonium for outpatient laparoscopy. Br J Anaesth 1986;58 Suppl 1:40S–43S.

27. Stevens JB, Walker SC, Fontenot JP. The clinical neuromuscular pharmacology of cisatracurium versus vecuronium during outpatient anesthesia. Anesth Analg 1997;85(6):1278–83.

28. Puhringer FK, Khuenl-Brady KS, Koller J, Mitterschiffthaler G. Evaluation of the endotracheal intubating conditions of rocuronium (ORG 9426) and succinylcholine in outpatient surgery. Anesth Analg 1992;75(1):37–40.

29. Lippmann M, Ginsburg R. Neuromuscular blockers in day-case surgery: is speed of onset more important than duration of action? Br J Anaesth 1993;70(2):235.

30. Bevan JC, Collins L, Fowler C, Kahwaji R, Rosen HD, Smith MF, et al. Early and late reversal of rocuronium and vecuronium with neostigmine in adults and children. Anesth Analg 1999;89(2):333–39.

31. Kaplan RF, Uejima T, Lobel G, Goudsouzian N, Ginsberg B, Hannallah R, et al. Intramuscular rocuronium in infants and children: a multicenter study to evaluate tracheal intubating conditions, onset, and duration of action. Anesthesiology 1999;91(3):633–38.

32. Wimberly JS. Neuromuscular blockade. In: Hurford WE, Bailin MT, Davison JK, Haspel KL, Rosow C (eds.), Clinical Anesthesia Procedures of the Massachusetts General Hospital, 5th ed. Philadelphia: Lippincott-Raven Publishers, 1998, pp. 181–203.

33. Watcha MF, Safavi FZ, McCulloch DA, Tan TS, White PF. Effect of antagonism of mivacurium-induced neuromuscular block on postoperative emesis in children. Anesth Analg 1995;80(4):713–17.

34. Fuchs-Buder T, Mencke T. Use of reversal agents in day care procedures (with special reference to postoperative nausea and vomiting). Eur J Anaesthesiol Suppl 2001;23:53–59.

35. Lubarsky DA, Sanderson IC, Gilbert WC, King KP, Ginsberg B, Dear GL, et al. Using an anesthesia information management system as a cost containment tool. Description and validation. Anesthesiology 1997;86(5):1161–69.

36. Lubarsky DA, Glass PS, Ginsberg B, Dear GL, Dentz ME, Gan TJ, et al. The successful implementation of pharmaceutical practice guidelines: analysis of associated outcomes and cost savings. SWiPE Group. Systematic Withdrawal of Perioperative Expenses. Anesthesiology 1997;86(5):1145–60.

Local Anesthetics and Adjuvants for Ambulatory Anesthesia

JOHN E. TETZLAFF

INTRODUCTION

Understanding the use of local anesthetics (LA) and adjuvants for ambulatory anesthesia begins with basic science, including the physiology of nerve cell function, the molecular basis for conduction block and an overview of the organic chemistry of local anesthetics. This basic information is used to explain the fundamental clinical properties of conduction block, including potency, duration of action, speed of onset, toxicity and allergy.

The issues associated with the clinical use of LA for ambulatory anesthesia include ambulation, urinary retention, nausea/vomiting, detection of neurological injury and the duration of postoperative analgesia. An overview of the clinical options for LA selection are presented by class (ester and amide) with the above issues as the perspective. The additives that can be added to LA solutions are presented in the context of the goal of the intervention and the suitability for ambulatory patients. The additives discussed include vasoconstrictors, alkalinization, compounding, opiates, adrenergic agents and miscellaneous additives that provide postoperative analgesia.

The final element of the discussion of LA and adjuvants for ambulatory anesthesia is a presentation of the common techniques of regional anesthesia that can apply to ambulatory surgery and how the LA choice can influence the outcome. Techniques presented include topical anesthesia, infiltration, peripheral nerve blocks, plexus blocks, central neuraxial blocks, intravenous regional anesthesia (IVRA), and other block techniques that are designed for prolonged postoperative analgesia.

Local anesthetics have an important role in surgical anesthesia and postoperative analgesia for ambulatory surgery patients. A rational decision for selection of a local anesthetic solution depends on an understanding of the basic science of nerve conduction, the organic chemistry of LA molecules and the unique properties of individual agents. One additional element for ambulatory anesthesia is the specific techniques of regional anesthesia and their suitability for outpatients.

BASIC SCIENCE

The Excitable Cell

The fundamental element of electrical signaling within the nervous system is the excitable membrane of the nerve cell axon. The specific elements that allow message transfer are the lipid membrane, ion-specific channels, and selective permeability. Potassium moves freely through potassium channels according to its electrical gradient. In contrast, sodium movement is restricted to open sodium channels. As a result, potassium is the predominant intracellular cation and sodium is the predominant extracellular cation. Because of the large amount of negatively charged axoplasmic proteins, the axoplasmic side is negatively charged in reference to the extracellular side, and this gradient (resting membrane potential) is determined by negatively charged proteins, fixed intracellularly by size, and potassium that moves freely down its electrochemical gradient. The result is a resting membrane potential of −70 mV. Because sodium has limited movement through sodium channels in the resting state, it has very little influence on the resting membrane potential.

When a signal is received, forward movement (conduction) occurs because of an alteration in the resting membrane potential. Sodium channels open, positively charged sodium cations move into the cell, and depolarization occurs. When the nerve cell membrane is rapidly depolarized from the resting state (−70 mV) to −20 mV, there is a large transient increase in sodium channel permeability. As permeability increases, sodium ion movement increases. The greater the depolarization, up to +20 mV, the greater the movement intracellularly of sodium. Beyond +20 mV, there is no greater increase in sodium conductance. Even with 80–90% of sodium channels blocked in a given area of axon, conduction continues, although the rate decreases as blockade increases. The electrical disturbance that occurs causes the adjacent sodium channels to open, and the signal is propagated. The baseline is restored first by passive movement of potassium followed by active, energy-dependent sodium transport.

Conduction Block

Propagation of a signal stops at a given point when a critical mass of sodium channels is blocked. Although sodium channels can be blocked on the axoplasmic and the extracellular side, they are reversibly blocked only on the axoplasmic side. When an ionic interaction between the axoplasmic opening of the sodium channel and the amine portion of a LA molecule occurs, the sodium channel is reversibly blocked. When a critical mass of sodium channels are blocked, signal propagation ceases (impulse extinction) and conduction block occurs until the association between the amine and the sodium channel ceases.

Organic Chemistry of Local Anesthetic Molecules

The molecules available for LA use in humans have a number of characteristics in common. Understanding the role of the component parts of these molecules helps to understand the important elements of LA action and the chemical basis for the difference between agents.

LA are all weak bases with a pKa between 7.6 and 9.3. They are amphipathic molecules, with a hydrophobic group connected to a hydrophilic group by an intermediate chain with an embedded covalent bond. The hydrophobic group is the primary determinant of lipid solubility, and because passage of the molecule through the lipid axon membrane is an essential component of LA action, this is a primary determinant of potency. The hydrophilic side determines the ionic behavior of the molecule and is responsible for the ionic bond with the axoplasmic opening of the sodium channel. The intermediate chain must be a critical length so that the chemically opposite poles of the molecule cause the correct alignment of the tertiary amine with the sodium channel. The covalent bond is one of two types—amide or ester—and this is the basis for the classification of LA, the amides (derived from aniline) and the esters (derived from paraminobenzoic acid). The covalent bond makes manufacture of the amphipathic molecule easier, determines metabolism and allergy (rare with amides, more frequent with esters), and influences toxicity. The ester LA are rapidly split into nontoxic metabolites by plasma cholinesterase. Even the most lipophillic agent, tetracaine, has a plasma metabolic half-life of 2.5–3.0 min, which significantly reduces potential toxicity. In contrast, the amide bond is relatively resistant to metabolism, and all of the amide LA have an initial termination of action by redistribution, and second-order metabolism at 45 min or longer. The potential for differential toxicity between amides and esters is obvious.

ELEMENTS OF LOCAL ANESTHETIC ACTION THAT DETERMINE SUITABILITY FOR AMBULATORY ANESTHESIA

There are a number of critical elements for appropriate anesthesia management for ambulatory patients. The impact of LA on these issues will determine the suitability of an agent or the concentration of an agent for ambulatory anesthesia. The choices are practical and include ambulation, urinary retention, detection of neurologic injury, duration of postoperative analgesia, and the incidence of nausea and vomiting.

Ambulation

Under most circumstances, the ambulatory patient must be able to walk out of the hospital. The decision to use LA and the specific choice of agent will influence this outcome. Where the LA is injected and the purpose must be considered. Delay in the interval to successful ambulation is undesirable after ambulatory anesthesia, and significantly increases the cost of care due to prolonged time in recovery.[1]

Some regional anesthesia techniques are totally appropriate under most circumstances for ambulatory patients. Topical anesthesia of mucous membranes (the eye, the rectum, etc.) and wound infiltration of the head, neck, and upper extremity (plexus and peripheral nerve blocks) have no impact on ambulation. Lower-extremity blocks, such as ankle, popliteal, femoral, sciatic, or psoas compartment block, render the leg incompetent to various degrees. Central neuraxial blocks (spinal, epidural, caudal) usually make ambulation unwise or impossible depending on the agent selected. The issue is the concern about the potential for falls, trauma to the limb, and the inability to ambulate. Despite this concern, discharge of ambulatory patients with insensate limbs was not associated with any injury or trauma in a large number of patients with either upper- or lower-extremity blocks.[2]

The goal of the LA must also be considered. When surgical anesthesia is the intended objective, complete sensory and motor block is usually required. For an upper-extremity procedure, this has no impact on ambulation. If central neuraxial block or complete peripheral nerve block of the lower extremities is necessary, a short-acting agent, such as 2-chloroprocaine or lidocaine, may be the best choice. When the LA is selected as a part of a surgical anesthetic, and one of the intended goals is postoperative pain control, the longer-acting agents (bupivacaine, ropivacaine, levobupivacaine) are better choices for maximum duration of anesthesia with prolonged analgesia; prolonged motor block could be an issue. If the role of the LA does not include dense motor block, a reduced concentration of the LA will provide analgesia with reduced motor block. The best example is bupivacaine, which is analgesic at concentrations of 0.25% and below with virtually no motor block. A caudal block with 0.125% bupivacaine in a child will provide extended analgesia without immobilization.

Urinary Retention

Although the absolute requirement to void prior to discharge has been eliminated in all but the high-risk patient, unfortunately, all patients who receive central neuraxial LA are high risk for urinary retention. The urge to void and the neuromuscular activity required to empty the bladder depend on coordinated activity of the autonomic nervous system. The preganglionic autonomic fibers for both the sympathetic and parasympathetic outflow are B-type fibers, which are small, fast-conducting neural structures and among all fiber types are the easiest to block with LA. As a result, these fibers are blocked at the lowest concentration of LA, have the most dense block, and are the last to be unblocked. Since the sympathetic outflow to the voiding process (lumbar) and the parasympathetic outflow (sacral) are exposed to maximum concentrations, the duration of block for any LA is longest for these fibers. The sensation of the urge to void is absent until central neuraxial block has regressed to the third sacral level[3] and the muscle strength and coordination to void is blocked even longer than the motor strength of the lower limbs.[4] If central neuraxial block is planned, especially in male patients, short-acting agents are essential.

If LA are used for procedures at risk for urinary retention, such as inguinal herniorrhaphy, there will be less urinary retention if the LA is used peripherally versus centrally.[5] In patients with low risk for urinary retention, discharge prior to voiding was safe after spinal or epidural anesthesia, as long as bladder ultrasound revealed less than 400 mL of urine in the bladder.[6] A small but significant number of males with a higher residual were unable to void without catheterization.

Detection of Neurologic Injury

Based more on tradition than reality, there is concern about discharge of ambulatory patients without recognition of neurologic injury. Dense conduction block can mask neurologic injury, as focal neurologic signs are indistinguishable from conduction block. This issue is in direct conflict with a primary role of local anesthesia in ambulatory anesthesia—postoperative analgesia. The optimum compromise is to have prolonged analgesia and evidence of neural function in the same dermatomes. Lower concentrations of long-acting LA will allow recovery of motor function while providing analgesia. In fact, higher concentrations of LA do not improve either quality or duration of analgesia. Recovery of motor function makes the probability of any neurologic injury low enough that discharge prior to further recovery is reasonable.[2] Compared to general anesthesia for ambulatory surgery, there is significantly less cognitive impairment with regional anesthesia, which theoretically decreases the risk of injury after surgery.[7]

Postoperative Analgesia

Because the ambulatory operating room places emphasis on efficiency, rapid-onset LA can be preferred on this basis. Those LA with prolonged analgesia uniformly have a slow onset and could be rejected based on efficiency. As an alternative, either compounding or double injection can be an option. Compounding of lidocaine with bupivacaine combines both needs—rapid onset of conduction block with prolonged analgesia. Alternatively, injection with a rapid-onset agent to achieve surgical anesthesia can be followed during surgery with repeated infiltration of a long-acting agent for sustained analgesia without concern for the latency to onset. Minor breast surgery can be rendered pain-free postoperatively with aggressive infiltration of the breast with bupivacaine.[8] Intercostal block with bupivacaine also creates a pain-free postoperative state,[8,9] but more technical effort is required, and the risk of pneumothorax, although small, is an issue for ambulatory patients. Preincisional wound infiltration with bupivacaine for adult inguinal herniorrhaphy creates a pain-free postoperative period for up to 24 hr.[10] Either field block or ilioinguinal block during pediatric herniorrhaphy under general anesthesia has the same effect, whether performed before or after the incision.[11] Interventions as simple as wound infiltration after surgery with dilute bupivacaine or application of gel lidocaine are effective postoperative adjuncts to ambulatory analgesia.[12] Infiltration and eutectic mixture of local anesthetics (EMLA) can be equivalent analgesic intervention, although use of EMLA requires the latency to onset (at least 30 min) to be considered.[13] Caudal block can provide profound postoperative analgesia after dilatation and curettage with minimal impact on ambulation when a short-acting local anesthetic is selected.[14] Even in procedures where monitored anesthesia care is the primary technique, the infiltration by the surgeon with LA is a component of postoperative analgesia as long as the surgeon can be convinced to use a long-acting LA.[15]

Postoperative Nausea and Vomiting

Because of the serious adverse impact of postoperative nausea and vomiting (PONV) in ambulatory surgery, LA have a significant role in operative anesthesia and postoperative analgesia. Because opioids and severe pain are both emetogenic, LA has a unique role because there is very little emetogenic potential.[15] The prominent role of LA in preemptive analgesia and as a component of a multimodal postoperative analgesia plan also has a direct impact on the reduction of PONV, because of opioid sparing.

LOCAL ANESTHETIC OPTIONS FOR AMBULATORY ANESTHESIA

For convenience, the agents are presented by class (ester or amide) and details relevant to ambulatory anesthesia are highlighted.

Ester Local Anesthetics

The ester LA have the attractive profile of low toxicity related to rapid metabolism by plasma cholinesterase. Although the overall risk of allergy to LA is very low, the majority of proven cases involved allergy to ester agents, due to a metabolite-para-aminobenzoic acid.

Procaine

Procaine has low potency, intermediate speed of onset, and short duration of action. Its use in ambulatory anesthesia is limited because of superior options for most applications. Historically, procaine has been used in the office setting for infiltration procedures requiring very large volumes. Tumescent application of lidocaine has replaced this use of procaine for virtually all cases, except neurosurgery. Neurosurgeons still occasionally infiltrate the scalp with large volumes (> 100 ml) of 0.5% procaine, although this is very uncommon in the ambulatory setting. Procaine also has a role in ambulatory spinal anesthesia. It provides a dense, short-duration subarachnoid block (SAB) and would be a reasonable choice for SAB for an outpatient with increased risk for urinary retention.[16]

2-Chloroprocaine

The chloride added to procaine to create chloroprocaine makes a short-duration agent with the highest pKa (9.3) of all the commercially available LA. Theoretically, the speed of onset should be slow, but the low potential for central nervous system (CNS) toxicity related to short plasma half-life (< 30 sec) allows the drug to be used in high concentrations (2–3%), and the result is a rapid onset of conduction block, ideally suited to ambulatory anesthesia.[17] Because of its hydrophilic chemistry, it is prepared commercially at a very acid pH (< 3.5) to achieve water solubility. Without alkalinization prior to injection, infiltration is a poor choice, owing to patient discomfort. With alkalinization, chloroprocaine is more comfortable for infiltration than plain lidocaine.[18] Chloroprocaine has been an attractive choice for ambulatory epidural anesthesia. A concentrated solution will create a dense sensory and motor block for surgical anesthesia, which fully resolves rapidly (60–90 min).

Use of chloroprocaine for ambulatory anesthesia has been associated with controversy. The original preparation of 2-chloroprocaine was stabilized and preserved with sodium metabisulfite (SMB). Because of disastrous outcomes, including adhesive arachnoiditis and profound neurologic deficits, after massive subarachnoid injection of this solution during attempted epidural blockade,[19–21] which were attributed first to 2-chloropaine[22] and later specifically to SMB,[23] the solution was changed to one with calcium disodium ethylenediamene tetra-acetic acid (EDTA). In addition to preservative and antioxidant properties, EDTA also chelates ionized calcium. While being injected into the epidural space, the solution makes contact with skeletal muscle within the paraspinous muscle groups by backtracking around the needle or catheter. The resulting chelation of ionized calcium causes a derangement of contraction and relaxation, which results in muscle spasm. When this preparation of 2-chloroprocaine was used for ambulatory epidural anesthesia, a high incidence of the patients developed debilitating back pain from muscle spasm after leaving the hospital that persisted for days in some cases.[24–27] The agent has been reformulated without any preservative, and no further problems have been reported with chloroprocaine so far.

Tetracaine

Tetracaine is a slow-onset, high-potency, long-duration LA. Although it is a versatile LA, some of the most common uses of tetracaine have a very limited role in ambulatory anesthesia. The toxicity of tetracaine has also limited the use of the LA, even though the concern has more basis in history than clinical fact. Because of the excellent topical anesthesia possible with liquid tetracaine, the agent rapidly became the most popular topical agent for eye surgery. Tetracaine also creates excellent topical anesthesia of mucous membranes of long duration. Unfortunately, plasma uptake is high, and when the dose is not controlled, toxicity is a potential. Early in the clinical experience with tetracaine, excessive doses used for topical anesthesia for upper GI and pulmonary endoscopy resulted in CNS toxicity. In the setting of minimal monitoring and, sometimes, very low light, disasters occurred and created a bad reputation for tetracaine.

In ambulatory anesthesia, tetracaine has a prominent role in a few applications. Topical anesthesia of the eye has been mentioned. Pain relief with acute ophthalmic injury is also most often achieved with tetracaine ophthalmic solution. When available, concentrated tetracaine gel or paste can achieve dense topical anesthesia of the skin,[28–33] although EMLA or intophoresis of lidocaine is a more common choice. Tetracaine added to other LA for peripheral nerve block or plexus block has some role in ambulatory anesthesia. The advantage is dense motor and sensory block with long-duration analgesia. The prolonged motor block can be a disadvantage with some proximal lower-extremity blocks. Tetracaine spinal anesthesia has very limited use in ambulatory anesthesia because of the long duration of the block, especially urinary retention. Topical anesthesia of the airway with tetracaine can also be unwise for ambulatory patients as it may suppress protective airway reflexes and delay safe discharge from the outpatient unit.

Cocaine

Cocaine has a very limited role in ambulatory centers because of toxicity and the issues with control and diversion. It has been reformulated as an alkaloid to make illicit use more difficult. The current role of cocaine in anesthesia is related to unique properties. Cocaine is an excellent topical anesthetic and has the unique property among LA of being an intense vasoconstrictor. When topically applied to mucous membranes, dense anesthesia and intensive vasoconstriction occur in contrast to other topical LA that causes vasodilation. The only other LA with vasoconstrictive action is ropivacaine, and the vasoconstriction is weak. This combined action makes cocaine an excellent choice for topical anesthesia of mucous membranes. The result of intranasal application is anesthesia and intense vasoconstriction that physically shrinks the tissue and creates ideal conditions for intranasal surgery.

The most serious toxicity issues with cocaine are cardiovascular effects. When it is properly applied in reasonable doses (less than 100 mg), the resulting plasma uptake can be minimal.[34] When plasma levels are achieved, cocaine blocks the reuptake of catecholamines and causes hypertension, tachycardia, and arrhythmia. Myocardial ischemia can result from catecholamine effects, interaction with anesthetic agents, or the unique potential of cocaine to induce coronary vasospasm.[35] As a result of the hyperdynamic effect of catecholamine release, arrhythmia, and/or coronary vasospasm, numerous serious cardiovascular events have been reported, including prolonged myocardial ischemia in patients without coronary artery disease,[36] myocardial infarction,[37,38] ventricular arrhythmia,[39] and pulmonary edema.[40,41] Because of these serious issues, especially in healthy patients, there is a high level of interest in alternate LA options and the combination of lidocaine and phenylephrine or epinephrine is the most common choice.[42,43]

Benzocaine

Benzocaine is a unique LA with low pKa (3.5) and a secondary amine structure. As such, its role is limited to topical anesthesia. Large doses (> 300 mg) can induce methemoglobinemia,[44–46] especially in children[47,48] and adults genetically predisposed to methemoglobinemia.

Amides

The amide LA options for ambulatory anesthesia in the United States includes lidocaine, mepivacaine, prilocaine, bupivacaine, ropivacaine, and levobupivacaine. Prilocaine has limited use and etidocaine has virtually disappeared from use. Dibucaine is also an amide agent used clinically outside the United States.

Lidocaine

Lidocaine is the most commonly used LA in the United States, primarily because of versatility. It has rapid onset, intermediate duration of action, and a favorable toxicity profile. It is an excellent choice for topical anesthesia of mucous membranes when applied as a liquid or gel. It is one of the two components of EMLA. Lidocaine is the most commonly selected LA for topical anesthesia as a liquid or gel. Topical anesthesia of the airway with lidocaine has a rapid onset and short-enough duration not to delay release from an ambulatory surgery center.

Lidocaine has a primary role in numerous forms of conduction block; 0.5% lidocaine is the most common LA for IVRA. Plexus and peripheral nerve blocks with lidocaine allows dense sensory and motor block with a reasonable recovery profile in cases where discharge requires full or near-full recovery. When used in the epidural space, rapid resolution of motor and sensory block occurs, although delayed recovery of the ability to void occurs as with all epidural LA.

Lidocaine has had a prominent place in ambulatory spinal anesthesia. Dilute hypobaric spinal anesthesia creates a brief subarachnoid block that can be ideal for some kinds of ambulatory surgery.[49] The hyperbaric solution (5% lidocaine in 7.5 % glucose) creates a rapid onset of a dense sensory and motor block with complete recovery typically in 2 hr or less. Use of lidocaine for spinal anesthesia has severely decreased because of the case reports and studies that have associated intrathecal lidocaine with cauda equina syndrome and transient neurologic symptoms (TNS).[50–52] Increased use of lower-concentration (1.5–2%) lidocaine has not eliminated concern with TNS.[51] Other factors such as obesity and use of the lithotomy position may be more contributory[51,53] than concentrated lidocaine.[54,55] This is particularly an issue for ambulatory patients because disturbing neurologic symptoms of TNS can present after discharge from the ambulatory surgery center (ASC).

Mepivacaine

Mepivacaine is very similar in action to lidocaine. Mepivacaine has been used for epidural anesthesia and peripheral nerve and plexus blocks. The longer duration may delay discharge compared to lidocaine, when complete recovery is a discharge criterion for central neuraxial blocks. Mepivacaine has made a return to spinal anesthesia, as an alternative to lidocaine, out of concern for TNS. The onset, density, and resolution are appropriate for some ambulatory anesthetics,[56] but could be prolonged excessively in patients taking clonidine.[57] It should be noted that mepivacaine has not been completely absolved from TNS.[58]

Prilocaine

Prilocaine was developed as an alternative to lidocaine, with more rapid metabolism and, theoretically, less toxicity. It may be an ideal agent for IVRA.[59] In low doses it has onset, action, and resolution that would be well suited to ambulatory spinal anesthesia, with lower, but not eliminated, risk of TNS compared to lidocaine.[60] Because of the incidence of methemoglobinemia with large doses, the clinical use of prilocaine has virtually disappeared, except for EMLA. Even though prilocaine has the most rapid elimination of all the amides, and methemoglobinemia is usually clinically silent and easily treated, the cyanosis is disconcerting and requires testing (measurement of methemoglobin) that may not be easily obtained in ASCs (arterial blood gas—ABG). Most disconcerting may be the risk with very low doses in children via either infiltration[61,62] or application of topical cream.[63,64]

Bupivacaine

The potency and toxicity of bupivacaine create a limited role for ambulatory anesthesia. Prolonged conduction block would be a serious issue with discharge if complete recovery is required. On the other hand, prolonged analgesia can be achieved with bupivacaine with limited motor block at lower concentrations (0.25% and below), an attractive property for ambulatory anesthesia. Postoperative pain control by infiltration with low-concentration bupivacaine can be an excellent component of sustained postoperative analgesia. Spinal and epidural anesthesia with bupivacaine in traditional doses will have a prolonged duration and has very limited use for ambulatory surgery.

Low-dose spinal anesthesia[65–67] and unilateral spinal anesthesia with low-dose bupivacaine,[68,69] both have recovery profiles that are reasonable for many ambulatory applications. Caudal blocks with bupivacaine may be reasonable in children because ambulation is not required. The selective cardiac toxicity with bupivacaine is an issue, but only for high-dose applications. The majority of the ambulatory applications do not require bupivacaine doses that approach potential toxicity.

Ropivacaine

Ropivacaine is a chemical derivative of bupivacaine designed to achieve the favorable clinical properties of bupivacaine with a reduction of the selective cardiac toxicity. Both LA are members of the pipecolylxylide family and are also chemically related to mepivacaine. The difference in these three agents is at one substitution of the tertiary amine. Mepivacaine (methyl, one carbon) has a very low potential for cardiac toxicity. Bupivacaine (butyl, four carbons) has high selective cardiac toxicity. Ropivacaine (propyl, three carbons) was manufactured to have the clinical properties of bupivacaine with reduced cardiac toxicity.

The clinical experience suggests that it is equally potent with bupivacaine although at this time it has been used at concentrations slightly higher than that of bupivacaine.[70] In animal models, the selective cardiac toxicity of ropivacaine appears to be intermediate between that of mepivacaine and bupivacaine.[71] The mortality with cardiac toxicity in animals is greatly reduced with ropivacaine compared to bupivacaine.[72] With intravenous infusion in human volunteers, ropivacaine produced less decrease in left ventricular contractility and less delay in electrical conduction compared to bupivacaine.[73] The quality of clinical block with ropivacaine appears to be very similar in onset, duration, and quality to that of bupivacaine[74] and has excellent analgesia postoperatively when used for wound infiltration or epidural infusion.[75] At 0.5%, there is a low level of motor block when injected in the epidural space.[76] At lower concentrations, there may be even less motor block than with bupivacaine at comparable analgesia.[70] When 0.1% and 0.2% ropivacaine is compared to the same concentrations of bupivacaine, the analgesia is equivalent between bupivacaine and ropivacaine, with no improved analgesia at the higher doses.[77]

The promise of reduced cardiac toxicity with ropivacaine also seems to be matched by the early clinical experience. The toxicity that has been reported more closely resembles that with mepivacaine, manifest by CNS symptoms, seizure activity, and no manifestation of cardiac toxicity.[78–82] Overall, early clinical evaluation reveals that ropivacaine has slightly less duration of action compared to bupivacaine, reduced motor block at equivalent concentration, and a unique property of weak vasoconstriction.[83,84]

The clinical role of ropivacaine in ambulatory anesthesia may be even more limited than that of bupivacaine because of comparable clinical action at considerably increased cost. The reduced cardiac toxicity is relevant only at higher doses. Ropivacaine has been used for ambulatory spinal anesthesia with comparable efficacy and no advantage over bupivacaine to justify the cost differential.[85,86] The vasoconstrictive properties could be an advantage for cutaneous procedures, unless end-organ blood supply is involved, which would be a relative contraindication. For prolonged postoperative analgesia, the total dose could be high. This would also be relevant if outpatient infusions via peripheral nerve catheters are considered.

Levobupivacaine

In the process of investigating selective cardiac toxicity with bupivacaine, it was identified that a unique property of bupivacaine was rapid entry into the sodium channels of the cardiac conducting system and slow exit, resulting in accumulation. Since egress occurs during diastole, time for egress decreases with heart rate and tachycardia potentiates accumulation. A further observation about bupivacaine is that it is a racemic mixture. Because there is a central, asymmetric carbon, bupivacaine is really two different mirror-image molecules—a dextro (right) and levo (left) rotatory form. Investigation into the causes of cardiac toxicity for bupivacaine revealed that the right-side (dextro) version had 3–4 times as much potential for cardiac toxicity due to slower exit from cardiac sodium channels during diastole compared to the left-sided (levo) molecule.[87] For this reason, ropivacaine was prepared from the start as a levo-isomer. This observation also led to the creation of L-bupivacaine, known as levobupivacaine.[88]

Animal studies have confirmed a reduction in cardiac effects of levobupivacaine compared to bupivacaine. In swine, ropivacaine and levobupivacaine have an equivalent reduction in lethal dose during intracoronary injection compared to bupivacaine.[89] An equivalent reduction in lethal dose was found with intravenous levobupivacaine in sheep compared to bupivacaine.[90] Also in sheep, a significant reduction in arrhythmia was noted at nonlethal infusion rates.[91] In human volunteers, less negative inotropy, less conduction delay, and less arrhythmia were found during intravenous infusion of levobupivacaine compared to bupivacaine.[92] In comparing levobupivacaine to ropivacaine and bupivacaine in isolated rabbit heart tissue, there was more prolongation of the QRS with bupivacaine, an intermediate prolongation with levobupivacaine, and the least prolongation in a ratio of 1.0/0.4/0.3 with ropivacaine.[93]

Just as the toxicity data are preliminary at this time, so is the evidence of the clinical performance of levobupivacaine compared to bupivacaine. Clinical studies reported to date find no difference in the clinical behavior of levobupivacaine compared to equivalent concentrations of bupivacaine.[92,94] Murdoch et al. evaluated levobupivacaine for postoperative epidural analgesia after orthopedic surgery, looking at 0.0625%, 0.0125%, and 0.25%, and found the best analgesia with 0.25% with no difference in motor block.[95]

As with ropivacaine, there is similar clinical performance to bupivacaine and a large cost differential. Except for cardiotoxicity, there does not seem to be any clinical difference between racemic bupivacaine and levobupivacaine. The cost differential limits the role of levobupivacaine to high-total-dose applications. Levobupivacaine may establish itself as a choice in continuous infusion for at-home analgesia after ambulatory surgery.

ADDITIVE OPTIONS FOR LOCAL ANESTHETIC SOLUTIONS FOR AMBULATORY ANESTHESIA

In addition to the choice of LA for ambulatory anesthesia, there are choices to be made about additives. Options include vasoconstrictors, alkalinization, opioids, and autonomically active agents, added to change some of the properties of a given LA.

Vasoconstrictors

Vasoconstrictors, including epinephrine, phenylephrine, ephedrine, and norepinephrine, have been added to LA solutions for a variety of purpose. Epinephrine is the most common choice and most extensively studied. Added epinephrine induces intense vasoconstriction at the site of the injection. This prevents uptake of the agent, keeping the LA in contact with target neural structures. This allows more uptake of the agent. Except for the most lipid-soluble agents where the effect is minimal, the result is a more dense block with longer duration, up to 50% with some agents (lidocaine). Another consequence is delayed plasma uptake of the LA. With large doses of LA, this has the favorable property of decreasing peak plasma levels and delaying the time to peak level, which further reduces toxicity. Epinephrine also has independent properties as an analgesic centrally and perhaps peripherally by interfering with nociceptive transmission at the interneuron level. Historically, ephedrine, phenylephrine, and norepinephrine also have been used to achieve some or all of these effects.

Because of the concern for toxicity with significant plasma levels of LA, many techniques have evolved to help identify intravenous injection. Epinephrine has been used for this purpose because of the strong adrenergic agonist properties and the easy recognition of beta-adrenergic response. When $15\mu g$ of epinephrine is injected rapidly intravenously, there is a predictable, transient (30–60 sec) 30–50% increase in heart rate. Epinephrine has a unique indication as the test dose of choice in most clinical situations to detect intravascular injection.

For ambulatory anesthesia, the decision to add a vasoconstrictor to LA solutions must be individualized to the indication. Concentrated phenylephrine can be added to lidocaine to achieve anesthesia and vasoconstriction of nasal mucous membranes in those practice settings where it is desirable to avoid cocaine. When epinephrine prolongs analgesia, it can be a good choice. When it delays recovery, such as urinary retention[96] or ambulation[97] after central neuraxial block, epinephrine can be a poor choice for ambulatory anesthesia. An additional disadvantage of vasoconstrictors, especially phenylephrine,[98] is that they may increase the incidence of TNS after ambulatory spinal anesthesia.

Alkalinization

Alkalinization of LA solutions is performed to alter a number of properties of conduction block. The LA is a weak base, but has poor solubility at alkaline pH. They are manufactured as a hydrochloride salt and bottled at pH 5.0–5.5. At this pH, the cation/base ratio is 1000:1. Because the target is an axon membrane (lipoprotein membrane), onset of conduction block is determined by the concentration of the base, as the cation has virtually no lipid solubility. When plain LA solutions are injected, buffering occurs with extracellular buffering systems, predominantly the bicarbonate system. This observation led to experiments with added sodium bicarbonate. When the LA solution is adjusted to physiologic pH (7.2–7.4), the cation/base ratio becomes 60:40 and the increased base concentration accelerates the speed of onset and can increase the density/quality of the block.

The clinical results of alkalinization of LA solutions have been extensively studied. Tables for optimum alkalinization have been published,[99] and the clinical efficacy is most pronounced for LA that can be alkalinized to a pH > 7.0. The most lipid-soluble agents, bupivacaine, ropivacaine, and levobupivacaine, cannot be alkalinized above pH 6.5 because of precipitation.

Alkalinization of LA solutions has a role in ambulatory anesthesia. Alkalinization prior to injection eliminates the pain on injection related to acidity.[99–103] This is highly relevant for injections in the face, urogenital areas, and breasts, and in children. In contrast to epinephrine, which prolongs conduction block, the increase in quality of conduction block with alkalinization does not delay recovery.[104] Improved motor block,[105] quality of epidural block[106,107] of large nerve roots (L5 or S1), and reduced tourniquet pain[108] are properties that can be relevant in planning an ambulatory anesthetic. The increased speed of onset[109] is an attractive advantage in the ambulatory setting, where turnover time is a premium issue.

Opioids

Opioids have been added to LA solutions to improve the quality of block achieved with central neuraxial blocks. The presence of opiate receptors at the spinal cord level explains the additive analgesia achieved with spinal or epidural opioids.[110] Additional work has shown sustained analgesic effects of opioids in the intra-articular space[111] and perhaps with plexus block.[112] Other spinal opiate receptor actions in addition to analgesia present some issues for ambulatory patients. Pruritus and PONV can result from opioid use and delay discharge.[113] Urinary retention can be an issue as it is with central axis LA.[114] The most ominous consequence of central opioids is respiratory depression.[115] Respiratory depression occurs when rostral spread of the opioid reaches the fourth ventricle. With the highly lipid-soluble opioids such as fentanyl or sufentanil, plasma uptake makes rostral spread from lumbar or low thoracic epidural or intrathecal injection very unlikely without overdose.[110] With more water-soluble opiates, such as morphine, rostral spread is likely and delayed onset of respiratory depression is a serious issue.[115] Because the onset of clinically significant respiratory depression can be delayed up to 18 hr after injection even with very low doses, central axis morphine is rarely used with LA solutions for ambulatory patients.

In contrast, intra-articular morphine provides sustained analgesia after arthroscopic knee,[116] shoulder,[117] and perhaps other intra-articular procedures. When iliac crest is a site for bone graft harvest, infiltration with bupivacaine and morphine provides excellent sustained analgesia.[118] Intrathecal fentanyl is very unlikely to cause delayed respiratory depression, but could extend the duration of urinary retention in a patient at risk.

Autonomic Drugs

Numerous agents with autonomic activity have been added to LA solutions, mainly to achieve postoperative analgesia. Clonidine is analgesic in the central axis by alpha-adrenergic action, but is less than ideal for ambulatory patients owing to extended urinary retention and orthostasis.[119] Use of clonidine may prolong peripheral analgesia with LA, without the undesired effects that occur centrally.[120,121] The alpha-2 selective agents, such as dexmedetomidine,[119] may offer the analgesia with a reduced side effect profile. Cholinergic agents have had trials as neuraxial analgesics. Neostigmine provides analgesia when administered intrathecally or epidurally, but with a side effect profile not acceptable for outpatient surgery.[122–124] Peripheral use of neostigmine combined with LA may have a more acceptable side effect profile for ambulatory patients.[125] N-methyl-D-aspartate (NMDA) receptor antagonists, such as ketamine,[126,127] have demonstrated analgesic activity interfering with interneuronal nociceptive signals. Ultimately, multimodal analgesia may focus on neuraxial "cocktails" designed to silence central nociceptive transmission with a side effect profile acceptable to ambulatory patients.

Compounding Local Anesthetics

One LA can be added to another to achieve a variety of goals. A rapid-onset agent can be added to one with slow onset and longer duration of action to achieve a compound with both profiles. An example of this choice would be a mixture of lidocaine and bupivacaine. Another choice for compounding is the addition of an agent designed for prolonged postoperative analgesia to an agent well suited to complete surgical anesthesia. Examples of this choice would be the addition of tetracaine to chloroprocaine, lidocaine, or mepivacaine. EMLA is compounded lidocaine and prilocaine (5% bases) mixed to achieve the potential for topical anesthesia of intact skin. Tetracaine-adrenaline-cocaine solution (TAC) is another mixture compounded for topical anesthesia of lacerations and mucous membranes.

Compounding may be less optimal in clinical practice than in theory. The toxicity of the solution is not reduced by compounding[128] although it is also not increased compared to the parent agents. Mixture of chloroprocaine with bupivacaine to increase the duration of the solution does not achieve the desired effect, because chloroprocaine reduces the duration of analgesia achieved with bupivacaine.[129,130]

Tetracaine-Epinephrine (Adrenaline)-Cocaine Solution for Topical Anesthesia

A mixture of tetracaine, cocaine, and epinephrine (TAC) has been used for topical anesthesia of wounds and mucous membrane.[131] The analgesia achieved is rapid and complete enough for minor procedures, especially lacerations of the face.[132] Variability in absorbance of the agents and liberal application have led to toxicity[133] and morbidity,[134,135] especially in children. Attempts to modify this toxicity have included reducing the cocaine concentration,[136] omitting tetracaine,[137] and replacing cocaine with lidocaine, which achieved equivalent analgesia to TAC.[138]

Eutectic Mixture of Local Anesthetics Cream

The creation of EMLA results from a mixture of lidocaine (5% base paste) with prilocaine (5% base paste), resulting in a 2.5% emulsion of both agents that has a unique property of penetrating intact dermis.[139] The depth of the anesthesia is proportional to the time of exposure, achieving anesthesia of the skin when properly applied. With proper advance preparation, EMLA can provide complete anesthesia for cutaneous procedures, minor otologic surgery,[140,141] perineal surgery,[142–144] genital procedures,[145–147] dialysis, or aspiration of bone marrow. It can also be a component of postoperative analgesia, with the attractive option of reapplication by the patient at home.[147] EMLA can be applied to the hands of pediatric patients to facilitate preoperative intravenous placement, allowing rapid induction of anesthesia and rapid emergence techniques (propofol, remifentanil) favored in the rapid-turnover ambulatory setting.[139] Application of EMLA cream prior to infiltration for aesthetic procedures in adults can make them more comfortable.[148]

COMMON USES OF LOCAL ANESTHESIA FOR AMBULATORY ANESTHESIA

Choice of LA for ambulatory anesthesia depends on the chemical activity of the LA and the type of regional anesthesia planned. Considerable variability in choice can be influenced by the site of injection and type of block.

Topical Anesthesia

The most commonly used LA for topical anesthesia is lidocaine. Used in a 1–4% concentration (liquid or gel), lidocaine achieves rapid topical anesthesia of mucous membrane with 30–60-min duration. Control of the total dose used is important because plasma uptake is high. Tetracaine can also be used for this purpose, achieving topical anesthesia for 2–3 hr or longer. The total dose of topical tetracaine must be carefully controlled because the potential for toxicity is high.

EMLA and lidocaine iontophoresis can achieve topical anesthesia of intact skin surfaces, both require time to achieve anesthesia, and in fact, the skin exposed to EMLA is hypersensitive prior to 30-min exposure time. TAC can achieve topical anesthesia with exposure, but the very high concentrations of the tetracaine and cocaine can create toxicity with plasma uptake from mucous membranes, lacerated wound edges, or disrupted skin (e.g., burns).

Infiltration

The LA selected for infiltration depends on the purpose and volume needed. In general, low concentrations are used, as motor block is never the objective. Lidocaine is the most common choice for simple infiltration at 0.5–1% concentrations. A special variation of infiltration anesthesia has been developed for aesthetic surgical procedures. Very dilute lidocaine (0.5% or less) and epinephrine (1:500,000 or less) are injected under pressure into the flesh of the hips and thighs for liposuction and lift procedures.[149] Referred to as tumescent technique,[150] apparently huge (35–50 mg/kg) doses of lidocaine can be used with surprisingly low plasma levels.[151] This is related to the low vascularity of the fatty tissues at the injection site, the pressurized injection that further decreases vascular uptake, and the suction removal of the tissue during liposuction, which removes considerable amounts of the agent.[152] Toxicity has been encountered with lidocaine,[153,154] and pulmonary edema from the injection of pressurized fluid in additional to the intravenous fluid administered has been reported.[155]

Infiltration into the intra-articular space is unique in outcome. Intra-articular analgesia requires large volumes, but plasma levels that result are low (approaching zero). Even in volumes as high as 60 mL in the knee, 0.25% bupivacaine resulted in very low plasma levels.[156] One possible exception is intra-articular injection after trauma, where intra-articular fractures could result in massive intervascular uptake.[157]

Plexus and Peripheral Nerve Blocks

When peripheral regional anesthesia is selected for surgical anesthesia for ambulatory patients, complete anesthesia and motor block are necessary. If the block is a part of a balanced anesthetic, and the LA is not required to provide motor block, low concentration may be a better choice to avoid motor block. Another element in the decision is the extent of recovery necessary before discharge. With upper-extremity procedures, minimal recovery may be required. A surgical anesthetic with 1.5% lidocaine or mepivacaine could be compounded with tetracaine to achieve prolonged (8–12 hr) analgesia. A dilute concentration of tetracaine (0.1%) will allow motor function to return early enough to verify neurologic integrity. If the block will be

used in conjunction with general anesthesia, 0.25% bupivacaine or ropivacaine will achieve even longer analgesia, without significant motor block.

For lower-extremity surgery, some centers are resistant to discharge with proximal motor block of the surgical limb. Proximal surgical anesthesia can be achieved with lidocaine (1–1.5%) or 2% chloroprocaine for even shorter duration. A more distal supplemental block where motor block is less relevant (ankle block) could be performed with a long-acting agent.

Intravenous Regional Anesthesia (IVRA)

IVRA is selected for brief soft-tissue procedures of the upper extremity or, less frequently, the lower extremity.[158] Most commonly, IVRA is performed with 50 mL of 0.5% lidocaine for the upper extremity and 75–100 mL for the lower extremity. Opioids, clonidine, and ketorolac have been evaluated as additives for IVRA with variable success.

Epidural Anesthesia

Single injection and continuous techniques have been used for ambulatory epidural anesthesia. In an effort to achieve dense surgical anesthesia with rapid recovery, chloroprocaine has some enthusiasm. The chloroprocaine solution preserved with EDTA resulted in lumbar muscle spasm cases. This has not been reported with the preservative-free reformulation. Alternatively, lidocaine (1–1.5%) will provide complete surgical anesthesia in the epidural space and fully resolve in 90–120 min.

Spinal Anesthesia

Early in the era of ambulatory surgery, spinal anesthesia was rarely selected. With newer needles (25–27 gauge/Whitacre, Sprotte) and interest in low-dose and unilateral spinal blocks, spinal anesthesia has returned to many ambulatory centers.[159,160] As previously mentioned, as intrathecal block is returning to ambulatory surgery, lidocaine is disappearing due to concerns for TNS. As an alternative, plain lidocaine (1–2%) is used by some at low total doses (30–50 mg) to achieve a block with 60–90 min total duration.[161] For those concerned with TNS, similar low doses of mepivacaine can be used with only slightly longer duration. Ropivacaine is acceptable on a clinical basis, but offers no distinct advantage over bupivacaine to justify the cost differential.[161] Very low doses of bupivacaine or tetracaine (3–5 mg) provide brief intrathecal block, but the block is shallow at best.[162,163] Hyperbaric technique and dependent position provide some degree of unilateral block that some consider reasonable for the ambulatory setting.

Prolonged Postoperative Analgesia

Peripheral nerve catheters,[164–166] intra-articular infusion,[167] epidural catheters,[15] and even wound infusion[168] have been placed for sustained analgesia in patients going home. Dilute bupivacaine (0.1% or less) has been the first choice, but the alternatives, ropivacaine or levobupivacaine, are attractive for their reduced cardiotoxicity. EMLA has the attractive property of allowing reapplication by the patient/family to extend analgesia in cases where it is relevant.

REFERENCES

1. Greenberg CP. Practical, cost-effective regional anesthesia for ambulatory surgery. J Clin Anesth 1995;7:614–21.

2. Klein SM, Nielsen KC, Greengrass RA, et al. Ambulatory discharge after long-acting peripheral nerve blockade: 2382 blocks with ropivacaine. Anesth Analg 2002;94:65–70.

3. Kamphuis ET, Ionescu TI, Kuipers PWG, et al. Recovery of storage and emptying functions of the urinary bladder after spinal anesthesia with lidocaine and with bupivacaine in men. Anesthesiology 1998;88:310–16.

4. Axelsson K, Mollefors K, Olsson G, et al. Bladder function in spinal anesthesia. Acta Anaesthesiol Scand 1985;29:315–21.

5. Jensen P, Mikkelsen T, Kehlet H. Postherniorrhaphy urinary retention-effect of local, regional and general anesthesia: a review. Reg Anesth Pain Med 2002;27:612–17.

6. Mulroy MF, Salinas FV, Larkin KL, et al. Ambulatory surgery patients may be discharged before voiding after short-acting spinal and epidural anesthesia. Anesthesiology 2002;97:315–19.

7. Tzabar Y, Asbury AJ, Millar K. Cognitive failures after general anaesthesia for day-case surgery. Br J Anaesth 1996;76:194–97.

8. Romm S, Kennell E, Berggren R. Patient acceptance of intercostal block anesthesia. Plast Reconstr Surg 1980;65:39–41.

9. Huang TT, Parks DH, Lewis SR. Outpatient breast surgery under intercostal block anesthesia. Plast Reconstr Surg 1979;63:299–303.

10. Lichtenstein IL, Shulman AG. Ambulatory outpatient hernia surgery. Including a new concept, introducing tension-free repair. Int Surg 1986;71:1–4.

11. Reid MF, Harris R, Phillips PD, et al. Day-case herniotomy in children: a comparison of ilio-inguinal nerve block and wound infiltration for postoperative analgesia. Anaesthesia 1987;42:658–61.

12. Davies P, Ogg T. Postoperative pain relief. Practitioner 1992;236:840–42.

13. Philip BK. Regional anaesthesia for ambulatory surgery. Can J Anaesth 1992;39:3–6.

14. Baker AB, Baker JE. Outpatient anaesthesia for dilation and curettage. Anaesth Intens Care 1979;7:362–66.

15. White PF. The role of non-opioid analgesic techniques in the management of pain after ambulatory surgery. Anesth Analg 2002;94:577–85.

16. Boucher C, Girard M, Drolet P, et al. Intrathecal fentanyl does not modify the duration of spinal procaine block. Can J Anaesth 2001;48:466–69.

17. Allen RW, Fee JPH, Moore J. A preliminary assessment of epidural chloroprocaine for day procedures. Anaesthesia 1993;48:773–75.

18. Marica LS, O'Day T, Janosky JE, et al. Chloroprocaine is less painful than lidocaine for skin infiltration anesthesia. Anesth Analg 2002;94:351–54.

19. Reisner LS, Hochman BN, Plumer MH. Persistent neurologic deficit and adhesive arachnoiditis following intrathecal 2-chloroprocaine injection. Anesth Analg 1980;59:452–54.

20. Moore DC, Spierdijk J, vanKleef, et al. Chloroprocaine neurotoxicity: four additional cases. Anesth Analg 1982;61:155–58.

21. Ravindran RS, Bond VK, Tasch MD, et al. Prolonged neural blockade following regional anesthesia with 2-chloroprocaine. Anesth Analg 1980;59:447–51.

22. Ravindran RS, Turner MS, Muller J. Neurologic effects of sub-

23. Wang BC, Hillman DE, Spielholz NI, et al. Chronic neurological deficits and nesacaine CE—an effect of the anesthetic, 2-chloroprocaine, or the antioxidant, sodium bisulfite? Anesth Analg 1984;63:445–47.

24. Stevens RA. Back pain following epidural anesthesia with 2-chloroprocaine. Reg Anesth 1997;22:299–302.

25. Drolet P, Veillette Y. Back pain following epidural anesthesia with 2-chloroprocaine (EDTA-free) or lidocaine. Reg Anesth 1997;22:303–7.

26. McLoughlin TM, DiFazio CA. More on back pain after nesacaine-MPF. Anesth Analg 1990;71:562–63.

27. Stevens RA, Urmey WF, Urquhart B, et al. Back pain after epidural anesthesia with chloroprocaine. Anesthesiology 1993;78:492–97.

28. Barfield JM, Lee FS, Raccio-Robak N, Salluzzo RF, et al. Topical tetracaine attenuates the pain of infiltration of buffered lidocaine. Acad Emerg Med 1996;3:1001–5.

29. Doyle E, Freeman J, Im NT, et al. An evaluation of a new self-adhesive patch preparation of amethocaine for topical anesthesia prior to venous cannulation in children. Anaesthesia 1993;45:1050–52.

30. McCafferty DF, Woolfson AD, Boston V. In vivo assessment of percutaneous local anaesthetic preparations. Br J Anaesth 1989;62:17–21.

31. McCafferty DF, Woolfson AD. New patch delivery system for percutaneous local anaesthesia. Br J Anaesth 1993;71:370–74.

32. Miller KJ, Goodwin SR, Westermann-Clark GB, et al. Evaluating of local anesthesia provided by transdermal patches containing different formulations of tetracaine. J Pharm Sci 1993;82:1123–25.

33. Molodecka J, Stenhouse C, Jones JM, et al. Comparison of percutaneous anaesthesia for venous cannulation after topical application of either amethocaine or EMLA cream. Br J Anaesth 1994;72:174–76.

34. Greinwald JH, Holtel MR. Absorption of topical cocaine in rhinologic procedures. Laryngoscope 1996;106:1223–25.

35. Lange RA, Cigarroa RG, Yancy CW, et al. Cocaine-induced coronary-artery vasoconstriction. N Engl J Med 1989;321:1557–62.

36. Laffey JG, Neligan P, Ormonde G. Prolonged perioperative myocardial ischemia in a young male: due to topical intranasal cocaine? J Clin Anesth 1999;11:419–24.

37. Chiu YC, Brecht K, DasGupta DS, et al. Myocardial infarction with topical cocaine anesthesia for nasal surgery. Arch Otolaryol Head Neck Surg 1986;112:988–90.

38. Minor RL, Scott BD, Brown DD, et al. Cocaine-induced myocardial infarction in patients with normal coronary arteries. Ann Intern Med 1991;115:797–806.

39. Lustik SJ, Wojtczak J, Chhibber AK. Wolff-Parkinson-White syndrome simulating inferior myocardial infarction in a cocaine abuser for urgent dilation and evacuation of the uterus. Anesth Analg 1999;89:609–12.

40. Singh PP, Dimich I, Shamsi A. Intraoperative pulmonary edema in a young cocaine smoker. Can J Anaesth 1994;41:961–64.

41. Bird DJ, Markey JR. Massive pulmonary edema in a habitual crack cocaine smoker not chemically positive for cocaine at the time of surgery. Anesth Analg 1997;84:1157–59.

42. Noorily AD, Noorily SH, Otto RA. Cocaine, lidocaine, tetracaine: which is the best for topical nasal anesthesia? Anesth Analg 1995;81:724–27.

43. Goodell JA, Gilroy G, Huntress JD. Reducing cocaine solution use by promoting the use of lidocaine-phenylephrine solution. Am J Hosp Pharm 1988;45:2510–13.

44. Kern K, Langevin PB. Methemoglobinemia after topical anesthesia with lidocaine and benzocaine for difficult intubation. J Clin Anesth 2000;12:167–72.

45. Udeh C, Bittikofer J, Sum-Ping STJ, et al. Severe methemoglobinemia on reexposure to benzocaine. J Clin Anesth 2001;13:128–30.

46. Cooper HA. Methemoglobinemia caused by benzocaine topical spray. South Med J 1997;90:946–48.

47. Townes PL, Geertsma MA, White MR. Benzocaine-induced methemoglobinemia. Am J Dis Child 1977;131:697–98.
48. Tush GM, Kuhn RJ. Methemoglobinemia induced by an over-the-counter medication. Ann Pharmacother 1996;30:1251–53.
49. Bodily MN, Carpenter RL, Ownes BD. Lidocaine 0.5% spinal anaesthesia: a hypobaric solution for short-stay perirectal surgery. Can J Anaesth 1992;39:770–73.
50. Schneider M, Ettlin T, Kaufmann M, et al. Transient neurologic toxicity after hyperbaric subarachnoid anesthesia with 5% lidocaine. Anesth Analg 1993;76:1154–57.
51. Freedman JM, Li DK, Drasner K, et al. Transient neurologic symptoms after spinal anesthesia. Anesthesiology 1998;89:633–41.
52. Hampl KF, Schneider MC, Ummenhofer W, et al. Transient neurologic symptoms after spinal anesthesia. Anesth Analg 1995;81:1148–53.
53. Pollock JE, Neal JM, Stephenson CA. Prospective study of the incidence of transient radicular irritation in patients undergoing spinal anesthesia. Anesthesiology 1996;84:1361–67.
54. Pollock JE, Liu SS, Neal JM. Dilution of spinal lidocaine does not alter the incidence of transient neurologic symptoms. Anesthesiology 1999;90:445–50.
55. Hodgson PS, Neal JM, Pollock JE, et al. The neurotoxicity of drugs given intrathecally (spinal). Anesth Analg 1999;88:797–809.
56. Pawlowski J, Sukhain R, Pappas AL, et al. The anesthetic and recovery profile of two doses (60 and 80 mg) of plain mepivacaine for ambulatory spinal anesthesia. Anesth Analg 2000;91:580–84.
57. Tagariello V, Bertini L. Unusually prolonged duration of spinal anesthesia following 2% mepivacaine. Reg Anesth Pain Med 1998;23:424–26.
58. Liguori GA, Zayas VM, Chisholm MF. Transient neurologic symptoms after spinal anesthesia with mepivacaine and lidocaine. Anesthesiology 1998;88:619–23.
59. Bader AM, Concepcion M, Hurley RJ, et al. Comparison of lidocaine and prilocaine for intravenous regional anesthesia. Anesthesiology 1988;69:409–12.
60. Hampl KF, Heinzmann-Wiedmer S, Luginbuehl I, et al. Transient neurologic symptoms after spinal anesthesia. Anesthesiology 1998;88:629–33.
61. Duncan PG, Kobrinsky N. Prilocaine-induced methemoglobinemia in a newborn infant. Anesthesiology 1983;59:75–76.
62. Klos CP, Hays GL. Prilocaine-induced methemoglobinemia in a child with Shwachman syndrome. J Oral Maxillofac Surg 1985;43:621–23.
63. Frayling IM, Addison GM, Chattergee K, et al. Methaemoglobinemia in children treated with prilocaine-lignocaine cream. Br Med J 1990;301:153–54.
64. Mandel S. Methemoglobinemia following neonatal circumcision. JAMA 1989;261:702.
65. Gentili M, Senlis H, Houssel P, et al. Single-shot spinal anesthesia with small doses of bupivacaine. Reg Anesth 1997;22:511–14.
66. Ben-David B, Levin H, Solomon E, et al. Spinal bupivacaine in ambulatory surgery: the effect of saline dilution. Anesth Analg 1996;83:716–20.
67. Kuusniemi KS, Pihlajamaki KK, Pitkanen MT, et al. A low-dose hypobaric spinal anesthesia for knee arthoscopies. Reg Anesth 1997;22:534–38.
68. Casat A, Fanelli G, Cappelleri G, et al. Low dose hyperbaric bupivacaine for unilateral spinal anesthesia. Can J Anaesth 1998;45:850–54.
69. Kuusniemi KS, Pihlajamaki KK, Pitkanen MT. A low dose of plain or hyperbaric bupivacaine for unilateral spinal anesthesia. Reg Anesth Pain Med 2000;25:605–10.
70. Zaric D, Axelsson K, Nydahl P-A, Phillipsson L, Larsson P, Jansson JR. Sensory and motor blockade during epidural analgesia with 1%, 0.75%, and 0.5% ropivacaine-a double blind study. Anesth Analg 1991;72:509–15.
71. Feldman HS, Arthur GR, Pitkanen M, Hurley R, Doucette AM, Covino BG. Treatment of acute systemic toxicity after the rapid in-

72. Dony P, Dewinde V, Vanderick B, Cuignet O, Gautier P, Legrand E, Lavand'homme P, De Kock M. The comparative toxicity of ropivacaine and bupivacaine at equipotent doses in rats. Anesth Analg 2000;91:1489–92.
73. Knudsen K, Beckman Suurkula M, Blomberg S, Sjovall J, Edvardsson N. Central nervous and cardiovascular effects of i.v. infusions of ropivacaine, bupivacaine and placebo in volunteers. Br J Anaesth 1997;78:507–14.
74. Wildsmith JAW. Peripheral nerve block and ropivacaine. Am J Anesthesiol 1997;24:14–17.
75. Kehlet H. Ropivacaine for postoperative pain relief and incisional anesthesia/analgesia. Am J Anesthesiol 1997;24:26–30.
76. Concepcion M, Arthur GR, Steele SM, Bader AM, Covino BG. A new local anesthetic, ropivacaine: its epidural effect in humans. Anesth Analg 1990;70:80–85.
77. SenArd M, Joris JL, Ledoux D, Toussaint JP, Lahaya-Goffart B, Lamy ML. A comparison of 0.1% and 0.2% ropivacaine and bupivacaine combined with morphine for postoperative patient-controlled epidural analgesia after major abdominal surgery. Anesth Analg 2002;95:444–49.
78. Thong WY, Pajel V, Khalil SN. Inadvertent administration of intravenous ropivacaine in a child. Paediatr Anaesth 2000;10:563–64.
79. Ala-Kokko TI, Lopponen A, Alahuhta S. Two instances of central nervous system toxicity in the same patient following repeated ropivacaine-induced brachial plexus block. Acta Anaesthesiol Scand 2000;44:623–26.
80. Klein SM, Benveniste H. Anxiety, vocalization, and agitation following peripheral nerve block with ropivacaine. Reg Anesth Pain Med 1999;24:175–78.
81. Borgeat A, Ruetsch YA, Jorg M. Convulsions induced by ropivacaine during interscalene plexus block. Anesth Analg 1998;87:497–98.
82. Mardirosoff C, Dumont L. Convulsions after the administration of high dose ropivacaine following an interscalene block. Can J Anaesth 2000;47:1263–65.
83. Kopacz DJ, Carpenter RL, Mackey DC. Effect of ropivacaine on cutaneous capillary blood flow in pigs. Anesthesiology 1989;71:69–74.
84. Ishiyama T, Dohi S, Iida H, et al. The effects of topical and intravenous ropivacaine on canine pial microcirculation. Anesth Analg 1997;85:75–81.
85. Gautier PE, De Kock M, Van Steenberge AV, et al. Intrathecal ropivacaine for ambulatory surgery. Anesthesiology 1999;91:1239–45.
86. De Kock M, Gautier P, Fanard L, et al. Intrathecal ropivacaine and clonidine for ambulatory knee arthroscopy. Anesthesiology 2001;94:574–78.
87. De Jong RH. Ropivacaine. White knight or dark horse? Reg Anesth 1995;20:474–81.
88. Nau C, Strichartz GR. Drug chirality in anesthesia. Anesthesiology 2002;97:497–502.
89. Morrison SG, Dominguez JJ, Frascarolo P, Reiz S. A comparison of the electrocardiographic cardiotoxic effects of racemic bupivacaine, levobupivacaine, and ropivacaine in anesthetized swine. Anesth Analg 2000;90:1308–14.
90. Chang DH, Ladd LA, Wilson KA, Gelgor L, Mather LE. Tolerability of large-dose intravenous levobupivacaine in sheep. Anesth Analg 2000;91:671–79.
91. Huang HF, Pryor ME, Mather LE, Veering AT. Cardiovascular and central nervous system effects of intravenous levobupivacaine and bupivacaine in sheep. Anesth Analg 1998;86:797–804.
92. Foster RH, Markham A. Levobupivacaine: a review of its pharmacology and use as a local anesthetic. Drugs 2000;59:551–79.
93. Mazoit JX, Decaux A, Bouaziz H, Edouard A. Comparative ventricular electrophysiologic effect of racemic bupivacaine, levobupivacaine, and ropivacaine on the isolated rabbit heart. Anesthesiology 2000;93:784–92.

94. McClellan KJ, Spencer CM. Levobupivacaine. Drugs 1998;56:355–62.

95. Murdoch JAC, Dickson UK, Wilson PA, Berman JS, Gad-Elrab RR, Scott NB. The efficacy and safety of three concentrations of levobupivacaine administered as a continuous epidural infusion in patients undergoing orthopedic surgery. Anesth Analg 2002;94:438–44.

96. Moore JM, Liu SS, Pollock JE, et al. The effect of epinephrine on small-dose hyperbaric spinal anesthesia: clinical implications for ambulatory surgery. Anesth Analg 1998;86:973–77.

97. Chiu AA, Liu SS, Carpenter RL, et al. The effects of epinephrine on lidocaine spinal anesthesia: a cross-over study. Anesth Analg 1995;80:735–39.

98. Sakura S, Sumi M, Sakaguchi Y, et al. The addition of phenylephrine contributes to the development of transient neurological symptoms after spinal anesthesia with 0.5% tetracaine. Anesthesiology 1997;87:771–78.

99. Ikuta PT, Raza SM, Durrani Z, et al. PH adjustment schedule for amide local anesthetics. Reg Anesth 1989;14:229–35.

100. Crose VW. Pain reduction in local anesthetic administration through pH buffering. J Indiana Dent Assoc 1991;70:24–25.

101. Martin AJ. PH-adjustment and discomfort caused by intradermal injection of lignocaine. Anaesthesia 1990;45:975–78.

102. McKay W, Morris R, Mushlin P. Sodium bicarbonate attenuates pain on skin infiltration with lidocaine, with or without epinephrine. Anesth Analg 1987;66:572–74.

103. Xia Y, Chen E, Tibbits DL, et al. Comparison of effects of lidocaine hydrochloride, buffered lidocaine, diphenhydramine, and normal saline after intradermal injection. J Clin Anesth 2002;14:339–43.

104. Copogna G, Celleno D, Tagariello V. The effect of pH adjustment of 2% mepivacaine on epidural anesthesia. Reg Anesth 1989;14:121–23.

105. Curatolo M, Petersen-Felix S, Arendt-Nielsen L, et al. Adding sodium bicarbonate to lidocaine enhances the depth of epidural blockade. Anesth Analg 1998;86:341–47.

106. Gosteli P, Van Gessel E, Gamulin Z. Effects of pH adjustment and carbonation of lidocaine during epidural anesthesia for foot or ankle surgery. Anesth Analg 1995;81:104–9.

107. Benzon HT, Toleikis JR, Dixit P, et al. Onset, intensity of blockade and somatosensory evoked potential changes of the lumbosacral dermatomes after epidural anesthesia with alkalinized lidocaine. Anesth Analg 1993;76:328–32.

108. Tetzlaff JE, Yoon HJ, Walsh M. Regional anaesthetic technique and the incidence of tourniquet pain. Can J Anaesth 1993;40:591–95.

109. Tetzlaff JE, Yoon HJ, O'Hara J, et al. Alkalinization of mepivacaine accelerates the onset of interscalene block for shoulder surgery. Reg Anesth 1990;15:242–44.

110. Cousins MJ, Mather LE. Intrathecal and epidural administration of opioids. Anesthesiology 1984;61:276–310.

111. Stein C, Comisel K, Haimeri E, et al. Analgesic effect of intraarticular morphine after arthroscopic knee surgery. N Engl J Med 1991;325:1123–26.

112. Reuben SS, Reuben JP. Brachial plexus anesthesia with verapamil and/or morphine. Anesth Analg 2000;91:379–83.

113. Martin R, Lamarche Y, Tetrault JP. Epidural and intrathecal narcotics. Can Anaesth Soc J 1983;30:662–73.

114. De Leon-Casasola OA, Lema MJ. Postoperative epidural opioid analgesia: what are the choices? Anesth Analg 1996;83:867–75.

115. Ready LB, Loper KA, Nessly M, et al. Postoperative epidural morphine is safe on surgical wards. Anesthesiology 1991;75:452–56.

116. Tetzlaff JE, Dilger JA, Abate J, Parker RD. Preoperative intraarticular morphine and bupivacaine for pain control after outpatient arthroscopic anterior cruciate ligament reconstruction. Reg Anesth Pain Med 1999;34:220–24.

117. Tetzlaff JE, Brems J, Dilger J. Intraarticular morphine and bupivacaine reduces postoperative pain after rotator cuff repair. Reg Anesth Pain Med 2000;25:611–14.

118. Todd BD, Reed SC. The use of bupivacaine to relieve pain at iliac graft donor sites. Int Orthop 1991;15:53–55.

119. Kamibayashi T, Maze M. Clinical use of alpha-2 adrenergic agonists. Anesthesiology 2000;93:1345–49.

120. Singelyn FJ, Dangoisse M, Bartholomee S, et al. Adding clonidine to mepivacaine prolongs the duration of anesthesia and analgesia after axillary brachial plexus block. Reg Anesth 1992;17:148–50.

121. Singelyn FJ, Gouverneur JM, Robert A. A minimum dose of clonidine added to mepivacaine prolongs the duration of anesthesia and analgesia after axillary brachial plexus block. Anesth Analg 1996;83:1046–50.

122. Lauretti GR, Lima ICPR. The effects of intrathecal neostigmine on somatic and visceral pain: improvement by association with a peripheral anticholinergic. Anesth Analg 1996;82:617–20.

123. Pan PM, Huang CT, Wei TT, et al. Enhancement of analgesic effect of intrathecal neostigmine and clonidine on bupivacaine spinal anesthesia. Reg Anesth Pain Med 1998;23:49–56.

124. Liu SS, Hodgson PS, Moore JM, et al. Dose-response effects of spinal neostigmine added to bupivacaine spinal anesthesia in volunteers. Anesthesiology 1999;90:710–17.

125. Gentili M, Enel D, Szymskiewicz O, et al. Postoperative analgesia by intraarticular clonidine and neostigmine in patients undergoing knee arthroscopy. Reg Anesth Pain Med 2001;26:342–47.

126. Carpenter KJ, Dickenson AH. NMDA receptors and pain—hopes for novel analgesics. Reg Anesth Pain Med 1999;24:506–8.

127. Arendt-Nielsen L, Petersen-Felix S, Fischer M, et al. The effect of N-methyl-d-aspartate agonist (ketamine) on single and repeated nociceptive stimuli: a placebo controlled experimental human study. Anesth Analg 1995;81:63–68.

128. de Jong RH, Bonin JD. Mixtures of local anesthetics are no more toxic than the parent drugs. Anesthesiology 1981;54:177–81.

129. Galindo A, Wicher T. Mixtures of local anesthetics: bupivacaine-chloroprocaine. Anesth Analg 1980;59:683–85.

130. Kim JM, Goto H, Arakawa K. Duration of bupivacaine intradermal anesthesia when the bupivacaine is mixed with chloroprocaine. Anesth Analg 1979;58:364–66.

131. Bonadio WA. TAC: a review. Ped Emerg Care 1989;5:128–30.

132. Ordog GJ, Ordog C. The efficacy of TAC (tetracaine, adrenaline, and cocaine) with various wound-application durations. Acad Emerg Med 1994;1:360–63.

133. Tipton GA, DeWitt GW, Eisenstein SJ. Topical TAC (tetracaine, adrenaline, cocaine) solution for local anesthesia in children: prescribing inconsistency and acute toxicity. South Med J 1989;82:1344–46.

134. Daya MR, Burton BT, Schleiss MR, et al. Recurrent seizures following mucosal application of TAC. Ann Emerg Med 1988;17:646–48.

135. Daily RH. Fatality secondary to misuse of TAC solution. Ann Emerg Med 1988;17:159–60.

136. Vinci RJ, Fish SS. Efficacy of topical anesthesia in children. Arch Pediatr Adolesc Med 1996;150:466–69.

137. Ernst AA, Crabbe LH, Winsemius DK, Bragdon R, Link R. Comparison of tetracaine, adrenaline and cocaine with cocaine alone for topical anesthesia. Ann Emerg Med 1990;19:51–54.

138. Schilling CG, Bank DE, Borchert BA, Klatzko MD, Uden DL. Tetracaine, epinephrine (adrenaline), and cocaine (TAC) versus lidocaine, epinephrine, and tetracaine (LET) for anesthesia of lacerations in children. Ann Emerg Med 1995;25:203–8.

139. Gajraj NM, Pennant JH, Watcha MF. Eutectic mixture of local anesthetics (EMLA) cream. Anesth Analg 1994;78:574–83.

140. Bingham B, Hawthorne M. The use of anaesthetic EMLA cream in minor otologic surgery. J Laryngol Otol 1988;102:517.

141. Sirimanna KS, Madden GJ, Miles S. Anaesthesia of the tympanic membrane: comparison of EMLA cream and iontophoresis. J Laryngol Otol 1990;104:195–96.

142. Byrne MA. Topical anaesthesia with lidocaine-prilocaine cream for vulval biopsy. Br J Obstet Gynecol 1989;96:497–99.

143. Rylander E, Sjoberg I, Lillieborg S, et al. Local anesthesia of the genital mucosa with lidocaine/prilocaine cream (EMLA) for laser treatment of condyloma acuminata: a placebo-controlled study. Obstet Gynecol 1990;75:302–6.

144. Ljunghall K, Rylander E, Sjoberg I, et al. Topical anaesthesia with lidocaine-prilocaine cream for vulval biopsy. Br J Obstet Gynaecol 1990;97:864–65.

145. MacKinlay GA. Save the prepuce: painless separation of preputial adhesions in the outpatient clinic. Br Med J 1988;297:590–91.

146. Lee JJ, Forrester P. EMLA for postoperative analgesia for day case circumcision in children. Anaesthesia 1992;47:1081–83.

147. McLeod D. EMLA cream for postcircumcision analgesia. Anaesthesia 1993;48:925–26.

148. Abenavoli FM, Corvelli L. Use of anesthetic cream before infiltration with local anesthesia in aesthetic surgery. Aesth Plast Surg 1995;19:555–56.

149. Hunstad JP. Tumescent and syringe liposculpture: a logical partnership. Aesth Plast Surg 1995;19:321–23.

150. Cohn MS, Seiger E, Goldman S. Ambulatory phlebectomy using tumescent technique for local anesthesia. Dermatol Surg 1995;21:315–18.

151. Klein JA. Tumescent technique for regional anesthesia permits lidocaine doses of 35 mg/kg for liposuction. J Dermatol Surg Oncol 1990;16:248–63.

152. Klein JA. Anesthesia for liposuction in dermatologic surgery. J Dermatol Surg Oncol 1988;14:1124–32.

153. Klein JA, Kassarjdian N. Lidocaine toxicity with tumescent liposuction. Dermatol Surg 1997;23:1169–74.

154. Klein JA, Kassarjdian N. Lidocaine toxicity with tumescent liposuction. A case report of probable drug interactions. Dermatol Surg 1997;23:1169–74.

155. Gilliland MD, Coates N. Tumescent liposuction complicated by pulmonary edema. Plastic Reconstr Surg 1997;99:215–19.

156. Weiker GG, Kuivila TE, Pippinger CE. Serum lidocaine and bupivacaine levels in local technique arthroscopy. Am J Sports Med 1991;19:499–502.

157. Sullivan SG, Abbott PJ. Cardiovascular toxicity associated with intraarticular bupivacaine. Anesth Analg 1994;79:591–593.

158. Dunlop DJ, Graham CM, Waldram MA. The use of Bier's block for day case surgery. J Hand Surg (Brit) 1995;20:679–80.

159. Liu SS. Optimizing spinal anesthesia for ambulatory surgery. Reg Anesth 1997;22:500–10.

160. Mulroy MF, Wills RP. Spinal anesthesia for outpatients: appropriate agents and techniques. J Clin Anesth 1995;7:622–27.

161. Buckenmaier CC, Nielsen KC, Pietrobon R, et al. Small-dose intrathecal lidocaine versus ropivacaine for anorectal surgery in an ambulatory setting. Anesth Analg 2002;95:1253–57.

162. Kuusniemi KS, Pihlajamaki KK, Pitkanen MT, et al. A low-dose hypobaric spinal bupivacaine anesthesia for knee arthroscopies. Reg Anesth 1997;22:534–38.

163. Gentili M, Senlis H, Houssel P, et al. Single-shot spinal anesthesia with small doses of bupivacaine. Reg Anesth 1997;22:511–14.

164. Nielsen KC, Greengrass RA, Pietrobon R, et al. Continuous interscalene brachial plexus blockade provides good analgesia at home after major shoulder surgery- report of four cases. Can J Anaesth 2003;50:57–61.

165. Grant SA, Nielsen KC, Greengrass RA, et al. Continuous peripheral nerve block for ambulatory surgery. Reg Anesth Pain Med 2001;26:209–14.

166. Rawal N, Allvin R, Axelsson K, et al. Patient-controlled regional analgesia (PCRA) at home. Anesthesiology 2002;96:1290–96.

167. Rawal N, Axelsson K, Hylander J, et al. Postoperative patient-controlled local anesthetic administration at home. Anesth Analg 1998;86:86–89.

168. Vintar N, Pozlep G, Rawal N, et al. Incisional self-administration of bupivacaine or ropivacaine provides effective analgesia after inguinal hernia repair. Can J Anaesth 2002;49:481–86.

Local Anesthetic Toxicity in the Ambulatory Setting

ÉTIENNE DE MÉDICIS • OSCAR A. DE LEON-CASASOLA

INTRODUCTION

The use of regional anesthesia techniques has been associated with a reduced mortality rate,[1] as well as a decreased incidence of deep vein thrombosis, pulmonary embolism, transfusion requirements, pneumonia, respiratory depression, myocardial infarction, and renal failure. In addition, the ability of regional anesthesia to block the stress response leads to reduced perioperative opiate use, nausea, vomiting, and ileus.[2] The recent advances in the new local anesthetic drugs and regional anesthesia equipment partly explain why regional anesthetic procedures have increased more than 10-fold in the past 20 years.[3]

Serious complications related to regional anesthesia procedures are very rare with an incidence of 3.5 per 10,000 procedures.[4,5] They can range from systemic local anesthetic toxicity, radiculopathy, cauda equina syndrome, and paraplegia to death. Less severe complications are the transient neurologic symptoms (TNS), initially described in 1993.[6] The objective of this review is to describe the cardiac toxicity and neurotoxicity of local anesthetics with special emphasis on the clinical differences between the newer drugs. Moreover, we will review their use in the ambulatory setting.

LOCAL ANESTHETIC CARDIAC TOXICITY

Bupivacaine

Bupivacaine is a long-acting amide local anesthetic commonly used for infiltration, nerve block, spinal and/or epidural anesthesia, or analgesia. It has a butyl side chain and is a racemic mixture of two enantiomers: R(+) and S(−).[7] The safety of bupivacaine in the perioperative setting is well documented,[8–10] although accidental intravenous injections have been associated with cardiac arrest and death.[11,12] Since the approval for epidural administration of 0.75% bupivacaine has been withdrawn, there has been a reported decrease in maternal death secondary from local anesthetic toxicity.[13]

Bupivacaine binds rapidly to sodium channel, yet unbinds slowly, thus potentially blocking a high fraction of these channels.[14] Blockage of the sodium channels in the myocardium leads to conduction blockade (increased PR and QRS intervals).[15] This phenomenon probably explains its dose-dependent cardiotoxicity. Bupivacaine blocks potassium and calcium channels at higher concentrations, leading to decreased inotropy, conduction block, and pulseless electrical activity.[16–19] Beyond the concentration needed for cardiac arrest, there is RyR2-calcium channel and beta-2 adrenergic blockade as well as mitochondrial metabolism inhibition explaining the difficulty in resuscitating patients with bupivacaine-induced cardiac toxicity.[20–23]

Lidocaine

The decreased cardiotoxity of lidocaine compared to bupivacaine is well established,[24–32] but its shorter duration of action may limit its clinical use. This has stimulated research into long-acting local anesthetics with less cardiotoxicity than bupivacaine. Through chirality[7] (the property of a carbon atom bounded by four different atoms or group of atoms leading to the potential of a molecule with a chiral carbon to exist in two different three-dimensional mirror-imaged configurations), it was discovered that the S(−) enantiomer of amide local anesthetic is less cardiotoxic; hence, the S(−) enantiomer of bupivacaine (levobupivacaine) and the S(−) enantiomer of an amide local anesthetic with a propyl side chain (ropivacaine), a side chain length intermediate between those of mepivacaine and bupivacaine, were developed.

Ropivacaine

The physicochemical properties of ropivacaine are essentially the same as those of bupivacaine except for lipid solubility (Table 20-1). This difference in lipid solubility im-

Table 20-1   Physicochemical Properties of Bupivacaine and Ropivacaine

	Bupivacaine	Ropivacaine
pKa	8.2	8.2
Octanol/buffer coefficient	346	115
Protein binding (%)	96	94

plies that bupivacaine is a more potent drug than ropivacaine, explaining, at least partially, why it is more cardiotoxic: the more lipid-soluble a drug is, the more likely it is to enter the cell and block the sodium channel.

Several studies have been performed comparing the cardiotoxic properties of lidocaine, bupivacaine, and ropivacaine.[33–38] All have shown reduced cardiotoxicity of ropivacaine compared to bupivacaine. For example, in a model of intracoronary local anesthetic injection in ventilated pigs, it was found that ropivacaine was about 50% less cardiotoxic.[36] In that model, arrhythmogenecity was determined at a dosage of 2:4.5:30 mg for bupivacaine, ropivacaine, and lidocaine, respectively. In another model, there were more fatal injections in the animals receiving bupivacaine (5/6) than ropivacaine (1/6) or lidocaine (2/6).[37] In the awake sheep, the ratio of fatal doses was found to be 1:2:9 (3.7:7.3:30.8 mg/kg) for bupivacaine, ropivacaine, and lidocaine, respectively.[38]

Ropivacaine has been extensively studied during single injection peripheral nerve block. In this setting, it appears roughly equipotent to bupivacaine with a slightly shorter duration of action.[39–41] It has been found comparable to bupivacaine for axillary blocks,[41–43] supraclavicular blocks,[44] interscalene blocks,[45] ilioinguinal nerve blocks,[46] lumbar plexus blocks,[47] and femoral/sciatic nerve blocks.[48] Interestingly, ropivacaine has been studied in intravenous regional anesthesia.[49–51] In comparison of equal volumes of lidocaine 0.5% and ropivacaine 0.2%, or ropivacaine 1.2 or 1.8 mg/mL versus lidocaine 3 mg/mL, it was found that there were fewer central nervous system (CNS) disturbances at deflation of the tourniquet and longer residual analgesia with ropivacaine, making it a useful anesthetic for intravenous regional anesthesia in the ambulatory patient.

Levobupivacaine

Levobupivacaine has the same basic physicochemical properties and the same molecular weight as bupivacaine. However, levobupivacaine is supplied differently than bupivacaine. The molar concentration on a weight-per-weight basis of solutions contains 13% more levobupivacaine than bupivacaine. Hence, the potency of levobupivacaine is 0.87 times the potency of bupivacaine as assessed by the minimum analgesic local anesthetic model.[52]

In early investigation, there were fewer arrhythmias with levobupivacaine than bupivacaine in an isolated rabbit heart model.[53] In the anesthetized rat, all animals receiving

R(+) bupivacaine died (12/12) versus only 2/12 in the levobupivacaine group.[54] In a sheep model, the total convulsive drug amount was higher in the levobupivacaine group versus the racemic bupivacaine group (100 mg vs. 75 mg) but levobupivacaine was associated with fewer deleterious arrhythmias at convulsive doses,[55] and a higher intravenous lethal dose of levobupivacaine was found than with racemic bupivacaine (227 mg vs. 156 mg, respectively).[56]

In a human volunteers study, a 10-min intravenous infusion of 40 mg of levobupivacaine was associated with less electroencephalographic CNS depression than a similar infusion of 40 mg of bupivacaine.[57] In another volunteer study, an intravenous infusion of levobupivacaine produced significantly less cardiac depression than a bupivacaine infusion.[58]

In clinical studies, levobupivacaine has shown to have similar local anesthetic characteristics compared to bupivacaine when used for epidural anesthesia[59,60] or for supraclavicular blocks.[61] It has also been showed to be safe for ilioinguinal/iliohypogastric nerve block in children.[62]

Ropivacaine versus Levobupivacaine

Many studies have compared the cardiotoxic potentials of levobupivacaine and ropivacaine.[63–69] A model of intravenous local anesthetics injection in the awake rat showed a dose-dependent increase of the QRS greater for bupivacaine and levobupivacaine than ropivacaine as well as a greater incidence of arrhythmias with bupivacaine and levobupivacaine.[63] In an intracoronary injection model in the anesthetized swine, it was found that higher doses of ropivacaine and levobupivacaine than bupivacaine were necessary to induce a QRS widening.[64] These results were duplicated in an isolated rabbit heart model.[65] In isolated rat ventricular muscle strips, ropivacaine induced less reduction in the muscle contractility than bupivacaine and levobupivacaine (no difference between the latter two).[66]

In a series of local anesthetic infusions in instrumented anesthetized dogs, the incidence of spontaneous or programmed electrical stimulation (PES)-induced ventricular tachycardia and ventricular fibrillation did not differ among the different local anesthetics studied. The incidence of PES-induced extrasystoles was more frequent during bupivacaine and levobupivacaine infusions when compared to similar ropivacaine or lidocaine infusion.[67] The concentrations in μg/mL to obtain a certain value of myocardial depression (based on different indices of myocardial function including left ventricular end diastolic pressure [LVEDP], isovolumic contraction [dP/dt], ejection fraction [EF], and fractional shortening [FS]) are provided in Table 20-2.[68]

It was also found that there was a difference in resuscitability of the dogs after cardiovascular collapse and application of the advanced cardiac life support protocol: 10% of the ropivacaine-infused and 0% of the lidocaine-infused dogs died compared to 50% and 30% for the bupivacaine-infused and the levobupivacaine-infused animals, respectively.[69]

Table 20-2   Effects of Bupivacaine, Levobupivacaine, and Ropivacaine Infusions on Myocardial Function

Local Anesthetic	LVEDP (EC_{50} for 125% base)	dP/dt (EC_{50} for 65% base)	EF (%) (EC_{50} for 65% base)	FS (%) (EC_{50} for 65% base)
Bupivacaine	2.20 (1.15–4.4)	2.30 (1.73–3.05)	3.22 (2.22–4.66)	2.12 (1.47–3.08)
Levobupivacaine	1.65 (0.87–3.13)	2.42 (1.88–3.12)	3.09 (1.44–2.87)	1.26 (0.89–1.79)
Ropivacaine	3.98[a] (2.1–7.54)	4.03[b] (3.13–5.19)	4.25 (2.07–4.19)	2.95[a] (3.06–8.32)

[a]ropivacaine > levobupivacaine $p < 0.05$.

[b]ropivacaine > levobupivacaine, bupivacaine $p < 0.05$.

Data represented are effective concentration for 50% population (EC_{50}) estimates with 95% confidence intervals.

SOURCE: Adapted from Groban L, Deal DD, et al. Does local anesthetic stereoselectivity or structure predict myocardial depression in anesthetized canines? Reg Anesth Pain Med 2002;27(5):460–68.

NEURAL TOXICITY OF LOCAL ANESTHETICS

2-Chloroprocaine

2-Chloroprocaine is an ester local anesthetic, and as such is metabolized by plasma cholinesterase. Its short duration of action makes it an ideal drug for brief procedures that can be performed under regional anesthesia and that do not require prolonged analgesia.[70,71] It was introduced in clinical practice in 1952 in a solution of 2-chloroprocaine dissolved in 0.9% sodium chloride (for peripheral nerve blocks) or 10% dextrose (for spinal anesthesia). In 1956, to prolong shelf life, methylparaben 1 mg/mL (as a preservative) and sodium bisulfite 2 mg/mL (as an antioxydant) were added to the solution; the pH of the solution was also lowered. In 1964, methylparaben was removed from the 2% and 3% solutions, which subsequently received an indication for caudal and epidural anesthesia as Nesacaine-CE.

In 1982, several cases of neurologic injuries were reported after accidental intrathecal injection of a large volume (10–20 mL) of 3% 2-chloroprocaine.[72] Investigations[73–75] determined that the low pH as well as the sodium bisulfite were the etiologies of the neurotoxicity. By 1987, the sodium bisulfite had been removed and was replaced by the chelating agent calcium disodium ethylenediamine tetraacetic acid (EDTA) and marketed as Nesacaine-MPF. Soon after, reports of severe back pain after epidural anesthesia emerged. Evaluations suggested that the combination of EDTA plus 2-chloroprocaine was the culprit as it may cause abnormal skeletal muscle contraction.[76] In 1996, all additives were removed from 2% and 3% 2-chloroprocaine solutions. However, there is still methylparaben and EDTA in the 1% and 2% 2-chloroprocaine solutions. Some recent generic 2-chloroprocaine have included sodium metabisulfite and have been associated with neural toxicity.[77]

Lidocaine

Five percent hyperbaric lidocaine was introduced in 1948 for clinical spinal anesthesia. Although it has been used for millions of spinals, it was only in 1991 that concerns about possible neurotoxicity emerged[78,79] with the initial reports of 11 cases of cauda equina syndrome (10 with lidocaine) after continuous spinal anesthesia leading to the removal of the spinal microcatheters from the market. Two years later, the first report of transient radicular irritation (later renamed TNS) after a single dose of 5% hyperbaric lidocaine was published.[6]

TNS is defined as unilateral or bilateral pain in the anterior or posterior thighs +/– extension into the legs +/– back pain. Its onset is 6–36 hr after spinal or epidural anesthesia and typically lasts 1–7 days.[80] An epidemiologic study demonstrated that lidocaine spinal anesthesia, lithotomy position, and ambulatory surgery were important predictors of TNS occurrence,[81] although one study showed no difference in TNS incidence between immediate and late (12 hr) postoperative ambulation.[82] Prospective, randomized, controlled studies[82–98] showed a very low incidence of TNS following nonlidocaine spinal anesthesia, and a TNS incidence varying from around 30% for patients in the lithotomy position and 20% for arthroscopic knee surgery patients to 5% for patients in the supine position with lidocaine spinal anesthesia.

The etiology of TNS is not clear. Laboratory models have proven that all local anesthetics can be neurotoxic.[99–104] Bupivacaine appears to be less neurotoxic than lidocaine or tetracaine. Lidocaine concentrations of less than 1% are not neurotoxic to nerves; hence, such concentrations should not cause TNS if neurotoxicity is the etiology of TNS. A study showed no difference in the incidence of TNS between the three spinal lidocaine groups: 2%, 1%, and 0.5%.[91] Moreover, a study with volunteers showed no abnormal electromyographic findings, nerve conduction studies, or somatosensory-evoked potential abnormalities at day 1 of TNS and at 4–6 weeks later.[105] There is a case report showing nerve root inflammation on magnetic resonance imaging (MRI) testing in a patient with TNS[106] but its significance is not clear as we do not have any controlled prospective studies of serial MRI after spinal and epidural anesthesia.[107] An alternative low-dose lidocaine spinal anesthesia combined with opioids has been proposed,[108] but further studies are needed to evaluate this alternative.[109]

INCIDENCE OF LOCAL ANESTHETIC TOXICITY

Two prospective surveys of regional anesthesia in France have been published recently.[4,5] In the first one, 103,730 procedures were performed using regional anesthetia.

- There were 23 seizures, for an incidence of 2.2/10,000. Four were associated with epidural, 3 with tourniquet release after intravenous regional block, and 16 with peripheral nerve blocks. None progressed to cardiovascular collapse.
- Twenty-four patients developed neurologic injury after spinal anesthesia (40,640) including 19 radiculopathies, and 5 cauda equina syndrome. Ten of the 24 spinal procedures with complications were performed with hyperbaric lidocaine, one of those with a continuous infusion of lidocaine 5%. Half of these patients had pain or paresthesia during drug injection. Hyperbaric lidocaine was used in only 1 of those 12 patients.
- There were 5 radiculopathies associated with epidural anesthesia (30,413) and one paraplegia probably due to spinal cord ischemia secondary to hypotension.
- There were 4 radiculopathies with peripheral nerve blocks (21,278).

In a second survey of 158,083 regional anesthesia procedures published five years later:

- Seven cases of seizure were related to systemic toxicity of local anesthetics and occured after epidural anesthesia (1/5,561) and peripheral nerve blocks (6/44,036). There were no arrhythmias.
- Twelve patients had a peripheral nerve injury (9/35,439) or cauda equina syndrome after spinal anesthesia. Nine patients had no pain on injection (5/9 received lidocaine), all of whom recovered within 3 weeks. In the 3 patients in whom paresthesia occurred during the procedure, neurologic sequelae were still present at 6 months.

There are many case reports of ropivacaine systemic toxicity after epidural anesthesia,[110,111] brachial plexus blocks,[112–116] and sciatic nerve blocks.[117,118] The latter one was associated with ventricular fibrillation that stopped spontaneously. In addition, there is one case report of an accidental intravenous injection of levobupivacaine with no cardiovascular collapse.[119]

AMBULATORY CONTINUOUS PERIPHERAL NERVE BLOCK INFUSIONS

Plexus and peripheral nerve blocks are excellent techniques to provide superb analgesia after limb surgery.[120] With the advance of catheter and pump technologies (both electronic and disposable), it is now possible not only to provide superior analgesia with continuous peripheral nerve blocks[121,122] but also to send patients home with an ambulatory perineural local anesthetic infusion.[123,124] Patients have been sent home with perineural, intra-articular, surgical wounds, and periosseous (e.g., supraperiostal and subalveolar) local anesthetic infusions.[125] There are now studies showing the efficacy and safety of ambulatory continuous interscalene blocks,[126,127] infraclavicular blocks,[128] axillary blocks,[129] sciatic nerve blocks,[130,131] femoral nerve blocks,[132] psoas compartment blocks,[133] and paravertebral blocks.[134]

SUMMARY

Several studies have shown that the use of regional anesthesia techniques is associated not only with improved quality of pain control in the perioperative period, but also better patient recovery. Thus, clinicians are using peripheral nerve catheters and continuous local anesthetic infusions to provide superior postoperative analgesia to patients who underwent surgery in the ambulatory setting. The newer local anesthetics have been shown to be useful in this setting as they provide a wider margin of safety.

REFERENCES

1. Rogers A, Walker N, Schug S, McKee A, Kehlet H, van Zundert A, Sage D, Futter M, Saville G, Clark T, MacMahon S. Reduction of postoperative mortality and morbidity with epidural and spinal anesthesia: results from overviews of randomised trials. Br Med J 2000;321:1–12.
2. Larsson S, Lundberg D. A prospective survey of postoperative nausea and vomiting with special regard to incidence and relations to patient characteristics, anesthetic routines and surgical procedures. Acta Anaesthesiol Scand 1995;39:539–45.
3. Clergue F, Auroy Y, Peguignot F, Jougla E, Lienhart A, Laxenaire MC. French survey of anesthesia in 1996. Anesthesiology 1999;99:1509–20.
4. Auroy Y, Narchi P, Messiah A, Litt Lawrence, Rouvier B, Samii K. Serious complications related to regional anesthesia. Anesthesiology 1997;87:479–86.
5. Auroy Y, Benhamou D, Bargues L, Eccofey C, Falissard B, Mercier F, Bouaziz H, Samii K. Major complications of regional anesthesia in France. Anesthesiology 2002;97:1274–80.
6. Schneider M, Ettlin T, Kauffman M, Schumacher P, Urwyler A, Hampl K, Von Hochstetter A. Transient neurologic toxicity after hyperbaric subarachnoid anesthesia with 5% lidocaine. Anesth Analg 1993;76:1154–57.
7. Nau C, Strichartz GR. Drug chirality in anesthesia. Anesthesiology 2002;97:497–502.
8. Scott DA, Beilby DSN, McClymont C. Postoperative analgesia using epidural infusions of fentanyl with bupivacaine. Anesthesiology 1995;83:727–37.
9. Liu SS, Allen HW, Olsson GL. Patient-controlled epidural analgesia with bupivacaine and fentanyl on hospital wards. Anesthesiology 1998;88:688–95.
10. de Leon-Casasola OA, Parker B, Lema MJ, Harrison P, Massey J. Postoperative epidural bupivacaine-morphine therapy. Anesthesiology 1994;81:368–75.
11. Albright GA. Cardiac arrest following regional anesthesia with etidocaine or bupivacaine. Anesthesiology 1979;51:285–87.

12. Long WB, Rosenblum S, Grady IP. Successful resuscitation of bupivacaine-induced cardiac arrest using cardiopulmonary bypass. Anesth Analg 1989;69:403–6.

13. Hawkins JL, Koonin MN, Palmer SK, Gibbs CP. Anesthesia-related deaths during obstetric delivery in the United States, 1979–1990. Anesthesiology 1997;86:277–84.

14. Clarkson CW, Hondeghem LM. Mechanisms for bupivacaine depression of cardiac conduction: fast block of sodium channels during the action potential with slow recovery from block during diastole. Anesthesiology 1985;62:396–405.

15. Valenzueal C, Snyders DJ, Bennett PB. Stereoselective block of cardiac sodium channels by bupivacaine in guinea pig ventricular myocytes. Circulation 1995;92:3014–24.

16. Valenzueal C, Delpon E, Tamkkun. Stereoselective block of human cardiac potassium channel (Kv1.5) by bupivacaine enantiomers. Biophys J 1995;69:418–27.

17. Coyle DE, Sperelakis N. Bupivacaine and lidocaine blockade of calcium-mediated slow action potentials in guinea pig ventricular muscle. J Pharmacol Exp Ther 1987;242:1001–5.

18. Zapata-Sudo G, Trachez MM, Sudo RT. Is comparative cardiotoxicity of S(−) and R(+) bupivacaine related to enantiomer-selective inhibition of L-type Ca^{2+} channels? Anesth Analg 2001;92:336–42.

19. Groban L, Dolinski SY. Differences in cardiac toxicity among ropivacaine, levobupivacaine, bupivacaine and lidocaine. Tech Reg Anesth Pain Manag 2001;5:48–55.

20. Butterworth JF IV, James RL, Grimes J. Structure-affinity relationships and stereospecificity of several homologous series of local anesthetics for the beta-2 adrenergic receptor. Anesth Analg 1997; 85:336–42.

21. Komai H, Lokuta AJ. Interaction of bupivacaine and tetracaine with sarcoplasmic reticulum Ca^{2+} release channels of skeletal and cardiac muscles. Anesthesiology 1999;90:835–43.

22. Stark F, Malgat M, Dabadie P: Comparison of the effects of bupivacaine and ropivacaine on heart cell mitochondrial bioenergetics. Anesthesiology 1998;88:1340–49.

23. Heavner JE. Cardiac toxicity of local anesthetics in the intact isolated heart model: a review. Reg Anesth Pain Med 2002;27:545–55.

24. Block A, Covino BG. Effect of local anesthetic agents on cardiac conduction and contractility. Reg Anesth Pain Med 1981;6:55–61.

25. Komai H, Rusy BF. Effects of bupivacaine and lidocaine on AV conduction in the isolated rat heart: modification by hyperkalemia. Anesthesiology 1981;3:281–85.

26. Tanz RD, Heskett T, Loehning RW, Fairfax CA. Comparative cardiotoxicity of bupivacaine and lidocaine in the isolated perfused mammalian heart. Anesth Analg 1984;63;549–56.

27. Pitkanen M, Feldman HS, Authur GR, Covino BG. Chronotropic and inotropic effects of ropivacaine, bupivacaine and lidocaine in the spontaneously beating and the electrically isolated, perfused rabbit heart. Reg Anesth Pain Med 1992;17:183–92.

28. Mazoit JX, Orhant EE, Boïco O, Kantelip J-P, Samii K. Myocardial uptake of bupivacaine: I. Pharmacokinetics and pharmacodynamics of lidocaine in the isolated perfused rabbit heart. Anesth Analg 1993;77:469–76.

29. Liu P, Feldman HS, Covino BM. Acute cardiovascular toxicity of intravenous amide local anesthetics in anesthetized ventilated dogs. Anesth Analg 1982;61:317–22.

30. Kotelko DM, Schneider SM, Dailey PA. Bupivacaine-induced cardiac arrhythmias in sheep. Anesthesiology 1984;60:10–18.

31. Chadwick HS. Toxic and resuscitation in lidocaine or bupivacaine-infused cats. Anesthesiology 1985;63:385–90.

32. Buffington CW. The magnitude and duration of direct myocardial depression following intracoronary local anesthetics: a comparison of lidocaine and bupivacaine. Anesthesiology 1989;70:280–87.

33. Dony P, Dewinde V, Vandrick B, et al. The comparative toxicity of ropivacaine and bupivacaine at equipotent doses in rats. Anesth Analg 2000;91:1489–92.

34. Santos AC, Arthur GR, Wlody D, et al. Comparative systemic toxicity of ropivacaine and bupivacaine in nonpregnant and pregnant ewes. Anesthesiology 1995;82:732–40.

35. Feldman HS, Arthur GR, Pitkanen M, et al. Treatment of acute systemic toxicity after rapid intravenous injection of ropivacaine and bupivacaine in the conscious dog. Anesth Analg 1989;69:276–83.

36. Reiz S, Haggmark S, Johansson G, et al. Cardiotoxicity of ropivacaine—a new amide local anaesthetic agent. Acta Anaesthesiol Scand 1989;33:93–98.

37. Feldman HS, Arthur GR, Covino BG. Comparative systemic toxicity of convulsants and supraconvulsants doses of intravenous ropivacaine, bupivacaine and lidocaine in the conscious dog. Anesth Analg 1989;69:794–801.

38. Nancarrow C, Ritten AJ, Runciman WB, Mather LE, Carapetis RJ, McLean CF, HipkinsSF. Myocardial and cerebral drug concentrations and the mechanisms of death after fatal intravenous doses of lidocaine, bupivacaine and ropivacaine in the sheep. Anesth Analg 89;69:276–83.

39. Bertini L, Benedetto BD. Equipotency of ropivacaine and bupivacaine in peripheral nerve block. Reg Anesth Pain Med 2000; 25:659–60.

40. Whiteside J. Regional anesthesia with ropivacaine. Reg Anesth Pain Med 2000;25:659.

41. Bertini L, Tagariello V, Mancini S, et al. 0.75% and 0.5% ropivacaine for axillary brachial block: a clinical comparison with 0.5% bupivacaine. Reg Anesth Pain Med 1999;24:514–18.

42. McGlade DP, Kalpokas MV, Mooney PH, et al. A comparison of 0.5% ropivacaine and 0.5% bupivacaine for axillary brachial plexus anaesthesia. Anaesth Intensive Care 1998;26:515–20.

43. Viho V, Ermo H, Teija, et al. A clinical and pharmacokinetic comparison of ropivacaine and bupivacaine in axillary plexus block. Anesth Analg 1995;81:534–38.

44. Vaghadia H, Chan V, Ganapathy S, et al. A multicentre trial of ropivacaine 7.5 mg/mL vs bupivacaine 5 mg/mL for supraclavicular brachial plexus anesthesia. Can J Anaesth 1999;46:946–51.

45. Klein S, Greengrass RA, Steele S, et al. A comparison of 0.5% bupivacaine and 0.75% ropivacaine for interscalene brachial plexus block. Anesth Analg 1998;87:1316–19.

46. Wulf H, Worthmann F, Behnke H, et al. Pharmacokinetics and pharmacodynamics of ropivacaine 2 mg/mL, 5 mg/mL or 7.5 mg/mL after ilioinguinal blockade for inguinal hernia repair in adults. Anesth Analg 1999;89:1471–74.

47. Greengrass RA, Klein SM, D'Ercole FJ, et al. Lumbar plexus block for knee arthroplasty: comparison of ropivacaine and bupivacaine. Can J Anaesth 1998;45:1094–96.

48. Fanelli G, Casati A, Beccaria P, et al. A double blind comparison of ropivacaine, bupivacaine and mepivacaine during sciatic and femoral nerve blockade. Anesth Analg 1998;87:597–600.

49. Chan VS, Weisbrod MJ, Kaszas Z, Dragomir C. Comparison of ropivacaine and lidocaine for intravenous regional anesthesia in volunteers. Anesthesiology 1999;90:1602–8.

50. Hartmannsgruber MWB, Silverman DG, Halaszinski TM, Bobart V, Brull SJ, Wilkerson C, Loepke A, Atanassoff PG. Comparison of ropivacaine 0.2% and lidocaine 0.5% for intravenous regional anesthesia in volunteers. Anesth Analg 1999;89:727–31.

51. Atanassoff PG, Ocampo CA, Bande MC, Hatmannsgruber MWB, Haszynski TM. Ropivacaine 0.2% and lidocaine 0.5% for intravenous regional anesthesia in outpatient surgery. Anesthesiology 2001;95:627–31.

52. Lyons G, Columb MO, Wilson RC, et al. Epidural pain relief in labour: potencies of levobupivacaine and racemic bupivacaine. Br J Anaesth 1998;81:899–901.

53. Mazoit JX, Noïco O, Samii K. Myocardial uptake of bupivacaine: II. Pharmacokinetics and pharmacodynamics of bupivacaine enantiomers in the isolated perfused rabbit heart. Anesth Analg 1993;77:477–82.

54. Denson DD, Behbahani MM, Gregg RV. Enantiomer-specific effects of an intravenously administered arrhythmogenic dose of bupivacaine on neuron of the nucleus tractus solitarius and the cardiovascular system in the anesthetized rat. Reg Anesth 1992;17:311–16.

55. Huang YF, Pryor ME, Mather LE, Veering BT. Cardiovascular and central nervous system effects of intravenous levobupivacaine and bupivacaine in sheep. Anesth Analg 1998;86:797–804.

56. Chang DH, Ladd LA, Wilson KA, et al. Tolerability of large-dose intravenous levobupivacaine in sheep. Anesth Analg 2000;91:671–79.

57. Van F, Rolan PE, Brennan N, Gennery B. Differential effects of levo- and racemic bupivacaine on the EEG of volunteers. Reg Anesth Pain Med 1998;23(S):35.

58. Bardsley H, Gristwood, Baker H, Watson N, Nimmo W. A comparison of the cardiovascular effects of levobupivacaine and racemic bupivacaine following intravenous administration to healthy volunteers. Br J Clin Pharmacol 1998;46:245–49.

59. Kopacz DJ, Allen HW, Thompson GE. A comparison of epidural levobupivacaine 0.75% with racemic bupivacaine for lower abdominal surgery. Anesth Analg 2000;90:642–48.

60. Cox CR, Faccenda KA, Gilooly C, Bannister J, Scott NB, Morisson LMM. Extradural S(−)-bupivacaine: comparison with racemic (RS)-bupivacaine. Br J Anaesth 1998;80:289–93.

61. Cox CR, Checketts, Mackenzie N, Scott NB, Bannister J. Comparison of S(−)-bupivacaine with racemic (RS)-bupivacaine in supraclavicular brachial plexus block. Br J Anaesth 1998;80:594–98.

62. Gunter JB, Gregg TL, Wittkugel EP, Varughese AM, Berlin RF, Ness D, Overbeck D. Ilioinguinal/iliohypogatric nerve block with levobupivacaine in children. Reg Anesth Pain Med 1998;23(S):54.

63. Ericson AC, Avesson M. Effects of ropivacaine, bupivacaine and S(−)-bupivacaine on the ECG after rapid IV injections to conscious rats. Int Monitor Reg Anaesth 1996;8:51.

64. Morrison SG, Dominguez JJ, Frascarolo P, et al. A comparison of the electrocardiographic cardiotoxic effects of racemic bupivacaine, levobupivacaine and ropivacaine in anesthetized swine. Anesth Analg 2000;90:1308–14.

65. Mazoit JX, Descaux A, Bouaziz H, Edouard A. Comparative ventricular electrophysiologic effect of racemic bupivacaine, levobupivacaine and ropivacaine on the isolated rabbit heart. Anesthesiology 2000;93:784–92.

66. Sudo RT, Trachez MM, Zapata-Sudo G. Comparative cardiac effects of R(+) and S(−) bupivacaine with ropivacaine. Anesthesiology 2000;93:A131.

67. Groban L, Deal DD, Vernon JS, James RL, Butterworth J. Ventricular arrhythmias with or without programmed electrical stimulation after incremental overdosage with lidocaine, bupivacaine, levobupivacaine and ropivacaine. Anesth Analg 2000;91:1103–11.

68. Groban L, Deal DD, et al. Does local anesthetic stereoselectivity or structure predict myocardial depression in anesthetized canines? Reg Anesth Pain Med 2002;27(5):460–68.

69. Groban L, Deal DD, Vernon JC, et al. Resuscitation after incremental overdosage with lidocaine, bupivacaine, levobupivacaine, and ropivacaine in anesthetized dogs. Anest Analg 2001;92:37–43.

70. Mulroy M, Larkin K, Hodgson P. A comparison of spinal, epidural and general anesthesia for outpatient knee arthroscopy. Anesth Analg 2000;91:860–64.

71. Neal J, Deck J, Kopacz D, Lewis M. Hospital discharge after ambulatory knee arthroscopy: a comparison of epidural 2-chloroprocaine versus lidocaine. Reg Anesth Pain Med 2001;26:35–40.

72. Moore DC, Spierdijk J, vanKleef JD, Coleman RL, Love GF. Chloroprocaine neurotoxicity: four additional cases. Anesth Analg 1982;61:155–59.

73. Kalichman MW, Powell HC, Resiner LS, Myers RR. The role of 2-chloroprocaine and sodium bisulfite in rat sciatic nerve edema. J Neuropathol Exp Neurol 1986;45:566–75.

74. Seravalli E, Lear E. Toxicity of chloroprocaine and sodium bisulfite on human neuroblastoma cells. Anesth Analg 1987;66:954–58.

75. Barsa J, Batra M, Fink BR, Sumi SM. A comparative in vivo study of local neurotoxicity of lidocaine, bupivacaine, 2-chloroprocaine, and a mixture of 2-chloroprocaine and bupivacaine. Anesth Analg 1982;61:96–67.

76. Stevens RA, Urmey WF, Urquhart BL, Kao TC. Back pain after epidural anesthesia with chloroprocaine. Anesthesiology 1993;78:492–97.

77. Winnie AP, Nader AM. Santayana's prophecy fulfilled. Reg Anesth Pain Med 2001;26:558–64.

78. Rigler M, Drasner K, Krejcie T, Yelich S, Scholnick F, Defontes J, Bohner D. Cauda equina syndrome after continuous spinal anesthesia. Anesth Analg 1991;72:275–81.

79. Schell R, Brauer F, Cole D, Applegate R. Persistent sacral root deficit after continuous spinal anesthesia. Can J Anaesth 1991;38:908–11.

80. Pollock JE. Transient neurologic symptoms: etiology, risk factors, and management. Reg Anesth Pain Med 2002;27:581–86.

81. Freedman J, Li D, Drasner K, Jaskela M, Larsen B, Wi S. Risk factors for transient neurologic symptoms after spinal anesthesia. Anesthesiology 1998;89:633–41.

82. Lindh A, Andersson AS, Westman L. Is transient lumbar pain after spinal anaesthesia with lidocaine influenced by early mobilisation? Acta Anaesthesiol Scand 2001;45:290–93.

83. Hampl KF, Schneider MC, Thorin D, Ummenhofer W, Drewe J. Hyperosmolarity does not contribute to transient radicular irritation after spinal anesthesia with hyperbaric 5% lidocaine. Reg Anesth Pain Med 1995;20:363–68.

84. Pollock JE, Neal JM, Stephenson CA, Wiley C. Prospective study of the incidence of transient radicular irritation in patients undergoing spinal anesthesia. Anesthesiology 1996;84:1361–67.

85. Hampl KF, Schneider MC, Pargger H, Gut J, Drewe J, Drasner K. A similar incidence of transient neurologic symptoms after spinal anesthesia with 2% and 5% lidocaine. Anesth Analg 1996;83:1051–54.

86. Liguori GA, Zayas VM, Chisholm M. Transient neurologic symptoms after spinal anesthesia with mepivacaine and lidocaine. Anesthesiology 1998;88:619–23.

87. Martiniez-Bourio R, Arzuaga M, Quintana JM, Aguiler L, Aguirre J, Saez-Equilaz J, Arizaga A. Incidence of transient neurologic symptoms after hyperbaric subarachnoid anesthesia with 5% lidocaine and 5% prilocaine. Anesthesiology 1998;88:619–23.

88. Hampl KF, Heinzmann-Wiedmer S, Luginbuehol I, Harms C, Seeberger M, Schneider M, Drasner K. Transient neurologic symptoms after spinal anesthesia. Anesthesiology 1998;88:629–33.

89. Salmela L, Aromma U. Transient radicular irritation after spinal anesthesia induced with hyperbaric solutions of cerebrospinal fluid-diluted lidocaine 50 mg/mL or bupivacaine 4 mg/mL. Acta Anaesthesiol Scand 1998;42:762–65.

90. Hiller A, Karjalainen K, Balk M, Rosenberg P. Transient neurologic symptoms after spinal anesthesia with hyperbaric 5% lidocaine or general anaesthesia. Br J Anaesth 1999;82:575–79.

91. Pollock J, Liu S, Neal J, Stephenson C. Dilution of spinal lidocaine does not alter the incidence of transient neurologic symptoms. Anesthesiology 1999;90:445–49.

92. Hodgson P, Liu S, Batra M, Gras T, Pollock J, Neal J. Procaine compared with lidocaine for incidence of transient neurologic symptoms. Reg Anesth Pain Med 2000;25:218–22.

93. Keld DB, Hein L, Dalgaard M, Krogh L, Rodt SA. The incidence of transient neurologic symptoms after spinal anaesthesia in patients undergoing surgery in the supine position: hyperbaric lidocaine 5% versus hyperbaric bupivacaine 0.5%. Acta Anaesthesiol Scand 2000;44:285–90.

94. Ostgaard G, Hallaraker O, Ulveseth OK, Flaatten H. A randomised study of lidocaine and prilocaine for spinal anaesthesia. Acta Anaesthesiol Scand 2000;44:436–40.

95. DeWeert K, Traksel M, Gielen M, Slappendel R, Weber E, Dirksen R. The incidence of transient neurologic symptoms after spinal anaesthesia with lidocaine compared to prilocaine. Anaesthesia 2000;55:1003–24.

96. Salazar F, Bogdanovitch A, Adalia R, Chabas E, Gomar C. Transient neurologic symptoms after spinal anaesthesia using isobaric 2% mepivacaine and isobaric 2% lidocaine. Acta Anaesthesiol Scand 2001;45:240–45.

97. Philip J, Sharma S, Gottumukkla V, Perez B, Slaymaker E, Wiley J. Transient neurologic symptoms after spinal anesthesia with lidocaine in obstetric patients. Anesth Analg 2001;92:405–9.

98. Aouad M, Siddick S, Jalbout M, Baraka A. Does pregnancy protect against intrathecal lidocaine-induced transient neurologic symptoms? Anesth Analg 2001;92:401–4.

99. Hodgson PS, Neal JM, Pollock JE, Liu SS. The neurotoxicity of drugs given intrathecally (spinal). Anesth Analg 1999;88:7 97–809.

100. Bainton C, Strichartz G. Concentration dependence of lidocaine-induced irreversible conduction loss in frog nerve. Anesthesiology 1994;81:657–67.

101. Kanai T, Katsuki H, Takasake M. Graded, irreversible changes in crayfish giant axon as manifestations of lidocaine neurotoxicity in vitro. Anesth Analg 1998;86:569–73.

102. Lambert L, Lambert D, Strichartz G. Irreversible conduction block in isolated nerve by high concentration of local anesthetics. Anesthesiology 1994;80:1082–93.

103. Johnson ME, Uhl CB, Saenz JA, DaSilva AD. Lidocaine is more neurotoxic than bupivacaine, with a different mechanism of cytoplasmic calcium elevation. Reg Anesth 1998;23:A30.

104. Johnson ME, Uhl CB. Toxic elevation of cytoplasmic calcium by high dose lidocaine in a neuronal cell line. Reg Anesth 1997:A68.

105. Pollock JE, Burkhaed D, Neal JM, Liu SS, Friedman A, Stephenson C, Polissar NL. Spinal nerve function in five volunteers experiencing transient neurologic symptoms after lidocaine subarachnoid anesthesia. Anesth Analg 2000;90:658–65.

106. Avidan A, Gomori M, Davidson E. Nerve root inflammation demonstrated by magnetic resonance imaging in a patient with transient neurologic symptoms after intrathecal injection of lidocaine. Anesthesiology 2002;97:257–58.

107. Aldrete A. Nerve root "irritation" or inflammation diagnosed by magnetic resonance imaging. Anesthesiology 2003;98:1294.

108. Ben-David B, Maryanosky M, Gurevitch A, Lucyk C, Solosko D, Frankel R, Volpin G, DeMeo PJ. A comparison of minidose lidocaine-fentanyl and conventionnal dose lidocaine spinal anesthesia. Anesth Analg 2000;91:865–70.

109. Pollock JE, Mulroy MF, Bent E, Polissar NL. A comparison of two regional anesthetic techniques for outpatient knee arthroscopy. Anesth Analg 2003;97:397–401.

110. Abouleish EL, Elias M, Nelson C. Ropivacaine-induced seizure after extradural anaesthesia. Br J Anaesth 1998;80:843–44.

111. Plowman AN, Bolsin S, Mather LE. Central nervous system toxicity attributable to epidural ropivacaine hydrochloride. Anaesth Intens Care 1998;26:204–6.

112. Korman B, Riley RH. Convulsions induced by ropivacaine during interscalene brachial plexus block. Anesth Analg 1997;85:1128–29.

113. Ala-Kokko TI, Löppönen A, Alahuta S. Two instances of central nervous system toxicity in the same patient following repeated ropivacaine-induced brachial plexus block. Acta Anaesthesiol Scand 2000;44:623–26.

114. Nüller M, Litz RJ, Hübler M, Albrecht DM. Grand mal convulsion and plasma concentrations after intravascular injection of ropivacaine for axillary brachial plexus blockade. Br J Anaesth 2001;87:784–87.

115. Mardirosoff C, Dumont L. Convulsions after the administration of high dose ropivacaine following an interscalene block. Can J Anaesth 2000;47:1263.

116. Raeder JC, Drosdahl S, Klaastad O, et al. Axillary brachial plexus block with ropivacaine 7.5 mg/mL: a comparative study with bupivacaine 5 mg/mL. Acta Anaesthesiol Scand 1999;43:794–98.

117. Rueetsch YA, Fattinger KE, Borgeat A. Ropivacaine-induced convulsions and severe cardiac dysrhythmia after sciatic block. Anesthesiology 1999;90:1784–86.

118. Klein SM, Pierce T, Rubin Y, Nielsen KC, Steele SM. Successful resuscitation after ropivacaine-induced ventricular fibrillation. Anesth Analg 2003;97:901–3.

119. Kopacz DJ, Allen HW. Accidental intravenous levobupivacaine. Anesth Analg 1999;89:1027–29.

120. Klein SM, Nielsen KC, Greengrass RA, Warner DS, Martin A, Steele SM. Ambulatory discharge after long-acting peripheral nerve blockade: 2382 blocks with ropivacaine. Anesth Analg 2002;94:65–70.

121. Liu SS, Salinas FV. Continuous plexus and peripheral nerve blocks for postoperative analgesia. Anesth Analg 2003;96:263–72.

122. Harrop-Griffiths W, Picard J. Continuous regional analgesia: can we afford not to use it? Anaesthesia 2001;56:299–301.

123. Ilfeld BM, Enneking FK. Ambulatory perineural local infusion. Tech Reg Anesth Pain Manag 2003;7:48–54.

124. Klein SM. Beyond the hospital: continuous peripheral nerve blocks at home. Anesthesiology 2002;96:1283–85.

125. Rawal N, Axelsson K, Hylander J, Allvin R, Amilon A, Lidegran G, Hallen J. Postoperative patient-controlled local anesthetic administration at home. Anesth Analg 1998;86:86–89.

126. Klein SM, Grant SA, Greengrass RA, Nielsen KC, Speer KP, White W, Warner DS, Steele SM. Interscalene brachial plexus block with a continuous catheter insertion system and a disposable infusion pump. Anesth Analg 2000;91:1473–78.

127. Ilfeld BM, Morey TE, Wright TW, Chidgey LK, Enneking FK. Continuous interscalene brachial plexus block for postoperative pain control at home: a randomized, double-blinded, placebo-controlled study. Anesth Analg 2003;96:1089–95.

128. Ilfeld BM, Morey TE, Enneking FK. Continuous infraclavicular brachial plexus block for postoperative pain control at home. Anesthesiology 2002;96:1297–304.

129. Rawal N, Allvin R, Axelsson K, Hallen J, Ekback G, Ohlsson T, Amilon A. Patient-controlled regional analgesia (PCRA) at home. Anesthesiology 2002;96:1290–96.

130. Illfeld BM, Morey TE, Wang RD, Ennekin FK. Continuous popliteal sciatic nerve block for postoperative pain control at home. Anesthesiology 2002;97:959–65.

131. Klein SM, Greengrass RA, Grant SA, et al. Ambulatory surgery for multi-ligament knee reconstruction with continuous dual catheter peripheral nerve blockade. Can J Anaesth 2001;48:375–78.

132. Chelley JE, Gebhard R, Coupe K, et al. Local anesthetic delivered via a femoral catheter by patient-controlled analgesia pump for pain relief after an anterior cruciate ligament outpatient procedure. Am J Anesthesiol 2001;28:192–94.

133. Illfeld BM, Morey TE, Enneking FK. Outpatient use of patient-controlled local anesthetic administration via a psoas compartment catheter to improve pain control and patient satisfaction after ACL reconstruction. Anesthesiology 2001;95:A38.

134. Buckenmaier CC II, Kamal A, Rubin Y, et al. Paravertebral block with catheter for breast carcinoma surgery and continuous paravertebral infusion at home. Reg Anesth Pain Med 2002;27:A47.

Analgesic Cyclooxygenase Inhibitors for Ambulatory Anesthesia

MARK DERSHWITZ

INTRODUCTION

History

The medications described in this chapter have in the past been termed "nonopioid analgesics" or "nonsteroidal antiinflammatory drugs." Since recent work can now ascribe inhibition of the enzyme cyclooxygenase (COX) to each of these medications, the term "COX inhibitor" is now preferred and will be used here.

COX inhibitors had been used as analgesics and antipyretics for many decades before the discovery that most of them inhibited COX and therefore the synthesis of prostaglandins. Sir John Vane shared the 1982 Nobel Prize for his work a decade earlier in which inhibition of COX by aspirin explained its pharmacologic effects.

In the early 1990s, two isozymes of COX were described and were named COX-1 and COX-2. COX-1 was described as a constitutive enzyme responsible for such physiologic roles as platelet adhesiveness and protection of the gastrointestinal (GI) tract against damage from acid. COX-2 was portrayed as an inducible enzyme that mediated the synthesis of prostaglandins that participated in the inflammatory response. When selective inhibitors of COX-2 were synthesized a few years later, it was thought that they would be nontoxic analgesic and antiinflammatory agents.

Inhibition of COX-1 or COX-2 could not, however, explain the excellent analgesic and antipyretic effects of acetaminophen, which interestingly has little, if any, antiinflammatory effects. The recent discovery of yet a third isozyme, named COX-3, that is inhibited by acetaminophen may now explain this drug's effectiveness.

Role of Prostaglandins

Figure 21-1 is a simplified pathway of prostaglandin biosynthesis and a brief list of some of the physiologic effects of specific prostaglandins. COX-1 is expressed in most tissues, while the expression of COX-2 may be stimulated by various growth factors, tumor promoters, hormones, bacterial endotoxin, and cytokines.[1] Prostaglandins are among the mediators of the inflammatory response and produce an increased sensitivity of peripheral nociceptors resulting in hyperalgesia. In addition, there is a central hyperalgesic action of prostaglandins at the level of the dorsal horn of the spinal cord.[2] Table 21-1 lists the organ-specific effects of prostaglandins according to which isozyme is responsible for their synthesis. It is clear that there is much overlap in the roles of COX-1 and COX-2 in maintaining normal homeostasis as well as in the response to injury. For example, maximal antinociceptive activity probably requires inhibition of COX-1 and COX-2 (and perhaps COX-3). Similarly, inhibition of either COX-1 or COX-2 may decrease the ability of the GI mucosa to protect itself from acid-mediated damage. Excellent recent reviews of the pathophysiologic roles of COX-1 and COX-2 have been published.[1,2]

Nonselective inhibitors of COX delay bone healing in both humans[3] and rats,[4] a finding of great concern to orthopedic surgeons whose patients often benefit from therapy with these agents. Recent evidence suggests that this potentially adverse effect is not produced by selective inhibitors of COX-2.[5]

COX-1 and COX-2 are coded by genes on different chromosomes. COX-3 is coded by the COX-1 gene but has an additional 30–34 amino acids (depending on species) and a very different pattern of inhibition. In humans, COX-3 is most abundant in cerebral cortex and heart. Its role in the heart is unknown.[6]

It is controversial whether a preemptive effect exists for giving a COX inhibitor prior to surgery. Many studies have attempted to measure such a preemptive effect in terms of decreased postoperative pain or decreased postoperative analgesic requirement; however, the results have been mixed.[7] In addition, even if a preemptive effect exists, if

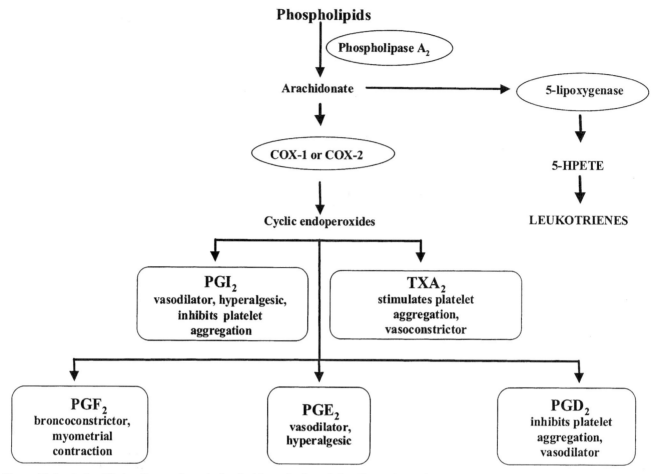

Figure 21-1   A simplified pathway of prostaglandin biosynthesis and the effects of specific prostaglandins. PG, prostaglandin; TX, thromboxane; 5-HPETE, 5-hydroperoxyeicosatetraenoic acid. (Reprinted with permission from Parente L, Perretti M. Advances in the pathophysiology of constitutive and inducible cyclooxygenases: two enzymes in the spotlight. Biochem Pharmacol 2003;65:153.)

the medication causing the effect inhibits COX-1, the potential increase in perioperative bleeding due to platelet inhibition must be factored into the decision of whether to give the drug preoperatively. This concern does not apply to the selective COX-2 inhibitors.

Pattern of COX Inhibition

The older and supposedly nonselective COX inhibitors are typified by medications such as aspirin and ibuprofen. While ibuprofen is a good inhibitor of all three COX isozymes, aspirin has inhibitory selectivity for COX-1 and COX-3 and is not an inhibitor of COX-2 at therapeutic concentrations. The newer and seemingly selective COX inhibitors, such as rofecoxib and valdecoxib, have great specificity for inhibiting COX-2 but not COX-1, defined primarily on the basis of their lack of ability to inhibit platelet thromboxane synthesis. Whether these agents inhibit COX-3 remains unknown. Acetaminophen does not inhibit COX-1 or COX-2 at therapeutic concentrations but does have inhibitory activity against COX-3. This new observation may explain why acetaminophen is an excellent

analgesic and antipyretic but a very poor antiinflammatory agent.[6]

COX Inhibitors as Analgesics

Comparing the analgesia produced by COX inhibitors to that produced by the opioids is difficult for several reasons. First, there is no ceiling effect with opioids. An adequate dose, individually titrated for a particular patient, will relieve virtually any pain, albeit at the cost of ventilatory depression and sedation. In contrast, COX inhibitors readily reach their ceiling effect in patients with severe pain. Second, since opioids have no intrinsic antiinflammatory effects, COX inhibitors work particularly well when the source of the pain has an inflammatory component. Third, in contrast to opioids, COX inhibitors do not decrease the intraoperative requirement for volatile anesthetics (i.e., there is no "MAC-sparing" effect, which is a reduction in the amount of volatile agent required to suppress somatic or hemodynamic reactions to noxious stimulation); however, they do decrease the postoperative requirements for opioids when given concomitantly (i.e.,

Table 21-1   Involvement of COX-1 and COX-2 in Various Physiologic Processes

COX-1	COX-2
Inflammation	*Inflammation*
	Resolution of inflammation
Nociception	Nociception
GI mucosal integrity	GI mucosal integrity
	GI adaptive cytoprotection
	Renal sodium balance
Glomerular filtration rate	
	Kidney development
Angiogenesis	*Angiogenesis*
Platelet TXA$_2$ synthesis	
Endothelial PGI$_2$ synthesis	Endothelial PGI$_2$ synthesis
	Protection against myocardial ischemic damage

Italic type indicates a major role in the function, standard type indicates a minor role.

Source: Adapted from Parente L, Perretti M. Advances in the pathophysiology of constitutive and inducible cyclooxygenases: two enzymes in the spotlight. Biochem Pharmacol 2003;65:153.

there is an opioid-sparing effect). Therefore, it is difficult to compare potencies of opioids and COX inhibitors; in most cases the COX inhibitor should be titrated to the usual ceiling dose or the maximum dose tolerated by the patient (that is often lower than the usual ceiling dose). If the patient still has inadequate analgesia, an opioid should be added to the regimen.

There may be a theoretical advantage to combining acetaminophen with another COX inhibitor in therapy, although definitive studies demonstrating this utility are still lacking. A higher ceiling effect of the combination may be achievable without an increase in overall toxicity.[8]

NONSELECTIVE COX INHIBITORS

Aspirin

The structures of the medications described in this chapter are shown in Figure 21-2. Aspirin is the prototypical COX inhibitor (see Table 21-2); however, its mechanism of inhibition is unique among the medications in this class. It inhibits COX-1 and COX-3 but not COX-2. Aspirin reacts covalently with COX, resulting in permanent inhibition of the enzyme. Its analgesic, antiinflammatory, and antipyretic effects are no longer in duration than those of ibuprofen, suggesting that new synthesis of COX molecules in most tissues occurs rapidly. Platelets, however, do not carry out protein synthesis and thus aspirin essentially

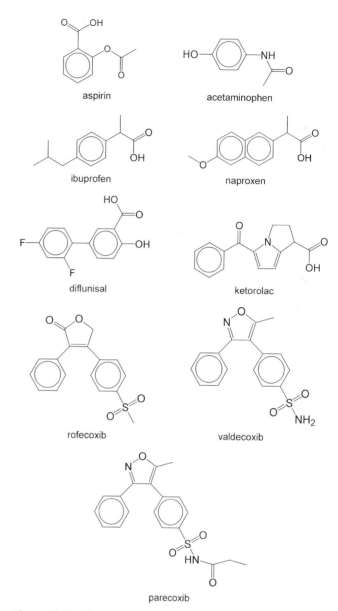

Figure 21-2   The structures of the medications discussed in this chapter. The counter ion for each medication (e.g., ketorolac tromethamine) is not shown.

kills platelets, rendering them unable to become sticky. Thus a single dose of aspirin will result in a measurable increase in bleeding time lasting for about a week.

The GI effects of aspirin may be divided into those that occur rapidly versus those that require days to weeks to become manifest. Heartburn, nausea, or vomiting may all occur soon after aspirin ingestion, and the emetic symptoms are due to both central and peripheral actions. Formation of ulcers in the GI tract takes longer to occur and may result in bleeding. Such bleeding is usually painless, often unnoticed by the patient, but in some cases may be of a magnitude to cause the patient to seek medical attention, especially if the patient is vomiting blood or passing melanotic stools.

At higher doses, aspirin often causes tinnitus. This is reversible upon discontinuation of the drug. Aspirin may also have deleterious effects on renal function; in the presence of

Table 21-2   Probable Maximum Doses and Dosing Intervals for the COX Inhibitors

Drug	Trade Name(s)	Dose	Interval
Aspirin		1200 mg	4 hr
Acetaminophen	Tylenol	1000 mg	4 hr
Ibuprofen	Motrin, Advil, Nuprin	800 mg	6 hr
Naproxen	Naprosyn, Anaprox, Aleve	500 mg	12 hr
Diflunisal	Dolobid	1000 mg	12 hr
Ketorolac	Toradol	30 mg	6 hr
Rofecoxib	Vioxx	50 mg	12 hr[a]
Valdecoxib[b]	Bextra	40 mg	12 hr[b]
Parecoxib[c]	Dynastat	40 mg	12 hr

[a]The package insert states that once-daily dosing is recommended; however, some patients may have better pain relief with two daily doses.

[b]Valdecoxib is not currently labeled for use in postoperative pain and this dose is higher than what is listed in the package insert. The safety of this dose is supported by several studies; in addition, this is essentially the amount of valdecoxib received when the patient is given parecoxib at its maximum recommended dose.

[c]Parecoxib is an investigational drug in the United States at the time of this writing, although it is available in many other countries.

hypovolemia, prostaglandins mediate renal vascular dilation. Thus aspirin decreases sodium excretion and may precipitate acute renal failure in a patient in whom renal perfusion is dependent upon a critical level of prostaglandins.[9]

A hypersensitivity-like reaction to aspirin can occur. Patients at highest risk are those with a history of asthma, nasal polyps, or urticaria. The manifestations may be as minor as rhinorrhea or resemble a full-blown anaphylactic reaction, although the mechanism is not immunologic. One reasonable hypothesis is that when COX is inhibited, in some persons arachidonic acid preferentially is converted to leukotrienes that mediate the observed effects. Persons having such a reaction to one COX inhibitor should avoid all other COX inhibitors except for acetaminophen.

A recent large review examined the studies of aspirin as a postoperative analgesic.[10] The results suggest that doses of 1000 mg or 1200 mg are needed for maximum effectiveness, and that aspirin is approximately equipotent with acetaminophen on a milligram basis. Aspirin has a short duration and usually needs to be given as often as every 4 hr. Aspirin is also available in combination with opioids such as codeine and oxycodone.

Ibuprofen

Ibuprofen is a reversible nonselective inhibitor of COX. Although it is certainly capable of causing GI toxicity, the in-

cidence and severity are less as compared with aspirin. Platelet inhibition is of short duration and platelet function returns to normal after the drug is discontinued.

Ibuprofen is available in the United States without a prescription for tablets containing 200 mg. Larger tablets (400 mg, 600 mg, 800 mg) require a prescription. Most patients with significant pain will require 600 mg or 800 mg given every 6 hr. Ibuprofen is also available in combination with hydrocodone.

Naproxen

Naproxen is similar to ibuprofen except for the fact that it has a longer duration and may be given twice daily. In the United States, tablets containing 200 mg may be obtained without a prescription, while larger tablets (375 mg, 500 mg) require a prescription. Most patients with significant pain will require 500 mg given every 12 hr.

Diflunisal

Diflunisal is similar to naproxen in that it may be given twice daily. Most patients with significant pain will require 1000 mg given every 12 hr.

Ketorolac

The introduction of ketorolac caused a significant change in how anesthesiologists and surgeons managed perioperative pain because for the first time an effective alternative to opioids was available that could be given parenterally. As with many new medications, there was also a period of learning during which ketorolac was given to some patients in too high a dose or for too long a time, resulting in significant toxicity. The present dosing guidelines strike a balance between achieving good analgesia while minimizing (but not eliminating) severe toxicity. Thus, when repeated doses are planned, ketorolac is given as 30-mg doses (intravenously or intramuscularly) as often as every 6 hr. The intramuscular (IM) route has a slower onset with the peak plasma concentration occurring about an hour after the injection as compared with 1–2 min after intravenous (IV) injection. However, the IM route also results in a more prolonged effect, potentially increasing the dosing interval. Ketorolac is also available in tablet form (10 mg), but the maximum recommended daily dose by the oral route is only 40 mg. To minimize severe toxicity, the use of ketorolac by any route should generally not exceed 5 days. The incidence of GI ulcers, even during only 5 days of therapy, is high. In one study in elderly volunteers who were given ketorolac 15 mg every 6 hr, 23% had endoscopically proven gastric or duodenal ulcers at the end of the study compared with none in the placebo group.[11]

Because of its effects on platelet function, ketorolac should generally not be given preoperatively. In considering intraoperative use, the desirability of having analgesia mediated by a COX inhibitor present at the end of surgery has to be balanced against the increased risk of surgical bleeding. Ketorolac delayed bone healing in rats in which experimental fractures were produced.[5]

Ketorolac was the first drug in this class that could reliably substitute for morphine in some subsets of patients with significant postoperative pain. It is difficult to compare potencies of medications that act via completely different mechanisms, but in many prospective blinded studies of postoperative pain, 30 mg of ketorolac was found to be superior to 6 mg morphine and similar to 12 mg morphine in a broad range of surgeries. In addition, in persons requiring opioids for postoperative pain management, the concurrent administration of ketorolac results in a decreased use of opioids by patient-controlled analgesia (PCA) typically by 50%. Interestingly, despite these effects, ketorolac cannot substitute for an opioid in decreasing intraoperative requirements for volatile anesthetics.

SELECTIVE COX-3 INHIBITORS

Acetaminophen

Acetaminophen is very similar to aspirin in terms of its analgesic and antipyretic effects (see Table 21-2). It differs from aspirin in that it has little, if any, antiinflammatory activity, and it has no adverse effects referable to inhibition of COX-1 or COX-2, such as platelet inhibition, GI ulceration, or renal impairment. It is also the only COX inhibitor that may be given during the third trimester of pregnancy because it is the only one that does not cause premature closure of the ductus arteriosus. Persons who have had hypersensitivity reactions to other COX inhibitors will not react similarly when given acetaminophen.

Acetaminophen may cause fatal hepatic necrosis; however, this effect invariably follows a deliberate overdose. The fatal dose in the average adult is in excess of 10 g taken all at once. The usual dose for postoperative pain is 1000 mg given every 4 hr. The maximum daily dose should probably not exceed 4 g or 5 g; however, even at these highest doses the adverse effects of acetaminophen are generally minor, if they occur at all.

As previously mentioned, acetaminophen and another COX inhibitor given concomitantly may produce superior analgesia to either medication given alone. Acetaminophen is also available in combination with opioids such as codeine, oxycodone, and hydrocodone.

SELECTIVE COX-2 INHIBITORS

Rofecoxib (See Table 21-2)

Celecoxib was the first selective COX-2 inhibitor that was marketed. Its absorption from the GI tract is slow and the time to the peak effect is a few hours. It was therefore marketed for the management of arthritis but not for acute pain. Rofecoxib was the second selective COX-2 inhibitor to be marketed. After oral administration, the onset of analgesia is within 30–45 min.

The overall long-term safety of rofecoxib has been compared with that of naproxen.[12] In more than 8000 patients treated for rheumatoid arthritis and followed for 9 months, the incidence of GI ulceration, perforation, or bleeding was measured. The incidence in the rofecoxib group was about half that in the naproxen group, yet the incidence in the rofecoxib group was still substantial (2.1 events per 100 patient-years). In addition, the same study showed that the rofecoxib group had more than twice as many thrombotic events and more than twice as many myocardial infarctions. These results demonstrate that selective inhibition of COX-2 decreases the concentrations of prostaglandins that are beneficial to the GI tract and the cardiovascular system (as suggested in Table 21-1). Because the duration of this study was long, these results cannot be used to predict the safety of rofecoxib in comparison to nonselective COX inhibitors when these drugs are used for the very short term (e.g., a day or a few days) management of postoperative surgical pain.

Rofecoxib has no effect on platelet function and does not increase surgical bleeding. Like the nonselective COX inhibitors, rofecoxib decreases sodium excretion and may cause acute renal failure in the hypovolemic patient.

Rofecoxib has been evaluated in many studies involving postoperative pain. In some studies it was given preoperatively in an attempt to demonstrate a preemptive effect; the results from these studies are mixed with some showing a decreased postoperative analgesic requirement and others showing no difference. What is unequivocal is that rofecoxib is an excellent perioperative analgesic. The optimum dose appears to be 50 mg; however, higher doses have not been studied in detail. In addition, no study has compared once-daily with twice-daily dosing; based on the numbers of patients who have needed supplemental analgesia is these studies, some patients may benefit from a second dose given 12 hr after the first. None of these individual studies has included enough patients to permit quantitation of the possible increased risk of cardiovascular events as described above.

Valdecoxib

Valdecoxib was the third selective COX-2 inhibitor to be marketed. As such, the experience with valdecoxib is about 3 years less than with rofecoxib. Valdecoxib is the active metabolite of parecoxib, the first parenteral selective COX-2 inhibitor (see below).

In a study that utilized typical postoperative analgesic doses, valdecoxib (40 mg twice daily) was compared with ibuprofen (800 mg four times daily) and placebo each given for a week, in terms of their effects on platelet function in elderly volunteers. Valdecoxib was indistinguishable from placebo, while ibuprofen decreased platelet aggregation and increased bleeding time.[13] Valdecoxib, like rofecoxib, decreases sodium excretion and may cause acute renal failure in the hypovolemic patient.

Since valdecoxib is a sulfonamide derivative, some persons allergic to the chemically similar antibacterial sulfonamides or to the sulfonamide diuretics may exhibit cross-sensitivity to valdecoxib. Toxic epidermal necrolysis has occurred in patients given valdecoxib who were also allergic to sulfonamides.

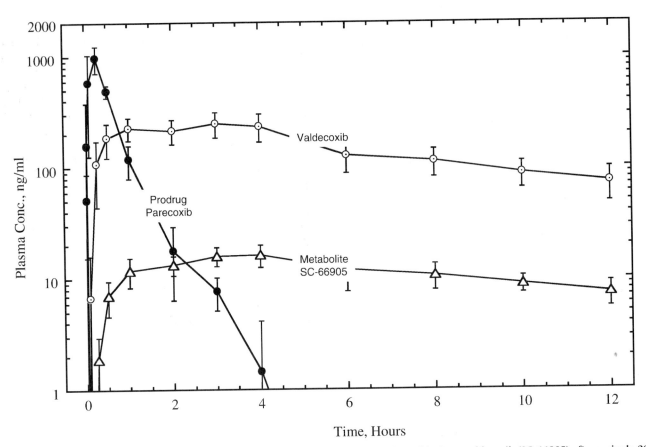

Figure 21-3   The time course of the plasma concentrations of parecoxib, valdecoxib, and hydroxyvaldecoxib (SC-66905) after a single 20-mg IM injection in normal volunteers. (Reprinted with permission from Karim A, Laurent A, Slater ME, et al. A pharmacokinetic study of intramuscular (IM) parecoxib sodium in normal subjects. J Clin Pharmacol 2001;41:1111.)

The current labeling for valdecoxib lists treatment of osteoarthritis and dysmenorrhea as its indications. The recommended doses for these indications are too low for the management of postoperative pain. Valdecoxib has been evaluated in numerous studies involving patients having outpatient dental, orthopedic, and gynecologic procedures. The recommended dose is 40 mg given every 12 hr. The indication for postoperative pain, recommending the aforementioned dose, is likely to be added to the medication's labeling in the future.

Parecoxib

Parecoxib is the first selective COX-2 inhibitor that is given parenterally. It is available in numerous countries, but at the time of this writing remains an investigational drug in the United States. This medication, like ketorolac before it, is likely to significantly change the perioperative pain management of patients. After IV or IM injection, parecoxib is rapidly and completely converted to valdecoxib. In addition, an oxidative metabolite of valdecoxib, resulting from hydroxylation of the methyl group on the isoxazoline ring, is active, although less so than valdecoxib. Figure 21-3 depicts the time course of the plasma concentrations of parecoxib, valdecoxib, and hydroxyvaldecoxib after the IM injection of a 20-mg dose.

In a study that utilized the typical postoperative analgesic dose of parecoxib but a low dose of ketorolac, parecoxib (40 mg twice daily for 7 days) was compared with ketorolac (15 mg four times daily for 5 days) and placebo in terms of their abilities to produce GI ulcers in elderly volunteers. As described previously, 23% of the persons given ketorolac had endoscopically proven gastric or duodenal ulcers at the end of the study compared with none in the parecoxib or placebo groups.[11] In contrast to ketorolac, parecoxib did not delay bone healing in rats in which experimental fractures were produced.[5]

Parecoxib has been evaluated in numerous studies involving patients having outpatient dental, orthopedic, and gynecologic procedures. The recommended dose is 40 mg given every 12 hr. Increasing the dose to 80 mg does not increase analgesic efficacy. Like rofecoxib, results from studies attempting to demonstrate a preemptive effect have been mixed.

COX INHIBITORS FOR PERIOPERATIVE ANALGESIA

In deciding which COX inhibitor to use as a perioperative analgesic, probably the most important question to consider is whether the nature of the patient's surgery contraindicates use of a nonselective COX inhibitor that impairs platelet function. This is a decision that should usually be made in consultation with the surgeon. The older COX inhibitors are generally available as relatively inexpensive generic products. If use of a nonselective COX inhibitor is planned, it is usually first given in the postanesthesia care unit when the patient is able to tolerate oral intake (or, in the case of ketorolac, given late in the case when the risk of increased bleeding is minimal). Acetaminophen may be safely given preoperatively, although its short duration of action may render it beneficial preoperatively only for very short cases.

The choice among the nonselective COX inhibitors is then usually made on the basis of kinetics. Aspirin is only rarely used today in outpatient surgery because of its long-lasting platelet effects. Naproxen and diflunisal have the advantage over ibuprofen of a substantially longer duration of action, at the cost of a slightly slower onset of action. Again, consider adding acetaminophen to the regimen if maximizing efficacy to avoid an opioid is a goal.

The selective COX-2 inhibitors rofecoxib and valdecoxib are much more expensive than their older counterparts; the eventual price of parecoxib in the United States is unknown but will certainly be higher than that of generic ketorolac. The total costs of using the nonselective versus the selective COX-2 inhibitors remain unknown; although rare events, a single patient having a postoperative GI bleed or a wound hematoma that may be due to the use of a nonselective COX inhibitor will add thousands of dollars to that patient's surgical cost and skew the average cost for the group. Similarly, if the use of nonselective COX inhibitors increases the incidence of nonhealing fractures as compared with selective COX-2 inhibitors, the average cost of managing fractures would be much higher in the group given the nonselective COX inhibitors for analgesia. Thus, large prospective studies with pharmacoeconomic outcome variables are needed to answer this question.

Because all three selective COX-2 inhibitors have long durations of action, there is probably nothing to be lost by giving them preoperatively. There may be no significant preemptive effect; however, there will still be substantial analgesia at the conclusion of surgery. Head-to-head comparisons have not yet been performed, but it is likely that parecoxib will be found to be superior to the other oral medications because oral absorption may be erratic and unreliable in some outpatients owing to their anxiety and increased sympathetic tone. There are no data thus far to suggest that either valdecoxib or rofecoxib has superior analgesic activity or a better overall safety profile. The ultimate choice among the two may depend on cost, factoring in whether rofecoxib may need to be given once or twice daily.

REFERENCES

1. Parente L, Perretti M. Advances in the pathophysiology of constitutive and inducible cyclooxygenases: two enzymes in the spotlight. Biochem Pharmacol 2003;65:153–59.

2. Hinz B, Brune K. Cyclooxygenase-2—10 years later. J Pharmacol Exp Ther 2002;300:367–75.

3. Giannoudis PV, MacDonald DA, Matthews SJ, et al. Nonunion of the femoral diaphysis: the influence of reaming and nonsteroidal antiinflammatory drugs. J Bone Joint Surg Br 2000;82:655–58.

4. Altman RD, Latta LL, Keer R, et al. Effect of nonsteroidal antiinflammatory drugs on fracture healing: a laboratory study in rats. J Orthop Trauma 1995;9:392–400.

5. Gerstenfeld LC, Thiede M, Seibert K. Differential inhibition of fracture healing by non-selective and cyclooxygenase-2 selective nonsteroidal anti-inflammatory drugs. J Orthop Res 2003;21:670–75.

6. Chandrasekharan NV, Dai H, Roos KLT, et al. COX-3, a cyclooxygenase-1 variant inhibited by acetaminophen and other analgesic/antipyretic drugs: cloning, structure, and expression. Proc Natl Acad Sci USA 2002;99:13926–31.

7. Souter AJ, Fredman B, White PF. Controversies in the perioperative use of nonsteroidal antiinflammatory drugs. Anesth Analg 1994;79:1178–90.

8. Hyllested M, Jones S, Pedersen JL, et al. Comparative effect of paracetamol, NSAID's or their combination in postoperative pain management: a qualitative review. Br J Anaesth 2002;88:199–214.

9. Galli G, Panzetta G. Do non-steroidal anti-inflammatory drugs and COX-2 selective inhibitors have different renal effects? J Nephrol 2002;15:480.

10. Edwards JE, Oldman AD, Smith LA, et al. Oral aspirin in postoperative pain: a quantitative systematic review. Pain 1999;81:289–97.

11. Stoltz RR, Harris SI, Kuss ME, et al. Upper GI mucosal effects of parecoxib sodium in healthy elderly subjects. Am J Gastroenterol 2002;97:65–71.

12. Bombardier C, Laine L, Reicin A, et al. Comparison of upper gastrointestinal toxicity of rofecoxib and naproxen in patients with rheumatoid arthritis: VIGOR Study Group. N Engl J Med 2000;343:1520–28.

13. Leese PT, Recker DP, Kent JD. The COX-2 selective inhibitor, valdecoxib, does not impair platelet function in the elderly: results of a randomized controlled trial. J Clin Pharmacol 2003;43:504–13.

14. Karim A, Laurent A, Slater ME, et al. A pharmacokinetic study of intramuscular (IM) parecoxib sodium in normal subjects. J Clin Pharmacol 2001;41: 1111–19.

Monitored Anesthesia Care for Ambulatory Surgery

JASON GREGORY • KATHRYN E. MCGOLDRICK

INTRODUCTION

Monitored anesthesia care (MAC) with intravenous (IV) sedation has become increasingly important in the ambulatory venue for a variety of cogent reasons. Advances in surgical technology have enabled many procedures to be performed through an endoscope rather than a surgical incision, and these procedures that previously required general or major regional anesthesia can now be accomplished with local anesthesia plus sedation. Similarly, technologic advances in the expanding area of diagnostics have created an augmented demand for MAC. In addition, demographic shifts have seen a steady growth in the proportion of geriatric patients with coexisting medical conditions that benefit from minimally invasive surgical and anesthetic techniques. Finally, as patients become more knowledgeable "consumers" they frequently request anesthetic techniques that will obviate the side effects associated with general or neuraxial anesthesia and that will facilitate the most rapid return to their normal activities. MAC nicely dovetails with these exigencies.

DEPTH OF SEDATION: DEFINITIONS

MAC is typically selected for patients who require supervision of vital signs and administration of sedative/anxiolytic drugs to supplement local infiltration or regional anesthesia, or to provide sedation during uncomfortable or unpleasant diagnostic procedures. In everyday clinical practice MAC usually connotes an anesthetic state ranging from conscious sedation to deep sedation. However, it is imperative to appreciate that sedation is a continuum, and it is not always possible to predict how an individual patient will respond to a given dose of drug. Moreover, it is incumbent upon the provider to recognize the characteristics of increasing depth of sedation (Table 22-1). Toward this end, we will briefly summarize the definitions of levels of sedation proffered by the American Society of Anesthesiologists (ASA) after approval by its House of Delegates in 1999.[1]

Minimal sedation or anxiolysis is a drug-induced state during which patients respond normally to verbal commands. Although cognitive function and coordination may be slightly impaired, ventilatory and cardiovascular functions are unaffected.

Moderate sedation, often referred to as "conscious sedation," is a drug-induced depression of consciousness during which patients respond purposefully to verbal commands, either spontaneously or accompanied by light tactile stimulation. Clearly, reflex withdrawal from a painful stimulus is not synonymous with a purposeful response. In this state no interventions are required to maintain a patent airway, and spontaneous respiration is adequate. Similarly, cardiovascular function is typically maintained. Although the concept of conscious sedation had its genesis in the practice of office-based dentistry and oral surgery,[2] the development of newer, short-acting pharmacologic agents and the evolution of noninvasive monitoring techniques acted as accelerants in promoting the adaptation of conscious sedation methods by anesthesiologists and other medical practitioners for both surgical and diagnostic procedures.

Deep sedation describes a drug-induced depression of consciousness during which patients cannot be easily aroused but respond purposefully after repeated or painful stimulation. The ability to independently maintain ventilatory function may be impaired. Although cardiovascular function is usually maintained, patients may require intervention to maintain a patent airway and spontaneous ventilation may require assistance.

General anesthesia is a drug-induced loss of consciousness during which patients are not arousable, even by painful stimulation. Patients frequently require assistance in maintaining a patent airway, and positive-pressure ventilation may be necessary owing to respiratory depression or drug-induced depression of neuromuscular function. Moreover, cardiovascular function may be affected.

Because sedation is a continuum, safety demands that practitioners intending to produce a given level of sedation should be able to rescue patients whose level of sedation

Table 22-1   Patient Responsiveness during Continuum of Depth of Sedation

Anxiolysis	Normal response to verbal stimulation
Moderate sedation ("Conscious sedation")	Purposeful response to verbal or tactile stimulation
Deep sedation	Purposeful response after repeated or painful stimulation
General anesthesia	Unarousable with painful stimulation

becomes deeper than initially intended. Therefore, individuals administering moderate sedation should be able to rescue patients who enter a state of deep sedation, while those administering deep sedation should be able to rescue patients who enter a state of general anesthesia.

GOALS

The major objective of outpatient anesthesia is to provide a balance between patient comfort and patient safety while preventing hemodynamic or respiratory instability, or delay in recovery. Sedation techniques encompass the use of sedatives, hypnotics, analgesics, and subanesthetic concentrations of inhalational anesthetics alone or in combination to supplement local or regional anesthesia. These classes of drugs, when combined, confer three important components of sedation: amnesia, anxiolysis, and analgesia.

MAC is most commonly conducted with IV drugs, alone or in combination, that can quickly foster a range of hypnotic states from anxiolysis to loss of consciousness without significant hemodynamic and respiratory compromise. Although the drugs are primarily administered intraoperatively via the IV route, one or more drugs may also be given as premedication via the oral (PO), transmucosal, intramuscular (IM), or rectal routes. These drugs in combination exert effects that, at the very least, are additive and may ultimately abolish protective reflexes, promote airway obstruction, and cause respiratory depression.

It is essential to appreciate that the technique of sedation is as much an art as a science, and facility is gained best through experience, sensitivity, and proper patient and surgeon selection. MAC is recommended for patients who fear or reject general anesthesia or who are at increased risk owing to age or certain coexisting medical conditions. MAC must be used with caution, however, for extremely anxious, impaired, or uncooperative patients. Similarly, MAC is not a panacea for certain types of medical problems. For example, patients with severe coronary artery disease or certain morbidly obese patients might be managed with a greater degree of control under general anesthesia. In addition, the surgeon must be comfortable operating on an awake patient and must be capable of working gently and with alacrity. The outpatient procedures that lend themselves to management with MAC include arthroscopy, biopsies, blepharoplasty and other types of superficial skin procedures, bronchoscopy, carpal tunnel repair and other types of upper-extremity surgery, cataract extraction as well as retina and vitrectomy surgery, cystoscopy, dilatation and curettage, dental surgery, gastrointestinal endoscopy, in vitro fertilization, insertion of lines and shunts, herniorrhaphy, rhinoplasty, and rhytidectomy. Similarly, many diagnostic cardiologic and radiologic procedures are conducted smoothly and expeditiously under MAC.

DRUG SELECTION: AN OVERVIEW

A broad spectrum of IV drugs have been used during MAC, including barbiturates, benzodiazepines, ketamine, and propofol, as well as opioid and nonopioid analgesics.

Thiopental and Methohexital

The most commonly used barbiturates for MAC are thiopental and methohexital. Although thiopental is the most familiar barbiturate used in general anesthetic practice, it has significant disadvantages in the ambulatory setting. Its fat solubility and large volume of distribution combine to produce a prolonged elimination half-life of 10–12 hr. Moreover, the agent, especially in larger doses, can produce adverse hemodynamic effects and respiratory depression, including apnea. It has also been associated with cough and laryngospasm. Owing to its alkalinity, thiopental may precipitate when given concomitantly with certain other drugs. Lacking analgesic properties, thiopental also has a relatively low therapeutic index. Although inexpensive, the drug does not have a niche in ambulatory surgery, for the aforementioned reasons.

Methohexital is a potent oxybarbiturate with a redistribution half-life and volume of distribution similar to those of thiopental. However, methohexital has a much more rapid clearance and briefer elimination half-life than the thiobarbiturate thiopental, thereby permitting its effective use as a continuous infusion. Recovery is more rapid compared with thiopental, especially with cumulative doses; patients emerge more quickly and have less pronounced drowsiness.[3] However, methohexital is associated with such adverse effects as pain on injection, excitatory movements, hiccups, cough, antianalgesic properties, and nausea and vomiting.[4] It is, nonetheless, cost-effective when compared with propofol.[5]

Ketamine

Ketamine, a phencyclidine derivative that is also a N-methyl-D-aspartate (NMDA) antagonist, produces a dissociative state characterized by catalepsy, catatonia, sedation, hypnosis, amnesia, and analgesia. Its administration, however, has been associated with a troubling incidence of side effects, including psychic disturbances. Delirium, bad dreams, and hallucinations may occur in as many as 30–40% of patients.[6] However, combining a benzodiazepine with ketamine typically attenuates the adverse psychomimetic effects of ketamine.[7] It is important to appreciate that ketamine is metabolized to norketamine, an active metabolite that is 30% as potent as ketamine and, therefore, can produce prolonged effects.[8]

The analgesic properties of ketamine are considerable and are thought to be mediated by noncompetitive antagonism at the NMDA and opioid receptors. Indeed, the analgesic properties of ketamine are discerned at plasma concentrations significantly lower (100–200 ng/mL) than those producing loss of consciousness (5–10 μg/kg/min infusion).[9] Low-dose ketamine has been used adjunctively during propofol sedation to enhance analgesia and to minimize the need for supplemental opioids.[10]

Midazolam

Midazolam, a potent, water-soluble benzodiazepine, produces sedation, amnesia, and anxiolysis. Its redistribution and elimination half-lives are much shorter than those of diazepam, and its metabolites have no significant pharmacologic activity. Midazolam is highly selective for amnesia, with its amnestic dose being one-tenth of the hypnotic dose.[11] Unlike diazepam and propofol, midazolam does not produce pain on injection. Although its clinical significance remains to be determined, the antiplatelet activity of midazolam in human patients should be acknowledged.[12]

Interpatient variability is marked with midazolam, and it is important to appreciate that some patients may be exquisitely sensitive to its pharmacologic effects. Indeed, when midazolam initially was introduced to clinicians, reports soon began to circulate of deaths from unrecognized airway obstruction, apnea, and hypoxia predominantly in older patients with concomitant respiratory or cardiovascular disease. The package insert was appropriately revised to include warnings about the necessity of careful monitoring, ability to manage the airway, and immediate availability of emergency resuscitation equipment. It is imperative to appreciate that midazolam depresses the slope of the carbon dioxide (CO_2) response curve, and attenuates the ventilatory response to hypoxia. Apnea is not uncommonly encountered. The apparent steepness of the dose-response curve seen with midazolam underscores the necessity for meticulous titration and careful monitoring. In geriatric or debilitated patients, elimination is slower and the dose should be adjusted downward. Moreover, effects are synergistic with opioids. Indeed, when midazolam is combined with barbiturates, opioids, or propofol, the dose should be reduced by at least 25% in young, healthy patients. This dose reduction should be much more marked (i.e., 50% or more) initially in elderly and frail individuals.

Typically midazolam is given IV as small, divided boluses of 0.02 mg/kg up to 0.1 mg/kg. Midazolam can also be administered as a titrated infusion during local and regional anesthesia.[13] After an incremental loading dose of 0.025–0.05 mg/kg, an infusion rate of 1–2 μg/kg/min provides adequate sedation for many clinical situations. The specific benzodiazepine receptor antagonist flumazenil may be used to reverse the central effects, including excessive residual somnolence, of benzodiazepines in a dose-

related manner.[14] Although flumazenil may have limited ability to reverse benzodiazepine-induced respiratory depression,[15] it is thought to have efficacy in reversing the benzodiazepine component of apnea associated with administration of midazolam-opioid combinations.[16] Because the half-life of flumazenil is approximately only 1 hr, the potential for resedation exists and has been reported. Therefore, it is incumbent upon clinicians to monitor patients carefully for at least 2 hr after administration of flumazenil.

Etomidate

Etomidate is a water-soluble imidazole compound whose chief advantage is hemodynamic stability. Despite its favorable pharmacokinetic profile, etomidate is seldom used in the ambulatory setting owing to its high incidence of adverse side effects. These include pain on injection, phlebitis, involuntary movements, emergence excitement, potential adrenocortical suppression, and considerable postoperative nausea and vomiting (PONV).

Propofol

There is increasing consensus that propofol, a sedative hypnotic of the alkyl phenol class, has become the drug of choice for induction of day-case anesthesia and the most widely used IV agent for ambulatory anesthesia. Its favorable pharmacokinetic and pharmacodynamic profiles, including its antiemetic properties,[17] make propofol an especially appropriate drug in the ambulatory venue. Propofol can be administered by intermittent boluses or as part of a continuous or target-controlled infusion (TCI) technique.

Propofol has a short context-sensitive half-life and a high plasma clearance that produce a rapid, clear-headed awakening when used as the sole agent even after prolonged continuous infusion. Propofol does, however, cause a dose-dependent reduction in arterial blood pressure and it should be used with caution, if at all, in hypovolemic patients. The respiratory effects of low-dose propofol are moderate. Ketamine has been used to advantage to attenuate propofol-induced hypoventilation and to enhance analgesia.[18] To avoid the unwanted hemodynamic side effects associated with relative overdosage, it is critical to reduce initial doses by approximately 40% in the elderly, even for conscious sedation.[19] In addition, it is important to appreciate that recovery of psychomotor function after propofol sedation is prolonged in geriatric patients.[20]

Pain on injection with propofol occurs very commonly (28% to more than 90% of patients)[21,22] even with the low doses of propofol often used for MAC. The etiology of this pain remains unconfirmed but two causes have been suggested. First, the phenol may cause immediate pain from a local irritant effect on the vein. This recedes when propofol in the aqueous phase is diluted by adding it to fat emulsion.[23] Second, delayed pain (after 10–20 sec) from an indirect action on the endothelium releasing kininogens may trigger painful stimuli in the nerve endings between the intima and the media of the vessel wall.[24] Administering a low dose of lidocaine attenuates the pain associated with propofol injection. Despite conflicting reports, it appears that doses as low as 0.1 mg/kg lidocaine are effective in reducing the incidence of propofol-induced pain on injection,[25] although typically doses of 20 mg are used. Lidocaine may be admixed with propofol or can be given as a pretreatment dose 20 sec before propofol injection. A meta-analysis of this clinical problem involving predominantly adult subjects suggested that the optimum treatment is to administer IV lidocaine 0.5 mg/kg while a tourniquet is applied to the arm for at least 30–120 sec before the injection of propofol.[21] This recommendation, however, is impractical in many respects, especially for the pediatric population. In addition, a recent investigation reported that a 3:1.2 volume admixture of 1% propofol and 2.5% thiopental was a practical and efficacious alternative to propofol-lidocaine admixtures in children.[26] This study did not, however, evaluate hemodynamic effects or the incidence of PONV associated with the propofol-thiopental admixture.

Fentanyl and Its Congeners

Fentanyl

Fentanyl, a phenylpiperidine derivative, is a popularly used opioid for ambulatory anesthesia and MAC that produces analgesia and sedation, but not amnesia. Fentanyl has a rather slow onset (4–5 min), and its time to peak effect may be as long as 10 min. As with all opioids, careful respiratory monitoring is essential. Although peak respiratory effect is at 30 min, respiratory depression comparable with that produced by morphine may last as long as 4 hr. Moreover, shift in the ventilatory response curve to CO_2 and depression of hypoxic ventilatory drive occur with doses too small to depress consciousness. In addition, fentanyl produces vagally mediated bradycardia, emesis, and chest wall rigidity.

Alfentanil and Sufentanil

Alfentanil is one-fifth as potent and its duration of action is approximately one-third that of fentanyl, in un-ionized form at physiologic pH. Alfentanil has a rapid onset (time to peak effect of 1.5 min) and redistribution. Moreover, its low lipid solubility, high protein binding, and small volume of distribution render it available for rapid elimination. For example, after a bolus infusion loading dose of 5–10 μg/kg, onset is typically within 1–2 min, and the effective duration of action is approximately 20 min. Although alfentanil is cumulative only after large doses or prolonged administration, clearance is reduced in the elderly, the obese, and in patients with hepatic disease. Similar to fentanyl, alfentanil produces vagally mediated bradycardia, rigidity involving the chest wall and larynx, and PONV.

Sufentanil, a thiamyl analogue of fentanyl, is extremely potent and has a rather long time (6 min) to peak effect. Sufentanil has a low ability to be titrated, and therefore—

combined with its cost, the potential risks associated with its potency, and its propensity to produce chest wall rigidity—has not attained popularity in the ambulatory setting.

Remifentanil

Remifentanil, the most recently introduced opioid and an ultrashort-acting fentanyl analog, has a truncated onset, resembling that of alfentanil, and a high metabolic clearance. Its most relevant advantage, however, is its brief context-sensitive half-life (approximately 3 min) that is independent of the duration of the infusion. Remifentanil's high lipid solubility and relatively high unbound un-ionized fraction at physiologic pH result in peak effect compartment concentration (C_e) within 1–2 min after bolus administration.[27,28] Likewise, distribution and widespread esterase metabolism of remifentanil allow for early offset and return of spontaneous ventilation.[29] Although remifentanil is unique among the opioids in terms of its metabolism and brief context-sensitive half-life, remifentanil shares the typical opioid-related side effects of bradycardia and potential to produce chest wall rigidity and PONV.

The effects of a wide range of remifentanil doses on loss of consciousness and muscle rigidity have been studied.[30] The results disclosed that the median dose of remifentanil required to achieve loss of consciousness when administered as a continuous infusion over 2 min was 12 μg/kg. None of the patients given a dose of 5 μg/kg or less lost consciousness. In terms of muscle rigidity, the chest wall, abdominal wall, and extremity muscle mobility were assessed. None of the patients receiving < 4 μg/kg developed severe muscle rigidity, but several did develop mild-to-moderate rigidity. In addition, preliminary work assessing the respiratory effects and analgesia of remifentanil bolus administration reported that no muscle rigidity was observed over a bolus dose range of 25–200 μg in volunteers.[31]

Although no work to date has examined the influence of midazolam on remifentanil-induced rigidity, the impact of midazolam on fentanyl-induced rigidity has been studied.[32] With fentanyl doses of 10 μg/kg or less, midazolam (75 μg/kg) prevented rigidity and at fentanyl doses of 15–20 μg/kg midazolam attenuated but did not prevent fentanyl-associated rigidity.

Nuances pertaining to dosing of remifentanil merit discussion. Elderly patients require less remifentanil owing to altered pharmacokinetics and pharmacodynamics that involve a substantial reduction in central compartment volume and clearance, and reduction in effective concentration for 50% population (EC_{50}) and the equilibration between plasma and its effect compartment (k_{eo}).[33] It has also been reported that adjusting pharmacokinetic models to lean body mass improves model performance.[33,34] These results suggest that the dosing of remifentanil should be adjusted to the lean body mass and that geriatric patients require as much as 50–70% dosage reduction.

Remifentanil can be administered as intermittent boluses or as a continuous infusion. Although use of continuous infusions (0.025–0.15 μg/kg/min) in patients undergoing ex-

Table 22-2 Recommended Doses of Commonly Used Sedative and Analgesic Drugs during MAC

Drug	Bolus Dosage	Infusion Rate
Sedative-Anxiolytics		
Midazolam	25–50 µg/kg (used alone)	0.25–2.0 µg/kg/min
	1–2 mg (when used with propofol)	
Propofol	0.25–1 mg/kg	10–75 µg/kg/min
Analgesics		
Alfentanil	5–10 µg/kg	0.25–1.0 µg/kg/min
Fentanyl	25–50 µg	
Remifentanil	0.10–0.35 µg/kg	0.025–0.15 µg/kg/min

tracorporeal lithotripsy afforded superior intraoperative analgesia, this approach was associated with a higher incidence of hypoxemia when compared with intermittent boluses (25 µg).[35] Remifentanil has been used effectively by bolus injection for intensely stimulating procedures of brief duration, such as awake laryngoscopy.[36] Owing to the relative absence of residual opioid effect, prudent use of remifentanil requires adjunctive analgesics to maintain satisfactory postoperative analgesia following painful procedures. This is often accomplished with a combination of nonopioid analgesics given well in advance of remifentanil discontinuation, often at or before induction or toward the completion of surgery. Examples of this multimodal approach to analgesia include preoperative oral administration of a cyclooxygenase-2 (COX-2) inhibitor followed by local infiltration of the wound with local anesthetic. Table 22-2 summarizes recommended doses of sedative and analgesic drugs most commonly used for MAC.

Inhalation Sedation

The inhalation anesthetic agents can be used in subanesthetic concentrations during MAC to provide sedation and analgesia. Advantages of inhaled anesthetics include rapid reversibility and relative ease of maintaining a constant end-tidal concentration. Nitrous oxide (N_2O) is frequently used at concentrations ranging from 30% to 50% in oxygen, reaching peak psychomotor effect in 5–7 min.[37] Concentrations greater than 30% may trigger excitement, nausea, and dizziness. Enflurane 0.5% produces psychomotor impairment and amnesia corresponding to that of 40% N_2O.[38] Isoflurane is a rather pungent agent that can produce respiratory irritation as well as headache and dizziness when administered at a concentration of 0.5%.[39] Desflurane, the least soluble inhalation agent, is associated with the most rapid uptake and elimination, as well as negligible metabolism and toxicity. It is, however, very pungent and can produce airway irritation in some patients even when administered at 1–2% concentration for sedation. Sevoflurane is a promising agent for sedation, owing to its lack of pungency and rapid onset and offset. Typical concentrations for sedation range from 0.3% to 0.6%.

METHODS OF ADMINISTRATION

The obvious objective of any form of administration is to maintain an appropriate concentration of anesthetic drug(s) at the site of action in the central nervous system (CNS). Intermittent bolus injections of drugs may produce a high peak plasma concentration as well as high concentrations at the effect site, with possible adverse occurrences (Fig. 22-1). Furthermore, significant accumulation can occur, depending on the type and amount of drug given as well as on the time intervals between boluses. Clearly, dur-

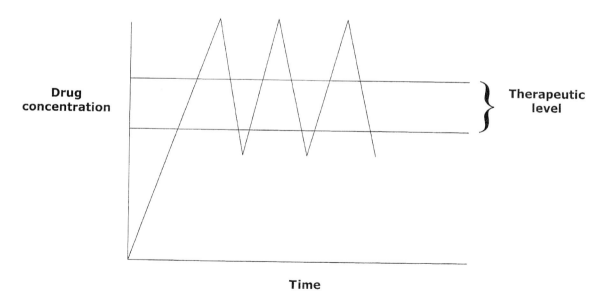

Figure 22-1 Intermittent bolus injections of a drug can result in excessive levels immediately after the bolus is administered (peaks) and inadequate levels during the period between bolus injections (valleys).

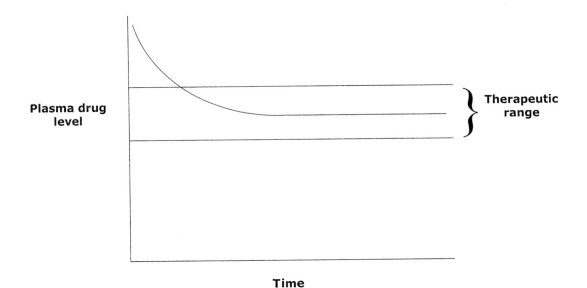

Figure 22-2   Simulated drug level curve when a continuing infusion is given after an adequate loading dose. This approach is designed to avoid the peaks and valleys associated with intermittent bolus doses.

ing day-case surgery, there will be impressive interindividual variability in patients' anxiety, age, ASA physical status, level of stimulation, and type of surgery. These differences demand a broad range of sedative/analgesic dosing requirements. Recently, patient-controlled sedation (PCS) devices have been introduced to accommodate this variability. PCS devices deliver a predefined bolus of IV drug during a defined interval, with or without a lockout period.[40]

Continuous infusions of short-acting drugs should allow sedation and analgesia to be maintained with impressive precision, titratability, and safety (Fig. 22-2). Administration may be directed by the findings from population studies that suggest infusion rates necessary to sustain a constant plasma or effect site concentration. Infusion rate requirements, naturally, will decrease over time as muscle and fat storage sites equilibrate with a specific plasma concentration. Assorted monitors, such as the bispectral index (BIS, Aspect Medical Systems, Natick, MA), may further guide infusion rates, perhaps permitting a reduction of hypnotic drug doses and earlier awakening.[41]

New TCI devices use pharmacokinetic models to predict the plasma and effect site concentrations and allow the anesthesiologist to target a chosen concentration. The device calculates the appropriate infusion scheme to attain this concentration, thereby enabling the anesthesiologist to deal directly with the concentration/effect relationship. TCI devices enable a predefined plasma or effect site concentration of the selected drug to be attained quickly and maintained consistently. Appropriate target concentrations will vary depending on specific patient characteristics and the type of surgery. Therefore, the desired clinical end point will guide selection of an appropriate target concentration. These innovative TCI devices have been approved for propofol administration, and it is anticipated that this approval will extend to other drugs in the future.

EVALUATION OF SEDATION AND MONITORING

Clinical methods of assessing sedation include tests based on the subject's self-assessment, evaluation of the patient by a trained observer, and measurement of objective signs by a clinician.

Aitken first described the use of analog scales to measure drug effects.[42] These scales typically consist of opposing adjectives at either end of a 100-mm line. Visual analog scores (VAS) also can be used by a trained observer. One of the more widely accepted scales for assessing sedation by an observer is the Observer's Assessment of Alertness/Sedation (OAAS) scale.[43] Other scales include the Ramsay score and the University of Michigan Sedation Scale (UMSS).[44]

Systematic measurement of objective signs is the method of assessment most commonly used intraoperatively by anesthesiologists during MAC. Continuous measurement of oxygen saturation by pulse oximetry is invaluable, and end-tidal CO_2 monitoring is also helpful, but lacks the precision associated with endotracheal intubation. Determination of vital signs at regular intervals is important because autonomic responses to anxiety include diaphoresis, tremor, increased muscle tension, hypertension, and tachycardia. As a patient becomes more deeply sedated, blood pressure and heart rate decrease, and the rate and depth of respiration change. Electroencephalographic (EEG) measurements show a reduction in alpha activity and an increase in delta activity.[45]

Monitoring the hypnotic component of anesthesia has undergone significant recent changes with the introduction of the bispectral index monitor. BIS is an empirically derived index dependent on a measure of "coherence" among EEG components. It provides a nondimensional number between 0 and 100 that purportedly correlates with the level of sedation and hypnosis. In patients who are awake, the BIS is between 90 and 100, while complete suppression of cortical activity results in a BIS of zero. BIS values below 70 are thought to generally indicate a low probability of recall and consciousness perception.[46–48] While BIS values between 40 and 60 are recommended as adequate targets to guide the administration of hypnotic drugs during general anesthesia, BIS values of 60–70 are often sought during MAC. However, no specific numeric threshold can guarantee "not aware" for the individual patient. Moreover, BIS thresholds are not independent of the combinations of anesthetic agents administered,[49] and variation in electrode montage will also alter derived BIS values. Indeed, the scientific literature does not support the notion that any commercially available monitor can prevent awareness with reliability.[50,51] BIS values are useful, however, for trend monitoring, and are thought to allow a reduction in drug dosing. For example, when used during propofol and alfentanil TCI, BIS monitoring allowed a significant reduction in propofol doses compared with standard clinical practice, and also afforded a faster recovery.[41] Clearly, the purported savings accrued from reduced drug costs achieved with BIS monitoring must be weighed against the cost of the disposable sensors needed to operate this apparatus.

SAFETY AND MEDICOLEGAL ISSUES

It is, perhaps, easy to be lulled into a false sense of security when one is involved in "only" a MAC procedure for a healthy patient. This misperception, combined with the production pressures inherent in contemporary clinical practice, can lead to tragic outcomes. Unfortunately, the literature is replete with reports of adverse events associated with sedation techniques.[52–54] Some of these catastrophes reflect performance in remote locations with inadequate monitoring and sedation administered by individuals not thoroughly trained in monitoring, pharmacology, airway management, and resuscitation.

Even in the skilled hands of an experienced anesthesiologist, MAC can be challenging. Patients expected to be most susceptible to the effects of these medications are those at the extremes of age, the obese, those given additive or synergistic drug combinations, and those with cardiopulmonary, renal, or hepatic disease.

According to data from the Food and Drug Administration (FDA), midazolam was implicated in at least 80 deaths during gastrointestinal endoscopy, which occurred mainly in the absence of monitoring by an anesthesiologist.[52] Respiratory events were responsible for the majority of the incidents, and most patients had also received an opioid.

Another area of grave concern occurs in the realm of pediatric "sedation," especially in the setting of dental offices. Coté and colleagues, using critical incident techniques, reviewed 118 adverse sedation-related techniques in pediatric patients from data supplied by the FDA, the *United States Pharmacopoeia*, and the results of a survey of pediatric specialists.[53,54] Ninety-five of these events provided sufficient information for the investigators to examine systems issues that contributed to the adverse out-

comes. They found that death and permanent neurologic injury were more likely to occur in children sedated in non-hospital-based venues, compared with hospital-based venues, despite the fact that the former group of patients were older and healthier. Nearly 80% of the events presented initially as respiratory compromise. Most of the subsequent unacceptable outcomes were ascribed to failure to rescue the patients. Inadequate resuscitation contributed to adverse outcomes more frequently in non-hospital-based venues. Inadequate and inconsistent physiologic monitoring (especially failure to use or respond appropriately to pulse oximetry) was another major factor contributing to poor outcome. Other issues included drug overdose and drug interactions, particularly when three or more drugs were used. Adverse outcome was associated with all routes of drug administration and all classes of medication, even those (such as chloral hydrate) thought to have minimal effect on respiration. Moreover, inadequate presedation medical evaluation as well as inadequate recovery procedures were also cited by the reviewers as contributing to death or permanent neurologic damage.

Children sedated for dental procedures in the office represented a high-risk group. They accounted for 32 events resulting in 29 patients suffering death or permanent neurologic injury (11 practitioners were oral surgeons, 17 were pedodontists, and 1 was a certified registered nurse anesthetist [CRNA] supervised by a dentist). The only apparent differences in the pattern of drug class selection by dental practitioners compared with those performing other procedures were the use of N_2O and the use of multiple sedating medications. A higher proportion of patients undergoing dental care received three or more sedating medications at the time of the severe adverse event (death or permanent neurologic injury) compared with all other specialties combined. Moreover, all 10 patients in the database who received N_2O were dental patients, and 9 of those suffered a negative outcome.

The investigators concluded that uniform specialty-independent guidelines for monitoring children during and after sedation are essential. Age- and size-appropriate equipment and medications for resuscitation must be immediately available regardless of the location where the child is sedated. All health care providers who sedate children, regardless of practice venue, should have advanced airway assessment and management training and be skilled in the resuscitation of infants and children so that they can successfully rescue their patient should an adverse sedation event occur.

In a study by Cohen et al. of 100,000 anesthetics, MAC morbidity was 208/10,000, higher than that associated with either general anesthesia or regional techniques.[55] In fact, during the 1990s, MAC medicolegal claims became more common, accounting for 6% of the cases in the Closed Claims database.[56] Sixty-five percent of the MAC patients involved were older, sicker (ASA physical status III to V) outpatients. In contradistinction to most ambulatory claims that tend to involve rather minor types of injuries in healthier patients,[57] the MAC claims reflected more severe injuries, with death (39%) and brain damage (15%) common. Moreover, payments were high (similar to that for general anesthesia), and the mechanism of injury was often respiratory (25%) or cardiovascular (14%). It is troubling that litigation from MAC-related injury increased during the 1990s, despite the use of pulse oximetry and other respiratory monitoring.

SUMMARY

The development of new short-acting pharmacologic agents and the impressive growth of minimally invasive surgical and diagnostic techniques have enabled anesthesiologists and other medical practitioners to utilize MAC for a broad spectrum of procedures both inside and outside the operating room. The goals of sedation are to provide a balance between patient comfort and safety by preventing cardiopulmonary perturbation and delayed recovery. The sine qua non of safety is that the provider must have a profound respect for the continuum from anxiolysis to unconsciousness. Adherence to uniform standards is critical. Patients receiving MAC should benefit from the same level of preoperative, intraoperative, and postoperative vigilance as patients receiving general anesthesia. Therefore, it is imperative that patients be monitored appropriately by qualified personnel who are knowledgeable about pharmacokinetics and pharmacodynamics and who are experienced in airway management and resuscitation.

The recent development of ultrashort-acting drugs such as remifentanil, new techniques of administration (e.g., PCS and TCI), and monitoring devices such as the BIS may further optimize intraoperative conditions and expedite recovery, thereby enhancing the safety, efficiency, and cost-effectiveness of ambulatory surgery.

REFERENCES

1. Continuum of depth of sedation: definition of general anesthesia and levels of sedation/analgesia. *American Society of Anesthesiologists 2001 Directory of Members.* Park Ridge, IL, 2001, p. 513.
2. Bennett CR. The spectrum of pain control. In: *Conscious Sedation in Dental Practice,* 2nd ed. St. Louis: Mosby, 1978, pp. 10–23.
3. Vickers MD. The measurement of recovery from anesthesia. Br J Anaesth 1965;37:296–302.
4. Doze VA, Westphal LM, White PF. Comparison of propofol with methohexital for outpatient anesthesia. Anesth Analg 1986;65:1189–95.
5. Sun R, Watcha MF, White PF, et al. A cost comparison of methohexital and propofol for ambulatory anesthesia. Anesth Analg 1999;89:311–16.
6. White PF, Way WL, Trevor AJ. Ketamine—its pharmacology and therapeutic uses. Anesthesiology 1982;56:119–36.
7. Deng XM, Xiao WJ, Luo MP, et al. The use of midazolam and small-dose ketamine for sedation and analgesia during local anesthesia. Anesth Analg 2001;93:1174–77.
8. Grant IS, Nimmo WS, McNicol LR, Clements JA. Ketamine disposition in children and adults. Br J Anaesth 1983;55:1107–11.
9. Idvall J, Ahlgren I, Aronsen KR, et al. Ketamine infusions: Pharmacokinetics and clinical effects. Br J Anaesth 1979;51:1167–73.
10. Badrinath S, Avramov MN, Shadrick M, et al. The use of a ketamine-propofol combination during monitored anesthesia care. Anesth Analg 2000;90:858–62.
11. Vinik HR, Bradley EL, Kissin I. Midazolam-alfentanil synergism for anesthetic induction in patients. Anesth Analg 1989;69:312–17.
12. Sheu JR, Hsiao G, Luk HN, et al. Mechanisms involved in the antiplatelet activity of midazolam in human platelets. Anesthesiology 2002;96:651–58.
13. White PF, Negus JB. Sedative infusions during local and regional anesthesia: a comparison of midazolam and propofol. J Clin Anesth 1991;3:32–39.
14. Ghouri AF, Ramirez-Ruiz MA, White PF. Effect of flumazenil on recovery after midazolam and propofol sedation. Anesthesiology 1994;81:333–39.
15. Mora CT, Torjman M, White PF. Sedative and ventilatory effects of midazolam infusion: effect of flumazenil reversal. Can J Anaesth 1995;42:677–84.
16. Rouiller M, Forster A, Gemperle M. Evaluation de l'efficacité et de la tolerance d'un antagoniste des benzodiazepines (Ro 15-1788). Ann Fr Anesth Reanim 1987;6:1–6.
17. Borgeat A. Subhypnotic doses of propofol possess direct antiemetic properties. Anesth Analg 1992;74:539–41.
18. Mortero RF, Clark LD, Tolan MM, et al. The effects of small-dose ketamine on propofol sedation: respiration, postoperative mood, perception, cognition, and pain. Anesth Analg 2001;92:1465–69.
19. Kazema T, Takeuchi K, Ikeda K, et al. Optimal propofol plasma concentration during upper gastrointestinal endoscopy in young, middle-aged, and elderly patients. Anesthesiology 2000;93:662–69.
20. Shinozaki M, Usui Y, Yamaguchi S, et al. Recovery of psychomotor function after propofol sedation is prolonged in the elderly. Can J Anaesth 2002;49:927–31.
21. Mangar D, Holak EJ. Tourniquet at 50 mmHg followed by intravenous lidocaine diminishes hand pain associated with propofol injection. Anesth Analg 1992;74:250–52.
22. Picard P, Tramèr MR. Prevention of pain on injection with propofol: A quantitative systematic review. Anesth Analg 2000;90:963–69.
23. Doenicke AW, Roizen MF, Rau J, et al. Reducing pain during propofol injection: the role of the solvent. Anesth Analg 1996;82:472–74.
24. Scott RP, Saunders DA, Norman J. Propofol: clinical strategies for preventing the pain of injection. Anaesthesia 1988;43:492–94.
25. Johnson RA, Harper NJN, Chadwick S, et al. Pain on injection of propofol: methods of alleviation. Anaesthesia 1990;45:439–42.
26. Pollard RC, Makky S, McFadzean J, et al. An admixture of 3 mg/kg of propofol and 3 mg/kg of thiopentone reduces pain on injection in pediatric anesthesia. Can J Anaesth 2002;49:1064–69.
27. Egan TD. The clinical pharmacology of the new fentanyl congeners. Anesth Analg 1997;84(Suppl):31–38.
28. Bailey PL, Egan TD, Stanley TH. Intravenous opioid anesthesia. In: Miller RD (ed.), *Anesthesia,* 5th ed. Philadelphia: Churchill Livingstone, 2000, pp. 273–376.
29. Egan TD. Remifentanil pharmacokinetics and pharmacodynamics: A preliminary appraisal. Clin Pharmacokinet 1995;29:80–94.
30. Jhaveri R, Joshi P, Batenhorst R, et al. Dose comparison of remifentanil and alfentanil for loss of consciousness. Anesthesiology 1997;87:253–59.
31. White JL, Kern SE, Egan TD. Analgesia and respiratory effects of remifentanil boluses in healthy elderly volunteers. Anesthesiology 1999;91(3A):A14.
32. Neidhart P, Burgener MC, Schwieger I, et al. Chest wall rigidity during fentanyl and midazolam-fentanyl induction: ventilatory and haemodynamic effects. Acta Anaesthesiol Scand 1989;33:1–5.
33. Minto CF, Schnider TW, Egan TD, et al. Influence of age and gender on the pharmacokinetics and pharmacodynamics of remifentanil. Anesthesiology 1997;86:10–23.
34. Egan TD, Huizinga B, Gupta SK, et al. Remifentanil pharmacokinetics in obese versus lean patients. Anesthesiology 1998;89:562–73.
35. Sa Rego MM, Inagaki Y, White PF. Remifentanil administration during monitored anesthesia care: are intermittent boluses an effective alternative to a continuous infusion? Anesth Analg 1999;88:518–22.
36. Johnson KB, Swenson JD, Egan TD, et al. Midazolam and remifentanil by bolus injection for intensely stimulating procedures of brief

duration: Experience with awake laryngoscopy. Anesth Analg 2002;
94:1241–43.

37. Korttila K, Ghoneim MM, Jacobs L, et al. Time course of mental and psychomotor effects of 30 percent nitrous oxide during inhalation and recovery. Anesthesiology 1981;54:220–26.

38. Abboud TK, Shnider SM, Wright RG, et al. Enflurane analgesia in obstetrics. Anesth Analg 1981;60:133–37.

39. Rodrigo MRC, Rosenquist JB. Isoflurane for conscious sedation. Anaesthesia 1988;43:369–75.

40. Ng, Kong CF, Nyam D. Patient-controlled sedation with propofol for colonoscopy. Gastrointest Endosc 2001;54:22–13.

41. Gan TG, Glass PS, Windsor A, et al. Bispectral index monitoring allows for faster emergence and improved recovery from propofol, alfentanil, and nitrous oxide anesthesia. BIS Utility Study Group. Anesthesiology 1997;87:808–15.

42. Aitken RCB. Measurement of feelings using visual analogue scales. Proc R Soc Med 1969;62:989–93.

43. Chernik DA, Gillings D, Laine H, et al. Validity and reliability of the Observer's Assessment of Alertness/Sedation scale: studies with intravenous midazolam. J Clin Psychopharmacol 1990;10:244–51.

44. Malviya S, Voepel-Lewis T, Tait AR, et al. Depth of sedation in children undergoing computed tomography: validity and reliability of the University of Michigan Sedation Scale (UMSS). Br J Anaesth 2002;88:241–45.

45. Liu J, Singh H, White PF. Electroencephalogram bispectral analysis predicts the depth of midazolam-induced sedation. Anesthesiology 1996;84:64–69.

46. Flaishon R, Windsor A, Sigl J, et al. Recovery of consciousness after thiopental or propofol: bispectral index and isolated forearm technique. Anesthesiology 1997;86:613–19.

47. Sebel PS, Lang E, Rampil IJ, et al. A multicenter study of bispectral electroencephalogram analysis for monitoring anesthetic effect. Anesth Analg 1997;84:891–99.

48. Glass PS, Bloom M, Kearse L, et al. Bispectral analysis measures sedation and memory effects of propofol, midazolam, isoflurane, and alfentanil in healthy volunteers. Anesthesiology 1997;86:836–47.

49. McDermott NB, VanSickle T, Motas D, et al. Validation of the bispectral index monitor during conscious and deep sedation in children. Anesth Analg 2003;97:39–43.

50. Drummond JC. Monitoring depth of anesthesia with emphasis on the application of the bispectral index and the middle latency auditory evoked response to the prevention of recall. Anesthesiology 2000;93:876–82.

51. Schneider G, Wagner K, Reeker W, et al. Bispectral index (BIS) may not predict awareness reaction to intubation in surgical patients. J Neurosurg Anesthesiol 2002;14:7–11.

52. Food and Drug Administration: Warning re-emphasized in midazolam labeling. FDA Drug Bull 1986;27:5.

53. Coté CJ, Notterman DA, Karl HW, et al. Adverse sedation events in pediatrics: a critical incident analysis of contributing factors. Pediatrics 2000;105:805–14.

54. Coté CJ, Karl HW, Notterman DA, et al. Adverse sedation events in pediatrics: analysis of medications used for sedation. Pediatrics 2000;106:633–44.

55. Cohen MM, Duncan PG, Tate RB. Does anesthesia contribute to operative mortality? JAMA 1988;260:2859–63.

56. Domino KB. Trends in litigation in the 1990s: MAC claims. ASA Newslett 1997;61:15–17.

57. Posner KL. Liability profile of ambulatory anesthesia. ASA Newslett 2000;64(6):10–12.

Fast-Track General Anesthesia and Ambulatory Discharge Criteria

GIRISH P. JOSHI • RALPH GERTLER

INTRODUCTION

With an increasing number of surgical procedures being performed on an outpatient basis, ambulatory surgical facilities have been forced to improve efficiency. This has increased emphasis on expeditious recovery and shorter hospital stay. Fast-tracking is a new recovery paradigm commonly referred to as transferring patients from the operating room directly to the phase II recovery area (i.e., bypassing the postanesthesia care unit [PACU]).[1,2] The process of fast-tracking can be further extended to achieving shorter phase II recovery unit stay, resulting in an early discharge home.[3] Although fast-tracking should reduce the hospital stay, premature discharge from the hospital may increase the incidence of postoperative complications and readmissions, and may have legal repercussions.

This chapter describes general anesthesia techniques and the discharge process that should consistently allow safe fast-tracking in patients undergoing ambulatory surgery.

ANESTHETIC TECHNIQUES FOR FAST-TRACKING

Local and regional anesthesia techniques probably allow the most rapid recovery,[4-6] but general anesthesia remains the most commonly utilized technique.[7] The modern balanced general anesthetic technique consists of the use of a combination of drugs to achieve amnesia (using hypnotic-sedatives), analgesia or hemodynamic stability (using analgesics such as opioids), and patient immobility (or muscle relaxation). The skillful use of anesthetic and analgesic drugs provides adequate anesthetic and surgical conditions while allowing rapid recovery. The currently available shorter-acting anesthetic and analgesic drugs has allowed a rapid emergence from general anesthesia such that most patients are awake and alert at the end of surgery and may fulfill the PACU discharge criteria in the operating room.[1,2]

INDUCTION OF GENERAL ANESTHESIA

Propofol remains the drug of choice for induction of anesthesia because of its unique recovery profile. Other advantages of propofol include its antiemetic properties and associated euphoria on emergence. Induction of anesthesia can also be achieved with sevoflurane, which allows more rapid emergence.[8] However, propofol induction is shorter and is preferred by most patients.[8] Therefore, sevoflurane induction is usually reserved for selected patients (e.g., "needle-phobic" patients or if spontaneous ventilation is preferred, such as for patients with anticipated difficult airway).[7]

Induction of anesthesia can be facilitated with supplementation of the hypnotic-sedative with remifentanil, an ultrashort-acting opioid. Use of remifentanil with propofol facilitates tracheal intubation without the use of muscle relaxants or with lower doses of these drugs.[9] Furthermore, remifentanil reduces the requirements of inhaled anesthetics, which allows for a rapid recovery.[10] However, there is a learning curve with the use of remifentanil.[11] Avoidance of bolus dosing and initial infusion rate of remifentanil of 0.25 μg/kg/min reduce the incidence of side effects (e.g., bradycardia and hypotension) while providing adequate conditions.[12] In addition, because of its shorter duration of action, it is imperative that other longer-acting analgesics (preferably with nonopioids) be used with remifentanil to provide postoperative analgesia.

INHALATION ANESTHESIA VERSUS TOTAL INTRAVENOUS ANESTHESIA (TIVA) FOR MAINTENANCE OF GENERAL ANESTHESIA

Anesthesia can be maintained with the newer shorter-acting volatile anesthetics (i.e., desflurane and sevoflurane) or a propofol infusion (i.e., TIVA). Propofol TIVA is increasingly utilized with the availability of newer delivery systems (e.g., target-controlled infusion) and the reports of lower incidence of postoperative nausea and vomiting (PONV).[13–15] In fact, propofol TIVA is preferred in patients at very high risk of PONV.[16]

However, inhalation anesthesia techniques remain the mainstay of modern anesthesia practice because of ease of titratibility, neuromuscular blocking effects, and a more rapid emergence from anesthesia.[7] Early emergence from inhalation anesthesia reduces the risks of postoperative complications (e.g., respiratory complications such as airway obstruction and hypoxemia)[17,18] and increases fast tracking.[19]

Apfelbaum et al.[20] reported faster recovery (e.g., eye opening and orientation) and ability to sit earlier after desflurane than after propofol anesthesia. Similarly, psychomotor tests 1 hr after desflurane anesthesia were superior when compared with propofol anesthesia.[20] Another study found that postural stability was achieved earlier after desflurane anesthesia than after propofol anesthesia.[21] Although inhalation anesthesia techniques allow fast-tracking with respect to bypassing the PACU, this may not translate into an earlier discharge home.[19,20,22]

Compared with sevoflurane, desflurane allows for a faster emergence.[19,23,24] Song et al.[19] assessed the recovery times and fast-track eligibility with desflurane, sevoflurane, or propofol. Compared with propofol TIVA, maintenance of anesthesia with desflurane or sevoflurane resulted in shorter times to awakening, tracheal extubation, and orientation. A larger percentage of patients who received desflurane for maintenance were considered fast-track eligible compared with sevoflurane and propofol (90% vs. 75% and 26%, respectively).[19]

Titration of anesthetic concentration using "depth of hypnosis" monitors (e.g., bispectral index [BIS] monitoring) has been shown to reduce anesthetic requirements and facilitate emergence after anesthesia.[25,26] Similarly, titration of hypnotic-sedatives to a predetermined BIS value has been reported to facilitate fast-tracking.[27,28] However, similar to the non-BIS-titrated studies, there were no differences in late recovery times.

Juvin et al.[29] evaluated the recovery characteristics among morbidly obese patients receiving desflurane, isoflurane, or propofol administered according to BIS values. Immediate recovery occurred faster and was more consistent, and oxygen saturations were higher after desflurane than after propofol or isoflurane. However, these differences persisted only in the early recovery phase (up to 2 hr after surgery). The same group investigated recovery characteristics in elderly patients and found similar results.[30]

A recent study in elderly patients evaluated the recovery from propofol TIVA, isoflurane, and desflurane anesthesia with 70% N_2O titrated to maintain a BIS value between 60 and 65.[24] A significantly larger percentage of patients receiving desflurane were judged to be fast-track eligible compared with those receiving either isoflurane or propofol (73% vs. 43% and 44%, respectively). In addition, the need for therapeutic interventions in the PACU was significantly less in the desflurane group.[24]

Nitrous Oxide

The amnestic and analgesic properties of nitrous oxide (N_2O) reduce anesthetic and analgesic requirements. In addition, the time to spontaneous breathing after equi-MAC (1.3 MAC) of sevoflurane is decreased with the use of N_2O.[31] However, many practitioners omit N_2O because of its potential for increased incidence of PONV. A large study comparing propofol-N_2O and propofol alone found that N_2O reduced propofol requirements by 20–25% without increasing the incidence of adverse events or the time to home readiness.[32] Furthermore, a meta-analysis of randomized controlled trials found that the emetic effect of N_2O is not significant.[33] Also, omitting N_2O may increase the risk of awareness.[33] In addition, because N_2O inhibits the N-methyl-D-aspartate (NMDA) receptors, it might improve postoperative pain control by reducing tolerance and hypersensitivity.[34] Thus, there is no convincing evidence to avoid N_2O.

Muscle Relaxants

Muscle relaxants are commonly used to facilitate tracheal intubation and improve surgical conditions. With increased emphasis on use of minimal dosages of hypnotic-sedatives (e.g., propofol and inhaled anesthetics), muscle relaxants are often used to ensure patient immobility. There is a perception that unlike hypnotic-sedatives, muscle relaxants do not have any deleterious effects on the recovery process. However, even a minor degree of residual neuromuscular blockade (not appreciated clinically) can cause distressing symptoms such as visual disturbances, inability to sit up without assistance, facial weakness, and generalized weakness, all of which may delay recovery.[35] Therefore, avoidance or minimization of muscle relaxants may facilitate recovery and increase the ability to fast-track.

If muscle relaxant use is deemed necessary, a drug with a short duration of action may be beneficial. In addition, because propofol and remifentanil depress laryngeal and pharyngeal reflex, tracheal intubation may be accomplished with lower doses of muscle relaxants.[9] Furthermore, inhaled anesthetics exert some neuromuscular blocking effect,[36] which may reduce the requirements of nondepolarizing muscle relaxants. In fact, a recent study reported that adequate surgical conditions were achieved in approximately two-thirds of the patients undergoing lower abdominal surgery without the use of muscle relaxants.[37] Importantly, muscle relaxants should be administered based on clinical needs rather on the train-of-four response.

Many practitioners avoid the use of reversal drugs because of their potential to increase the incidence of PONV. However, recent studies report that the incidence of PONV and the need for antiemetics do not increase with the use of neostigmine for reversal of residual muscle paralysis.[38,39] Because of the potential for detrimental effects of residual neuromuscular paralysis, particularly in an outpatient setting, it is necessary that reversal drugs be used (in appropriate doses) without hesitation.

Laryngeal Mask Airway

One of the major advances that facilitate recovery after ambulatory surgery is the availability of the laryngeal mask airway (LMA).[40] Compared with the tracheal tube, the LMA is easy to place and does not require muscle relaxation and laryngoscopy. In addition, the LMA is tolerated at lower anesthetic concentrations than the tracheal tube and is associated with reduced hemodynamic changes during placement and emergence from general anesthesia. With the patient breathing spontaneously, analgesics (i.e., opioid or nonopioid) can be administered based on the respiratory rate while hypnotic anesthetics (i.e., intravenous [IV] or inhaled) can be administered based on BIS values. This practice should allow earlier emergence from anesthesia.

Sevoflurane is generally considered the inhaled anesthetic of choice for patients breathing spontaneously through an LMA. However, recent studies suggest that desflurane can be safely used with the LMA.[23,26,41–43] Avoiding rapid increase in concentrations and use of concentrations of less than 6% as well as small doses of opioids (e.g., fentanyl 1 μg/kg) can prevent the airway irritation from desflurane.

PREVENTION OF POSTOPERATIVE COMPLICATIONS

A key to success of fast-tracking after ambulatory surgery is prevention of postoperative complications such as dizziness, drowsiness, pain, and PONV.[44,45] Prevention of these side effects should facilitate recovery and fast-tracking.

Postoperative Pain

One of the factors that affect our ability to fast-track after ambulatory surgery is adequacy of postoperative pain management.[46] Although opioids are effective analgesics, their usefulness is limited by side effects such as drowsiness, dizziness, nausea, vomiting, and respiratory depression.[47] Therefore, nonopioids (e.g., acetaminophen, nonsteroidal anti-inflammatory drugs [NSAIDs], and local anesthetics) are preferred in an outpatient setting. It is increasingly apparent that combination of analgesics provides more effective pain relief with fewer side effects.[48] Furthermore, preoperative administration of nonopioid analgesics has numerous benefits, including reassurance of patients, reduced intraoperative opioid requirements, and improved postoperative analgesia.

After discharge from an outpatient facility, acetaminophen is commonly used often combined with less potent opioids (e.g., codeine, oxycodone, and hydrocodone). A recent study reported that the analgesic efficacy of oral ibuprofen 800 mg is equivalent to acetaminophen 800 mg plus codeine 60 mg when given every 8 hr for 3 days after ambulatory surgery.[49] Furthermore, use of ibuprofen results in significantly less constipation and better overall patient satisfaction. However, concerns have been raised regarding the potential side effects of NSAIDs, such as impaired coagulation and gastric irritation. The limitations of NSAIDs prevent their use even when they would otherwise be desirable.

Conventional NSAIDs nonspecifically inhibit the cyclooxygenase (COX) enzyme, which has two isoforms, COX-1 and COX-2.[50] It is believed that the therapeutic activity of NSAIDs is primarily through the inhibition of the COX-2 isoform, whereas the adverse effects on platelet function and gastrointestinal function result from the inhibition of the COX-1 isoform. The currently available drugs with ability to specifically inhibit COX-2 enzyme include celecoxib, rofecoxib, and valdecoxib. These drugs have analgesic efficacy similar to the conventional NSAIDs but without their potential side effects.[51]

Parecoxib is a parenterally administered inactive prodrug that undergoes rapid amide hydrolysis to pharmacologically active COX-2 inhibitor valdecoxib.[52] Recent studies suggest that preoperative parecoxib 40 mg IV followed by valdecoxib reduced opioid requirements, improved pain relief, and reduced recovery after ambulatory surgery.[53] To provide optimal analgesia, it is imperative that these analgesics are administered on a regular "around-the-clock" basis to minimize the occurrence of breakthrough pain with opioids used as "rescue" analgesics.

Postoperative Nausea and Vomiting

Another limiting factor in the early discharge after ambulatory surgery is PONV. Although prophylactic antiemetic therapy has been shown to reduce the incidence of PONV, routine use of prophylactic antiemetics in all outpatients is not cost-effective.[54,55] Recently published guidelines provide comprehensive, evidence-based recommendations for the management of patients at risk for PONV.[16] In patients at risk for PONV, the baseline risk factors should be decreased (e.g., with the use of regional anesthesia, propofol TIVA, minimal opioids, and adequate hydration). Prophylactic antiemetics either alone or in combination should be considered for patients at moderate risk for PONV. Double- or triple-antiemetic prophylaxis (e.g., dexamethasone, metoclopramide, and 5-Hydroxytryptamine 3 (5-HT$_3$) receptor antagonists with or without nonpharmacologic techniques) is recommended for patients at high risk for PONV.

SAFETY AND FEASIBILITY OF FAST-TRACKING

It is imperative that safety be primarily considered before implementing a fast-tracking program in routine clinical practice. Although there are numerous studies evaluating fast-track eligibility as a surrogate for fast-tracking (i.e., actually bypassing the PACU), there are only a few randomized studies evaluating the safety and feasibility of fast-tracking.

A multicenter observational study, the largest outcome study to date on fast-track anesthesia, found that the PACU bypass rate after implementation of a fast-track program after general anesthesia increased from 0.4% (4 of 1151) to 31.8% (361 of 1136) without increasing the incidence of adverse events.[5] Patel et al.[56] performed a randomized trial to determine the feasibility and benefits of fast-tracking children after outpatient surgery. In this study, 155 children undergoing surgical procedures of less than 90 min who met predefined recovery criteria in the operating room were randomized to be transferred either to the PACU or to the phase II recovery unit.[56] There were no clinically significant adverse events. The investigators concluded that fast-tracking is feasible, safe, and beneficial when specific selection criteria are utilized.

DISCHARGE CRITERIA

An important step in improvement in efficiency of an ambulatory facility is to change practice from traditional time-based to clinical-based discharge from the PACU and home readiness (Tables 23-1 and 23-2). The use of appropriate

Table 23-1   Modified Aldrete Scoring System for Determining Discharge from the Postanesthesia Care Unit

Activity: able to move voluntarily or on command	
4 extremities	2
2 extremities	1
0 extremities	0
Respiration	
Able to deep breathe and cough freely	2
Dyspnea, shallow or limited breathing	1
Apneic	0
Circulation	
Blood pressure ± 20 mmHg of preanesthetic level	2
Blood pressure ± 20–50 mmHg of preanesthetic level	1
Blood pressure ± 50 mmHg of preanesthetic level	0
Consciousness	
Fully awake	2
Arousable on calling	1
Not responding	0
Oxygen saturation	
Able to maintain $SaO_2 > 92\%$ on room air	2
Needs supplemental oxygen to maintain $SaO_2 > 90\%$	1
$SaO_2 < 90\%$ even with supplemental oxygen	0

Score ≥ 9 required for discharge.

SOURCE: Aldrete JA. The post-anesthesia recovery score revisited. J Clin Anesth 1995;7:89.

Table 23-2   Modified Postanesthesia Discharge Scoring System for Determining Home Readiness

Vital signs	
Blood pressure and pulse within 20% of preoperative value	2
Blood pressure and pulse 20–40% of preoperative value	1
Blood pressure and pulse > 40% of preoperative value	0
Activity level	
Steady gait, no dizziness, or meets preoperative level	2
Requires assistance	1
Unable to ambulate	0
Nausea and/or vomiting	
Minimal: successfully treated with oral medication	2
Moderate: successfully treated with intramuscular medication	1
Severe: continues after repeated treatment	0
Pain	
Acceptable	2
Not acceptable	1
Surgical bleeding	
Minimal: does not require dressing change	2
Moderate: up to two dressing changes required	1
Severe: more than three dressing changes required	0

Score ≥ 9 required for discharge.

SOURCE: Marshall SI, Chung F. Discharge criteria and complications after ambulatory surgery. Anesth Analg 1999;88:508.

discharge criteria allows early discharge and prevents postoperative complications and readmission.[57–59] If the criteria for PACU discharge are met in the operating room, it may be appropriate to consider bypassing the PACU. In addition to PACU discharge criteria, patients' ability to move unassisted from the operating table may be used to determine the ability to fast-track.

The postanesthesia discharge scoring system has been commonly used to determine home readiness.[58] However, the need for mandatory oral intake and voiding before discharge has been challenged in recent years.[59] It is suggested that eliminating these criteria would significantly decrease hospital stay in 10–20% of outpatients without increasing adverse events.

A large prospective, randomized study compared the effect of mandatory oral intake and voluntary drinking in children undergoing ambulatory surgery.[60] The investigators found that the voluntary drinkers had a shorter length of stay in the PACU as well as the phase II recovery unit. In addition, the incidence of PONV was significantly lower in this group of patients. Importantly, no child required readmission for problems resulting from this liberal oral intake policy. Jin et al.[61] verified these findings in the adult population. Although the mandatory drinkers in this study had a longer duration of hospital stay, there was no difference in the incidence of PONV between the mandatory drinkers and elective drinkers. Of note, the patients in these studies were allowed oral intake until 2 hr prior to surgery and the adult patients received a large bolus infusion (20 mL/kg) of crystalloid, intraoperatively. Current consensus is that outpatients should not be required to drink and that discharge policy should be adapted accordingly.[59]

Another area of debate is the need to void before discharge home. The reason for insistence on voiding is the concern of urinary retention and subsequent complications after discharge home. The risk factors for postoperative urinary retention include prior history of urinary retention, anesthetic technique (e.g., central neuraxial blocks), and type of surgical procedure (e.g., hernia and anorectal procedures). Pavlin et al.[62] evaluated the need for voiding prior to discharge home. Patients at low risk of postoperative urinary retention were discharged home without being required to void, while the high-risk patients were required to void or catheterized. Based on the postoperative bladder volumes, measured using ultrasound, the authors concluded that patients at low risk of urinary retention can be safely discharged home, even those who received large crystalloid infusion intraoperatively.[62] In contrast, the patients at high risk of urinary retention should be required to void or their bladder evacuated prior to discharge. Furthermore, these patients should receive perioperative fluids judiciously. Importantly, all patients should be cautioned to return to the medical facility if they are unable to void within 8–12 hr after discharge.

SUMMARY

Fast-track anesthesia grants a paradigm shift in postanesthesia care after ambulatory surgery. Current concept of fast-track anesthesia (i.e., accelerated postoperative course) includes bypassing the PACU. However, there is a need to expand this concept to early discharge home as well as early return to normal living function.

The choice of general anesthesia techniques improves our ability to consistently achieve rapid recovery, particularly emergence from anesthesia. Achieving early emergence from general anesthesia allows bypassing the PACU while prevention of common side effects should allow early discharge from the hospital, thus reducing the overall hospital stay.

Although fast-tracking may reduce the recovery time and overall hospital stay, it is necessary to assure a smooth and safe transition to the home setting. Simple, clear, objective criteria should be used to guide safe discharge of outpatients. Requirement for oral intake and voiding before discharge home should not be a part of a discharge protocol and may be necessary only in selected patients. Importantly, patients should be given clear instructions and cautioned against performing functions that require complete recovery of cognitive function.

With the application of benchmarking and timely feedback to clinicians and administrators on patient and process outcomes, fast-tracking can be realistically implemented at any type of surgical center, including community hospitals and freestanding ambulatory surgical centers, without increasing the complication rate.

REFERENCES

1. Joshi GP. Fast tracking in outpatient surgery. Curr Opin Anaesthesiol 2001;14:635.
2. Joshi GP, Twersky RS. Fast tracking in ambulatory surgery. Ambul Surg 2000;8:185.
3. Joshi GP. New concepts in recovery after ambulatory surgery. Ambul Surg 2003;10:167.
4. Joshi GP. Recent developments in regional anesthesia for ambulatory surgery. Curr Opin Anaesthesiol 1999;12:643.
5. Apfelbaum JL, Walawander CA, Grasela TH, et al. Eliminating intensive postoperative care in same-day surgery patients using short-acting anesthetics. Anesthesiology 2002;97:66.
6. Williams BA, Kentor ML, Williams JP, et al. PACU bypass after outpatient knee surgery is associated with fewer unplanned hospital admissions but more phase II nursing interventions. Anesthesiology 2002;97:981.
7. Joshi GP. Inhalational techniques in ambulatory anesthesia. Anesthesiol Clin North Am 2003;21:263.
8. Joo HS, Perks WJ. Sevoflurane versus propofol for anesthetic induction: a meta-analysis. Anesth Analg 2000;91:213.
9. Schlaich N, Mertzlufft F, Soltesz S, Fuchs-Buder T. Remifentanil and propofol without muscle relaxants or with different doses of rocuronium for tracheal intubation in outpatient anesthesia. Acta Anaesthesiol Scand 2000;44:720.
10. Breslin DS, Reid JE, Mirakhur RK, et al. Sevoflurane-nitrous oxide anaesthesia supplemented with remifentanil: effect on recovery and cognitive function. Anaesthesia 2001;56:114.
11. Joshi GP, Jamerson BD, Roizen MF, et al. Is there a learning curve associated with the use of remifentanil? Anesth Analg 2000;91:1049.
12. Joshi GP, Warner DS, Twersky RS, Fleisher LA. A comparison of remifentanil and fentanyl adverse effect profile in a multicenter phase IV study. J Clin Anesth 2002;14:494.
13. Sneyd JR, Carr A, Byrom WD, Bilski AJ. A meta-analysis of nausea and vomiting following maintenance of anaesthesia with propofol or inhalational agents. Eur J Anaesth 1998;15:433.
14. Tramer M, Moore A, McQuay H. Propofol anaesthesia and postoperative nausea and vomiting: quantitative systematic review of randomized controlled studies. Br J Anaesth 1997;78:247.
15. Visser K. Hassink EA, Bonsel GJ, et al. Randomized controlled trial of total intravenous anesthesia with propofol versus inhalation anesthesia with isoflurane-nitrous oxide: postoperative nausea with vomiting and economic analysis. Anesthesiology 2001;95:616.
16. Gan TJ, Meyer T, Apfel CC, et al. Consensus guidelines for managing postoperative nausea and vomiting. Anesth Analg 2003;97:62.
17. Georgiou LG, Vourlioti AN, Kremastinou FI, et al. Influence of anesthetic technique on early postoperative hypoxemia. Acta Anaesthesiol Scand 1996;40:75.
18. Fredman B, Nathanson MH, Smith I, et al. Sevoflurane for outpatient anesthesia: a comparison with propofol. Anesth Analg 1995;81:823.
19. Song D, Joshi GP, White PF. Fast-track eligibility after ambulatory anesthesia: a comparison of desflurane, sevoflurane, and propofol. Anesth Analg 1998;86:267.
20. Apfelbaum JL, Lichtor JL, Lane BS, et al. Awakening, clinical recovery, and psychomotor effects after desflurane and propofol anesthesia. Anesth Analg 1996;83:721.
21. Song D, Chung F, Wong J, Yogendran S. The assessment of postural stability after ambulatory anesthesia: a comparison of desflurane with propofol. Anesth Analg 2002;94:60.
22. Raeder J, Gupta A, Pedersen FM. Recovery characteristics of sevoflurane- or propofol-based anaesthesia for day-care surgery. Acta Anaesthesiol Scand 1997;41:988.

23. Mahmoud NA, Rose DJA, Laurence AS. Desflurane or sevoflurane for gynaecological day-case anaesthesia with spontaneous respiration? Anaesthesia 2001;56:171.

24. Fredman B, Sheffer O, Zohar E, et al. Fast-track eligibility of geriatric patients undergoing short urologic surgery procedures. Anesth Analg 2002;94:560.

25. Song D, Joshi GP, White PF. Titration of volatile anesthetics using bispectral index facilitates recovery after ambulatory anesthesia. Anesthesiology 1997;87:842.

26. Gan TJ, Glass PS, Windsor A, et al. Bispectral index monitoring allows faster emergence and improved recovery from propofol, alfentanil, and nitrous oxide anesthesia. Anesthesiology 1997;87:808.

27. Song D, van Vlymen J, White PF. Is the bispectral index useful in predicting fast-track eligibility after ambulatory anesthesia with propofol and desflurane? Anesth Analg 1998;87:1245.

28. Tang J, White PF, Wender RH, et al. Fast-track office-based anesthesia: a comparison of propofol versus desflurane with antiemetic prophylaxis in spontaneously breathing patients. Anesth Analg 2001;92:95.

29. Juvin P, Vadam C, Malek L, et al. Postoperative recovery after desflurane, propofol, or isoflurane anesthesia among morbidly obese patients: a prospective, randomized study. Anesth Analg 2000;91:714.

30. Juvin P, Servin F, Giraud O, Desmonts JM. Emergence of elderly patients from prolonged desflurane, isoflurane, or propofol anesthesia. Anesth Analg 1997;85:647.

31. Einarsson S, Bengtsson A, Stenqvist O, Bengtson JP. Decreased respiratory depression during emergence from anesthesia with sevoflurane/N_2O than with sevoflurane alone. Can J Anaesth 1999;46:335.

32. Arellano RJ, Pole ML, Rafuse SE, et al. Omission of nitrous oxide from a propofol-based anesthetic does not affect the recovery of women undergoing outpatient gynecological surgery. Anesthesiology 2000;93:332.

33. Tramer M, Moore A, McQuay H. Omitting nitrous oxide in general anaesthesia: meta-analysis of intraoperative awareness and postoperative emesis in randomized controlled trials. Br J Anaesth 1996;76:186.

34. Jevtovic-Todorovic V, Todorovic SM, Mennerick S, et al. Nitrous oxide (laughing gas) is an NMDA antagonist, neuroprotectant, and neurotoxin. Nat Med 1998;4:460.

35. Kopman AF, Yee PS, Neuman GG. Relationship of the train-of-four fade ratio to clinical signs and symptoms of residual paralysis in awake volunteers. Anesthesiology 1997;86:765.

36. Eriksson LI. The effects of residual neuromuscular blockade and volatile anesthetics on control of ventilation. Anesth Analg 1999;89:243.

37. King M, Sujirattanawimol N, Danielson DR, et al. Requirements for muscle relaxants during radical retropubic prostatectomy. Anesthesiology 2000;93:1392.

38. Joshi GP, Garg SA, Hailey A, Yu SY. Effects of antagonizing residual neuromuscular blockade by neostigmine and glycopyrrolate on nausea and vomiting after ambulatory surgery. Anesth Analg 1999;89:628.

39. Tramer MR, Fuchs-Buder T. Omitting antagonism of neuromuscular block: effect on postoperative nausea and vomiting and risk of residual paralysis: a systemic review. Br J Anaesth 1999;82:379.

40. Joshi GP. The use of laryngeal mask airway devices in ambulatory anesthesia. Semin Anesth, Periop Med Pain 2001;20:257.

41. Goodwin AP, Rowe WL, Ogg TW. Day case laparoscopy: a comparison of two anaesthetic techniques using the laryngeal mask during spontaneous breathing. Anaesthesia 1992;47:892.

42. Ashworth J, Smith I. Comparison of desflurane with isoflurane or propofol in spontaneously breathing ambulatory patients. Anesth Analg 1998;87:312.

43. Eshima RW, Maurer A, King T, et al. A comparison of airway responses during desflurane and sevoflurane administration via a laryngeal mask airway for maintenance of anesthesia. Anesth Analg 2003;96:701.

44. Chung F, Mezei G. Factors contributing to a prolonged stay after ambulatory surgery. Anesth Analg 1999;89:1352.

45. Pavlin DJ, Rapp SE, Polissar NL, et al. Factors affecting discharge time in adult outpatients. Anesth Analg 1998;87:816.

46. Joshi GP. Pain management after ambulatory surgery. Ambul Surg 1999;7:3.

47. Kehlet H, Rung GW, Callesen T. Postoperative opioid analgesia: time for a reconsideration? J Clin Anesth 1996;8:441.

48. Kehlet H. Multimodal approach to control postoperative pathology and rehabilitation. Br J Anaesth 1997;78:606.

49. Raeder JC, Steine S, Vatsgar TT. Oral ibuprofen versus paracetamol plus codeine for analgesia after ambulatory surgery. Anesth Analg 2001;92:1470.

50. Jackson LM, Hawkey CJ. COX-2 selective nonsteroidal anti-inflammatory drugs: do they really offer any advantages? Drugs 2000;59:1207.

51. Ormond D, Wellington K, Wagstaff AJ. Valdecoxib. Drugs 2002;62:2059.

52. Cheer SM, Goa KL. Parecoxib (parecoxib sodium). Drugs 2001;61:1133.

53. Joshi GP, Viscusi E, Gan TJ, et al. Effective treatment of laparoscopic cholecystectomy pain with intravenous followed by oral COX-2 specific inhibitor. Anesth Analg 2004;98:336–42.

54. Watcha MF. The cost-effective management of postoperative nausea and vomiting. Anesthesiology 2000;92:931.

55. Apfel CC, Laara E, Koivuranta M, et al. A simplified risk score for predicting postoperative nausea and vomiting. Anesthesiology 1999;91:693.

56. Patel RI, Verghese ST, Hanallah RS, et al. Fast-tracking children after ambulatory surgery. Anesth Analg 2001;92:918.

57. Aldrete JA. The post-anesthesia recovery score revisited. J Clin Anesth 1995;7:89.

58. Marshall SI, Chung F. Discharge criteria and complications after ambulatory surgery. Anesth Analg 1999;88:508.

59. Practice guidelines for postanesthesia care: a report by the American Society of Anesthesiologists Task Force on postanesthesia care. Anesthesiology 2002;96:742.

60. Schreiner MS, Nicholson SC, Martin T, et al. Should children drink before discharge from day surgery? Anesthesiology 1992;76:528.

61. Jin FL, Norris A, Chung F. Should adult patients drink fluids before discharge from ambulatory surgery? Can J Anaesth 1998;87:306.

62. Pavlin DJ, Pavlin EG, Fitzgibbon DR, et al. Management of bladder function after outpatient surgery. Anesthesiology 1999;91:42.

General Anesthesia for Modern Ambulatory Surgery

DONALD M. MATHEWS • REBECCA S. TWERSKY

INTRODUCTION

With the decision to administer general anesthesia to an ambulatory patient, the anesthesiologist is faced with a series of choices. While any one of a number of techniques will allow the patient to survive the surgery and eventually be discharged home, each decision that the anesthesiologist makes should be designed to give the patient the greatest chance of being able to leave the ambulatory facility in a timely manner. This involves understanding the complications that delay patient discharge and making choices that are intended to avoid them. It also involves understanding the pharmacologic properties of the available anesthetic agents so that the anesthetic delivered has the greatest chance of returning the patient quickly to his/her preoperative physiologic and neuropsychologic state. In addition, patients who are highly satisfied with their care may return more quickly to their level of preoperative functioning. The anesthesiologist should therefore consider factors that promote rapid and safe recovery from general anesthesia.

OPTIMAL GENERAL ANESTHETIC

When designing a general anesthetic, the ambulatory anesthesiologist should make choices that will return the patient to the preoperative level of functioning as quickly as possible. Clinical investigations in this area of study tend to compare one anesthetic regimen with another utilizing some measure of outcome. This research is complicated by a lack of agreement about what should be measured in order to ideally assess outcome. Many studies describe the timing of emergence from anesthesia and recovery milestones such as time to eye opening, extubation, and meeting a set of discharge criteria. Another approach is to measure neuropsychologic parameters preoperatively and determine how quickly they return to baseline after surgery. While a series of tests, such as the Mini-Mental Status Exam (MMSE), the Digit-Symbol Substitution Test

(DSST), and the Color Trail Making Test, are utilized in a variety of studies, no test or group of tests has been determined to be a definitive assessment of neuropsychologic recovery. Other studies measure functional recovery by assessing patient balance or performance in a car simulator. In a pilot study in volunteers, the investigators found no significant difference in postanesthetic driving skills at 2, 3, and 4 hr postanesthesia and the corresponding control session.[1] Another approach is to determine the timing of recovery milestones after discharge, such as ability to eat, drink, and perform other activities of daily living. Return to gainful economic activity, perhaps the most important measure of recovery, is not often utilized in these investigations.

Despite the limitations caused by a variety of outcome data, some observations can be made about how choices made by an anesthesiologist affect the patient's recovery. In particular, choices pertaining to use of "depth of hypnosis" monitoring, use of anxiolytic premedication, choice of airway device, choice of induction agent, and choice of maintenance agent can be addressed.

"Depth of Hypnosis" Monitors

A series of monitors are now available that have been investigated in the ambulatory patient. These monitors utilize differing parameters of central nervous system (CNS) electroencephalographic (EEG) measurement in an attempt to quasi-linearize the complicated relationship between the hypnotic agent and CNS function. In these studies patients are cared for using either traditional care, where the caregiver is blinded to information generated by the monitor, or titrated care, where the amount of hypnotic agent administered is guided by information generated by the monitor. Milestone recovery parameters and drug utilization are then compared between the two groups.

The most widely studied of the monitors is the bispectral index monitor (BIS, Aspect Medical System, Natick,

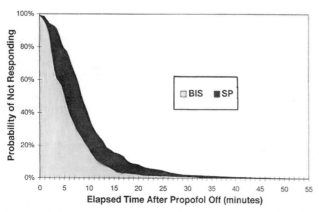

Figure 24-1   The comparison of probability of not responding following a propofol-alfentanil-nitrous oxide anesthestic with care given by standard practice (SP) or guided by the bispectral index monitor (BIS). (From Gan TJ, Glass PS, Windsor A, et al. Bispectral index monitoring allows faster emergence and improved recovery from propofol, alfentanil, and nitrous oxide anesthesia. BIS Utility Study Group. Anesthesiology 1997;87:808–15. Used with permission.)

MA). A number of studies utilizing the BIS monitor have been conducted and, in general, they agree with the initial studies of propofol-alfentanil-nitrous oxide[2] or inhalation agent[3] anesthetics and found decreased drug usage, faster early recovery milestones, and increased incidence of postanesthesia care unit (PACU) bypass eligibility in the BIS-guided groups (Fig. 24-1). Similar results have been reported during a propofol-alfentanil-nitrous oxide anesthetic both with the Patient State Index Monitor (PSA-4000, Physiometrix, North Billerica, MA)[4] and with a monitor of the entropy of the EEG signal (D-O Entropy, Datex-Ohmeda, Madison, WI).[5] The Audio Evoked Potential Index Monitor (AAI, Danmeter A/S, Odense, Denmark) showed similar efficacy when guiding the administration of a desflurane anesthetic compared to a group given traditional care.[6]

Critics of this type of monitoring argue that their usage may result in a higher incidence of intraoperative awareness as caregivers may, in an attempt to titrate the hypnotic agent to a particular number, decrease the hypnotic agent to a degree that a subsequent stimulation might be more likely to result in awareness than had the stimulation occurred during traditional care.[7] Preliminary studies, however, indicate that the utilization of BIS monitoring results in a decreased incidence of awareness in the care of both high-risk[8] and average-risk[9] patient groups. It is also noted that in most of the utility studies of these monitors, the monitored group typically is not discharged from the facility sooner despite faster early recovery milestones. This may reflect inefficiencies in the discharge process rather than a valid criticism of the technology.

While the exact role of these monitors in ambulatory surgery is yet to be determined, their use results in faster early recovery, higher percentage of PACU-bypass-eligible patients, and offers the possibility of improved "throughput" to practitioners who can streamline their center's traditional postoperative discharge process.

Premedication

Oral premedication with a benzodiazepine can provide a lowered anxiety state in the ambulatory patient. Also, administration resulted in lower "stress response" as measured by urinary cortisol and noradrenaline in patients who received a benzodiazepine compared to those who did not.[10] Not every patient, however, requires these medications. A survey of practice in the United Kingdom revealed that only 2% of adults received benzodiazepine premedication prior to urologic and orthopedic surgery.[11] An appropriate question is, if these agents are utilized, will they delay the recovery and discharge process? A recent meta-analysis found that most studies showed no significant effect between premedication and delayed discharge.[12] Studies that showed any effect on psychomotor functioning utilized relatively large oral doses of benzodiazepines: midazolam 7.5 mg[13] and 15 mg,[14] and diazepam 10 mg.[15] Oral midazolam 5–10 mg should not be withheld from anxious patients or those who request an anxiolytic out of the anesthesiologist's concern for delaying discharge.

Choice of Airway Device

The laryngeal mask airway (LMA) has greatly changed airway management in ambulatory surgery. There are multiple advantages in utilizing an LMA compared with an endotracheal tube (ETT). The insertion of an LMA is significantly less stimulating and requires less induction agent to blunt the hemodynamic stimulation to placement. In both normotensive and hypertensive patients endotracheal intubation was associated with increased hemodynamic response compared with LMA insertion.[16] In another study of the comparison between ETT and LMA, the LMA group had significantly less hemodynamic response to airway placement, less coughing upon removal, and less analgesic requirement in the PACU.[17] In a large multicenter study concerned with the effect of LMA use on ambulatory surgery center (ASC) efficiency, the LMA was associated with shorter PACU times and time to ambulation with a significantly lower incidence of sore throat.[18] ETT use also resulted in significantly greater postoperative laryngeal swelling compared with the LMA.[19] In addition, both neuromuscular blocking drugs and their reversal agents, with their attendant possible side effects, morbidities, and complications, can be avoided. Analysis of the causes of anaphylaxis during surgery repeatedly shows neuromuscular blocking drugs in general, and rocuronium and succinylcholine in particular, to be the most common etiologies.[20]

Concerns about increased risk for aspiration with LMA use have proven unfounded; the risk is about the same as that associated with ETT use.[21] When barium was instilled into the pharynx after LMA placement, none could be subsequently found in the trachea.[17] Measurements of pH in the hypopharynx during LMA use in spontaneously breathing patients showed no evidence of regurgitation of stomach contents.[22] While some are concerned that positive-pressure ventilation possibly adds to the risk of aspiration,[23] others disagree[24] and a survey of LMA use found it to be a common practice.[25] The Pro-Seal LMA was developed to allow greater positive-pressure ventilation and decrease the incidence of aspiration.[26] Comparison between the Pro-Seal LMA and the original LMA showed the Pro-Seal to be more difficult to insert, but to allow greater positive-pressure ventilation.[27] Case reports of both aspiration[28] and prevention of aspiration[29] during Pro-Seal LMA utilization have appeared in the literature.

The uses for the LMA continue to expand. It is a highly effective device during difficult intubations to maintain oxygenation and is in the American Society of Anesthesiologists (ASA) difficult-airway algorithm. Its use has been described in the prone position,[30] during endoscopic retrograde cholangiopancreatography (ERCP),[31] and for cesarean section.[32] New uses will continue to be investigated by innovative clinicians.

Although these uses are notable, the true advantage of the LMA resides in the more mundane use in the daily practice of the individual ambulatory anesthesiologist. Through the advantages listed above, patient care is significantly improved by utilizing a LMA instead of an ETT. Unless there is a clear contraindication to LMA use, it should be chosen rather than an endotracheal tube.

Induction of Anesthesia

Studies of induction of anesthesia for ambulatory surgery focus on the speed of induction, incidence of hemodynamic perturbation, incidence of apnea, and cost. While these issues are of concern, they are not highly correlated with the primary goal of rapid return to preoperative functional level.

Intravenous versus Inhalation Induction

Modern ambulatory anesthetics are induced with either intravenous agents, most often propofol, or inhalation agents, most often sevoflurane. Studies that compare these approaches have mixed results. With a protocol of increasing sevoflurane by 0.5% every three breaths, an inhalation induction took longer than propofol administered at a rate of 1% per second of the calculated induction dose.[33] However, a vital capacity breath of 8% sevoflurane from a primed circuit resulted in a faster induction than intravenous propofol 2 mg/kg, with similar side effects.[34] LMA insertion was more rapid and required fewer attempts after propofol 3 mg/kg compared to a vital capacity induction with 8% sevoflurane.[35] In the elderly, an induction of 8% sevoflurane was equally rapid as propofol administered at 10 mL/min; both were faster than sevoflurane increased 1% every three breaths.[36]

In these studies, there tended to be a greater incidence of apnea and hypotension in the propofol group, which was of limited clinical significance. The choice of induction agent is often determined by the planned maintenance anesthetic. Obviously, a propofol total intravenous anesthesia (TIVA) technique will be induced with propofol. An inhalation sevoflurane anesthetic can be induced with either, although a sevoflurane induction results in more postoperative nausea and vomiting (PONV).[37] An inhalation anesthetic with another agent could be induced with any intravenous agent.

Intravenous Induction

A recent comprehensive review of anesthetic technique for ambulatory surgery found that the psychomotor recovery from propofol was superior compared with other intravenous induction agents.[38] Doses range from 2.0 to 2.5 mg/kg but can be reduced by coinduction with midazolam and/or opiate (see below). Thiopental, compared with propofol, has an unattractive recovery profile.[39]

Despite the apparent superiority of propofol, some practitioners continue to utilize methohexital for reasons of economics or personal preference. Comparative studies that focus on quality of induction tend to find "smoother" inductions with propofol caused by more excitatory movement and hiccupping in the methohexital group.[40] Differences in recovery profile are probably not clinically significant.[41] Induction with methohexital may be less expensive than with propofol[42] in part because the induction dose, 1.5 mg/kg, is usually somewhat smaller, and some authors question whether the increased expense of propofol is justified.[43] Outcome from induction with mixture of equal volumes of 1% propofol and 0.5% methohexital is not clinically different from that with propofol alone.[44] Caution should perhaps be exercised in the asthmatic patient, however, as an increased incidence of wheezing has been reported following induction with methohexital compared with propofol.[45]

Coinduction

Induction doses of hypnotic agents can be decreased with the concomitant administration of benzodiazepines, usually midazolam, and/or opiate. During induction, propofol interacts synergistically with both midazolam and alfentanil. In the presence of midazolam and alfentanil, the 50% effective dose of propofol, the ED_{50}, was decreased by 52% and 73%, respectively.[46] In the presence of both midazolam and alfentanil, the ED_{50} of propofol was decreased by 82%. Further analysis of the same data found that the point of maximal synergy associated with a 95% chance of hypnosis in a 50-kg woman was midazolam 3.2 mg, alfentanil 1.8 mg, and propofol 6.9 mg.[47] While this was one-twelfth the dose of propofol alone that resulted in a 95% chance of hypnosis, 86 mg, the resultant average length of hypnosis, 14.4 min, was almost four times longer than that with propofol alone.

Coinduction may decrease the cost of propofol during induction and, in certain combinations, may decrease the hemodynamic consequences of hypnotic induction. To prevent the induction agents from delaying recovery parameters, the length of the resultant hypnosis needs to be taken into consideration, particularly for short procedures. While some information about various combinations of these agents is available, more knowledge is necessary to determine the ideal combinations for ambulatory surgery.

Midazolam. Propofol induction following midazolam has been investigated in several studies. The pharmacokinetics of midazolam suggests that peak effect is achieved in 4 min. When midazolam 3 mg was administered between 1 and 10 min before propofol induction, the ED_{50} of propofol was decreased by 34–67% with no statistical difference caused by the timing of midazolam.[48] In addition, patients who received midazolam had less recollection of events surrounding induction and recalled the induction experience as being more pleasant than those who did not receive midazolam. In another study, small doses of midazolam, 10 μg/kg, significantly decreased the propofol dose and induction time compared with placebo without delaying emergence parameters.[49] In a study of patients over 70 years of age, midazolam 20 μg/kg significantly decreased the necessary propofol dose but did not ameliorate the resultant hemodynamic depression.[50] After fentanyl 0.75 μg/kg, the administration of midazolam, both 25 and 50 μg/kg, resulted in decreased propofol requirements that were significantly more profound in elderly compared to younger patients.[51] The propensity of propofol to cause apnea or hemodynamic depression was not altered in either group by the propofol dose reduction achieved through midazolam coadministration. Postoperatively, after coinduction with midazolam 30 μg/kg, patients demonstrated decreased concentration but increased vigilance and accuracy as measured by neuropsychologic testing compared to patients who received no midazolam.[52]

Opiates.   Opiate utilization during induction not only decreases hypnotic agent requirement but also blunts the hemodynamic response to and improves conditions for airway instrumentation. Conditions for the insertion of an LMA are greatly improved by the coadministration of doses of remifentanil as small as 0.25[53] or 0.3 μg/kg,[54] or alfentanil 5 μg/kg.[55] For tracheal intubation with muscle relaxants, remifentanil 0.5 μg/kg or 1 μg/kg was found to have a similar effect as fentanyl 1 μg/kg.[56] After induction with propofol 2 mg/kg and without muscle relaxants, remifentanil 2 μg/kg[57] or alfentanil 40 μg/kg[58] was found to be required for acceptable intubating conditions. Other studies found that remifentanil doses of 3 μg/kg[59] or 4 μg/kg[60] were required for good or excellent conditions for intubation.

Maintenance of Anesthesia

A myriad of studies have compared maintenance anesthetics considering a variety of recovery parameters. In general, they found that the newer, less soluble agents desflurane[61–64] and sevoflurane [65,66] were superior to isoflurane. However, there are several studies that did not find a commendable difference.[67–69] Propofol TIVA was also superior to isoflurane in terms of discharge time and nausea rate, however at more than three times the cost.[70] Superiority of one agent over the other when comparing desflurane, sevoflurane, and propofol TIVA, however, is less clear because of contradictory information.

Desflurane Versus Sevoflurane

The blood/gas coefficient, or solubility, of desflurane, 0.45, is less than that of sevoflurane, 0.65, and therefore should result in faster recovery parameters. This is borne out in some, but not all, studies that compare the agents. In one study, desflurane resulted in faster awakening and extubation times, with no difference in further recovery milestones, neuropsychologic testing, or incidence of side effects.[71] Another study found faster emergence times and improved early psychomotor recovery, but no difference in discharge time, with desflurane utilization.[72] A third study, of gynecologic patients, found faster awakening and discharge, and a greater percentage of return to function on postoperative day one, in desflurane patients.[73] In another study, however, sevoflurane patients tended toward faster discharge, with one significantly superior neuropsychologic test result, compared to desflurane patients.[74] Prior concern about airway irritability demonstrated during desflurane inhalation inductions[75] was demonstrated to be unfounded when the agent was utilized for anesthetic maintenance with an LMA.[76]

Ultimately, there is probably not much difference in clinical outcome between the utilization of these two agents.[38] Clinicians seem to prefer one to the other, as do some authors.[77]

Propofol versus Desflurane or Sevoflurane

Studies that compared propofol-nitrous oxide or propofol-TIVA to desflurane or sevoflurane yield conflicting data. This is probably because the studies were conducted in a variety of different types of surgery and the criteria used to judge "depth of anesthesia" between the two groups differed. Of note, none of the studies utilized "depth of hypnosis" monitoring as most were performed before these criteria were widely clinically available.

In office-based plastic surgery patients, utilization of desflurane-nitrous oxide compared to propofol-nitrous oxide resulted in faster emergence and time to standing and ambulation, but no statistically significant difference in time to discharge readiness.[78] In patients undergoing laparoscopy, emergence times were faster with desflurane-nitrous oxide compared to propofol-nitrous oxide, but time to discharge was similar and there was less PONV in the propofol group.[79] In orthopedic patients, desflurane-nitrous oxide had similar emergence and discharge times and psychometric test results when compared to propofol-nitrous oxide.[80] A meta-analysis of six studies found that patients cared for with propofol were discharged home 17 min faster than patients given desflurane.[81] However, in a different study, when assessed for postural stability, a desflurane-treated group performed significantly better than a propofol-treated group.[82]

In a European multicenter study, emergence and discharge times were not different between groups cared for with sevoflurane-nitrous oxide or propofol-nitrous oxide; and PONV was lower in the propofol patients.[83] Another study found emergence times to be faster in sevoflurane-nitrous oxide-treated patients, but no difference in discharge times or incidence of PONV.[84] A third study found no difference in recovery parameters between the two groups, but a higher incidence of PONV in the sevoflurane group.[85] When compared to sevoflurane-nitrous oxide, use of propofol-nitrous oxide in an office-based plastic surgery population resulted in similar emergence times but significantly faster times to ambulation, toleration of fluids, and discharge.[86] In a study of patients undergoing knee arthroscopy, patients who received sevoflurane-nitrous oxide could follow commands significantly more quickly and had better early psychomotor testing than patients who received propofol-nitrous oxide.[87] There was no difference, however, in time to home readiness or actual discharge, and higher rates of PONV were found in the sevoflurane group. In a study that considered "fast-track" eligibility after laparoscopic tubal ligation, patients who received desflurane-nitrous oxide or sevoflurane-nitrous oxide were significantly more likely to be bypass-eligible than patients who received propofol-nitrous oxide: 90%, 75%, and 26%, respectively (Fig. 24-2).[88]

Propofol TIVA may prove to be superior to either desflurane or sevoflurane. When compared to sevoflurane-nitrous oxide, propofol TIVA with remifentanil resulted in similar early recovery times but faster times to discharge readiness.[89] In a study that compared propofol-remifentanil to both desflurane-nitrous oxide and sevoflurane-nitrous oxide, the propofol patients emerged significantly more quickly than patients given either inhalation agent.[90] The propofol patients performed better on psychomotor testing during the first hour; the difference between propofol and sevoflurane was greater than that between propofol and desflurane (Fig. 24-3). At 90 min, however, there were no discernible differences.

Consideration of all of this data does not demonstrate a clearly superior agent. As will be discussed, patients at risk for PONV probably benefit from either a propofol-nitrous oxide or a propofol-TIVA anesthetic. In plastic sur-

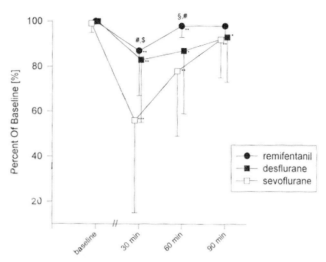

Figure 24-3   Percent change from baseline for the digit symbol substitution test following three anesthetic techniques. $^*p < 0.05$, $^{**}p < 0.01$, $^{***}p < 0.001$ value versus previous value. $^ap < 0.05$ remifentanil-propofol versus sevoflurane. $^bp < 0.05$ desflurane versus sevoflurane. $^cp < 0.05$ remifentanil-propofol versus desflurane. (From Larsen B, Seitz A, Larsen R. Recovery of cognitive function after remifentanil-propofol anesthesia: a comparison with desflurane and sevoflurane anesthesia. Anesth Analg 2000;90:168–74. Used by permission.)

gery patients, there is no difference in PONV between the two.[91] Studies that standardize the comparison of "depth of anesthesia" by utilizing hypnosis monitoring may help further clarify this issue.

Opiates

Opiates are utilized during the maintenance of anesthesia to exploit their synergistic relationship with hypnotic agents. The minimum alveolar concentration (MAC), the minimum alveolar concentration for blunting sympathetic responses after surgical incision (MAC_{BAR}) of inhalation agents, and the equivalent plasma concentrations of propofol are greatly decreased by the addition of relatively small amounts of opiate. This allows the anesthesia care team to maintain the anesthetic state of the patient with significantly less hypnotic agent than would otherwise be required if the hypnotic agent were used alone. When done skillfully, this allows the patient to emerge more quickly from the hypnotic state. Interestingly, these goals can also be met through an esmolol infusion, which has been shown to be as effective as either a remifentanil[92] or an alfentanil[93] infusion.

The choice of opiate and style of dosing, through either bolus or infusion techniques, is perhaps the most widely varied, and least studied, element of modern ambulatory anesthesia. The choice of opiate and dosing style should be guided by the expected length of the procedure, the desired relative "intensity" of the opiate's contribution to the anesthetic state, and the anticipated degree of postoperative pain. The practitioner needs to integrate all of these factors into the opiate management choices to achieve a predictably smooth and timely recovery. For example, a

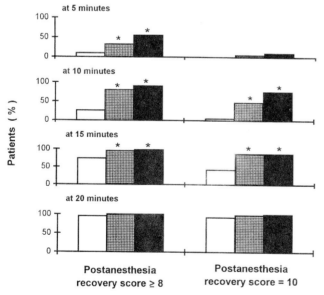

Figure 24-2   Percentage of patients achieving a postanesthesia recovery score of ≥ 8 and 10 at various times after the discontinuation of anesthesia. Desflurane group is represented by dark boxes, sevoflurane by shaded boxes, and propofol by white boxes ($^*p < 0.05$ compared with the propofol group). (From Song D, Joshi GP, White PF. Fast-track eligibility after ambulatory anesthesia: a comparison of desflurane, sevoflurane, and propofol. Anesth Analg 1998;86:267–73. Used by permission.)

remifentanil anesthetic that initially appears perfect because of ideal intraoperative stability is ultimately imperfect if the patient requires a prolonged postoperative stay because of pain.

The utility of studies that compare opiate techniques is often limited because equipotent doses were not compared. This is usually manifested in the observation that one technique led to more intraoperative hemodynamic stability than the other. It is therefore difficult to compare the effect of these techniques on postoperative recovery parameters. Nonetheless, useful information can be discerned.

Bolus versus infusion techniques. Administration of opiate by infusion is a technique that has advantages compared with the administration of opiates by intermittent boluses. The peaks and troughs of effect-site opiate level caused by boluses can be thereby avoided. This is particularly effective when the opiate infusion is titrated to specific anesthetic parameters rather than set at a "cookbook" infusion rate. For instance, if the nature of the procedure allows the patient to breathe spontaneously, titrating the opiate infusion to the patient's respiratory rate can be very effective. While this approach would predictably cause some respiratory depression and elevated end-tidal carbon dioxide (CO_2) levels, by definition the opiate dose so delivered is less than that which would otherwise result in apnea upon emergence. Computer-controlled infusion pumps, which deliver opiates according to pharmacokinetic modeling, are available for research purposes. They can be programmed to achieve either a predicted plasma or effect-site level of the infused agent. Investigators are currently developing closed-feedback loop algorithms for these devices, which may, someday, allow physiologic data from the patient to determine the opiate infusion schema.

The shorter the context-sensitive half-time, the more attractive is the opiate for infusion; relative overdosages are less likely to have significant consequences. This is especially true for remifentanil, which has a context-sensitive half-time of about 5 min. The practice of simply running high infusion rates of remifentanil without regard to titration should probably be avoided out of concern for the development of tolerance to opiates.[94] Even an opiate with a relatively long context-sensitive half-time, such as fentanyl, can benefit from administration by infusion. In a study in which patents were given only 70% nitrous oxide after thiopental induction, administration of a continuous fentanyl infusion adjusted to signs of anesthetic depth resulted in significantly less drug usage and faster emergence and discharge times compared to a technique of administrating fentanyl 50-μg boluses in response to similar signs.[95] Prolonged infusion of fentanyl without titration to clinical parameters may result in accumulation of effect as, theoretically, the context-sensitive half-time is significantly increased by prolonged infusion.[96]

Opiate with inhalation agents. In a study comparing infusions of equipotent doses of fentanyl, sufentanil, and alfentanil during an isoflurane–nitrous oxide anesthetic, there was no difference in the PACU time or overall discharge time between the agents.[97] Compared to fentanyl, there was less PONV following discharge from the PACU in the alfentanil group. In a study utilizing 0.8% isoflurane, patients who received an alfentanil infusion returned to spontaneous respiration and were extubated more quickly than those who received remifentanil.[98] However, the infusions were not equipotent as the remifentanil group had significantly less intraoperative response to noxious stimulation. Despite this, neuropsychologic testing favored the remifentanil group at 30, 60, and 90 min after surgery. Compared with simply increasing the desflurane in response to noxious stimulation, the administration of remifentanil averaging 0.07 ± 0.03 μg/kg/min resulted in significantly faster emergence and time to achieve PACU discharge.[99] There was no difference in PONV or need for antiemetic agents. In a study of 2438 patients (61% ambulatory) and either a propofol or sevoflurane anesthetic, patients who received a remifentanil regimen of 0.5-μg/kg bolus followed by an infusion of 0.25 μg/kg/min were compared to those who received fentanyl administered by usual clinical parameters.[100] Remifentanil patients were given additional opiates to transition them to PACU care. The remifentanil patients responded to verbal command, left the operating room, and were discharged home sooner than fentanyl-treated patients. In the first 24 hr, they scored significantly higher on four of nine assessments of functional recovery: walking without dizziness, thinking clearly, concentration, and communicating effectively.[101]

Opiates and propofol TIVA. Opiate infusion plays a particularly important role in the administration of TIVA. Alfentanil and remifentanil are usually utilized for this purpose. A study of patients undergoing laparoscopy comparing the two opiates during propofol TIVA found similar emergence times with similar home readiness times.[102] However, the alfentanil patients were eligible for PACU discharge sooner and required additional analgesics later than the remifentanil patients. In another study comparing the two, remifentanil patients had significantly shorter times to response to verbal commands, extubation, and achieving an Aldrete score greater than or equal to 9.[103] Home readiness times were the same, however, the remifentanil patients had more postoperative pain.

An interesting study was done on the infusion rates of propofol and alfentanil in the presence of 60% nitrous oxide, which examined the relationship between the two drugs and the effect of various combinations on recovery parameters.[104] A synergistic relationship between the two was described and early recovery times varied inversely with the targeted alfentanil concentration. For example, the time to extubation was 20.2, 7.4, 5.2, and 3.8 min in patients whose intraoperative target predicted alfentanil concentration was 0, 50, 100, and 150 ng/mL, respectively. The 150-ng/mL group, however, required a PACU stay of 30 min longer than the 50- or 100-ng/mL group, supporting the conclusion that the ideal combination was found in the 100-ng/mL group. The infusion schedule for alfentanil and the median required propofol infusion rates in this group were described (Table 24-1). Ten min before the conclusion of the case the alfentanil was discontinued; 5 min before the conclusion, the propofol was discontinued.

Table 24-1 An Infusion Schedule for TIVA with Alfentanil and Propofol That Yielded the Best Combination of Emergence Time and Time to PACU Discharge

Time Postinduction (min)	Alfentanil Bolus (μg/kg)	Alfentanil Infusion (μg/kg/min)	Propofol Bolus (mg/kg)	Median Propofol Infusion Rate for Adequate Anesthesia (μg/kg • min)
0	19		2	
0–5		1.01		0
5–15		0.92		95
15–30		0.80		74
30–60		0.67		73

The alfentanil is calculated to yield an effect site level of 100 ng/mL. The propofol infusion rate is the median rate for the population studied.

SOURCE: Pavlin DJ, Arends RH, Gunn HC, et al. Optimal propofol-alfentanil combinations for supplementing nitrous oxide for outpatient surgery. Anesthesiology 1999;91:97–108. Used by permission.

These infusion rates are a good reference point for those who want to practice TIVA with alfentanil. Similar propofol infusion rates can be utilized with a remifentanil infusion of 0.1–0.2 μg/kg/min. By using higher infusion rates of remifentanil, 0.2–0.3 μg/kg/min, the required propofol dose can be decreased even further, to 35–50 μg/kg/min. The utilization of depth-of-hypnosis monitors is especially useful in TIVA cases.

Anesthetic Techniques for Minimizing PONV

Anesthetic technique can influence the incidence of PONV, particularly for those at high risk. In a randomized clinical trial of patients at all levels of risk for PONV, inhalation agents were associated with 15–17 times increase in relative risk for PONV in the first two postoperative hours compared to propofol.[105] The risk for PONV with inhalation anesthesia increased with increased anesthetic duration (Fig. 24-4). Meta-analysis of studies that compared propofol to inhalation anesthesia in the moderate-to-high-risk patient demonstrated that induction and maintenance with propofol compared with inhalational agent maintenance resulted in a significantly lower incidence of PONV[106] and that propofol maintenance compared with inhalational agent maintenance resulted in less PONV regardless of induction agent or use of nitrous oxide or opiates.[107] Utilization of nitrous oxide is associated with increased PONV in the high-risk patient and should probably be avoided, particularly if inhalational agents are utilized.[108,109] Avoidance of large doses of neuromuscular-blocking-reversal agents also decreases the risk for PONV.[110] Opiates can cause PONV, but their avoidance is not always possible as they are often required for successful postoperative pain management. Opiates in appropriate doses have been demonstrated to not increase PONV.[111]

TIVA with propofol and a judicious amount of an appropriate opiate is a technique that is very attractive for the prevention of PONV in the high-risk patient and may ultimately be the technique of choice. For example, in middle ear surgery, TIVA with propofol and remifentanil resulted in less PONV and antiemetic requirements in the

PACU compared to an inhalation technique using isoflurane and fentanyl.[112]

It is not clear whether the technique of choice for the high-risk patient is inhalation anesthesia with combination PONV prophylaxis or TIVA with propofol. A recent study compared inhalation anesthesia plus dolasetron to TIVA with and without dolasetron in ambulatory gynecologic patients. It was found that propofol TIVA, with or without dolasetron, reduced postoperative nausea, but not perioperative vomiting or antiemetic requirement, when compared with inhalation anesthesia plus dolasetron.[113] Further work is needed in this area to determine the superior approach.

The clinical practice of the authors for high-risk patients is to utilize a propofol TIVA technique with triple prophylactic PONV therapy. This approach has generated

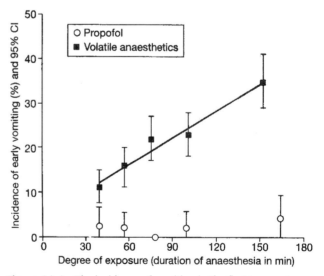

Figure 24-4 The incidence of vomiting in the first two postoperative hours compared with the length of exposure to either volatile agents or propofol. (From Apfel CC, Kranke P, Katz MH, et al. Volatile anaesthetics may be the main cause of early but not delayed postoperative vomiting: a randomized controlled trial of factorial design. Br J Anaesth 2002;88:659–68. Used by permission.)

a series of thankful letters from patients with history of severe PONV who greatly preferred their TIVA to whatever they had previously received.

PACU BYPASS

The final ingredient in a modern ambulatory anesthesia is the appropriate disposition of the patient. By utilizing short-acting agents and through careful titration techniques, a percentage of patients meet PACU discharge criteria within a few min of the end of surgery. Taking these patients to the high-acuity environment of the PACU is unnecessary and leads to inefficiencies of the recovery process. In even the most streamlined PACU processes, there are inevitable systemic factors, paperwork, telephone calls, and transport issues that delay the process. A very useful scale to determine bypass eligibility is the White modification of the Aldrete score (Table 24-2).[114] In the authors' experience, patients who are comfortable and can move themselves onto a gurney or into a wheelchair can bypass the PACU.

Implementation of PACU bypass protocols requires education and agreement among surgeons, anesthesiologists, and nursing staff. A study of five centers showed that by implementing a bypass program without change in anesthetic technique, bypass rates for general anesthesia patients were increased from 0.4% to 31.8% without change in outcome.[115] A large study of knee arthroscopy patients who received either general anesthesia or nerve blocks showed that 87% could bypass the PACU.[116]

An alternative strategy is to simply discharge patients home from the PACU, thereby skipping the step of transport to the PACU second-stage area. In a recent study of 1380 patients, 952 patients were triaged to a PACU "fast-track" area.[117] Eighty-eight percent of those patients were discharged to home within an hour, which compared favorably with patients who bypassed the PACU.

Those who are currently designing a post-ambulatory-surgery recovery-and-discharge process should strongly consider implementing a one-stop process with the ability to care for the increasingly rare patient who requires intensive and prolonged recovery care.

SUMMARY

The modern ambulatory anesthesiologist who is administering a general anesthetic attempts to do everything within his/her power to return the patient to the preoperative level of functioning as soon as possible. This involves utilization of judicious amounts of faster-acting anesthetic agents and PACU bypass in the appropriate patients, and consideration of utilizing "depth of hypnosis" monitors. Minimizing undesirable side effects, such as postoperative pain and PONV, need also to be factored into the anesthetic choices made. It should further be the goal of the ambulatory anesthesiologist to educate anesthetic colleagues, nurses, surgeons, and other ASC health professionals as to how to change their current practice to incorporate these principles. Finally, clinical practice guidelines based on tri-

Table 24-2 The White Modification of the Aldrete Postoperative Score

Category/Criteria	Score
Level of consciousness	
Awake and oriented	2
Arousable with minimal stimulation	1
Responsive only to tactile stimulation	0
Physical activity	
Able to move all extremities on command	2
Some weakness in movement of extremities	1
Unable to voluntarily move extremities	0
Hemodynamic stability	
Blood pressure < 15% of baseline mean arterial pressure (MAP) value	2
Blood pressure 15–30% of baseline MAP value	1
Blood pressure > 30% below baseline MAP value	0
Respiratory stability	
Able to breathe deeply	2
Tachypnea with good cough	1
Dyspneic with weak cough	0
Oxygen saturation status	
Maintains value > 90% on room air	2
Requires supplemental oxygen (nasal prongs)	1
Saturation < 90% with supplemental oxygen	0
Postoperative pain assessment	
None or mild discomfort	2
Moderate to severe pain	1
Persistent severe pain	0
Postoperative emetic symptoms	
None to mild nausea with no active vomiting	2
Transient vomiting or retching	1
Persistent moderate to severe nausea and vomiting	0
Total score	14

The patient may be considered for PACU bypass if the score is at least 12 of 14.

SOURCE: White PF, Song D. New criteria for fast-tracking after outpatient anesthesia: a comparison with the modified Aldrete's scoring system. Anesth Analg 1999;88:1069–72.

als that demonstrate these principles should be incorporated into daily ambulatory anesthesia practice.

REFERENCES

1.   Sinclair DR, Chung F, Smiley A. General anesthesia does not impair simulator driving skills in volunteers in the immediate recovery period- a pilot study. Can J Anaesth 2003;50:238–45.

2. Gan TJ, Glass PS, Windsor A, et al. Bispectral index monitoring allows faster emergence and improved recovery from propofol, alfentanil, and nitrous oxide anesthesia. BIS Utility Study Group. Anesthesiology 1997;87:808–15.

3. Song D, Joshi GP, White PF. Titration of volatile anesthesics using bispectral index facilitates recovery after ambulatory surgery. Anesthesiology 1997;87:842–48.

4. Drover DR, Lemmens HJ, Pierce ET, et al. Patient State Index: titration of delivery and recovery from propofol, alfentanil, and nitrous oxide anesthesia. Anesthesiology 2002;97:82–89.

5. Yli-Hankala A, Vakkuri A, Sandin R, et al. EEG entropy monitoring decreases propofol consumption and shortens early recovery times. Eur J Anaesthesiol 2000;17:83.

6. Recart A, White PF, Wang A, et al. Effect of auditory evoked potential index monitoring on anesthetic drug requirements and recovery profile after laparoscopic surgery: a clinical utility study. Anesthesiology 2003;99:813–18.

7. Kalkman CJ, Drummond JC. Monitors of depth of anesthesia, quo vadis? Anesthesiology 2002;96:784–87.

8. Myles P, Leslie K. A large randomized trial of BIS monitoring to prevent awareness in high risk patients. Anesthesiology 2003;99:A-320.

9. Lennmarken C, Ekman A. Incidence of awareness using BIS monitoring. Anesth Analg 2003;96:S–133.

10. Duggan M, Dowd N, O'Mara D, et al. Benzodiazepine premedication may attenuate the stress response in daycase anesthesia: a pilot study. Can J Anaesth 2002;49:932–35.

11. Payne K, Moore EW, Elliott RA, et al. Anaesthesia for day case surgery: a survey of adult clinical practice in the UK. Eur J Anaesthesiol 2003;20:311–24.

12. Smith AF, Pittaway AJ. Premedication for anxiety in adult day surgery (Cochrane Review). The Cochrane Library, Issue 1, 2003. Oxford: Update Software.

13. Ahmed N, Khan FA. Evaluation of oral midazolam as premedication in day care surgery in adult Pakistani patients. J Pak Med Assoc 1995;45:239–41.

14. Raybould D, Bradshaw EG. Premedication for day case surgery: a study of oral midazolam. Anaesthesia 1987;42:591–95.

15. Dyck JB, Chung F. A comparison of propanolol and diazepam for preoperative anxiolysis. Can J Anaesth 1991;38:704–9.

16. Fujii Y, Tanaka H, Toyooka H. Circulatory responses to laryngeal mask airway insertion or tracheal intubation in normotensive and hypertensive patients. Can J Anaesth 1995;42:32–36.

17. Cork RC, Depa RM, Standen JR. Prospective comparison of use of the laryngeal mask and endotracheal tube for ambulatory surgery. Anesth Analg 1994;79:719–27.

18. Joshi GP, Inagaki Y, White PF, et al. Use of the laryngeal mask airway as an alternative to the tracheal tube during ambulatory anesthesia. Anesth Analg 1997;85:573–77.

19. Tanaka A, Isono S, Ishikawa T, et al. Laryngeal resistance before and after minor surgery: endotracheal tube versus laryngeal mask airway. Anesthesiology 2003;99:252–58.

20. Mertes PM, Laxenaire MC, Alla F, et al. Anaphylactic and anaphylactoid reactions occurring during anesthesia in France in 1999–2000. Anesthesiology 2003;99:536–45.

21. Brimacombe JR, Berry A. The incidence of aspiration associated with the laryngeal mask airway: a meta-analysis of published literature. J Clin Anesth 1995;7(4):297–305.

22. Joshi GP, Morrison SG, Okonkwo NA, White PF. Continuous hypopharyngeal pH measurements in spontaneously breathing anesthetized outpatients: laryngeal mask airway versus tracheal intubation. Anesth Analg 1996;82:254–57.

23. Sidaras G, Hunter JM. Is it safe to artificially ventilate a paralysed patient through the laryngeal mask? The jury is still out. Br J Anaesth 2001;86:749–53.

24. Verghese C, Jago R. Is it safe to artificially ventilate paralysed patients through a laryngeal mask? Br J Anaesth 2002;88:149–51.

25. Verghese C, Brimacombe JR. Survey of laryngeal mask airway usage in 11,910 patients: safety and efficacy for conventional and nonconventional usage. Anesth Analg. 1996;82:129–33.

26. Brimacombe J, Keller C. The ProSeal laryngeal mask airway. Anesthesiol Clin North Am 2002;20:871–91.

27. Cook TM, Nolan JP, Verghese C, et al. Randomized crossover comparison of the proseal with the classic laryngeal mask airway in unparalysed anaesthetized patients. Br J Anaesth 2002;88:527–33.

28. Brimacombe J, Keller C. Aspiration of gastric contents during use of a ProSeal laryngeal mask airway secondary to unidentified foldover malposition. Anesth Analg 2003;97:1192–94.

29. Mark DA. Protection from aspiration with the LMA-ProSeal after vomiting: a case report. Can J Anaesth 2003;50:78–80.

30. Ng A, Raitt DG, Smith G. Induction of anesthesia and insertion of a laryngeal mask airway in the prone position for minor surgery. Anesth Analg 2002;94:1194–98.

31. Osborn IP, Cohen J, Soper RJ, Roth LA. Laryngeal mask airway—a novel method of airway protection during ERCP: comparison with endotracheal intubation. Gastrointest Endosc 2002;56:122–28.

32. Han TH, Brimacombe J, Lee EJ, Yang HS. The laryngeal mask airway is effective (and probably safe) in selected healthy parturients for elective Cesarean section: a prospective study of 1067 cases. Can J Anaesth 2001;48:1117–1121.

33. Thompson S, Drummond GB. Loss of volition and pain response during induction of anaesthesia with propofol or sevoflurane. Br J Anaesth 2001;87:283–86.

34. Philip BK, Lombard LL, Roaf ER, et al. Comparison of vital capacity induction with sevoflurane to intravenous induction with propofol for adult ambulatory anesthesia. Anesth Analg 1999;89:623–27.

35. Ti LK, Chow MY, Lee TL. Comparison of sevoflurane with propofol for laryngeal mask airway insertion in adults. Anesth Analg 1999;88:908–12.

36. Kirkbride DA, Parker JL, Williams GD, Buggy D. Induction of anesthesia in the elderly ambulatory patient: a double-blinded comparison of propofol and sevoflurane. Anesth Analg 2001;93:1185–87.

37. Elliott RA, Payne K, Moore JK, et al. Clinical and economic choices in anaesthesia for day surgery: a prospective randomised controlled trial. Anaesthesia 2003;58:412–21.

38. Pollard BJ, Elliott RA, Moore EW. Anaesthetic agents in adult day case surgery. Eur J Anaesthesiol 2003;20:1–9.

39. Raeder JC, Misvaer G. Comparison of propofol induction with thiopentone or methohexitone in short outpatient general anaesthesia. Acta Anaesthesiol Scand 1988;32:607–13.

40. Gold MI, Abraham EC, Herrington C. A controlled investigation of propofol, thiopentone and methohexitone. Can J Anaesth 1987;34:478–83.

41. Boysen K, Sanchez R, Ravn J, et al. Comparison of induction with and first hour of recovery from brief propofol and methohexital anesthesia. Acta Anaesthesiol Scand 1990;34:212–15.

42. Sun R, Watcha MF, White PF, et al. A cost comparison of methohexital and propofol for ambulatory anesthesia. Anesth Analg 1999;89:311–16.

43. Cade L, Morley PT, Ross AW. Is propofol cost-effective for daysurgery patients? Anaesth Intens Care 1991;19:201–4.

44. Thompson N, Robertson GS. Comparison of propofol and a propofol-methohexitone mixture for induction of day-case anaesthesia. Br J Anaesth 1996;77:213–16.

45. Pizov R, Brown RH, Weiss YS, et al. Wheezing during induction of general anesthesia in patients with and without asthma: a randomized, blinded trial. Anesthesiology 1995;82:1111–16.

46. Short TG, Plummer JL, Chui PT. Hypnotic and anaesthetic interactions between midazolam, propofol and alfentanil. Br J Anaesth 1992;69:162–67.

47. Minto CF, Schnider TW, Short TG, et al. Response surface model for anesthetic drug interactions. Anesthesiology 2000;92:1603–16.

48. Ong LB, Plummer JL, Waldow WC, Owen H. Timing of midazolam and propofol administration for co-induction of anaesthesia. Anaesth Intens Care 2000;28:527–31.

49. Adachi YU, Watanabe K, Higuchi H, Satoh T. A small dose of midazolam decreases the time to achieve hypnosis without delaying emergence during short-term propofol anesthesia. J Clin Anesth 2001;13:277–80.

50. Jones NA, Elliott S, Knight J. A comparison between midazolam co-induction and propofol predosing for the induction of anaesthesia in the elderly. Anaesthesia 2002;57:649–53.

51. Cressey DM, Claydon P, Bhaskaran NC, Reilly CS. Effect of midazolam pretreatment on induction dose requirements of propofol in combination with fentanyl in younger and older adults. Anaesthesia 2001;56:108–13.

52. Tighe KE, Warner JA. The effect of co-induction with midazolam upon recovery from propofol infusion anaesthesia. Anaesthesia 1997;52:1000–4.

53. Lee MP, Kua JS, Chiu WK. The use of remifentanil to facilitate the insertion of the laryngeal mask airway. Anesth Analg 2001;93:359–62.

54. Grewal K, Samsoon G. Facilitation of laryngeal mask airway insertion: effects of remifentanil administered before induction with target-controlled propofol infusion. Anaesthesia 2001;56:897–901.

55. Ang S, Cheong KF, Ng TI. Alfentanil co-induction for laryngeal mask insertion. Anaesth Intensive Care 1999;27:175–58.

56. Song D, Whitten CW, White PF. Use of remifentanil during anesthetic induction: a comparison with fentanyl in the ambulatory setting. Anesth Analg 1999;88:734–36.

57. Grant S, Noble S, Woods A, et al. Assessment of intubating conditions in adults after induction with propofol and varying doses of remifentanil. Br J Anaesth 1998;81:540–43.

58. Scheller MS, Zornow MH, Saidman LJ. Tracheal intubation without the use of muscle relaxants: a technique using propofol and varying doses of alfentanil. Anesth Analg 1992;75:788–93.

59. Stevens JB, Wheatley L. Tracheal intubation in ambulatory surgery patients: using remifentanil and propofol without muscle relaxants. Anesth Analg 1998;86:45–49.

60. Erhan E, Ugur G, Alper I, et al. Tracheal intubation without muscle relaxants: remifentanil or alfentanil in combination with propofol. Eur J Anaesthesiol 2003;20:37–43.

61. Tsai SK, Lee C, Kwan WF, Chen BJ. Recovery of cognitive functions after anaesthesia with desflurane or isoflurane and nitrous oxide. Br J Anaesth 1992;69:255–58.

62. Smiley RM, Ornstein E, Matteo RS. Desflurane and isoflurane in surgical patients: comparison of emergence time. Anesthesiology 1991;74:425–28.

63. Ghouri AF, Bodner M, White PF. Recovery profile after desflurane-nitrous oxide versus isoflurane-nitrous oxide in outpatients. Anesthesiology 1991;74:419–24.

64. Fletcher JE, Sebel PS, Murphy MR, et al. Psychomotor performance after desflurane anesthesia: a comparison with isoflurane. Anesth Analg 1991;73:260–65.

65. Philip BK, Kallar SK, Bogetz MS, et al. A multicenter comparison of maintenance and recovery with sevoflurane or isoflurane for adult ambulatory anesthesia. The Sevoflurane Multicenter Ambulatory Group. Anesth Analg 1996;83:314–19.

66. Ebert TJ, Robinson BJ, Uhrich TD, et al. Recovery from sevoflurane anesthesia: a comparison to isoflurane and propofol anesthesia. Anesthesiology 1998;89:1524–31.

67. Gupta A, Kullander M, Ekberg K, et al. Anaesthesia for day-care arthroscopy: a comparison between desflurane and isoflurane. Anaesthesia 1996;51:56–62.

68. Elcock DH, Sweeney BP. Sevoflurane vs. isoflurane: a clinical comparison in day surgery. Anaesthesia 2002;57:52–56.

69. Karlsen KL, Persson E, Wennberg E, Stenqvist O. Anaesthesia, recovery and postoperative nausea and vomiting after breast surgery: a comparison between desflurane, sevoflurane and isoflurane anaesthesia. Acta Anaesthesiol Scand 2000;44:489–93.

70. Visser K, Hassink EA, Bonsel GJ, et al. Randomized controlled trial of total intravenous anesthesia with propofol versus inhalation anesthesia with isoflurane-nitrous oxide: postoperative nausea with vomiting and economic analysis. Anesthesiology 2001;95:616–26.

71. Nathanson MH, Fredman B, Smith I, White PF. Sevoflurane versus desflurane for outpatient anesthesia: a comparison of maintenance and recovery profiles. Anesth Analg 1995;81:1186–90.

72. Naidu-Sjosvard K, Sjoberg F, Gupta A. Anaesthesia for videoarthroscopy of the knee. A comparison between desflurane and sevoflurane. Acta Anaesthesiol Scand 1998;42:464–71.

73. Mahmoud NA, Rose DJ, Laurence AS. Desflurane or sevoflurane for gynaecological day-case anaesthesia with spontaneous respiration. Anaesthesia 2001;56:171–74.

74. Tarazi EM, Philip BK. A comparison of recovery after sevoflurane or desflurane in ambulatory anesthesia. J Clin Anesth 1998;10:272–77.

75. Zwass MS, Fisher DM, Welborn LG, et al. Induction and maintenance characteristics of anesthesia with desflurane and nitrous oxide in infants and children. Anesthesiology 1992;76:373–78.

76. Eshima RW, Maurer A, King T, et al. A comparison of airway responses during desflurane and sevoflurane administration via a laryngeal mask airway for maintenance of anesthesia. Anesth Analg 2003;96:701–5.

77. Ghatge S, Lee J, Smith I. Sevoflurane: an ideal agent for adult day-case anesthesia. Acta Anaesthesiol Scand 2003;47:917–31.

78. Tang J, White PF, Wender RH, et al. Fast-track office-based anesthesia: a comparison of propofol versus desflurane with antiemetic prophylaxis in spontaneously breathing patients. Anesth Analg 2001;92:95–99.

79. Van Hemelrijck J, Smith I, White PF. Use of desflurane for outpatient anesthesia: a comparison with propofol and nitrous oxide. Anesthesiology 1991;75:197–203.

80. Rapp SE, Conahan TJ, Pavlin DJ, et al. Comparison of desflurane with propofol in outpatients undergoing peripheral orthopedic surgery. Anesth Analg 1992;75:572–79.

81. Dexter F, Tinker JH. Comparisons between desflurane and isoflurane or propofol on time to following commands and time to discharge. A metaanalysis. Anesthesiology 1995;83:77–82.

82. Song D, Chung F, Wong J, Yogendran S. The assessment of postural stability after ambulatory anesthesia: a comparison of desflurane with propofol. Anesth Analg 2002;94:60–64.

83. Smith I, Terhoeve PA, Hennart D, et al. A multicentre comparison of the costs of anaesthesia with sevoflurane or propofol. Br J Anaesth 1999;83:564–70.

84. Jellish WS, Lien CA, Fontenot HJ, Hall R. The comparative effects of sevoflurane versus propofol in the induction and maintenance of anesthesia in adult patients. Anesth Analg 1996;82:479–85.

85. Fredman B, Nathanson MH, Smith I. Sevoflurane for outpatient anesthesia: a comparison with propofol. Anesth Analg 1995;81:823–28.

86. Tang J, Chen L, White PF. Recovery profile, costs, and patient satisfaction with propofol and sevoflurane for fast-track office-based anesthesia. Anesthesiology 1999;91:253–61.

87. Raeder J, Gupta A, Pedersen FM. Recovery characteristics of sevoflurane- or propofol-based anaesthesia for day-care surgery. Acta Anaesthesiol Scand 1997;41(8):988–94.

88. Song D, Joshi GP, White PF. Fast-track eligibility after ambulatory anesthesia: a comparison of desflurane, sevoflurane, and propofol. Anesth Analg 1998;86:267–73.

89. Montes FR, Trillos JE, Rincon IE, et al. Comparison of total intravenous anesthesia and sevoflurane-fentanyl anesthesia for outpatient otorhinolaryngeal surgery. J Clin Anesth 2002;14:324–28.

90. Larsen B, Seitz A, Larsen R. Recovery of cognitive function after remifentanil-propofol anesthesia: a comparison with desflurane and sevoflurane anesthesia. Anesth Analg 2000;90:168–74.

91. Tang J, Chen L, White PF, et al. Use of propofol for office-based anesthesia: effect of nitrous oxide on recovery profile. J Clin Anesth 1999;11:226–30.

92. Coloma M, Chiu JW, White PF, Armbruster SC. The use of esmolol as an alternative to remifentanil during desflurane anesthesia for fast-track outpatient gynecologic laparoscopic surgery. Anesth Analg 2001;92:352–57.

93. Smith I, Van Hemelrijck J, White PF. Efficacy of esmolol versus alfentanil as a supplement to propofol-nitrous oxide anesthesia. Anesth Analg 1991;73:540–46.

94. Vinik HR, Kissin I. Rapid development of tolerance to analgesia during remifentanil infusion in humans. Anesth Analg 1998;86:1307–11.

95. White PF. Use of continuous infusion versus intermittent bolus administration of fentanyl or ketamine during outpatient anesthesia. Anesthesiology 1983;59:294–300.

96. Shafer SL, Varvel JR. Pharmacokinetics, pharmacodynamics, and rational opioid selection. Anesthesiology 1991;74:53–63.

97. Langevin S, Lessard MR, Trepanier CA, Baribault JP. Alfentanil causes less postoperative nausea and vomiting than equipotent doses of fentanyl or sufentanil in outpatients. Anesthesiology 1999;91:1666–73.

98. Cartwright DP, Kvalsvik O, Cassuto J, et al. A randomized, blind comparison of remifentanil and alfentanil during anesthesia for outpatient surgery. Anesth Analg 1997;85:1014–19.

99. Song D, White PF. Remifentanil as an adjuvant during desflurane anesthesia facilitates early recovery after ambulatory surgery. J Clin Anesth 1999;11:364–67.

100. Twersky RS, Jamerson B, Warner DS, et al. Hemodynamics and emergence profile of remifentanil versus fentanyl prospectively compared in a large population of surgical patients. J Clin Anesth 2001;13:407–16.

101. Fleisher LA, Hogue S, Colopy M, et al. Does functional ability in the postoperative period differ between remifentanil- and fentanyl-based anesthesia? J Clin Anesth 2001;13:401–6.

102. Philip BK, Scuderi PE, Chung F, et al. Remifentanil compared with alfentanil for ambulatory surgery using total intravenous anesthesia. The Remifentanil/Alfentanil Outpatient TIVA Group. Anesth Analg 1997;84:515–21.

103. Alper I, Erhan E, Ugur G, Ozyar B. Remifentanil versus alfentanil in total intravenous anaesthesia for day case surgery. Eur J Anaesthesiol 2003;20:61–64.

104. Pavlin DJ, Arends RH, Gunn HC, et al. Optimal propofol-alfentanil combinations for supplementing nitrous oxide for outpatient surgery. Anesthesiology 1999;91:97–108.

105. Apfel CC, Kranke P, Katz MH, et al. Volatile anaesthetics may be the main cause of early but not delayed postoperative vomiting: a randomized controlled trial of factorial design. Br J Anaesth 2002;88:659–68.

106. Tramer M, Moore A, McQuay H. Propofol anaesthesia and postoperative nausea and vomiting: quantitative systematic review of randomized controlled studies. Br J Anaesth 1997;78:247–55.

107. Sneyd JR, Carr A, Byrom WD, Bilski AJ. A meta-analysis of nausea and vomiting following maintenance of anaesthesia with propofol or inhalational agents. Eur J Anaesthesiol 1998;15:433–45.

108. Tramer M, Moore A, McQuay H. Omitting nitrous oxide in general anaesthesia: meta-analysis of intraoperative awareness and postoperative emesis in randomized controlled trials. Br J Anaesth 1996;76:186–93.

109. Divatia JV, Vaidya JS, Badwe RA, Hawaldar RW. Omission of nitrous oxide during anesthesia reduces the incidence of postoperative nausea and vomiting: a meta-analysis. Anesthesiology 1996;85:1055–62.

110. Tramer MR, Fuchs-Buder T. Omitting antagonism of neuromuscular block: effect on postoperative nausea and vomiting and risk of residual paralysis: a systematic review. Br J Anaesth 1999;82:379–86.

111. Cepeda MS, Gonzalez F, Granados V, et al. Incidence of nausea and vomiting in outpatients undergoing general anesthesia in relation to selection of intraoperative opioid. J Clin Anesth 1996;8:324–28.

112. Mukherjee K, Seavell C, Rawlings E, Weiss A. A comparison of total intravenous with balanced anaesthesia for middle ear surgery: effects on postoperative nausea and vomiting, pain, and conditions of surgery. Anaesthesia 2003;58:176–80.

113. Paech MJ, Lee BH, Evans SF. The effect of anaesthetic technique on postoperative nausea and vomiting after day-case gynaecological laparoscopy. Anaesth Intens Care 2002;30:153–59.

114. White PF, Song D. New criteria for fast-tracking after outpatient anesthesia: a comparison with the modified Aldrete's scoring system. Anesth Analg 1999;88:1069–72.

115. Apfelbaum JL, Walawander CA, Grasela TH, et al. Eliminating intensive postoperative care in same-day surgery patients using short-acting anesthetics. Anesthesiology 2002;97:66–74.

116. Williams BA, Kentor ML, Williams JP, et al. PACU bypass after outpatient knee surgery is associated with fewer unplanned hospital admissions but more phase II nursing interventions. Anesthesiology 2002;97:981–88.

117. White PF, Rawal S, Nguyen J, Watkins A. PACU fast-tracking: an alternative to "bypassing" the PACU for facilitating the recovery process after ambulatory surgery. J Perianesth Nurs 2003;18:247–53.

SPECIFIC AMBULATORY PROCEDURES

Ambulatory Anesthesia for Head and Neck Surgery

KAREN C. NIELSEN • SUSAN M. STEELE

INTRODUCTION

A large variety of ophthalmic surgical procedures as well as ear, throat, and nose surgeries are now being performed in the ambulatory setting. Anesthetic management is critical for the success or failure of head and neck surgery. This chapter will review optimal anesthetic management to ensure improved patient outcomes in this outpatient population.

ANESTHESIA FOR EAR SURGERY

General anesthesia is used for the majority of ear surgical procedures, including tympanoplasty, mastoidectomy, and myringotomy. Local anesthetic infiltration with intravenous sedation is used for procedures such as stapedectomy or stapedotomy, and simple middle ear surgery of short duration (60–120 min).

Local Anesthesia with Monitored Anesthesia Care

Light sedation is usually used to keep the patient calm, cooperative, and comfortable during a surgical procedure. Intravenous propofol (0.5–0.8 mg/kg) is used during local anesthetic injection. Small doses of intravenous midazolam (0.02–0.04 mg/kg) and fentanyl (0.05–0.2 µg/kg) can be titrated during the procedure.

Four nerves provide the sensory innervation of the ear: the auriculotemporal nerve, the great auricular nerve, the tympanic nerve, and the auricular branch of the vagus nerve. The auriculotemporal nerve is a branch of the mandibular division of the trigeminal nerve, which supplies the outer auditory meatus. The great auricular nerve is a branch of the cervical plexus that supplies the medial and lower aspect of the auricle as well as part of the external auditory meatus. The tympanic nerve, branch of the glossopharyngeal nerve, supplies the tympanic cavity. Fi-

nally, the auricular branch of the vagus also supplies the external auditory meatus and the concha. Two mL of long-acting local anesthetic can be used (e.g., 0.5% ropivacaine) for each of the four nerves.

General Anesthesia

Several aspects of general anesthesia can influence ear surgery outcomes including the use of nitrous oxide (N_2O), facial nerve preservation, control of intraoperative bleeding, and prevention of postoperative nausea and vomiting (PONV).

Middle Ear Pressure and Nitrous Oxide

The middle ear is a cavity containing air that intermittently is vented by the opening of the eustachian tube. When N_2O is used, which is 34 times more soluble in blood than nitrogen, this gas diffuses much more rapidly into the middle ear via mucosal blood vessels than the nitrogen can leave. In a fixed cavity such as the middle ear, the result is an increase in pressure. In a normal ear, passive venting by the eustachian tube occurs at a pressure of 200–300 mmHg. In a diseased ear, the passive venting is compromised and middle ear pressure can reach 375 mmHg within 30 min of the start of the administration of N_2O.

Negative pressure can also occur after discontinuation of N_2O owing to its rapid diffusion out of the middle ear.[1] Subatmospheric middle ear pressure has been implicated in transient hearing loss in the postoperative period and may contribute to the development of serous otitis.[1,2] Increased middle ear pressures due to N_2O may lead to PONV, tympanic membrane rupture, and temporary deterioration of middle ear function.

The rate of pressure changes in the middle ear is directly related to the N_2O concentration.[3] However, there is no support that using $\leq 50\%$ of N_2O for tympanoplasty surgery will interfere with the graft placement and surgical outcome. N_2O should be avoided 15 min prior to the middle ear closure.

Preservation of Facial Nerve

Surgical identification and preservation of the facial nerve are critical during otologic surgery. For this reason many anesthesiologists avoid the use of neuromuscular blockers during surgery. If muscle relaxants are used, constant monitoring should be used to guarantee that at least 10–20% of muscle response remains for surgical assessment.

Intraoperative Bleeding

During microsurgery of the ear even minor bleeding can make the procedure difficult. Injection of an epinephrine-containing solution or topical application of epinephrine is one of the primary measures to control bleeding via vasoconstriction. Elevation of the head (10–15 degrees) increases venous drainage, decreasing bleeding. The use of volatile anesthetics helps to control the blood pressure. The use of induced hypotension during ear surgery is controversial. Eltringham et al.[4] found no correlation between hypotension and quality of surgical field during middle-ear surgery. In addition, various complications of hypotensive techniques have been reported, especially in the elderly.[5]

Modified hypotensive techniques based on controlled ventilation with volatile agents have been reported to provide successful anesthesia for ear surgery, maintaining the systolic blood pressure around 80–85 mmHg.[6]

Postoperative Nausea and Vomiting

Postoperative nausea and vomiting can severely affect the results of microscopic ear surgery. Antiemetics should be used for prophylaxis.

ANESTHESIA FOR NASAL SURGERY

Ambulatory nasal surgery consists in cosmetic or functional restoration of the airway procedures including septoplasty, rhinoplasty, and septorhinoplasty. These procedures can be performed under local anesthesia with intravenous sedation or general anesthesia. Because the nasal mucosa is extremely vascular, surgeons typically use topical 4% cocaine solution into the nasal cavity as well as local infiltration of 1% lidocaine with 1:100,000 epinephrine to ensure vasoconstriction and minimize bleeding. Head positioning of 30 degrees should also be used to decrease intraoperative bleeding. When general anesthesia is used, an endotracheal tube (ETT) oral RAE or flexible laryngeal mask airway (LMA) may be used to facilitate surgical access.

ANESTHESIA FOR ENDOSCOPIC SINUS SURGERY

Endoscopic techniques have been successfully used for several types of sinus surgery in the outpatient setting. In addition, reconstructive and cosmetic nasal surgeries (e.g., septoplasty) are frequently performed in the ambulatory setting.

Successful use of general or local/regional anesthesia techniques for nasal and endoscopic sinus surgery (ESS) has been reported.[7–10] Regional anesthesia (e.g., infraorbital nerve block) has been effectively used for maxillary sinus surgery as well as frontoethmoidal recess, anterior and posterior ethmoid cells.[11] Fedok and colleagues[7] demonstrated that patients undergoing local anesthesia with sedation presented shorter operative and recovery times when compared to general anesthesia. In addition, these authors also reported that the incidence of PONV and epistaxis was reduced, as well as unplanned hospital admissions, in patients undergoing local anesthesia with sedation.

One of the main considerations in sinus surgery, especially endoscopic, is blood loss because the mucosa is highly vascular. Studies have shown that controlled hypotension with potent vasodilators (e.g., sodium nitroprusside) does not improve surgical conditions or decrease blood loss during this type of surgery.[12] Interestingly, Ji and colleagues[13] performed a regression analysis reporting that general anesthesia significantly increased blood loss during ESS when compared to local anesthesia. This is in agreement with the Gittelman and colleagues[14] study where they demonstrated that general anesthesia considerably increased blood loss. Positive ventilation pressure and vasodilatation associated with some general anesthetic agents are suggested causes for increasing the potential for blood loss and consequently decreased visibility under general anesthesia.

As local anesthesia should be used only for selected patients and for selected types of surgery, anesthesiologists can use general anesthesia and vasoactive agents to reduced impact on surgical blood loss. Decreased blood pressure during general anesthesia is usually accomplished with potent inhalational anesthetics and/or intermittent boluses of vasoactive drugs (e.g., labetolol 0.1–0.3 mg/kg, esmolol 0.3–1 mg/kg). In addition, propofol can be used to improve operating conditions during ESS. Pavlin et al.[15] exemplified this point when they compared isoflurane versus propofol for EES. They reported that there is no difference in blood loss between propofol and isoflurane, but propofol improved operating conditions, particularly for ethmoid and sphenoid sinuses. Ideally systolic blood pressure must be lower than 100 mmHg and median arterial pressure (MAP) equal to 60–70 mmHg, unless contraindicated owing to medical comorbidities.

Appropriate airway management can be achieved by using endotracheal intubation or flexible LMA. A flexible LMA instead of an ETT offers significant advantages, including reduced airway reactivity and increased mucociliary clearance.[16]

ANESTHESIA FOR TONSILLECTOMY AND/OR ADENOIDECTOMY

Tonsillectomy and adenoidectomy are common ambulatory procedures, especially in the pediatric population. In adults, these procedures may be related to obstructive sleep apnea (OSA), which may be related to difficult mask ventilation and difficult intubation.

Endotracheal tube or flexible LMA can be used for airway management. It has been documented that the use of flexible LMA instead of an ETT safely protects the airway during adenotonsillectomy and reduces the incidence of postextubation complications in adults and children.[17] However, its use for this procedure has never become popular in the United States.

Secondary blood drainage into the stomach is common with secondary PONV, occurring in up to 70% of patients.[18] Prophylactic use of antiemetics is indicated as well as general anesthetic techniques that can potentially minimize PONV. Dexamethasone has been successfully used for PONV prophylaxis, including the pediatric population.[19] Postextubation laryngospasm after adenotonsillectomy is common. Topical lidocaine can be applied to the glottic and supraglottic areas before intubation which can minimize the incidence of laryngospasm. Of greater concern is the risk of postobstructive pulmonary edema, which may develop after relief of a long-standing, compensated upper airway obstruction. The removal of the obstruction, superimposed on a baseline increase in intrathoracic pressure, can lead to a rapid increase in pulmonary hydrostatic pressure, causing transudation of fluid into the pulmonary interstitium. A similar outcome may follow an inspiratory effort against an obstruction, as occurs, for example, in laryngospasm.[20]

Bleeding Tonsil

Postoperative bleeding is one of the main complications after tonsillectomy. Bleeding usually occurs at a slow speed and large volumes of blood may be swallowed before its detection. Rapid sequence induction with endotracheal intubation must be performed in this patient population.

ANESTHESIA FOR LARYNGOSCOPY, ESOPHAGOSCOPY, AND BRONCHOSCOPY

Patients undergoing laryngoscopy, esophagoscopy, and bronchoscopy often present difficult airway management. History of neck surgery, trauma, or radiotherapy, as well as presence of anatomic characteristics including decreased cervical spine range of motion, large tongue, and receding jaw, is common in this patient population. Anesthesiologists should be prepared to manage a difficult airway.

These surgical procedures are performed under general anesthesia with endotracheal intubation. Small-diameter 5.0–6.0 mm-cuffed ETT is used to facilitate larynx visualization. Jet ventilation may be necessary when ETT cannot be used (e.g., supraglottic and subglottic lesions).

Laser Surgery

Carbon dioxide (CO_2) and neodymium-yttrium aluminum garnet (Nd:YAG) lasers are frequently used for microsurgery of the upper airway and trachea. CO_2 is mainly used for throat surgery. Fire is a major risk. Special precautions should be taken to avoid problems with fire during laser surgery. To reduce the hazard of fire on the airway, not more than 30% oxygen in nitrogen, air, or helium should be used in the gas mixture. N_2O should be avoided as it supports combustion as oxygen. The use of special metal ETT (e.g., Lasertubus for Nd:YAG, Mallinkrodt LaserFlex for CO_2 laser) is mandatory. Methylene-blue-colored normal saline should be used to inflate the ETT cuffs to immediately alert the surgeon when one of the cuffs has been ruptured.

ANESTHESIA FOR RECONSTRUCTIVE SURGERY FOR SLEEP-DISORDERED BREATHING

Surgical procedures to the upper airway to relieve obstruction performed in the ambulatory setting include uvulopalatopharyngoplasty (UPPP), uvulopalatal flap (UPF), lingual-plasty, laser midline glossectomy, hyoid myotomy and suspension (HM), and inferior sagittal mandibular osteotomy and genioglossal advancement (MOGA), among others. Patients undergoing this type of surgery usually have a positive history for OSA and often present with a large variety of related medical conditions. These may range from chronic fatigue to an increased risk of sudden death. In addition, morbid obesity is frequently associated with OSA. Before induction of anesthesia, consideration must be given if a difficult airway is anticipated.

Typically these procedures are performed under general anesthesia with endotracheal intubation. However, selected patients undergoing MOGA, HM, and UPF may only require intravenous sedation or monitored anesthesia care (MAC). Patients should remain intubated until sufficiently awake to maintain airway reflexes avoiding complete loss of airway or laryngospasm secondary to premature extubation. Postoperative opioids should be minimized to avoid or reduce excessive postoperative sedation in this high-risk patient population for airway compromise or obstruction.

ANESTHESIA FOR THYROID SURGERY

General anesthesia is the technique of choice for patients undergoing thyroidectomy. The successful use of bilateral superficial and/or deep cervical plexus block for postoperative analgesia has been reported for thyroidectomy.[21,22] Dieudonne et al.[21] reported that the use of bilateral superficial cervical plexus blocks reduced pain scores after thyroid surgery. Aunac and colleagues[22] found similar findings when they reported that a combination of superficial and deep cervical plexus blocks decreased intra- and postoperative opioid requirements. These authors also alert for the possibility of performing thyroid surgery under regional anesthesia as the technique of choice for the majority of the patients in the future.[23]

The most common perioperative complications after this type of surgery include compressing hematoma leading to airway obstruction, and recurrent or superior laryngeal nerve paralysis. To address the recurrent laryngeal nerve paralysis, Scheuller and Ellison[24] reported the use of LMA with intraoperative fiberoptic laryngoscopy to effectively identify and preserve the recurrent laryngeal nerve via direct visualization of vocal cord movement. This would be a viable alternative to decrease the incidence of postoperative recurrent laryngeal nerve injury.

ANESTHESIA FOR PAROTIDECTOMY AND SUBMANDIBULAR GLAND EXCISION

Superficial and total parotidectomy as well as submandibular gland excision are usually performed in the outpatient setting. General anesthesia with endotracheal intubation is the technique of choice. Anesthesiologists should discuss surgeon's preference regarding muscle relaxation and facial nerve monitoring prior to induction of anesthesia. Surgeons usually request avoidance of neuromuscular blockade to allow facial nerve monitoring during procedure. In addition, rapid emergence is preferable to allow surgeons to assess facial nerve function with patient cooperation.

ANESTHESIA FOR EYE SURGERY

The Oculocardiac Reflex

Bernard Aschner and Giuseppe Dagnini first described the oculocardiac reflex (OCR) in 1908.[25] The OCR is a trigeminal reflex that is induced by pressure on the eye globe or traction of the extraocular muscles, especially the medial rectus, resulting in bradycardia, atrioventricular block, ventricular fibrillation, or asystole. The OCR is more common in children during strabismus surgery and occasionally at the time of injection for retrobulbar block.

Regional Anesthesia for Eye Surgery

Local anesthetics for eye surgery can be administered through either injection (retrobulbar, peribulbar, subconjunctival, medial canthus episcleral, etc.) or the use of topical anesthesia (local anesthetic drops). Regional anesthesia techniques combined with MAC can be used for several ambulatory ophthalmic surgical procedures (Table 25-1). Currently there is no consensus as to the optimal approach to regional anesthesia. The choice of the regional anesthetic technique should be based on (1) the ability to produce akinesia, (2) the patient's discomfort or pain during block performance, (3) the quality of analgesia, and (4) the complications associated with the technique. In addition, patient and surgeon's preference of different techniques should be considered. Boezaart et al.[26] studied this topic comparing topical versus regional anesthesia for cataract surgery. These authors reported that patients who experienced both techniques clearly preferred the regional block to topical anesthesia. In addition, surgeons judged that it was more difficult and more painful to perform the operation under topical anesthesia. This finding is in accordance with previous reports.[27,28]

Table 25-1 Ambulatory Ophthalmologic Surgical Procedures Performed under Regional Anesthesia Techniques

Cataract surgery
Vitreoretinal surgery
Anterior/posterior segment surgery
Glaucoma surgery
Corneal surgery
Strabismus surgery
Enucleations/eviscerations

Retrobulbar Block

Retrobulbar block has been used for a long time in ophthalmic surgery.[29,30] The goal is to deposit local anesthetic into the cone formed by the extraocular muscles. Traditionally, this block was performed with the patient looking upward and inward (Atkinson's technique), which theoretically would facilitate needle introduction and injection. Lately, preference has been given to a safer maneuver—straight-ahead positioning of the eyeball (primary gaze)—owing to its safety. This was demonstrated by Unsold and colleagues[31] in a study performed in cadavers using computerized tomography. They demonstrated that the Atkinson's globe position displaces the optic nerve downward and outward, and the needle (35 mm) inserted in the lower eyelid would pass near the ophthalmic artery, superior ophthalmic vein, and the posterior limit of the globe.

Block performance. To minimize complications the globe should not be positioned as described by Atkinson's classic technique (up and in) but in the primary gaze position. The needle entry site is located on the inferotemporal border of the orbita at the junction of the lateral one-third and the medial two-thirds. A skin wheal must be performed before needle introduction. The needle (25–27 gauge, 1.5") is first directed straight back, until the tip is beyond the globe. Then, the needle is redirected toward the apex of the orbita and inserted to a depth of 25–35 mm. This is a low-volume technique, usually requiring 4 mL of local anesthetic solution. Rapid onset time is expected (3–5 min).

A compression balloon should be used after regional anesthesia techniques for eye surgery for 10–20 min to assist the spread of the local anesthetic solution, thus achieving akinesia of periorbital muscles. This balloon also facilitates the lowering of the intraocular pressure (IOP) after injection.

Side effects, complications, and safety. Potential but not uncommon complications related to retrobulbar block include subarachnoid injection with possible brain stem anesthesia, maxillary sinus penetration,[32] penetration or perforation of the globe, postoperative ptosis mainly due to local anesthesic myotoxicity,[33-35] optic nerve atrophy, retina ischemia, spread of the anesthetic to the contralateral orbit, and OCR triggering. Subarachnoid injection is a rare complication but requires prompt recognition and management owing to life-threatening respiratory and cardiac depression. The spread to the subarachnoid space occurs via the optic nerve sheath. The clinical presentation of brain stem anesthesia includes agitation, confusion, breathing difficulties or respiratory arrest, unconsciousness, dysphagia, impaired hearing, hypertension, tachycardia, cyanosis, contralateral amaurosis, shivering, and numb throat.[36-38] The treatment is mainly supportive.

Peribulbar Block

Peribulbar anesthesia has been used as the technique of choice for the majority of ophthalmic surgery because it is safer than retrobulbar block owing to needle insertion outside of the extraocular muscle cone.[39] Several techniques are described to perform peribulbar block, including transcutaneous single- or double-injection technique. This following section discusses the technique described by Bloomberg.[40]

Block performance.   The patient should look straight ahead (primary gaze position) during block performance to avoid entering the cone, thus decreasing the risk of retrobulbar hemorrhage, optic nerve injury, or spread of the local anesthetic to the central nervous system (CNS) via the optic nerve sheath.

The most common technique used to perform peribulbar block involves two injections above and below the globe. Bloomberg's technique[40] consists of two injections depositing the local anesthetic solution more superficially outside the muscle cone, approximately 18 mm from the skin surface. Five milliliters of local anesthetic is injected into the superonasal orbit and an additional 5 mL inferotemporally between the lateral third and medial two-thirds of the lower orbital margin using a 25–27 gauge, 25-mm needle.

Side effects, complications, and safety.   Akinesia can be achieved in 95% of the patients receiving peribulbar block.[41] Despite its benefits, there are disadvantages reported in the literature, including slower onset. In addition, large volumes of local anesthetic (5–6 mL) are necessary to perform peribulbar blocks, causing increase in IOP.[42] In addition, conjunctival edema is very common after peribulbar injections. Potential complications are inadvertent brain stem anesthesia,[43] postoperative ptosis,[35] myotoxicity of local anesthetics on inferior rectus muscle causing temporary or permanent vertical diplopia,[33,34] and globe perforation.

Medial Canthus Episcleral (Sub-Tenon) Block

Retrobulbar and peribulbar blocks are commonly used for ophthalmic surgery with great success. While providing excellent conditions for operating on the eye, these techniques are associated with serious but uncommon complications. Medial canthus episcleral anesthesia (sub-Tenon) technique was developed to avoid such complications. Re-

cent reports suggest that the use of sub-Tenon block is becoming more common by anesthesiologists and ophthalmologists.[44]

Block performance.   Sub-Tenon technique consists of the direct injection of local anesthetic into the posterior aspect of the sub-Tenon space. The local anesthetic spreads along the extraocular muscles and diffuses into the retrobulbar space.[45,46] A 25-gauge short-bevel needle is inserted to contact the conjunctiva between the eyeball and the semilunaris fold, at a depth of less them 1 mm. The bevel of the needle should be directed toward the globe. The needle is then shifted slightly, medially displacing the semilunaris fold and caruncle away from the eyeball. The needle is then advanced in an anteroposterior direction with the globe directed slightly medially by the needle until a "click" is perceived, at a mean depth of 15–20 mm. At this point, which is considered to be the depth marker confirming the episcleral location of the needle tip, the globe is returned to the primary position. After careful aspiration, local anesthetic solution is slowly injected. The injection should be stopped at the first sign of chemosis. Ocular compression can be applied for 10–20 min to lower IOP and resorb chemosis.

Sub-Tenon block is almost painless, thus reducing sedation requirements and being particularly advantageous in the ambulatory setting.[47] In addition, total akinesia can be achieved in 86.5% of patients after first puncture.[48]

Side effects, complications, and safety.   Sub-Tenon block is recognized as a safe regional anesthesia technique for ophthalmic surgery.[48,49] A reported side effect related to this technique includes edema of the conjunctiva (chemosis).[48,50] Complications are infrequent, including subconjunctival hemorrhage (32–56%),[50] retrobulbar hemorrhage,[48,51] CNS spread, and global perforation.[52] The use of large volumes of local anesthetic should be avoided because it can induce retinal damage due to decrease in pulsatile blood flow.[53] Increase in intraorbital and intraocular pressures was also reported.[54]

For patients receiving anticoagulants sub-Tenon anesthesia is often considered to be the technique of choice.[55,56]

Local Anesthetics and Adjuvants

Local anesthetics.   A local anesthetic mixture consisting of equal amounts of 2% lidocaine and 0.5–0.75% bupivacaine has been largely used for ophthalmic surgery. The rational for this mixture is to promote rapid onset with lidocaine and prolong the duration of analgesia with bupivacaine. Other local anesthetics have been successful when used as an alternative to this mixture.

Articaine is an amide local anesthetic with short duration, rapid onset of action, and low toxicity profile. It has been shown to be safe and effective for eye regional anesthesia.[57-59] When compared to the traditional lidocaine 2%/ bupivacaine 0.5% mixture without hyaluronidase, it has been reported to be more advantageous, including lower pain scores during injection.[60]

Ropivacaine is an amide local anesthetic that has been successfully used in regional anesthesia for eye surgery.[61]

Ropivacaine should be preferred over bupivacaine owing to its safety profile.

Adjuvants.   Hyaluronidase (3 U/mL of local anesthetic) can be added to the local anesthetic solution to increase tissue diffusion[62–64] and decrease the need for repeated injections, especially with the use of peribulbar block.

When compared to the retrobulbar block, the onset of akinesia is slower with the peribulbar block. Kucukyavuz and Arici[65] have reported that the addition of atracurium to the local anesthetic mixture decreases the onset time of akinesia.

Clonidine has also been used when performing regional anesthesia of the eye. Barioni et al.[66] demonstrated that the addition of 30 μg of clonidine to the local anesthetic solution decreased the onset time of anesthesia, while 15 and 30 μg prolonged the time to first rescue analgesics in patients under peribulbar block. No increase in the frequency of adverse events was noted. Cautious use of clonidine must be observed for outpatients because of potential side effects.

Sedation and Monitoring

Sedation is critical during insertion of regional anesthesia for eye surgery. Combinations including midazolam (0.015 mg/kg), alfentanil (5 μg/kg), and/or propofol (0.15 mg/kg) are indicated for outpatient surgery. Standard monitoring, including electrocardiogram (ECG), pulse oximetry, and arterial blood pressure measurements, is essential during and after block performance to promptly detect any potential complications.

General Anesthesia for Eye Surgery

General anesthesia is also used for outpatient ophthalmic surgery, especially for strabismus surgery in the pediatric population. Although enucleations and eviscerations can be performed under regional anesthesia,[67] general anesthesia is commonly used for these procedures. General anesthetic agents have different effects on IOP (Table 25-2). It is important to avoid drugs that can potentially increase the IOP when performing ophthalmologic anesthesia. In addition, laryngoscopy and endotracheal intubation are also common reasons to significantly increase IOP (10–20 mmHg).

Commonly Used Ophthalmic Drugs and Their Systemic Effects

It is important that anesthesiologists are aware of the eyedrops used by ophthalmologists and their systemic effects on patients, especially in the elderly population. Table 25-3 presents the most common eye medications used as well as their systemic side effects.

Table 25-2   Anesthetic Drugs and Their Effects on Intraocular (IOP) Pressure

Effect on Intraocular Pressure	Anesthetic Agents
Increase IOP	Ketamine Succinylcholine
Decrease IOP	Barbiturates (e.g., thiopental, pentobarbital) Etomidate Propofol Intravenous benzodiazepines (midazolam, diazepam) Inhalational agents Nondepolarizing muscle relaxants
Maintain IOP	Antisialogogues (atropine, glyco-pyrrolate, scopolamine) Neostigmine

Table 25-3   Commonly Used Ophthalmic Drugs and Their Systemic Effects

Ophthalmic Drugs	Systemic Side Effects
Phenylephrine	Significant hypertension, dysrhythmias, myocardial ischemia, and headaches
Timolol	Bradycardia, hypotension, congestive heart failure, exacerbation of asthma, and myasthenia gravis
Ecothiophate	Decrease in plasma cholinesterase activity prolonging succinylcholine muscle relaxation; 4–6 weeks are required to recover activity of this enzyme
Cyclopentolate	Central nervous system toxicity (e.g., seizures, psychotic reactions, dysarthria, disorientation)
Betaxolol	Additive effects to systemic beta-blockers
Acetylcholine	Bradycardia, hypotesion, bronchospasm, increased salivation, and bronchial secretions
Atropine	Central anticholinergic syndrome (dry mouth, agitation, tachycardia, hallucinations, delirium, and unconsciousness)
Acetazolamide	Diuresis and hypokalemic metabolic acidosis
Epinephrine	Tachyarrhythmias, premature ventricular beats
Scopolamine	Disorientation and hallucinations

SUMMARY

There are several anesthesia techniques that can be successfully used for head and neck surgery performed in the outpatient setting. Careful patient and anesthesia technique selection is critical to improve patient outcomes.

REFERENCES

1. Waun JE, Sweitzer RS, Hamilton WK. Effect of nitrous oxide on middle ear mechanics and hearing acuity. Anesthesiology 1967;28(5):846–50.

2. Blackstock D, Gettes MA. Negative pressure in the middle ear in children after nitrous oxide anaesthesia. Can Anaesth Soc J 1986;33(1):32–35.

3. Doyle WJ, Banks JM. Middle ear pressure change during controlled breathing with gas mixtures containing nitrous oxide. J Appl Physiol 2003;94(1):199–204.

4. Eltringham RJ, Young PN, Fairbairn ML, Robinson JM. Hypotensive anaesthesia for microsurgery of the middle ear: a comparison between enflurane and halothane. Anaesthesia 1982;37(10):1028–32.

5. Condon HA. Deliberate hypotension in ENT surgery. Clin Otolaryngol 1979;4(4):241–46.

6. Donlon JVJ. Anesthesia for eye, ear, throat, and nose surgery. In: Miller RD (ed.), Anesthesia, 5th ed. Philadelphia: Churchill Livingstone, 2000, pp. 2173–98.

7. Fedok FG, Ferraro RE, Kingsley CP, Fornadley JA. Operative times, postanesthesia recovery times, and complications during sinonasal surgery using general anesthesia and local anesthesia with sedation. Otolaryngol Head Neck Surg 2000;122(4):560–66.

8. Gao M, Fang H. [Choice of anesthetic method and prevention of ophthalmic complication in sphenoid sinus endoscopic surgery]. Lin Chuang Er Bi Yan Hou Ke Za Zhi 2002;16(8):416–17.

9. Thaler ER, Gottschalk A, Samaranayake R, Lanza DC, Kennedy DW. Anesthesia in endoscopic sinus surgery. Am J Rhinol 1997;11(6):409–13.

10. Lee WC, Kapur TR, Ramsden WN. Local and regional anesthesia for functional endoscopic sinus surgery. Ann Otol Rhinol Laryngol 1997;106(9):767–69.

11. Keles N, Ilicali OC, Deger K. Objective and subjective assessment of nasal obstruction in patients undergoing endoscopic sinus surgery. Am J Rhinol 1998;12(5):307–9.

12. Jacobi KE, Bohm BE, Rickauer AJ, Jacobi C, Hemmerling TM. Moderate controlled hypotension with sodium nitroprusside does not improve surgical conditions or decrease blood loss in endoscopic sinus surgery. J Clin Anesth 2000;12(3):202–7.

13. Ji X, Liang C, Wu X, Xie J. [Evaluation on hemorrhage factors secondary to endoscopic sinus surgery with multiple stepwise regression analysis]. Lin Chuang Er Bi Yan Hou Ke Za Zhi 2002;16(8):404–6.

14. Gittelman PD, Jacobs JB, Skorina J. Comparison of functional endoscopic sinus surgery under local and general anesthesia. Ann Otol Rhinol Laryngol 1993;102(4 Pt 1):289–93.

15. Pavlin JD, Colley PS, Weymuller EA, Jr., Van Norman G, Gunn HC, Koerschgen ME. Propofol versus isoflurane for endoscopic sinus surgery. Am J Otolaryngol 1999;20(2):96–101.

16. Nair I, Bailey PM. Review of uses of the laryngeal mask in ENT anaesthesia. Anaesthesia 1995;50(10):898–900.

17. Webster AC, Morley-Forster PK, Dain S, Ganapathy S, Ruby R, Au A, et al. Anaesthesia for adenotonsillectomy: a comparison between tracheal intubation and the armoured laryngeal mask airway. Can J Anaesth 1993;40(12):1171–77.

18. Ferrari LR, Donlon JV. Metoclopramide reduces the incidence of vomiting after tonsillectomy in children. Anesth Analg 1992;75(3):351–54.

19. Elhakim M, Ali NM, Rashed I, Riad MK, Refat M. Dexamethasone reduces postoperative vomiting and pain after pediatric tonsillectomy. Can J Anaesth 2003;50(4):392–97.

20. DeDio RM, Hendrix RA. Postobstructive pulmonary edema. Otolaryngol Head Neck Surg 1989;101(6):698–700.

21. Dieudonne N, Gomola A, Bonnichon P, Ozier YM. Prevention of postoperative pain after thyroid surgery: a double-blind randomized study of bilateral superficial cervical plexus blocks. Anesth Analg 2001;92(6):1538–42.

22. Aunac S, Carlier M, Singelyn F, De Kock M. The analgesic efficacy of bilateral combined superficial and deep cervical plexus block administered before thyroid surgery under general anesthesia. Anesth Analg 2002;95(3):746–50.

23. Saxe AW, Brown E, Hamburger SW. Thyroid and parathyroid surgery performed with patient under regional anesthesia. Surgery 1988;103(4):415–20.

24. Scheuller MC, Ellison D. Laryngeal mask anesthesia with intraoperative laryngoscopy for identification of the recurrent laryngeal nerve during thyroidectomy. Laryngoscope 2002;112(9):1594–97.

25. Dagnini G. Intorno ad un riflesso provocato in alcuni emiplegici collo stimolo della cornea e colla pressione sul bulbo oculare. Bull Sci Med 1908;8:380.

26. Boezaart A, Berry R, Nell M. Topical anesthesia versus retrobulbar block for cataract surgery: the patients' perspective. J Clin Anesth 2000;12(1):58–60.

27. Patel BC, Burns TA, Crandall A, Shomaker ST, Pace NL, van Eerd A, et al. A comparison of topical and retrobulbar anesthesia for cataract surgery. Ophthalmology 1996;103(8):1196–203.

28. Roman S, Auclin F, Ullern M. Topical versus peribulbar anesthesia in cataract surgery. J Cataract Refract Surg 1996;22(8):1121–24.

29. Atkinson WS. The development of ophthalmic anesthesia. Am J Ophthalmol 1961;51:1–14.

30. Knapp H. Further observations on the use of cocaine. Med Record 1884;26:656.

31. Unsold R, Stanley JA, DeGroot J. The CT-topography of retrobulbar anesthesia: anatomic-clinical correlation of complications and suggestion of a modified technique. Albrecht Von Graefes Arch Klin Exp Ophthalmol 1981;217(2):125–36.

32. Tsilimbaris MK, Karabekios S, Kozobolis VP, Velegrakis G, Pallikaris IG. Needle entrance into the maxillary sinus during retrobulbar anesthesia. Ophthal Surg Lasers 1998;29(7):602–5.

33. Rainin EA, Carlson BM. Postoperative diplopia and ptosis: a clinical hypothesis based on the myotoxicity of local anesthetics. Arch Ophthalmol 1985;103(9):1337–39.

34. Rao VA, Kawatra VK. Ocular myotoxic effects of local anesthetics. Can J Ophthalmol 1988;23(4):171–73.

35. Feibel RM, Custer PL, Gordon MO. Postcataract ptosis: a randomized, double-masked comparison of peribulbar and retrobulbar anesthesia. Ophthalmology 1993;100(5):660–65.

36. Hamilton RC. Brain stem anesthesia following retrobulbar blockade. Anesthesiology 1985;63(6):688–90.

37. Javitt JC, Addiego R, Friedberg HL, Libonati MM, Leahy JJ. Brain stem anesthesia after retrobulbar block. Ophthalmology 1987;94(6):718–24.

38. Lee DS, Kwon NJ. Shivering following retrobulbar block. Can J Anaesth 1988;35(3(Pt 1)):294–96.

39. Grizzard WS, Kirk NM, Pavan PR, Antworth MV, Hammer ME, Roseman RL. Perforating ocular injuries caused by anesthesia personnel. Ophthalmology 1991;98(7):1011–16.

40. Bloomberg LB. Administration of periocular anesthesia. J Cataract Refract Surg 1986;12(6):677–79.

41. Davis DB, 2nd, Mandel MR. Efficacy and complication rate of 16,224 consecutive peribulbar blocks: a prospective multicenter study. J Cataract Refract Surg 1994;20(3):327–37.

42. Morgan JE, Chandna A. Intraocular pressure after peribulbar anaesthesia: is the Honan balloon necessary? Br J Ophthalmol 1995;79(1): 46–49.

43. Hamilton RC. Brain-stem anesthesia as a complication of regional anesthesia for ophthalmic surgery. Can J Ophthalmol 1992;27(7): 323–25.

44. Eke T, Thompson JR. The National Survey of Local Anaesthesia for Ocular Surgery. I. Survey methodology and current practice. Eye 1999;13(Pt 2):189–95.

45. Ripart J, Lefrant JY, Lalourcey L, Benbabaali M, Charavel P, Mainemer M, et al. Medial canthus (caruncle) single injection periocular anesthesia. Anesth Analg 1996;83(6):1234–38.

46. Ripart J, Lefrant JY, Vivien B, Charavel P, Fabbro-Peray P, Jaussaud A, et al. Ophthalmic regional anesthesia: medial canthus episcleral (sub-Tenon) anesthesia is more efficient than peribulbar anesthesia: a double-blind randomized study. Anesthesiology 2000;92(5): 1278–85.

47. Canavan KS, Dark A, Garrioch MA. Sub-Tenon's administration of local anaesthetic: a review of the technique. Br J Anaesth 2003; 90(6):787–93.

48. Nouvellon E, L'Hermite J, Chaumeron A, Mahamat A, Mainemer M, Charavel P, et al. Ophthalmic regional anesthesia: medial canthus episcleral (sub-Tenon) single injection block. Anesthesiology 2004; 100(2):370–74.

49. Guise PA. Sub-Tenon anesthesia: a prospective study of 6,000 blocks. Anesthesiology 2003;98(4):964–68.

50. Roman SJ, Chong Sit DA, Boureau CM, Auclin FX, Ullern MM. Sub-Tenon's anaesthesia: an efficient and safe technique. Br J Ophthalmol 1997;81(8):673–76.

51. Olitsky SE, Juneja RG. Orbital hemorrhage after the administration of sub-Tenon's infusion anesthesia. Ophthal Surg Lasers 1997; 28(2):145–46.

52. Frieman BJ, Friedberg MA. Globe perforation associated with sub-Tenon's anesthesia. Am J Ophthalmol 2001;131(4):520–21.

53. Pianka P, Weintraub-Padova H, Lazar M, Geyer O. Effect of sub-Tenon's and peribulbar anesthesia on intraocular pressure and ocular pulse amplitude. J Cataract Refract Surg 2001;27(8):1221–26.

54. Mein CE, Woodcock MG. Local anesthesia for vitreoretinal surgery. Retina 1990;10(1):47–49.

55. O'Reilly J, Logan P. Sub-Tenon's anaesthesia. Br J Ophthalmol 1998;82(5):589–90.

56. Kollarits CR, Jaweed S, Kollarits FJ. Comparison of pain, motility, and preoperative sedation in cataract phacoemulsification patients receiving peribulbar or sub-Tenon's anesthesia. Ophthal Surg Lasers 1998;29(6):462–65.

57. Gouws P, Galloway P, Jacob J, English W, Allman KG. Comparison of articaine and bupivacaine/lidocaine for sub-Tenon's anaesthesia in cataract extraction. Br J Anaesth 2004;92(2):228–30.

58. Allman KG, McFadyen JG, Armstrong J, Sturrock GD, Wilson IH. Comparison of articaine and bupivacaine/lidocaine for single medial canthus peribulbar anaesthesia. Br J Anaesth 2001;87(4):584–87.

59. Allman KG, Barker LL, Werrett GC, Gouws P, Sturrock GD, Wilson IH. Comparison of articaine and bupivacaine/lidocaine for peribulbar anaesthesia by inferotemporal injection. Br J Anaesth 2002; 88(5):676–78.

60. Ozdemir M, Ozdemir G, Zencirci B, Oksuz H. Articaine versus lidocaine plus bupivacaine for peribulbar anaesthesia in cataract surgery. Br J Anaesth 2004;92(2):231–34.

61. Gioia L, Prandi E, Codenotti M, Casati A, Fanelli G, Torri TM, et al. Peribulbar anesthesia with either 0.75% ropivacaine or a 2% lidocaine and 0.5% bupivacaine mixture for vitreoretinal surgery: a double-blinded study. Anesth Analg 1999;89(3):739–42.

62. Dempsey GA, Barrett PJ, Kirby IJ. Hyaluronidase and peribulbar block. Br J Anaesth 1997;78(6):671–74.

63. Henderson TR, Franks W. Peribulbar anaesthesia for cataract surgery: prilocaine versus lignocaine and bupivacaine. Eye 1996;10(Pt 4):497–500.

64. Nicoll JM, Acharya PA, Ahlen K, Baguneid S, Edge KR. Central nervous system complications after 6000 retrobulbar blocks. Anesth Analg 1987;66(12):1298–302.

65. Kucukyavuz Z, Arici MK. Effects of atracurium added to local anesthetics on akinesia in peribulbar block. Reg Anesth Pain Med 2002; 27(5):487–90.

66. Barioni MF, Lauretti GR, Lauretti-Fo A, Pereira NL. Clonidine as coadjuvant in eye surgery: comparison of peribulbar versus oral administration. J Clin Anesth 2002;14(2):140–45.

67. Burroughs JR, Soparkar CN, Patrinely JR, Kersten RC, Kulwin DR, Lowe CL. Monitored anesthesia care for enucleations and eviscerations. Ophthalmology 2003;110(2):311–13.

Ambulatory Anesthesia Techniques for Orthopedic Surgery

RALF E. GEBHARD

INTRODUCTION

Ambulatory orthopedic surgery was initially introduced primarily for procedures of short duration and little invasive character, such as diagnostic knee arthroscopy or hardware removal.[1,2] However, the constant search for increased efficiency and decreased hospital length of stay, combined with advancements in surgical technique, has led to an increased number of major orthopedic surgeries performed on an outpatient basis.[3] In addition, there is a trend to include more and more patients with severe coexisting morbidity.[4] Individuals whose anesthetic risk is preoperatively classified as American Society of Anesthesiologists (ASA) Classes III or IV are now considered candidates for ambulatory orthopedic procedures, provided their medical conditions are controlled. Currently, efforts are being made to extend the ambulatory character of orthopedic surgery to procedures such as major joint replacements, that until recently were thought to require several days of hospitalization.[5] Further innovations in surgical techniques, such as the introduction of the minimal invasive approach for total hip replacement and the concept of immediate postoperative mobilization, have made these advances possible. However, performance of more invasive procedures on an ambulatory basis increases the demand for adequate perioperative pain management as severe pain may be present for several days after discharge. In the past, these demands have not been met with traditional anesthetic methods. Further, pain, together with nausea and vomiting, has been shown to be the limiting factor for timely discharge.[6] Altogether, these developments introduce new challenges to the field of anesthesiology. Modern anesthetic techniques for ambulatory orthopedic surgery will have to extend beyond the hospital or ambulatory surgery center not only to allow for fast postoperative recovery, but also to provide efficient postoperative pain control during rest and exercise for extended periods of time.[7] The modern "ambulatory orthopedic anesthesiologist" will be expected to be capable of performing a single anesthetic technique or a combination of different anesthetic techniques that facilitates achieving these goals.

GENERAL CONSIDERATIONS

It is important to choose an anesthetic technique for outpatient orthopedic procedures that is as simple and safe as possible, while at the same time providing efficient intraoperative anesthesia and perioperative analgesia, as needed. This requires an insight into surgical and perioperative pain-related requirements, as well as appropriate physiologic and anatomic knowledge. Given the characteristic of ambulatory surgery, techniques that may be associated with a significant risk of serious complications (e.g., the potential development of a pneumothorax after supraclavicular brachial plexus block) should only be chosen after serious consideration and in the absence of safer alternatives. In addition, the patient's requests, comprehension, and his or her specific living situation at home need to be reflected in the development of a specific anesthetic plan.

ANESTHETIC TECHNIQUES

General Anesthesia

General anesthesia techniques remain very popular for ambulatory orthopedic procedures.[8,9] While the introduction of new anesthetic agents with low-solubility characteristics allows for early awakening after surgery, there is still a high incidence of postoperative nausea and vomiting (PONV) associated with general anesthesia.[10] Total intravenous anesthesia with propofol has been shown to lower the incidence of PONV[11] but this represents a fairly expensive option.[12] More importantly, general anesthesia techniques alone provide very little postoperative pain control. Therefore, if general anesthesia is chosen as the intraoperative anesthetic method for ambulatory orthopedic surgery, other postoperative pain management concepts, such as peripheral nerve blocks or local infiltration by the surgeon, are often necessary to control postoperative pain. This is of special importance when the orthopedic procedure is associated with moderate to severe postoperative pain, or when the pain is expected to last for more than 24 hr after surgery. Another disadvantage associated with general anesthesia is the fact that most patients need to be admitted to a Phase I postanesthesia care unit (PACU) until they meet discharge criteria to a Phase II PACU.

Central Neuraxial Blocks

Spinal and epidural anesthesia represent an alternative to general anesthesia for ambulatory orthopedic surgery[13] and are associated with a lower incidence of PONV.[14] However, they do not decrease the overall hospital length of stay after these procedures.[9] In addition, concerns regarding the possibility of serious complications for patients receiving anticoagulation have led to extensive recommendations and regulations,[15] making these techniques less attractive for the ambulatory setting.

Spinal Anesthesia

Spinal anesthesia provides rapid onset, good surgical anesthesia, and relatively reliable duration. Although the introduction of small-gauge pencil-point needles and Whitacre needles has reduced the frequency of postdural puncture headache, this risk still exists along with the occurrence of postspinal transient radicular irritation and the rare, but devastating, cauda equina syndrome. Since radicular irritation and cauda equina syndrome have been mainly, but not exclusively, associated with lidocaine,[16] bupivacaine in different concentrations has been suggested as an alternative. However, while higher concentrations of bupivacaine (0.75%) result in prolonged motor blockade and delayed discharge,[17] lower concentrations offer only insufficient quality or duration of analgesia. Unilateral spinal anesthesia with hyperbaric concentrated bupivacaine provides good-quality surgical anesthesia and reliable duration, while limiting motor blockade to one leg.[18] As a result, unilateral spinal anesthesia is associated with fewer cardiovascular side effects than bilateral spinal anesthesia[19] but does not shorten discharge time after ambulatory orthopedic surgery.[20]

Epidural Anesthesia

Epidural anesthesia has been advocated for outpatient and office-based orthopedic surgery.[21] Although it provides efficient surgical anesthesia for knee procedures, there has been some controversy regarding the quality for foot and ankle surgery.[22] In addition, increased performance time and slower onset, when compared to spinal anesthesia, represent considerable disadvantages. Similar to spinal anesthesia, patients need to be admitted to a phase I PACU after surgery and cannot be discharged until their motor function has completely recovered, and they have voided. Discharge times can be shortened when 2-chloroprocaine is chosen as the local anesthetic for epidural anesthesia.[23]

Combined Spinal Epidural Anesthesia

Combined spinal epidural (CSE) anesthesia offers fast onset and dense surgical anesthesia associated with spinal anesthesia, while allowing adjustable duration of anesthesia as needed. However, the same disadvantages as described for spinal and epidural anesthesia regarding contraindications, postoperative recovery, and discharge criteria apply.

Peripheral Nerve Blocks

Peripheral nerve blocks represent an interesting alternative as the sole anesthetic technique or in combination with either intraoperative sedation or general anesthesia for ambulatory orthopedic surgery. These techniques have been shown to significantly reduce duration of hospitalization after inpatient[24] as well as outpatient orthopedic surgery,[25,26] and reduce unscheduled admissions after ambulatory surgery and the overall costs of surgery.[27] If these techniques are chosen as the sole anesthetic technique or in combination with mild to moderate sedation, most patients can be admitted directly to a Phase II PACU immediately after ambulatory orthopedic surgery. Peripheral nerve blocks are ideally performed prior to surgery in a specifically dedicated area, such as a "block area." This allows for sufficient onset time and completion of incomplete nerve blocks without delaying the start of surgery. It is essential that patients be monitored with ASA standard monitors during block performance, and that emergency intubation and resuscitation equipment is readily available to treat potential complications.

Single-Injection Peripheral Nerve Blocks

Single-injection peripheral nerve blocks with long-acting local anesthetic agents, such as ropivacaine, are especially indicated for ambulatory orthopedic procedures associated with moderate postoperative pain not expected to last more than 24 hr after surgery. Examples include diagnostic shoulder or knee arthroscopies or knee meniscectomies. These blocks have been demonstrated to significantly reduce pain after ambulatory orthopedic surgery.[28] Patients can routinely be discharged safely with residual motor blockade after receiving specific instructions.[29]

Continuous Peripheral Nerve Blocks

Continuous peripheral nerve blocks are useful if the pain after orthopedic outpatient surgery is moderate to severe and likely to last for more than 24 hr. After placement of an initial nerve block to achieve surgical anesthesia for the intraoperative period, a perineural catheter is placed through the same nerve block needle. It has been demonstrated that continuous infusions of low concentrations of

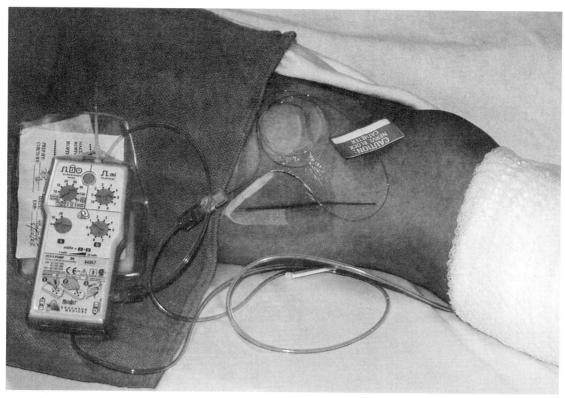

Figure 26-1   Ambulatory pump connected to lateral sciatic nerve catheter for postoperative pain management after outpatient ankle surgery.

ropivacaine (0.2%) via these catheters can provide efficient and safe analgesia several days after discharge from ambulatory orthopedic surgery.[30] Numerous ambulatory pumps are currently available allowing for continuous or patient-controlled infusion modes (Fig. 26-1). Patients should be carefully selected and should receive a contact phone number. Suggested inclusion criteria include appropriate comprehension and availability of a caretaker.

Intravenous Regional Anesthesia (Bier Block)

Intravenous injection of local anesthetics utilizing a tourniquet (Fig. 26-2) has been described as an anesthetic technique for orthopedic procedures of the upper and lower extremities.[31,32] While it provides adequate intraoperative analgesia in the majority of cases, normal sensory function returns almost immediately once the tourniquet is deflated.[33] Therefore, this technique offers very little postoperative pain control. This disadvantage, together with the potential for tourniquet pain in procedures lasting longer than 30 min, limits the use of intravenous regional anesthesia to an intervention of short-duration and mild perioperative pain.

Monitored Anesthesia Care

Monitored anesthesia care (MAC) alone, or in combination with local anesthetic infiltration, can be chosen for short ambulatory orthopedic surgeries with limited trauma, such as the removal of an external fixator.

Local Anesthetic Infiltration

Surgical site infiltration or intra-articular application of local anesthetics has been successfully utilized for ambulatory knee arthroscopies.[34] However, it is important to observe the maximum dosage to avoid potential side effects. In addition, intra-articular bupivacaine has been demonstrated to be less effective for "high-inflammatory" knee procedures, such as anterior cruciate ligament (ACL) repair.[35] Local anesthetic infiltration provides efficient perioperative analgesia for orthopedic procedures associated with minimal trauma, such as single screw removals or excision of ganglion cysts.

PERIOPERATIVE PAIN CONTROL

Pain control for patients undergoing ambulatory orthopedic procedures ideally starts preoperatively, continues during the intraoperative period, and lasts during recovery in the facility and at home until the pain associated with the specific procedure has subsided. When surgery is more extensive and moderate to severe pain is expected to last several days postoperatively, it is necessary to develop a pain management plan involving the patient, surgeon, anesthesiologist, nursing staff, potential caregivers, and other individuals involved in the recovery process, such as physical therapists. Effective perioperative pain control, together with good prophylaxis of PONV, is crucial for early discharge avoiding unplanned admission. Unfortu-

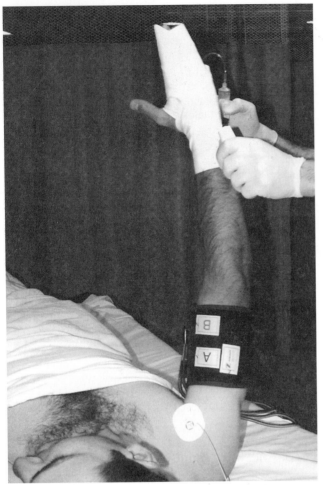

Figure 26-2 Preparation for upper-extremity intravenous anesthesia (Bier block).

proach has been demonstrated to positively impact discharge times after ambulatory surgery or to improve patient outcome.[38]

Multimodal Approach

In contrast to the monomodal approach, the multimodal approach combines several methods of pain therapy, targeting different receptors in an effort to maximize pain control and to minimize the unwanted side effects of each component. Combining agents from different classes allows limiting dosage of each component to an amount where side effects such as nausea, itching, or sedation become rare, while achieving efficient pain relief. Such an approach has been demonstrated not only to provide safe and efficient pain control after orthopedic surgery, but also to allow for earlier discharge after inpatient and ambulatory surgery.[24,26] Ideally this technique combines medical and nonmedical techniques, such as cooling or resting the operated extremity. Medications include the application of local anesthetics either to peripheral nerves, into joints, or locally to the incision site, together with the oral or parenteral use of opioids and nonsteroidal analgesics or cyclooxygenase-2 (COX-2) inhibitors. The latter class of drugs represents an interesting alternative to the prescription of nonsteroidal analgesics. Selective inhibition of the COX-2 isoenzyme results in reduction of anti-inflammatory and analgesic effects while platelet and kidney function are preserved and gastric mucosa protection is not compromised.[39] COX-2 inhibitors, as part of a multimodal pain management concept for ambulatory orthopedic surgery, have also been associated with preemptive analgesic and opioid-sparing effects.[40] Table 26-1

nately, in many ambulatory centers, little attention is given to optimizing perioperative pain control, and physicians responsible for prescribing pain medications often lack formal training or extensive experience in pain management.[36] There are two different approaches to control perioperative pain after ambulatory orthopedic surgery:

Monomodal Approach

The monomodal approach relies on one single method for postoperative pain management. Popular examples include patient-controlled analgesia (PCA) with intravenous opioids, traditionally used for inpatients, or prescriptions of acetaminophen with or without opioids for ambulatory patients. While the latter concept may be efficient for patients undergoing minor ambulatory orthopedic procedures with little postoperative pain, it has been clearly demonstrated that this approach is insufficient for the majority of outpatient orthopedic surgeries.[36,37] In addition, the excessive use of nonsteroidal analgesic agents carries the risks of side effects and harm to the patient. Moreover, by itself, no monomodal ap-

Table 26-1   Multimodal Pain Management for Ambulatory ACL Repair

Perioperative Period	Pain Management Components
Preoperative	Rofecoxib 50 mg PO 1 hr prior to surgery
Intraoperative	Continuous femoral nerve block (bolus injection of 15 mL 1.5% mepivacaine and 15 mL 0.75% ropivacaine)
	Single-injection sciatic nerve block (15 mL 1.5% mepivacaine plus 15 mL 0.75% ropivacaine)
Postoperative	Continuous femoral nerve block infusion (0.2% ropivacaine, 10 mL/hr),
	Rofecoxib 50 mg PO every morning for the next 4 days
	Oxycodone 5–10 mg PO, every 4–6 hr, PRN

shows a multimodal pain management concept for ambulatory ACL repair.

SPECIFIC ORTHOPEDIC PROCEDURES

It is important to recognize that anesthetic techniques recommended for specific orthopedic procedures in this chapter do not represent a "gold standard." Anesthetic requirements for even the most commonly performed orthopedic procedures, such as knee arthroscopies, can vary greatly depending on the skill and experience of the surgeon and on patient-related factors such as comorbidities and the patient's expectations. In addition, education and experience of the anesthesiologist also influence decision making regarding the ideal anesthetic technique. Therefore, a certain anesthetic concept for a specific orthopedic procedure may not be suitable for all patients, surgeons, or anesthesiologists. An individualized plan, taking into consideration the given circumstances and requirements, should be developed prior to each procedure to achieve a satisfying result for all involved parties.[41]

Shoulder Procedures

Since no tourniquet can be used for these procedures, patients are frequently placed in a lateral or beach chair position in an attempt to minimize blood loss and create optimal operating conditions, especially for arthroscopic shoulder surgery. In addition, some orthopedic surgeons may also prefer mild to moderate controlled hypotension. Consequently, to control the patient's airway and to facilitate blood pressure control, general anesthesia is often the preferred intraoperative technique for ambulatory shoulder surgeries. While diagnostic shoulder arthroscopies are associated with only mild to moderate pain of relatively short duration, rotator cuff repair, and especially subacromial decompression and distal clavicle resection, represent a much larger challenge for effective perioperative pain management. Consequently, interscalene, intra-articular, and intra-bursal application of local anesthetics, either as single-injection or as continuous infusion, has been suggested.[42–44] In this regard, single-injection or continuous interscalene brachial plexus blocks appear to offer the most effective approach for more painful surgeries,[45] while intra-articular infusion is effective only after less invasive procedures, such as diagnostic shoulder arthroscopies.[46] A single-injection interscalene brachial plexus block, as compared to general anesthesia, has been demonstrated to result in a significantly shorter stay in a Phase I PACU and with a significant decrease in the number of patients hospitalized following rotator cuff repair.[47] Table 26-2 presents recommendations for anesthetic management for ambulatory shoulder surgery.

Elbow Procedures

Examples of ambulatory orthopedic procedures of the elbow include elbow arthroscopies, bursectomies, and ulnar nerve

Table 26-2   Recommended Anesthetic Techniques for Ambulatory Shoulder Surgery

Procedure	Anesthetic Technique
Arthroscopy	S^a interscalene block + GA^b or S^a interscalene block + intraoperative sedation
Rotator cuff repair	C^c interscalene block + GA^b or C^c interscalene block + intraoperative sedation
Subacromial decompression	C^c interscalene block + GA^b or C^c interscalene block + intraoperative sedation
Distal clavicle resection	C^c interscalene block + GA^b or C^c interscalene block + intraoperative sedation

S^a, single injection.

GA^b, general anesthesia.

C^c, continuous.

transposition. Pain after surgery is usually mild to moderate and limited in duration. Therefore, single-injection peripheral nerve blocks combined with intraoperative sedation represent an efficient anesthetic method. Axillary brachial plexus blocks have been demonstrated to provide satisfactory perioperative analgesia for elbow surgery.[48] Alternatively, infraclavicular brachial plexus blocks (coracoid approach)[49] are preferred over supraclavicular approaches to the brachial plexus as they carry a smaller risk of pneumothorax. The chosen anesthetic technique needs to include tourniquet coverage if the procedure lasts more than 30 min. Table 26-3 lists suggested anesthetic methods for outpatient elbow procedures.

Table 26-3   Recommended Anesthetic Techniques for Ambulatory Elbow Surgery

Procedure	Anesthetic Technique
Arthroscopy	S^a axillary block + intraoperative sedation or S^a infraclavicular block + intraoperative sedation
Radial head resection	S^a axillary block + intraoperative sedation
Bursectomy	S^a axillary block + intraoperative sedation or S^a infraclavicular block + intraoperative sedation

S^a, single injection.

Forearm, Wrist, and Hand Procedures

A large variety of these procedures are currently performed on an outpatient basis. Suggested anesthetic techniques include general anesthesia, interscalene, supraclavicular, infraclavicular, axillary, humeral, elbow, and wrist nerve blocks, as well as intravenous regional anesthesia and local or intra-articular anesthesia.[50] In the majority of cases, single-injection peripheral nerve blocks provide sufficient perioperative analgesia and should be chosen when possible. While interscalene and supraclavicular brachial plexus blocks are effective for these procedures, they carry the risk of specific complications, such as phrenic nerve paralysis and pneumothorax. In contrast, axillary brachial plexus and humeral blocks are extremely efficient, easy to perform, and are not associated with specific complications.[51] Therefore, these blocks should be preferred, especially given the ambulatory character of the planned surgery. Alternatively, an infraclavicular brachial plexus block utilizing the coracoid approach can be considered.[49] If the anticipated duration of the procedure extends beyond 30 min, the chosen anesthetic technique needs to provide sufficient coverage for tourniquet pain. Elbow or wrist blocks provide sufficient perioperative anesthesia and analgesia for shorter procedures that are limited to a small area, such as removal of a ganglion cyst, carpal tunnel release, or fixation of single digital fractures. In addition, wrist blocks for carpal tunnel release (Fig. 26-3) have been demonstrated to provide superior intraoperative cardiovascular

stability and faster discharge times when compared to general anesthesia and intravenous regional anesthesia.[26] Recommended anesthetic methods for ambulatory orthopedic procedures of the forearm, wrist, and hand are listed in Table 26-4.

Knee Procedures

Arthroscopic knee procedures were among the first orthopedic interventions to be performed in an ambulatory setting. Local anesthesia has been advocated as providing efficient perioperative analgesia for diagnostic knee arthroscopies and meniscectomies,[52] while general anesthesia, as the sole anesthetic technique, is associated with delayed patient recovery.[53] However, intra-articular injection of even long-acting local anesthetics provides good postoperative pain control only in the immediate postoperative period prior to discharge.[54] Spinal or epidural anesthesia has been suggested, but discharge time after spinal anesthesia, even with short-acting lidocaine, varies from 3–5 hr[55] and is associated with an approximately 12% risk of transient neurologic symptoms.[56] Epidural anesthesia with 3% 2-chloroprocaine reduces discharge times to approximately 2–3 hr,[23] but does not provide postoperative analgesia after more invasive surgery. Femoral nerve blocks, alone or in combination with sciatic nerve blocks, have been shown to reduce the risk of unplanned admission af-

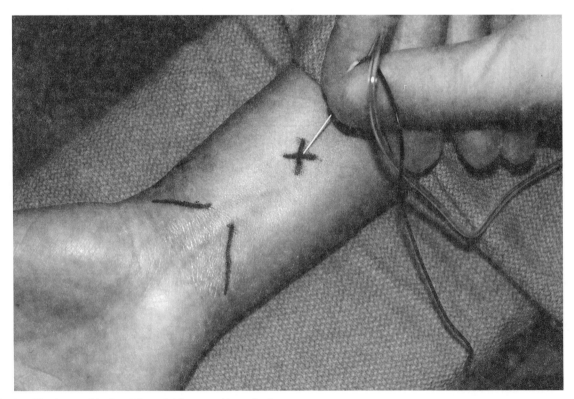

Figure 26-3   Distal nerve blocks at the wrist for carpal tunnel release.

Table 26-4   Recommended Anesthetic Techniques for Ambulatory Wrist and Hand Surgery

Procedure	Anesthetic Technique
Arthroscopy	S[a] axillary block + intraoperative sedation
Distal radius open reduction and internal fixation (ORIF)	S[a] axillary block + intraoperative sedation
Carpal tunnel release	Distal peripheral nerve blocks at the wrist + intraoperative sedation or local anesthesia + intraoperative sedation
Metacarpal ORIF	S[a] axillary block + intraoperative sedation
Finger ORIF	Peripheral nerve blocks at the elbow + intraoperative sedation or S[a] axillary block + intraoperative sedation

S[a], single injection.

Table 26-5   Recommended Anesthetic Techniques for Ambulatory Knee Surgery

Procedure	Anesthetic Technique
Arthroscopy	S[a] femoral nerve block + intraoperative sedation or local anesthesia + intraoperative sedation or GA[b] with short-acting agents
ACL repair (patella tendon graft)	C[c] femoral nerve block + S[a] sciatic nerve block + intraoperative sedation
ACL repair (hamstring graft)	C[c] femoral nerve block + C[c] sciatic nerve block + intraoperative sedation
Multiligament repair	C[c] femoral nerve block + C[c] sciatic nerve block + intraoperative sedation
Patella ORIF	C[c] femoral nerve block + S[a] sciatic nerve block

S[a], single injection.
GA[b], general anesthesia.
C[c], continuous.

ter more complex outpatient knee procedures.[27] If single- or multiligament knee reconstruction is performed, continuous peripheral nerve blocks are more effective than local anesthesia and are indicated to manage perioperative pain. ACL repair performed on an outpatient basis has been shown to reduce costs almost 60% when compared to inpatient procedures. ACL repair is associated with extensive postoperative pain and requires effective management. The procedure can be performed utilizing a combination of peripheral nerve block techniques with "light" general anesthesia or intraoperative sedation.

It is important to recognize that both femoral and sciatic nerves need to be blocked to achieve sufficient perioperative analgesia. Since postoperative pain after ACL repair with patella tendon graft usually lasts longer in the femoral nerve territory, a continuous infusion of local anesthetics for the femoral nerve is indicated, while the sciatic nerve block is performed in a single-injection technique. If the surgeon uses a hamstring graft to repair the ACL, a continuous sciatic nerve block may be needed in addition to the continuous femoral nerve block. A combination of continuous catheters for both nerves has also been suggested for multiligament repair,[57] especially when the posterior cruciate ligament is involved. The role of the obturator nerve for knee procedures remains controversial. In contrast to the classic three-in-one concept, it is now widely accepted that the femoral nerve block rarely affects the obturator nerve.[58] Consequently, some authors have suggested a single-injection or continuous lumbar plexus block to include the obturator nerve territory in the anesthetized area.[59] However, the sensory innervation of the obturator nerve at the inner aspect of the thigh varies widely in individuals,[60] and its importance for postoperative analgesia is questionable. In addition, lumbar plexus blocks are associated with specific complications such as development of a retroperitoneal hematoma[61] or kidney or ureter puncture. Therefore, it may be safer to perform femoral nerve blocks on ambulatory patients. Table 26-5 shows suggested anesthetic techniques for ambulatory knee surgery.

Foot and Ankle Procedures

Often performed by the orthopedic surgeons themselves, ankle or midfoot nerve blocks have, in the past, been the anesthetic technique of choice for forefoot procedures. These blocks, in combination with general anesthesia or intraoperative sedation, have been shown to be efficient in controlling perioperative pain for these procedures of limited extent.[62,63] Alternatively, intravenous regional anesthesia is a safe, reliable method for minor ankle and foot surgery of short duration. However, ambulatory ankle procedures and foot surgery of higher complexity require a different approach. In this regard, continuous or single-injection sciatic nerve blocks, in combination with a single-injection saphenous nerve block, allow for satisfactory perioperative analgesia and have been shown to reduce opioid consumption after ankle surgery.[64] Proposed anesthetic methods for ambulatory ankle and foot surgery are presented in Table 26-6.

Table 26-6   Recommended Anesthetic Techniques for Ambulatory Foot and Ankle Surgery

Procedure	Anesthetic Technique
Arthroscopy	S^a sciatic nerve block + S^a saphenous nerve block
Ankle ORIF	C^c sciatic nerve block + S^a saphenous nerve block
Metatarsal ORIF	S^a sciatic nerve block + S^a saphenous nerve block
Bunionectomy	Ankle block
Hallux valgus correction	Midfoot block *or* ankle block
Achilles tendon repair	S^a sciatic nerve block + S^a saphenous nerve block

S^a, single injection.

C^c, continuous.

Other Orthopedic Procedures

Hardware Removal

Depending on the amount and location of the hardware to be removed, anesthetic requirements differ greatly. Removal of single screws or external fixators can usually be performed under MAC and is usually associated with only mild postoperative pain. Single-injection peripheral nerve blocks with short-acting local anesthetics represent an alternative, but block performance and onset time can significantly prolong these extremely short procedures. More extensive hardware removal, such as removal of a femoral plate, takes longer and produces moderate pain that is normally limited to less than 24 hr. In this scenario, single-injection peripheral nerve blocks are recommended in combination with mild conscious sedation or general anesthesia for the intraoperative period.

Joint Manipulation

These interventions are indicated to mobilize joints such as frozen shoulders. Although of extremely brief duration, these procedures usually require general anesthesia as the orthopedic surgeon will request complete neuromuscular blockade to achieve a maximum degree of initial joint mobilization. It is important to realize that these surgeries are associated with significant perioperative pain, especially if the mobilization is continued by a physical therapist during the following days. In this scenario, a perineural catheter should be placed and either continuously infused or a bolus of a local anesthetic should be given approximately 1 hr prior to the planned physical therapy session. The latter approach allows utilizing a higher local anesthetic concentration in an attempt to achieve better motor blockade during this intervention.

FUTURE DEVELOPMENTS

Until most recently, patients undergoing total joint replacement surgery were hospitalized for several days. Modern multimodal perioperative pain management concepts with continuous peripheral nerve blocks as the main component are now combined with ambulatory physical therapy and home nursing in an effort to perform these procedures on an ambulatory basis.

Minimal Invasive Total Hip Arthroplasty

This fairly new procedure utilizes a two-incision minimal invasive technique and is thought to be associated with less perioperative blood loss and reduced levels of postoperative pain. In contrast to the conventional total hip replacement, this procedure can be performed in the supine position. This allows spinal anesthesia to be a very suitable intraoperative anesthetic technique without the difficulties associated with the potential need for airway management in the lateral decubitus position. General anesthesia, utilizing short-acting agents, can be chosen as an alternative. Effective postoperative pain management is of paramount importance for the ambulatory character of this procedure. Recent data show that a combination of a continuous lumbar plexus block with a single-injection sciatic nerve block, as part of a multimodal perioperative pain management concept, allowed for discharge of the majority of patients within 24 hr after surgery.[5] Therefore, this combination is recommended for postoperative pain management in patients undergoing minimal invasive total hip arthroplasty.

Ambulatory Total Knee Arthroplasty

Total knee arthroplasty is associated with severe postoperative pain lasting at least 48–72 hr. The concept of early mobilization utilizing continuous passive motion requires active pain management, not only at rest, but also during mobilization. Anesthetic techniques need to take these requirements into consideration. Continuous femoral nerve blocks, combined with single-injection sciatic nerve blocks, have been demonstrated to reduce hospital length of stay and improve outcome after inpatient total knee replacement. Research is currently being performed to investigate whether these anesthetic techniques as part of a multimodal pain management concept, together with physical therapy and nursing at home, will facilitate ambulatory total knee replacement.

SUMMARY

The number of orthopedic procedures performed on an outpatient basis will continue to grow. While general anesthesia and central neuraxial blockade are still important and popular anesthetic methods for these types of surgery, a shift away from these techniques toward peripheral nerve blocks is very likely to continue in the future. Peripheral nerve block techniques offer encouraging features, such as reduced discharge times, bypass of PACU, efficient perioperative analgesia for extended time periods, and reduction in opioid demand, which should be included in anesthetic management whenever possible. However, it is important to recognize that the key to successful performance of regional anesthesia techniques for ambulatory orthopedic surgery is proper training and equipment, as well as acceptance by the patient and the surgeon.

REFERENCES

1. Hazlett JW. Orthopedic outpatient surgery. Can J Surg 1978;21:446–47.
2. Older J. The first four years' experience of day case orthopaedic surgery in a district general hospital. Ann R Coll Surg Engl 1988;70:21–23.
3. Pregler JL, Kapur PA. The development of ambulatory anesthesia and future challenges. Anesthesiol Clin North Am 2003;21:207–28.
4. Prabhu A, Chung F. Anaesthetic strategies towards developments in day care surgery. Eur J Anaesthesiol Suppl 2001;23:36–42.
5. Chelly JE, Mears D, Scott J, et al. Acute postoperative management for ambulatory MIS total hip arthroplasty. Anesthesiology 2003;99:A18.
6. Pavlin DJ, Chen C, Penalozza DA, et al. Pain as a factor complicating recovery and discharge after ambulatory surgery. Anesth Analg 2002;95:627–34.
7. Klein SM. Beyond the hospital: continuous peripheral nerve blocks at home. Anesthesiology 2002;96:1283–85.
8. Mulroy MF, Larkin KL, Hodgson PS, et al. A comparison of spinal, epidural, and general anesthesia for outpatient knee arthroscopy. Anesth Analg 2000;91:860–64.
9. Payne K, Moore EW, Elliott RA. Anaesthesia for day case surgery: a survey of adult clinical practice in the UK. Eur J Anaesthesiol 2003;20:311–24.
10. Stadler M, Bardiau F, Seidel L, et al. Difference in risk factors for postoperative nausea and vomiting. Anesthesiology 2003;98:46–52.
11. Siler JN, Horrow JC, Rosenberg H. Propofol reduces prolonged outpatient PACU stay. An analysis according to surgical procedure. Anesthesiol Rev 1994;21:129–32.
12. Dolk A, Cannerfelt R, Anderson RE, et al. Inhalation anaesthesia is cost-effective for ambulatory surgery: clinical comparison with propofol during elective knee arthroscopy. Eur J Anaesthesiol 2002;19:88–92.
13. Salinas FV, Liu SS. Spinal anaesthesia: local anaesthetics and adjuncts in the ambulatory setting. Best Pract Res Clin Anaesthesiol 2002;16:195–210.
14. Borgeat A, Ekatodramis G, Schenker CA. Postoperative nausea and vomiting in regional anaesthesia: a review. Anesthesiology 2003;98:530–47.
15. Horlocker TT, Wedel DJ, Benzon H, et al. Regional anesthesia in the anticoagulated patient: defining the risks (the second ASRA Consensus Conference on Neuraxial Anesthesia and Anticoagulation). Reg Anesth Pain Med 2003;28:1726–97.
16. Hiller A, Rosenberg PH. Transient neurological symptoms after spinal anaesthesia with 4% mepivacaine and 0.5% bupivacaine. Br J Anaesth 1997;79:301–5.
17. Imarengiaye CO, Song D, Prabhu AJ, et al. Spinal anesthesia: functional balance is impaired after clinical recovery. Anesthesiology 2003;98:511–15.
18. Casati A, Fanelli G. Unilateral spinal anesthesia: state of the art. Minerva Anestesiol 2001;67:855–62.
19. Casati A, Fannelli G, Beccaria P, et al. Block distribution and cardiovascular effects of unilateral spinal anaesthesia by 0.5% hyperbaric bupivacaine: a clinical comparison with bilateral spinal block. Minerva Anestesiol 1998;64:307–12.
20. Fannelli G, Borghi B, Casati A, et al. Unilateral bupivacaine spinal anesthesia for outpatient knee arthroscopy. Italian Study Group on Unilateral Spinal Anesthesia. Can J Anaesth 2000;47:746–51.
21. Kopacz DJ, Mulroy MF. Chloroprocaine and lidocaine decrease hospital stay and admission rate after outpatient epidural anesthesia. Reg Anesth 1990;15:19–25.
22. Gosteli P, Van Gessel E, Gamulin Z. Effects of pH adjustment and carbonation of lidocaine during epidural anesthesia for foot and ankle surgery. Anesth Analg 1995;81:104–9.
23. Neal JM, Deck JJ, Kopacz DJ, et al. Hospital discharge after ambulatory knee arthroscopy: a comparison of epidural 2-chloroprocaine versus lidocaine. Reg Anesth Pain Med 2001;26:35–40.
24. Chelly JE, Greger J, Gebhard R, et al. Continuous femoral blocks improve recovery and outcome of patients undergoing total knee arthroplasty. J Arthroplasty 2001;16:436–45.
25. Casati A, Cappelleri G, Berti M, et al. Randomized comparison of remifentanil-propofol with a sciatic-femoral nerve block for outpatient knee arthroscopy. Eur J Anaesthesiol 2002;19:109–14.
26. Gebhard RE, Al-Samsam T, Greger J, et al. Distal nerve blocks at the wrist for outpatient carpal tunnel surgery offer intraoperative cardiovascular stability and reduce discharge time. Anesth Analg 2002;95:351–55.
27. Williams BA, Kentor ML, Vogt MT, et al. Femoral-sciatic nerve blocks for complex outpatient knee surgery are associated with less postoperative pain before same-day discharge; a review of 1,200 consecutive cases from the period 1996–1999. Anesthesiology 2003;98:1206–13.
28. Gebhard RE, Pivalizza EG, Warters RD, et al. Pain after discharge from ambulatory surgery-orthopedic patients benefit from peripheral nerve blocks. Anesthesiology 2002;A-25.
29. Klein SM, Nielsen KC, Greengrass RA, et al. Ambulatory discharge after long-acting peripheral nerve blockade: 2382 blocks with ropivacaine. Anesth Analg 2002;94:65–70.
30. Ilfeld BM, Morey TE, Wright TW, et al. Continuous interscalene brachial plexus block for postoperative pain control at home: a randomized, double-blinded, placebo-controlled study. Anesth Analg 2003;26:1089–95.
31. Chan KM, Ma GF, Chow YN, et al. Intravenous regional anaesthesia in hand surgery—experience with 632 cases. Hand 1981;13:1926–28.
32. Fagg PS. Intravenous regional anaesthesia for lower limb orthopaedic surgery. Ann R Coll Surg Engl 1987;69:274–75.
33. Atanassoff PG, Ocampo CA, Bande MC, et al. Ropivacaine 0.2% and lidocaine 0.5% for intravenous regional anesthesia in outpatient surgery. Anesthesiology 2001;95:627–31.
34. Klein W, Schulitz KP: Outpatient arthroscopy under local anesthesia. Arch Orthop Trauma Surg 1980;96:131–34.
35. Marchal JM, Delgado-Martinez AD, Poncela M, et al. Does the type of arthroscopic surgery modify the analgesic effect of intraarticular morphine and bupivacaine? A preliminary study. Clin J Pain 2003;19:240–46.
36. Gebhard RE, Pivalizza EG, Warters RD, et al. Acute pain after discharge from ambulatory surgery. ASRA 2002;PD-48.
37. Rawal N, Hylander J, Nydahl PA, et al. Survey of postoperative analgesia following ambulatory surgery. Acta Anaesthesiol Scand 1997;41:1017–22.
38. Jorris J. Efficacy of nonsteroidal anti-inflammatory drugs in postoperative pain. Acta Anaesthesiol Belg 1996;47:115–23.
39. Stichtenoth DO, Frolich JC. The second generation of COX-2 inhibitors: what advantages do the newest offer? Drugs 2003;63:33–45.
40. Reuben SS, Bhopatkar S, Maciolek H, et al. The preemptive analgesic effect of rofecoxib after ambulatory arthroscopic knee surgery. Anesth Analg 2002;94:55–59.
41. Horlocker TT, Hebl JR. Anesthesia for outpatient knee arthroscopy: is there an optimal technique? Reg Anesth Pain Med 2003;28:58–63.
42. D'Alessio JG, Rosenblum M, Shea KP, et al. A retrospective comparison of interscalene block and general anesthesia for ambulatory surgery shoulder arthroscopy. Reg Anesth 1995;20:626–28.
43. Klein SM, Nielsen KC, Martin A, et al. Interscalene brachial plexus

block with continuous intraarticular infusion of ropivacaine. Anesth Analg 2001;93:601–5.

44. Park JY, Lee GW, Kim Y, et al. The efficacy of continuous intrabursal infusion with morphine and bupivacaine for postoperative analgesia after subacromial arthroscopy. Reg Anesth Pain Med 2002;27: 145–49.

45. Laurila PA, Lopponen A, Kanga-Saarela T, et al. Interscalene brachial plexus block is superior to subacromial bursa block after arthroscopic surgery. Acta Anaesthesiol Scand 2002;46:1031–36.

46. Klein SM, Steele SM, Nielsen KC, et al. The difficulties of ambulatory interscalene and intra-articular infusions for rotator cuff surgery: a preliminary report. Can J Anaesth 2003;50:65–69.

47. Chelly JE, Greger J, Al Samsam T, et al. Reduction of operating and recovery room times and overnight hospital stays with interscalene blocks as sole anesthetic technique for rotator cuff surgery. Minerva Anestesiol 2001;67:613–19.

48. Schroeder LE, Horlocker TT, Schroeder DR. The efficacy of axillary block for surgical procedures about the elbow. Anesth Analg 1996; 83:747–51.

49. Desroches J. The infraclavicular brachial plexus block by the coracoid approach is clinically effective: an observational study of 150 patients. Can J Anaesth 2003;50:253–57.

50. Brown AR. Anaesthesia for procedures of the hand and elbow. Best Pract Res Clin Anaesthesiol 2002;16:227–46.

51. Koscielniak-Nielsen ZJ, Rotboll-Nielsen P, Rassmussen H. Patients experiences with multiple stimulation axillary block for fast-track ambulatory hand surgery. Acta Anaesthesiol Scand 2002;46:789–93.

52. Fried A, Lotem M. Local infiltration anesthesia for meniscectomy. Clin Orthop 1972;87:204–5.

53. Junger A, Klasen J, Hartmann B, et al. Shorter discharge time after regional or intravenous anaesthesia in combination with laryngeal mask airway compared with balanced anaesthesia with endotracheal intubation. Eur J Anaesthesiol 2002;19:119–24.

54. Tivonen J, Pitko VM, Rosenberg PH. Comparison between intra-articular bupivacaine with epinephrine and epinephrine alone on short and long-term pain after knee arthroscopic surgery under general anesthesia in day-surgery. Acta Anaesthesiol Scand 2002;46: 435–40.

55. Breebaart MB, Vercauteren MP, Hoffmann VL, et al. Urinary bladder scanning after day-case arthroscopy under spinal anaesthesia: comparison between lidocaine, ropivacaine, and levobupivacaine. Br J Anaesth 2003;90:309–13.

56. Pollock JE, Mulroy MF, Bent E, et al. A comparison of two regional anesthetic techniques for outpatient knee arthroscopy. Anesth Analg 2003;97:397–401.

57. Klein SM, Greengrass RA, Grant SA et al. Ambulatory surgery for multi-ligament knee reconstruction with continuous dual catheter peripheral nerve blockade. Can J Anaesth 2001;48:375–78.

58. Marhofer P, Nasel C, Sitzwhol C, et al. Magnetic resonance imaging of the distribution of local anesthetics during the three-in-one block. Anesth Analg 2000;90:119–24.

59. Jankowski CJ, Hebl JR, Stuart MJ, et al. A comparison of psoas compartment block and spinal and general anesthesia for outpatient knee arthroscopy. Anesth Analg 2003;97:1003–9.

60. Bouaziz H, Vial F, Jochum D, et al. An evaluation of the cutaneous distribution after obturator nerve block. Anesth Analg 2002;94: 445–49.

61. Weller RS, Gerancher JC, Crews JC, et al. Extensive retroperitoneal hematoma without neurologic deficit in two patients who underwent lumbar plexus block and were later anticoagulated. Anesthesiology 2003;98:581–85.

62. Needoff M, Radford P, Costigan P. Local anesthesia for postoperative pain relief after foot surgery: prospective clinical trial. Foot Ankle Int 1995;16:11–13.

63. Ptaszek AJ, Morris SG, Brodsky JW. Midfoot field block anesthesia with monitored intravenous sedation in forefoot surgery. Foot Ankle Int 1999;20:583–86.

64. Chelly JE, Greger J, Casati A, et al. Continuous lateral sciatic blocks for acute postoperative pain management after major ankle and foot surgery. Foot Ankle Int 2002;23:749–52.

Anesthesia for Ambulatory Upper-Extremity Surgical Procedures

MATTHEW OLDMAN   •   VINCENT W.S. CHAN

INTRODUCTION

Ambulatory upper-limb surgery, the majority of which are orthopedic and plastic-surgical procedures, may be performed under general or regional anesthesia. The choice of anesthetic is often determined by the preferences of the patient, anesthesiologist, and surgeon and influenced by the patient's physical status. Upper-limb surgery lends itself to a variety of regional anesthetic techniques because the nerve supply to the upper limb, derived from the brachial plexus, may be blocked at the level of the plexus or its terminal branches. Regional anesthesia may be used alone or in conjunction with general anesthesia.

There is a perception among anesthesiologists that regional anesthesia is safer and superior to general anesthesia because it can improve postoperative analgesia,[1,2] reduce side effects,[1,2] and increase patient satisfaction.[2] By avoiding tracheal intubation, and minimizing intraoperative opioid and muscle relaxant use, length of stay can be reduced.[3] However, unlike general anesthesia, not all anesthesiologists are familiar with regional anesthesia and thus it may be less reliable, and slower to administer.[4] The longer-term benefits of regional anaesthesia are unknown. Recent data suggest that there may be little difference between regional and general anesthesia after discharge.[5]

This chapter will concentrate on the application of regional anesthetic procedures to upper-limb ambulatory surgery. Details of suitable general anesthetic techniques may be found elsewhere in this book.

ORGANIZATIONAL CONSIDERATIONS

Most patients will consent to regional anesthesia when given a clear explanation and time to make a balanced decision (e.g., several days before the proposed surgery). The surgeon can play a valuable role by explaining the option of regional anaesthesia, where appropriate, at the preoperative consult. Regional blocks may be placed before surgery in a separate induction room or in the patient preoperative holding area. The effects may then be evaluated, with enough time for block supplementation if required. A dedicated block room may be advantageous if the workload is sufficient to support it, and has the added advantage of concentrating training for anesthesia trainees.[6] Many surgeons may be wary that regional anesthesia may delay their schedule or that the success may be unpredictable when compared with general anesthesia.[7] These concerns can best be addressed by careful organization and early placement of blocks.

PRACTICAL CONSIDERATIONS

Proper patient selection is essential for safe conduct of regional anaesthesia. Needle-phobic patients, those with learning disorders, or those with severe psychiatric disorders are probably best managed with general anesthesia unless contraindicated. Children should not be denied the benefits of regional anesthesia, and it may be safer to place a block in a motionless anesthetized child than in one who is moving owing to fear. The safety of this practice in children is supported by the literature, provided the anesthesiologist possesses adequate skill and training.

The choice of regional block performed will be largely determined by the surgical procedure and the anesthesiologist's skill with an individual technique. It is best discussed with the surgeon before block placement. Regional anesthetic technique should address concern over the ability to test postoperative neurologic function. Short procedures distal to the elbow are perhaps best accomplished by the use of intravenous regional anesthesia (IVRA). Longer procedures with significant postoperative pain lend themselves to a brachial plexus block with or without catheter placement.

A significant number of patients experience discomfort during block placement,[8] and sedation during block procedure is important to improve patient acceptance and satisfaction. Midazolam 1–2 mg and fentanyl 50 µg increments can provide sedation without adversely affecting patient discharge readiness. Sedation during surgery can be further provided by incremental intravenous (IV) boluses of midazolam or low-dose IV propofol infusion. Monitoring with pulse oximetry, noninvasive blood pressure, and electrocardiogram (ECG) is the minimum requirement during block performance. A suitably trained assistant and full resuscitation equipment should be available.

The choice of local anesthetic is determined by the type of procedure, duration of block desired, and local availability. Popular agents (e.g., lidocaine, mepivacaine, bupivacaine, and ropivacaine) differ with respect to their latency and duration of action (Table 27-1). Many anesthesiologists use a drug mixture that combines the benefits of both short- and long-acting solutions and allows slightly larger doses of each agent to be administered. Additives (e.g., epinephrine) may be mixed with the local anesthetic to alter its effects. Epinephrine increases the duration of action of lidocaine by up to 90%, and bupivacaine by 50%, and additionally acts as a marker of intravascular injection. Clonidine can provide analgesic benefit with minimal adverse effects in doses up to 150 µg.[9] The role of other agents is still to be determined, but some (e.g., ketamine) appear to be promising.[10]

Accuracy in nerve localization determines block success, and the two principal methods of localization are eliciting paresthesia and nerve stimulation. Neither technique has been conclusively shown to be superior or safer to the other. When nerve stimulation is employed, a short-beveled insulated needle should be used. Stimulation at ≤ 0.5 mA is generally considered adequate for the majority of brachial plexus blocks and indicates close proximity to the nerve. Lower currents may increase the risk of nerve injury.[11]

Table 27-1 Properties of Commonly Used Local Anesthetic Agents

Agent	Usual Duration of Action	Recommended Maximum Safe Dose for Single Administration
Lidocaine	1–3 hr	5 mg/kg 9 mg/kg with epinephrine
Mepivacaine	2–3 hr	5 mg/kg 9 mg/kg with epinephrine
Bupivacaine	4–12 hr	2 mg/kg 3 mg/kg with epinephrine
Levobupivacaine	4–12 hr	150 mg[a]
Ropivacaine	4–8 hr	250 mg[a]

[a]Manufacturers' data. Insufficient data exist to recommend a mg/kg maximum dose.

ANESTHETIC TECHNIQUES

Interscalene Brachial Plexus Block

Interscalene block, which anesthetizes mainly the lower cervical plexus and the upper trunks of the brachial plexus, is most suited to providing analgesia for shoulder surgery. The lower trunk of the brachial plexus (C8–T1) is often not blocked,[12] making it less suitable for procedures below the elbow. Either nerve stimulation or paresthesia techniques may be used. The classic interscalene approach described by Winnie suggested that only paresthesia below the shoulder should be accepted. More recent studies using nerve stimulation suggest proximal motor responses in the biceps, triceps, deltoid,[13] or pectoralis major[14] are equally successful end points, with success rates ranging from 92% to 95%. However, motor response to nerve stimulation is not always apparent, as demonstrated in a study by Urmey and Stanton, who found only 30% of the patients had a motor response to electrical stimulation despite eliciting sensory paresthesia (73% occurring in the shoulder) and producing clinically successful blocks in 100% of patients.[15] Shoulder analgesia after interscalene brachial plexus block is dose-dependent, with higher local anesthetic concentrations increasing anesthetic efficacy at the expense of increased motor and sensory block distal to the elbow. To block the entire brachial plexus 50–60 mL is generally required. For selective shoulder analgesia a low-dose technique (e.g., 15 mL of 0.125% bupivacaine with epinephrine 1:400,000) can reduce analgesic consumption while producing minimal motor and sensory block after 3 hr.[16]

Nerve localization may take several attempts. Current thinking suggests that inability to obtain an appropriate motor response at a current of < 0.5mA implies the needle is outside the interscalene groove. Phrenic nerve stimulation, resulting in diaphragmatic contraction, indicates too-anterior needle placement. Trapezius muscle contraction due to spinal accessory nerve stimulation suggests the needle should be repositioned more anteriorly. Use of a more caudal and lateral needle angulation to approach the plexus along the long axis, rather than perpendicularly, may increase the likelihood of plexus contact and facilitate catheter insertion.

Neurologic complications have been reported after interscalene brachial plexus block (up to 14% at 10 days but with less than 0.4% experiencing long-term complications).[17] Other complications include total spinal anesthesia, epidural anesthesia, intravascular injection, phrenic nerve palsy (100% incidence), Horner's syndrome, recurrent laryngeal nerve palsy, and pneumothorax (0.2% in a recent series[17]). Unilateral phrenic nerve palsy is usually asymptomatic except in individuals with poor respiratory reserve. Intravascular injection into the vertebral artery will result in loss of consciousness and seizure.

Supraclavicular Brachial Plexus Block

Supraclavicular brachial plexus block is effective for hand or arm surgery. Blockade of the brachial plexus at the trunk/proximal division level, where it is compactly arranged, produces a faster onset and more complete block than many other techniques. Classic supraclavicular brachial plexus block[18] is generally not recommended for ambulatory patients because the incidence of pneumothorax is up to 6% in some series[19] and clinical manifestation of pneumothorax may not present for 6–12 hr, by which time ambulatory surgical patients will have likely been discharged home.

Variations of the classic supraclavicular approach, including the subclavian perivascular approach and the plumb bob technique, have reduced but not eliminated the risk of pneumothorax. The recently described intersternocleidomastoid approach, as described by Pham-Dang et al., appears promising.[20] The dorsal and lateral needle angulation directs the needle anterior and superior to the dome of the pleura, reducing the chance of pneumothorax, and offers a tangential approach to the plexus, facilitating catheter placement.

Infraclavicular Brachial Plexus Block

Infraclavicular techniques block the cords of the brachial plexus as they run between the clavicle and the axilla. Potential advantages include the ability to perform the block without special positioning of the arm, and the ease of fixation of indwelling catheters to the chest wall. The vertical infraclavicular approach and the coracoid approach both have easily identified landmarks.

The vertical infraclavicular technique is performed with a puncture site immediately below the clavicle, halfway between the ventral apophysis of the acromion and the midpoint of the jugular notch. Success rates of up to 88% have been reported.[21] To avoid complications, strict adherence to correct technique is necessary—the needle should be advanced no farther than 3 cm and strict perpendicular angulation to the skin should be maintained. There is a 30% incidence of inadvertent vascular puncture, and a low, but potential, pneumothorax risk.

The coracoid approach has even simpler landmarks. The puncture site is 2 cm medial and 2 cm caudad to the tip of the coracoid process on the anterior chest wall. The cords of the plexus should be encountered at a mean depth of 4 cm as they surround the axillary artery. Success rates may be increased by accepting only distal stimulation,[22] and by using a multistimulation technique, targeting individual cords.[23] Musculocutaneous nerve stimulation (lateral cord) should not be accepted, and suggests that the needle should be redirected inferiorly. For coracoid approach, stimulation at < 0.4 mA is required to consistently achieve a reliable block. Recent advances have turned toward the use of ultrasound in the performance of this block.[24]

Axillary Brachial Plexus Block

The axillary block of the terminal branches of the brachial plexus is most commonly used for hand and arm surgery about or below the elbow. It is a safe technique, without the risk of pneumothorax. Techniques available for axillary brachial plexus block include paresthesia, nerve stimulation, and the transarterial (TA) approach. These all rely on consistent nerve-artery anatomic relationships, with the musculocutaneous, median, ulnar, and radial nerves lying in four quadrants around the axillary artery. The nerves are grouped closest together at the proximal edge of the axilla (lateral edge of pectoralis minor) and steadily diverge from the artery as they run distally. The median, ulnar, and radial nerves are enclosed together with the axillary artery within a sheath derived from the connective tissue of the prevertebral fascia and the scalene muscles. Discrete fascial septae enclose each component of the neurovascular bundle. These are functionally incomplete, but may still limit spread of injected local anesthetic solution.[25] The musculocutaneous nerve leaves the fascial sheath of the brachial plexus high in the axilla and runs within the coracobrachialis muscle. Thus accepting biceps muscle twitch during a single injection technique will predictably result in a high failure rate and, conversely, failure to block the musculocutaneous nerve is common.

The TA technique is popular in North America. The axillary artery is deliberately punctured, and the needle advanced until it is just through the posterior arterial wall before 40–50 mL of local anesthetic is injected behind the artery with intermittent aspiration. Epinephrine-containing solutions allow identification of intravascular placement by producing an increase in heart rate and blood pressure, or blanching of the hand. Injection of a proportion of the local anesthetic anterior to the artery, although popular with some anesthesiologists, does not increase speed of onset or success compared with a single posterior injection.[26] The success of the TA approach is similar to that of other axillary approaches. Stan et al. demonstrated a complete block in 89% of cases, incomplete block requiring supplemental local anesthesia in 10% of cases, and a complete block failure in 1.2%.[27] Complications in this series included sensory paresthesia (0.2%), reflex sympathetic dystrophy (0.2%), arterial spasm (1%), unintentional intravascular injection (0.2%), and hematoma formation (0.2%).

Nerve stimulation techniques are more popular in Europe. A good working knowledge of the orientation of the four main nerves around the axillary artery aids needle placement. If a single injection is to be performed, it is prudent to seek stimulation of the nerve whose sensory supply covers the surgical site. Musculocutaneous nerve stimulation should not be accepted as the nerve may have already left the sheath and a higher incidence of block failure may result. Needle position is optimized until maximal contraction is achieved at a current of < 0.5mA. Forty to fifty mL of local anesthetic is required for a single-injection technique. Stimulating more than one nerve and splitting administration of the anesthetic dose between the sites can improve success rate and block latency. Two-nerve stimulation increased success rate from 52% in the single-nerve stimulation group to 92% in the double-nerve stimulation group.[28] Three-nerve stimulation (where one of the nerves blocked is the musculocutaneous) is more successful than two-nerve stimulation.[29] However, four-nerve stimulation does not further increase success. Omission of ulnar nerve block does not affect the latency of block onset or extent of block, but does reduce block performance time and pain during block.[30] Multiple-nerve stimulation (MNS) compares favorably to TA axillary brachial plexus block, taking on average 3 min longer to perform but significantly reducing block latency (median 30 min TA and 10 min MNS) and supplementation rate (36% TA and 6% MNS).[31]

Humeral Block ("Midhumeral Block")

This is a recently described technique[32] whereby the four main nerves of the upper extremity are blocked separately at the junction of the upper third and middle third of the arm using a peripheral nerve stimulator. At this level the four nerves are anatomically well separated, allowing selective administration of different local anesthetics on the various nerves. By utilizing a longer-acting agent for the nerve covering the surgical site, postoperative analgesia may be enhanced without causing unwanted residual block in other nerve distributions. In addition, the humeral approach is an ideal site to supplement other brachial plexus blocks that are inadequate for surgery, without the risk of inserting the needle near a partially anesthetized nerve.

Published success rates for this block range from 82% to 96.9% and are comparable to four-nerve-stimulation axillary brachial plexus block.[33] A threshold current of < 0.6 mA should be adequate to achieve good success rates for each of the nerves.[34] Complication rates are low and adverse events usually minor.[34] The following sequence of nerve blockade has been proposed based on onset time: median, ulnar, radial, musculocutaneous.[35] Eight to ten mL of local anesthetic is required for each nerve.

Nerve Blocks at the Elbow

Blockade at the elbow is mainly indicated for rescue of an inadequate brachial plexus block, and for postoperative analgesia. It is also a suitable technique for procedures such as median nerve decompression, and most hand surgery, including nerve, tendon, and soft-tissue repair, and manipulation of fractured digits. Tourniquet pain in the arm will not be blocked and this may limit the use of this technique. Although not essential, the nerve stimulation technique can localize the median, ulnar, and radial nerves accurately. Generally 5 mL of local anesthetic is adequate for each nerve, noting that excessive volume may cause nerve compression, particularly the ulnar nerve over the medial epicondyle.

Nerve Blocks at the Wrist

Nerve blocks at the wrist can supplement incomplete surgical blocks or provide postoperative analgesia. The median and ulnar nerves may be easily blocked with 3–5 mL of local anesthetic. One should be aware of the theoretic risk of nerve compression because these nerves pass through relatively restricted fascial compartments. The ra-

dial nerve has a less constant anatomic location, and divides into multiple small cutaneous branches. It is best blocked by a subcutaneous injection of 5–10 mL of local anesthetic.

Digital Nerve Block

This simple block, also known as a ring block, is performed for minor finger procedures. Epinephrine-containing local anesthetic solutions are contraindicated as digital artery ischemia may occur. Excessive volumes should be avoided to prevent nerve compression. A similar technique may be performed at the midpoint of the metacarpal for anesthesia of the proximal finger, but may be less efficacious than digital block.[36]

Intravenous Regional Anesthesia

Intravenous regional anesthesia is an excellent technique for open or closed surgical procedures lasting less than 30 min. IVRA is a low-cost technique offering rapid patient recovery and reduction of postoperative nursing care and hospital discharge time compared to both general anesthesia and brachial plexus block.[4] Local anesthetic toxicity is a major potential risk with IVRA but can be minimized by slow local anesthetic injection into a vein distal to the tourniquet (e.g., in the dorsum of the hand and not in the antecubital veins). Careful tourniquet application is also recommended to prevent local anesthetic leakage by inflating the tourniquet 100 mmHg above the limb occlusion pressure. This minimal tourniquet pressure required to occlude arterial blood flow past the cuff not only prevents local anesthetic leakage, but also prevents a "venous tourniquet" where arterial flow into the limb is not abolished. This results in a poor operative block and a congested limb with troublesome surgical bleeding. Slow injection of local anesthetic is advised to avoid rapid increases in pressure within the venous system that may overcome tourniquet cuff pressure to allow leakage. Surgical anesthesia is usually complete within 10 min. Generally speaking, tourniquet inflation should not exceed 90 min, owing to the risk of ischemic nerve and muscle injury. The cuff may be deflated in one step 20 min after the injection of lidocaine.

Lidocaine 0.5% is the most commonly used local anesthetic in North America. The maximal-dose of lidocaine for IVRA is 3 mg/kg. Lidocaine concentrations greater than 0.5% predispose to toxic levels even if the same maximum dose is administered, and their use cannot be recommended. Prilocaine is a popular agent for IVRA in Europe, but is no longer available in North America owing to concerns over methemoglobinemia. Preservative-free chloroprocaine is also popular in Europe. Ropivacaine has been investigated for IVRA in 0.2% and 0.375% concentrations[37,38] and may be associated with fewer central nervous system side effects than lidocaine. Bupivacaine is contraindicated after reported cases of severe systemic local anesthetic toxicity and death.

Adjuncts added to IVRA can improve block efficacy, prolong duration of postdeflation analgesia, and reduce the incidence of tourniquet pain, as summarized in a recent review.[39] Ketorolac added to local anesthetic in doses up to 20 mg, reduces postoperative pain and analgesic consumption.[40] Tenoxicam 20 mg and acetylsalicilate 90 mg also appear to offer some improvement in postoperative analgesia. Clonidine 1 μg/kg increases tolerance to tourniquet pain[41] and reduces postoperative pain.[42] Larger doses may result in sedation and hypotension on tourniquet deflation. Muscle relaxants (e.g., atracurium 2 mg), improve limb paralysis and surgical operating conditions for fracture manipulation.[43] Ketamine 0.1 mg/kg slows the onset of tourniquet pain and decreases analgesic consumption for tourniquet pain relief, but up to 50% of patients may develop mild pyschomimetic side effects, limiting its clinical application.[44]

Tourniquet pain typically begins 30–45 min after inflation and may require general anesthesia if the patient is severely distressed despite sedation. There is no consistent relationship between tourniquet pain and tourniquet pressure or cuff width. A newer strategy to lengthen the duration of tourniquet tolerance (by up to 50 min) is the inflation of a separate distal forearm cuff and deflation of the original proximal arm cuff when severe tourniquet pain arises.[45] To further reduce the potential for local anesthetic toxicity, one can consider IVRA with a forearm tourniquet alone, which provides effective surgical anesthesia despite a 50% local-anesthetic dose reduction.[46]

Local Anesthetic Infiltration

Local anesthetic infiltration may be used either for surgical anesthesia for smaller surgical procedures, or for postoperative analgesia. Surgery under local anesthetic infiltration alone requires a surgeon who is both skilled enough and willing to perform the procedure under local anesthesia. Adequate time must be given for the local anesthetic solution to work, and extra local anesthetic should be available for intraoperative supplementation. Sedatives such as midazolam combined with monitored anesthetic care (MAC) may be used to improve patient comfort.

The benefits of incisional local anesthetic infiltration for postoperative analgesia in upper-limb surgery have not been established, but it is unlikely that the practice causes any harm.

Intra-articular Local Anesthetics

Intra-articular infusions of local anesthetic have been shown to be effective for postoperative analgesia after shoulder surgery under general anesthesia and interscalene brachial plexus block. Intra-articular catheters may be easily placed by the surgeon and deliver local anesthetic directly to the operative site. Patients may be discharged home with either a constant-infusion or patient-controlled boluses via an intra-articular infusion system. A peripheral analgesic effect has been demonstrated for morphine 1 mg combined with bupivacaine after rotator cuff repair.[47]

Subacromial bursa block with local anesthetic containing epinephrine is a simple and safe technique often performed by orthopedic surgeons during arthroscopic surgery to reduce both perioperative bleeding and postoperative pain. However, its analgesic benefit is no better than that provided by interscalene brachial plexus block.[48]

POSTOPERATIVE MANAGEMENT

One of the advantages of regional anesthesia is that it may facilitate bypass of the postanesthetic care unit (PACU), thus minimizing nursing requirements and increasing throughput through the unit. Scoring systems such as the modified Aldrete score can be used to identify patients suitable for PACU bypass. To safely bypass the PACU the patient should not have received sedatives or opioids in the preceding 30 min, and should achieve a modified Aldrete score greater than 9. Recovery of motor and sensory function is no longer essential prior to discharge home. The anesthetized limb must be protected in a sling and the patient advised of the risk of injury. Patients should be instructed to seek medical advice if they experience persistent numbness, weakness, or paresthesia. It should also be emphasized that driving and manual tasks are contraindicated until normal power and sensation have returned.

The incidence of severe postoperative pain is significant after ambulatory surgery, and is particularly common with orthopedic procedures.[49] The analgesic benefits of single-injection regional techniques are limited by the duration of local-anesthetic action, typically 13–14 hr if long-acting agents such as bupivacaine or ropivacaine are used. Failure to employ other analgesics at an early stage may result in a patient who was comfortable at discharge experiencing considerable discomfort later at home when regional block resolution occurs. While simple analgesics may be adequate for minor procedures, for more extensive surgery the use of IV opiates such as fentanyl or additional methods of analgesia, such as continuous peripheral nerve blocks, may be necessary.

Continuous Peripheral Nerve Block Techniques

Continuous peripheral nerve blocks extend the benefits of single-injection blocks into the postoperative period. In addition, the ability to supplement the block during surgery makes many longer surgical procedures amenable to regional techniques. Upper extremity catheters can decrease postoperative pain and opiate consumption and increase patient satisfaction.[50] Careful patient selection and education is required to achieve good success rates. These techniques also require more advanced skills from the anesthesiologist, and a learning curve is associated with their use. Most of the published studies use a peripheral nerve stimulator to localize the plexus and leave 5–10 cm of catheter in situ, depending on the site. The incidence of primary block failure (failure after initial local-anesthetic dose) with continuous peripheral nerve blocks is approximately 6%[50] and that of secondary block failure (failure once infusion commences) may be up to 37%.[51]

There are many varieties of continuous catheter delivery systems. These are either catheter-over-needle or catheter-through-needle systems. Recently, stimulating catheters have been introduced that allow confirmation that the catheter lies next to the nerves of the plexus. Theoretically this may help reduce secondary catheter failure, although there are currently no published data to support this. The median current needed to elicit a motor response may be up to 3.5 times greater for a stimulating catheter compared with the needle.[51] The key principle of plexus catheterization is to introduce the catheter parallel to the nerves to facilitate threading and reduce kinking. This may require modification of the approach usually used to perform a particular nerve block.

The optimal local-anesthetic solution for continuous peripheral nerve blocks has not been determined. Bupivacaine and ropivacaine are the most commonly used agents postoperatively. Ropivacaine produces less motor block than bupivacaine, which is more desirable in the ambulatory setting, and is also less cardiotoxic. Administration of a short-acting local anesthetic agent for surgical anesthesia (e.g., lidocaine) and a longer-acting agent for postoperative analgesia (e.g., ropivacaine) can facilitate surgical testing of nerve function after surgery (e.g., axillary nerve testing after shoulder surgery).

Postoperative perineural analgesia may be provided by repeat bolus administration, continuous infusion, or patient-controlled techniques. Although more convenient for patients, continuous infusions do not necessarily provide superior analgesia to intermittent boluses for axillary brachial plexus catheters,[52] and may result in higher plasma local-anesthetic concentrations. For shoulder surgery a continuous infusion with patient-controlled anelgesia boluses offers optimum analgesia, while minimizing local anesthetic consumption.[53] Continuing upper limb regional anesthesia in the home environment has been demonstrated to reduce analgesic consumption and reduce sleep interruption.[54–55] Disposable infusion devices are now marketed that employ continuous infusions at a variety of preset rates, with some devices offering patient-controlled boluses. The system should be carefully explained to patients and their caregivers prior to discharge, and written instructions provided, including an emergency contact number. Specifically, patients should be instructed to wear a sling at all times to protect the anesthetized limb, and not to drive. Catheter removal may be successfully performed by another health care provider or, more radically, by the patient caregiver with telephone supervision.[56]

It is important not to depend on continuous peripheral nerve block catheters as the sole postoperative analgesic agent. A multimodal analgesic strategy is essential, with appropriate rescue analgesia available in the event of secondary catheter failure. Although up to 90% of catheters remain functional at 24 hr, a high proportion of patients may still require IV or oral opiates in the first 24-hr period.[50]

SUMMARY

Orthopedic procedures are associated with a high incidence of postoperative pain. A number of techniques may be employed for successful anesthesia of the upper limb. The choice of general, regional, or combined general-regional anesthesia will be determined by surgical procedure, patient, surgeon, and anesthesiologist preference. The choice of regional anesthetic technique is determined by the site of surgery and the skill and preference of individual anesthesiologists. Multimodal analgesia combined with either single-injection or continuous regional anesthetic techniques is recommended.

REFERENCES

1. Singelyn FJ, Deyaert M, Joris D, et al. Effects of intravenous patient-controlled analgesia with morphine, continuous epidural analgesia, and continuous three-in-one block on postoperative pain and knee rehabilitation after unilateral total knee arthroplasty. Anesth Analg 1998 Jul;87(1):88–92.
2. Borgeat A, Schappi B, Biasca N, et al. Patient-controlled analgesia after major shoulder surgery: patient-controlled interscalene analgesia versus patient-controlled analgesia. Anesthesiology 1997 Dec; 87(6):1343–47.
3. Junger A, Klasen J, Benson M, et al. Factors determining length of stay of surgical day-case patients. Eur J Anaesthesiol 2001 May; 18(5):314–21.
4. Chan VW, Peng PW, Kaszas Z, et al. A comparative study of general anesthesia, intravenous regional anesthesia, and axillary block for outpatient hand surgery: clinical outcome and cost analysis. Anesth Analg 2001 Nov;93(5):1181–84.
5. Brull RT, von Schroeder H, Anastakis D, et al. Regional anesthesia versus general anesthesia for ambulatory hand surgery. Reg Anesth Pain Med 2003;28:A1.
6. Martin G, Lineberger CK, MacLeod DB, et al. A new teaching model for resident training in regional anesthesia. Anesth Analg 2002 Nov;95(5):1423–27.
7. Oldman M, McCartney C, Perlas A, et al. A survey of surgeons' attitudes to regional anesthesia. Reg Anesth Pain Med 2003;28:A12.
8. Koscielniak-Nielsen ZJ, Rotboll-Nielsen P, Rassmussen H. Patients' experiences with multiple stimulation axillary block for fast-track ambulatory hand surgery. Acta Anaesthesiol Scand 2002 Aug;46(7): 789–93.
9. Murphy DB, McCartney CJ, Chan VW. Novel analgesic adjuncts for brachial plexus block: a systematic review. Anesth Analg 2000 May; 90(5):1122–28.
10. McCartney CJ, Chan VW, Sanandaji K, et al. Small dose ketamine 0.5mg/kg produces a peripheral preventive analgesic effect when added to interscalene block for major shoulder surgery. Reg Anesth Pain Med 2003;28:A4.
11. Auroy Y, Benhamou D, Bargues L, et al. Major complications of regional anesthesia in France: the SOS Regional Anesthesia Hotline Service. Anesthesiology 2002 Nov;97(5):1274–80.
12. Lanz E, Theiss D, Jankovic D. The extent of blockade following various techniques of brachial plexus block. Anesth Analg 1983 Jan; 62(1):55–58.
13. Silverstein WB, Saiyed MU, Brown AR. Interscalene block with a nerve stimulator: a deltoid motor response is a satisfactory endpoint for successful block. Reg Anesth Pain Med 2000 Jul-Aug;25(4): 356–59.
14. Tonidandel WL, Mayfield JB. Successful interscalene block with a nerve stimulator may also result after a pectoralis major motor response. Reg Anesth Pain Med 2002 Sep-Oct;27(5):491–93.
15. Urmey WF, Stanton J. Inability to consistently elicit a motor response following sensory paresthesia during interscalene block administration. Anesthesiology 2002 Mar;96(3):552–54.

16. Al-Kaisy A, McGuire G, Chan VW, et al. Analgesic effect of inter-scalene block using low-dose bupivacaine for outpatient arthro-scopic shoulder surgery. Reg Anesth Pain Med 1998 Sep-Oct;23(5):469–73.

17. Borgeat A, Ekatodramis G, Kalberer F, et al. Acute and non acute complications associated with interscalene block and shoulder sur-gery: a prospective study. Anesthesiology 2001 Oct;95(4):875–80.

18. Kulenkampff D, Persky MA. Brachial plexus anesthesia: Its indica-tions, technic, and dangers. Ann Surg 1928;87:883.

19. Harley N, Gjessing J. A critical assessment of supraclavicular brachial plexus block. Anaesthesia 1969 Oct;24(4):564–70.

20. Pham-Dang C, Gunst JP, Gouin F, et al. A novel supraclavicular ap-proach to brachial plexus block. Anesth Analg 1997 Jul;85(1):111–16.

21. Neuberger M, Kaiser H, Rembold-Schuster I, et al. Vertical infra-clavicular brachial plexus blockade: a clinical study of the reliabil-ity of a new method for plexus anaesthesia of the upper extremity. Anaesthetist 1998;47:595–99.

22. Borgeat A, Ekatodramis G, Dumont C. An evaluation of the infra-clavicular block via a modified approach of the Raj technique. Anesth Analg 2001 Aug;93(2):436–41.

23. Gaertner E, Estebe JP, Zamfir A, et al. Infraclavicular plexus block: multiple injection versus single injection. Reg Anesth Pain Med 2002 Nov-Dec;27(6):590–94.

24. Sandhu NS, Capan LM. Ultrasound-guided infraclavicular brachial plexus block. Br J Anaesth 2002 Aug;89(2):254–59.

25. Klaastad O, Smedby O, Thompson GE, et al. Distribution of local anesthetic in axillary brachial plexus block: a clinical and magnetic resonance imaging study. Anesthesiology 2002 Jun;96(6):1315–24.

26. Desbordes J, Mille FX, Adnet P, et al. Brachial plexus anesthesia via an axillary route for emergency surgery: comparison of three ap-proach methods. Ann Fr Anesth Reanim 1998;17(7):674–80.

27. Stan TC, Krantz MA, Solomon DL, et al. The incidence of neu-rovascular complications following axillary brachial plexus block using a transarterial approach: a prospective study of 1,000 con-secutive patients. Reg Anesth 1995 Nov-Dec;20(6):486–92.

28. Inberg P, Annila I, Annila P. Double-injection method using pe-ripheral nerve stimulator is superior to single injection in axillary plexus block. Reg Anesth Pain Med 1999 Nov-Dec;24(6):509–13.

29. Sia S, Lepri A, Ponzecchi P. Axillary brachial plexus block using pe-ripheral nerve stimulator: a comparison between double- and triple-injection techniques. Reg Anesth Pain Med 2001 Nov-Dec;26(6):499–503.

30. Sia S, Bartoli M. Selective ulnar nerve localization is not essential for axillary brachial plexus block using a multiple nerve stimula-tion technique. Reg Anesth Pain Med 2001 Jan–Feb;26(1):12–16.

31. Koscielniak-Nielsen ZJ, Nielsen PR, Nielsen SL, et al. Comparison of transarterial and multiple nerve stimulation techniques for axil-lary block using a high dose of mepivacaine with adrenaline. Acta Anaesthesiol Scand 1999 Apr;43(4):398–404.

32. Dupré LJ. Brachial plexus block through humeral approach. Cah Anesthesiol 1994;42:767–69.

33. Sia S, Lepri A, Campolo MC, et al. Four-injection brachial plexus block using peripheral nerve stimulator: a comparison between ax-illary and humeral approaches. Anesth Analg 2002 Oct;95(4):1075–79.

34. Carles M, Pulcini A, Macchi P, et al. An evaluation of the brachial plexus block at the humeral canal using a neurostimulator (1417 patients): the efficacy, safety, and predictive criteria of failure. Anesth Analg 2001 Jan;92(1):194–98.

35. Gaertner E, Kern O, Mahoudeau G, et al. Block of the brachial plexus branches by the humeral route: a prospective study in 503 ambulatory patients. Proposal of a nerve-blocking sequence. Acta Anaesthesiol Scand 1999 Jul;43(6):609–13.

36. Knoop K, Trott A, Syverud S. Comparison of the digital versus metacarpal blocks for repair of finger injuries. Ann Emerg Med 1994;23(6):1296–300.

37. Atanassoff PG, Hartmannsgruber MW. Central nervous system side effects are less important after iv regional anesthesia with ropiva-caine 0.2% compared to lidocaine 0.5% in volunteers. Can J Anaesth 2002 Feb;49(2):169–72.

38. Peng PW, Coleman MM, McCartney CJ, et al. Comparison of anes-thetic effect between 0.375% ropivacaine versus 0.5% lidocaine in forearm intravenous regional anesthesia. Reg Anesth Pain Med 2002 Nov–Dec;27(6):595–599.

39. Choyce A, Peng P. A systematic review of adjuncts for intravenous regional anesthesia for surgical procedures. Can J Anaesth 2002 Jan;49(1):32–45.

40. Steinberg RB, Reuben SS, Gardner G. The dose-response relation-ship of ketorolac as a component of intravenous regional anesthe-sia with lidocaine. Anesth Analg 1998;86:791–93.

41. Lurie SD, Reuben SS, Gibson CS, et al. Effect of clonidine on up-per extremity tourniquet pain in healthy volunteers. Reg Anesth Pain Med 2000;25:502–5.

42. Reuben SS, Steinberg RB, Klatt JL, et al. Intravenous regional anes-thesia using lidocaine and clonidine. Anesthesiology 1999;91:654–58.

43. McGlone R, Heyes F, Harris P. The use of a muscle relaxant to sup-plement local anaesthetics for Bier's blocks. Arch Emerg Med 1988;5:79–85.

44. Gorgias NK, Maidatsi PG, Kyriakidis AM, et al. Clonidine versus ketamine to prevent tourniquet pain during intravenous regional anesthesia with lidocaine. Reg Anesth Pain Med 2001 Nov–Dec;26(6):512–17.

45. Perlas A, Peng PW, Plaza MB, et al. Forearm rescue cuff improves tourniquet tolerance during intravenous regional anesthesia. Reg Anesth Pain Med 2003 Mar-Apr;28(2):98–102.

46. Reuben SS, Steinberg RB, Maciolek H, et al. An evaluation of the analgesic efficacy of intravenous regional anesthesia with lidocaine and ketorolac using a forearm versus upper arm tourniquet. Anesth Analg 2002 Aug;95(2):457–60.

47. Tetzlaff JE, Brems J, Dilger J. Intraarticular morphine and bupiva-caine reduces postoperative pain after rotator cuff repair. Reg Anesth Pain Med 2000 Nov–Dec;25(6):611–14.

48. Laurila PA, Lopponen A, Kanga-Saarela T, et al. Interscalene brachial plexus block is superior to subacromial bursa block after arthroscopic shoulder surgery. Acta Anaesthesiol Scand 2002 Sep;46(8):1031–36.

49. Chung F, Ritchie E, Su J. Postoperative pain in ambulatory surgery. Anesth Analg 1997 Oct;85(4):808–16.

50. Grant SA, Nielsen KC, Greengrass RA, et al. Continuous peripheral nerve block for ambulatory surgery. Reg Anesth Pain Med 2001 May–Jun;26(3):209–14.

51. Pham-Dang C, Kick O, Collet T, et al. Continuous peripheral nerve blocks with stimulating catheters. Reg Anesth Pain Med 2003 Mar–Apr;28(2):83–88.

52. Mezzatesta JP, Scott DA, Schweitzer SA, et al. Continuous axillary brachial plexus block for postoperative pain relief. Intermittent bo-lus versus continuous infusion. Reg Anesth 1997 Jul–Aug;22(4):357–62.

53. Singelyn FJ, Seguy S, Gouverneur JM. Interscalene brachial plexus analgesia after open shoulder surgery: continuous versus patient-controlled infusion. Anesth Analg 1999 Nov;89(5):1216–20.

54. Ilfeld BM, Morey TE, Wright TW, et al. Continuous interscalene brachial plexus block for postoperative pain control at home: a ran-domized, double-blinded, placebo-controlled study. Anesth Analg 2003 Apr;96(4):1089–95.

55. Ilfeld BM, Morey TE, Enneking FK. Continuous infraclavicular brachial plexus block for postoperative pain control at home: a ran-domized, double-blinded, placebo-controlled study. Anesthesiology 2002 Jun;96(6):1297–304.

56. Ilfeld BM, Esener DE, Morey TE, et al. Ambulatory perineural in-fusion: the patients' perspective. Reg Anesth Pain Med 2003 Sep–Oct;28(5):418–23.

Anesthesia for Ambulatory Lower-Extremity Surgical Procedures

JEAN-LOUIS HORN • CHRISTOPHER SWIDE • PAMELA CAMPBELL

INTRODUCTION

Ambulatory surgery is a rapidly expanding specialty of anesthesia practice. Because of the lower cost of outpatient care, economic pressure is pushing for the widespread applicability of invasive lower-extremity surgery to the outpatient setting where minimal postoperative pain and complications are expected.[1–3] As a result, surgical techniques have transformed invasive surgeries into less traumatic procedures to minimized unplanned admissions.[4,5] The expansion of endoscopic procedures to include major surgeries like rotator cuff repair and, in particular, anterior cruciate ligament (ACL) repair exemplifies this surgical evolution.[6] Specialized techniques in ambulatory anesthesia have evolved alongside surgical progress. Anesthesia techniques to facilitate ambulatory surgery have used regional anesthesia (RA) as a mainstay in the multimodal approach to control pain and perioperative complications. RA and especially peripheral nerve block (PNB) have seen tremendous progress over the last decade. Recent developments include vast improvements of catheters and needles, as well as a better understanding of nerve localization.[7,8] Newer, safer local anesthetics, such as ropivacaine and levobupivacaine, have also furthered the practice of RA.[9,10] The controversial debate of general anesthesia (GA) versus RA has become irrelevant as regional techniques are often used to facilitate postoperative recovery and can therefore be combined, when indicated, with GA or sedation.[11] Uncontrolled pain and nausea, the major causes of unplanned admissions after ambulatory surgery, can be significantly decreased by systematic application of multimodal pain management (MPM), where RA and particularly PNB play key roles.[12–14]

The purpose of this chapter is to address the recent progress of anesthetic patient care for ambulatory surgery of the lower extremity focusing on several key aspects of MPM. The chapter will review in more details the role of RA in MPM, including site-specific surgeries.

MULTIMODAL ANESTHESIA FOR LOWER-EXTREMITY SURGICAL PROCEDURES

Improvements in surgical techniques and anesthesia practice have increased the ability to perform lower-extremity surgical procedures in the outpatient setting. Economic pressures continue to push for more cost-effective operations and shorter hospital stays.[1–3] As a result, the last 20 years have witnessed a change in applicability of outpatient surgery from relatively simple procedures to major surgery like rotator cuff or ACL reconstruction.[6,15] Better understanding of perioperative pain control has allowed more patients to safely undergo moderate to major surgery in the ambulatory setting.[16] Although the overall level of postoperative pain has been markedly reduced, published data continue to confirm that postoperative pain control is poorly managed in the home setting, demonstrating that there is opportunity for further improvement in postoperative pain control.[17,18] One method of improvement is to achieve a better, more precise understanding of the criteria involved in choosing a particular anesthesia technique. The choice of technique should be tailored to the surgery, the patient, and the institution. It has been well established that bone surgery and extensive soft-tissue procedures cause more pain than simpler soft-tissue surgeries or superficial interventions.[14] The condition of the patient is also directly linked to pain severity and, thus, to pain control methodologies. Patients with high pain sensitivity, depression, anxiety, chronic pain, or chronic opioid use may require more complex management to achieve satisfactory postoperative pain control.[19] Regional anesthesia techniques are strongly suggested for patients with chronic pain and those at risk for it in the future, such as those undergoing amputations or with reflex sympathetic dystrophy.[20]

Unplanned hospital admissions and/or discharge delays are expensive. Those are due to uncontrolled pain, intractable postoperative nausea and vomiting (PONV), or both.[12–14] The utilization of PNB addresses those issues by dramatically reducing PONV and uncontrolled postoperative pain. Because the anesthesiologist's field of expertise has, over the years, shifted from *intra*operative to *perioperative* medicine, his or her role in postoperative care has become increasingly important for good outcome. Appropriate anesthesia techniques with proper drug selection and administration can dramatically improve the perioperative course when combined with MPM.[21–23]

Multimodal Pain Management and Perioperative Care

MPM combines the use of a variety of anesthesia/analgesia methods to enhance postoperative pain control and outcome (Table 28-1). A combination of several methods will decrease the potential individual side effects, improve the overall efficacy with synergistic actions of each method, and minimize central sensitization of pain pathways, thus preventing hyperalgesia.[22–24] Though still controversial for human surgeries, the concept of preemptive analgesia appears most appropriate to operations on the limbs and should be implemented before surgery.[25] By pretreating pain before the surgical insult, we intend to improve the postoperative course through prevention of central sensitization.[25] Regional anesthesia techniques play a significant role in this venue, and can be as simple as local wound infiltration by a surgeon before incision or may involve prolonged perineural infusion with a catheter. Using a single-injection PNB with wound infiltration can enhance its efficiency and provide prolonged postoperative pain control.[26] For more painful procedures of the lower extremity, continuous PNBs should be at the core of the pain treatment plan for the early postoperative period.[27–30] In addition to RA techniques, many classes of drugs have been utilized in MPM. These includes nonsteroidal anti-inflammatory drugs (NSAIDs), cyclooxygenase-2 (COX-2) inhibitors, acetaminophen, supplemental and time-release opioids, and N-methyl-D-aspartate (NMDA) antagonists (e.g., ketamine).[31–34] The choice of techniques and adjuvant analgesics needs to be tailored to the unique profile of each patient, including special health conditions, drug intolerance and/or contraindication, previous pain experience, and expected surgical pain. Some analgesic agents, i.e., NSAIDs, COX-2 inhibitors, and acetaminophen, should be given on a fixed schedule;[35,36] others, i.e., opioids,[36] should only be given as circumstances require (PRN).

PERIPHERAL NERVE BLOCKS

The Use of Peripheral Nerve Blocks

PNBs should be the mainstay of MPM for lower extremity outpatient surgery. Unfortunately, many practitioners do not employ these techniques or use them infrequently.[37,38] Lower-extremity blocks are considered by many to be more challenging than upper-extremity blocks as two separate plexuses must be blocked for complete anesthesia.[39] In addition, anesthesia providers may worry that patients without pain will not protect their insensate limb and, because of the lack of proprioception, patients will not be able to care for themselves, ambulate, or may fall.[37,40] As with PNB for the upper extremity, concerns remain that patients may develop out-of-control pain after block resolution at home and consequently this will reduce patient satisfaction.[1,40] But a recent study by Klein et al. reports high patient satisfaction in 2382 patients who had lower-extremity blocks and were discharged home.[10] Other obstacles include lack of support from surgeons who commonly blame RA for delaying their surgery. Although surgery delay is real, it is often minimal and well compensated by an accelerated re-

Table 28-1   Multimodal Pain Management Options

Treatment Option	Preemptive	Fixed Schedule	PRN	Single Injection	Continuous Infusion
NSAIDs/ COX-2 inhibitors	x	x	x		
Acetaminophen	x	x	x		
Ketamine	x				
Time-release opioids	x	x			
Opioids			x		
Wound infiltration	x			x	x
PNBs	x			x	x
Spinal/epidural	x				

Depending on the severity of the expected postoperative pain and the patient condition (chronic pain patients, etc.), providers would likely choose one or more modalities from this table. Options for preemptive analgesics must start before the surgical procedure. Other analgesics are to be taken after the procedure on a fixed schedule and to be used in combination with PRN (as needed) opioids for breakthrough pain. Wound infiltration and PNBs play a major role for painful surgeries.

covery with diminished anesthesia-related complications.[41] Some patients fear being awake or in pain during the surgery. Their comfort can be guaranteed with sedation or GA. In fact, heavy sedation or GA is a good combination with PNBs for potentially uncomfortable and lengthy surgical procedures.

Aside from current strategies used to extend the life of a "single-injection" block, ambulatory anesthesia providers are investigating the use of continuous-delivery devices. The proven safety and efficacy of continuous PNBs for inpatients has triggered a recent move for patients to be sent home with a peripheral nerve catheter attached to an infusion pump.[27–30,42] This has resulted in excellent postoperative analgesia and much improved recovery.[28–30,42] In the inpatient population, studies of continuous PNB compared with traditional modes of pain relief, such as epidural and intravenous (IV) patient-controlled analgesia (PCA), show that PNB reduces PONV, pruritus, and sedation. Patients will ambulate and meet physical therapy targets earlier. Postoperative pain seems to be better controlled with fewer pain-related sleep disturbances. Patients experience less urinary retention, usually seen with epidural or spinal anesthesia.[43–47] Continuous popliteal sciatic nerve block has been studied in ambulatory patients having below-the-knee orthopedic surgery. Patients receiving patient-controlled regional analgesia (PCRA) had less pain, consumed less opiods, and had 10 times fewer sleep disturbances when compared with the saline group.[29] Overall, studies have shown that PNBs are safe with improved pain control, fewer side effects, and accelerated rehabilitation.

Organization

Regional Anesthesia Selection

Because each regional block is individualized to accommodate a specific surgery, surgeon, patient, and institution, several different factors are pertinent in block selection and technique.[48] Anatomic factors include specific innervation for the surgical site (see below), in which anatomic abnormalities that may complicate landmark identification and/or patient positioning should be taken into account.[48] Although aging does not appear to be a factor in patient selection,[49] the elderly may experience a prolonged duration of action from local anesthetics as evidenced by single-injection techniques on the brachial plexus.[50] In addition, pathophysiologic conditions such as infection in the desired block location, coagulopathy, and preexisting neuropathy, especially with patients diagnosed with multiple sclerosis and diabetes mellitus, can influence anesthesia selection and should thus be taken into consideration.[48]

In the case of coagulopathy, the American Society of Regional Anesthesia (ASRA) has published guidelines for each class of anticoagulation therapy for central neuraxial techniques.[51] The risk of complication after PNB in a coagulopathic patient depends on the severity of the condition and/or the antithrombotic medications involved. In general, RA techniques must be decided on a case-by-case basis depending on both the specific condition of the patient, the timing of anticoagulation dosage and catheter removal.

As aforementioned, preexisting nerve injury is also a concern. Common sense would tell us that a patient with a currently evolving or worsening nerve injury might be a poor choice for PNB, which would prevent neurologic examination and may be implicated to contribute to the patient's decline. Patients with stable neurologic deficits would be better candidates as long as a comprehensive neurologic history and physical examination with informed consent is obtained prior to block placement. Other classes of disease that feature progressive neurologic decline should be approached with caution. For example, arguments can be made against performing a nerve block on multiple sclerosis patients since symptoms wax and wane; however, one may argue in favor of a continuous PNB, which may prevent surgical stress that could worsen these patients' condition. Informed consent is particularly important for these patients, and both the pros and cons of RA should be presented to them before surgery. The same approach should be taken with diabetic patients.

Chronic pain patients are often considered good candidates for PNB. These patients tend to be difficult to manage postoperatively owing to their low pain threshold and high tolerance to pain medications.[49]

In addition, RA techniques may be able to facilitate the perioperative course of the many American Society of Anesthesiologists (ASA) physical status III patients who are now being scheduled for outpatient surgery. Stevens et al.'s study compared patients for total hip arthroplasty with and without a lumbar plexus block and indicated that the unilateral lower-extremity nerve blockade had a minimal effect on blood pressure.[52]

The use of RA for patients suffering from various psychologic/psychiatric conditions must be decided based on individual circumstances. Although performing routine RA under heavy sedation or GA is not recommended, certain circumstances may emerge where the risk/benefit ratio will be in favor of a RA technique. As such, disoriented and demented patients would most likely be excluded for home perineural catheter infusion unless a mature, well-informed caretaker is present throughout the infusion period at home.

Preparation for Regional Anesthesia

Efficacious use of PNBs as a part of MPM for lower-extremity procedures requires collaboration among patients, surgeons, and anesthesiologists. The surgeons are the first to introduce anesthesia options to the patient and thus strongly influence the patient's eventual selection. Surgeon collaboration and sometimes education are critical for efficient perioperative MPM.

For successful and safe usage of continuous PNBs at home, comprehensive patient education with proper instructions is crucial. Table 28-2 illustrates the key roles and subsequent actions that address the facilitation of continuous RA at home. In particular, three important issues are to be addressed to the patient: (1) education about the signs of systemic toxicity with clear instructions including an emergency contact number available 24 hr a day, 7 days a week; (2) instruction about careful protection of the in-

Table 28-2   Care Team and Patient Education

Target group	Role	Specific Actions
Surgeon	Patient selection	Recommendation to patient
Patient	Suspect toxicity	Contact procedure with number
	Protect insensate limb	Pressure point prevention
	Plan for ambulation	Preoperative education and training
Nursing	Examine patient and catheter	Daily home visit and/or phone call

For safe and efficient use of continuous PNBs at home, surgeons, patients, and nurses must understand and collaborate with the team. Education and support around the clock is paramount.

sensate limb; and (3) a clear plan for ambulation after surgery. This last item may represent a serious challenge for some patients after a lower extremity PNB, and preoperative training with crutches may be necessary. Since confusion is an early sign of local anesthetic toxicity, daily contact with patients through nurse visits and/or follow-up phone calls should be organized.[53]

A complete preoperative assessment of patients undergoing surgical procedures of the lower extremity is essential to facilitate the perioperative course, minimize complications, and assure optimal patient comfort with the most efficient anesthesia technique. As with GA, when RA is selected, a preoperative patient evaluation and plan must be completed, including backup plans in case of block failure/complication, local anesthetic toxicity, or patient agitation. Early identification and planning for the case of a difficult airway is paramount as urgent intubation may be required.[54] The plan should be discussed in detail with the patient and informed consent must be obtained through a discussion of RA complications, including the possibility of block failure and neurologic complications.[49,54] A separate consent form for the anesthesiologist may be a good course of action when RA is selected.

During block placement, standard ASA monitoring should be employed with supplemental oxygen and resuscitation equipment readily available. Conscious sedation can facilitate block placement with a relaxed patient and may improve the patient's overall experience of the procedure.

Perioperative Management with Regional Anesthesia

The anesthesiologist will need to adapt his/her practice for the safe and efficient placement of PNBs for lower-extremity surgery. Because lower-extremity blocks often require the injection of two separate plexi, time efficiency in block placement could be a challenge. However, a short

delay at the start of the operation is often compensated at the end by shortened emergence, reduced recovery time, and increased fast-tracking.[29,41] In a perfect clinical setting sufficient manpower would allow placement of the next block while the previous surgery is still in progress. Although this could be very time-efficient, its cost effectiveness has not yet been established.[2] For better time efficiency, creative organization could be implemented. In outpatient surgery centers with fast turnovers and short surgeries, one could place two or three blocks before the first surgery begins; then, during room turnover, the next block can be prepared. This will maximize block success by allowing plenty of time for the targeted nerves to "soak" in the anesthetic. For the safety of this last option, a well-trained and organized staff in a block area with monitoring is mandatory. Because many practices will not have the luxury of these options, the use of local anesthetics with rapid onset is often recommended.

Strategy for local anesthetic selection depends on the choice of the anesthesia technique. When RA is performed to minimize postoperative pain,[11,55] an anesthetic with a slow onset but long duration has become more desirable, especially for single-injection techniques in painful surgery.[15,37] When GA is selected with a PNB, a long-acting local anesthetic is again favored. Other options include the placement of a perineural catheter with an initial injection of a short-acting local anesthetic, and then, before discharge, a long-lasting local anesthetic is reinjected through the catheter, which can be removed or connected to an infusion pump. In selected cases, patients could be scheduled for a 23-hr stay with catheter reinjection before discharge. It is important to remember that the effective length of action of local anesthetics depends on the site of injection. For instance, similar doses of local anesthetic to the epidural space can last 4 hr whereas they may last as long as 28–36 hr in lower-extremity blocks.[56] In addition, while high concentrations of drugs are needed to produce a dense block in the epidural space, lower concentrations are needed in the PNB where volume is the main mechanism of a successful block. In ambulatory patients, Mulroy et al. have shown that higher concentrations of drugs in single-injection lower-extremity blocks do not significantly extend the life of the block. In this prospectively randomized blinded study, postoperative femoral nerve block lasted approximately 23.2 hr after injection of 25 mL of bupivacaine 0.25% and 25.7 hr after injection of bupivacaine 0.5%. Both concentrations had a similar onset time of approximately 20 min after injection.[57]

Aside from block selection and placement, intraoperative management should include the placement of adequate IV access[49] and communication with the surgical team regarding the timing of anticoagulation if required. Record keeping should include documentation and description of block placement, including the following: adherence to sterile technique, size and type of needle and/or catheter placed, location and approach, milliamperage of loss of stimulation, blood return, and paresthesias. If the patient is awake in the operating room, query the patient for signs of local anesthetic toxicity. Full ASA standard monitoring should be employed, including electrocardiogram monitoring. Since the most important role of RA is to facilitate recovery from anesthesia and surgery, the combination of RA with heavy sedation or GA is often appropriate. Adequate sedation ranges from small doses of midazolam or short-acting opioid, to propofol and/or remifentanil infusions, to GA.[58,59]

Anatomy (Figs. 28-1 and 28-2)

The nerve distribution to the lower extremity is divided between two major nerve bundles. The sciatic nerve derived from L4–S3 nerve roots and L1, L2, L3, and L4 nerve roots of the lumbar plexus. The lumbar plexus gives three main nerves to the leg: medially the obturator nerve innervates the inner thigh, the anterior hip joint, the medial femur, and the medial knee joint; laterally the lateral femoral cutaneous nerve (LFC) innervates the lateral

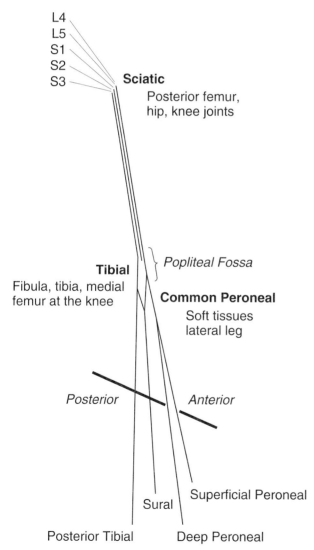

Figure 28-1   Schematic description of the sciatic nerve innervating part of the leg. Nerve structures are in bold, anatomic landmarks in italic.

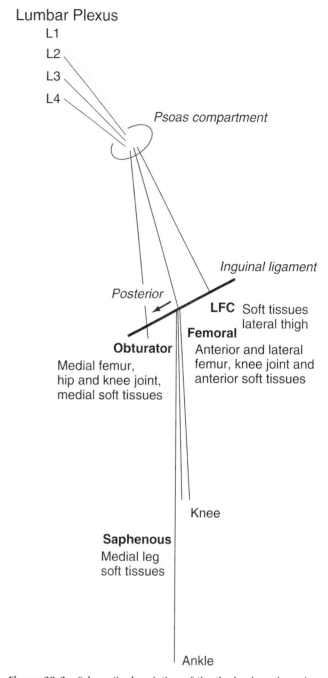

Figure 28-2   Schematic description of the the lumbar plexus innervating part of the leg. Nerve structures are in bold, anatomic landmarks in italic.

thigh; and in the middle the femoral nerve gives off branches to the medial and anterior thigh, to the anterior femur, and to the hip and knee joints. Its medial branch below the knee forms the saphenous nerve. The sciatic nerve innervates the posterior femur, thigh, and hip joint. The sciatic nerve also innervates most of the leg below the knee except for a small medial area in which the innervation comes from the saphenous nerve.[39] Those two nerve bundles should be used in combination when indicated by the surgical site.[49]

Applications

There are two approaches for the lumbar plexus blockade: the femoral nerve block (anterior) and the psoas compartment block (posterior). The femoral nerve block is efficient for postoperative analgesia after thigh and knee surgery.[49] However, only the psoas compartment approach of the lumbar plexus will provide a reliable blockade of its three main nerves. For surgical anesthesia of the knee, the psoas compartment approach should be used in combination with a sciatic nerve block.[60]

The sciatic nerve innervates the posterior thigh as well as the leg and foot below the knee; however, it misses the medial aspect of the leg that is innervated by the saphenous nerve. The sciatic nerve block must be placed above the level of the intended surgery, and must be combined with the lumbar plexus block for thigh or knee surgery.[38] A popliteal approach to the sciatic nerve must be combined with either the femoral or the saphenous nerve for surgical anesthesia of leg below the knee or may be used exclusively for surgical procedures of the foot. Individual injections at the ankle may be used alone for foot surgery.[39,49]

SITE-SPECIFIC PERIPHERAL NERVE BLOCKS

Hip

The hip joint is innervated anteriorly by the obturator nerve, an early branch off the lumbar plexus that is only blocked reliably through a posterior lumbar plexus approach.[60] The femoral nerve innervates the hip joint posteriorly. Skin over the upper lateral hip is innervated from as high up as T12 and will not be included in the lumbar plexus block. The lumbar plexus and sciatic nerve innervate the skin around the thigh anteriorly and posteriorly, respectively. A lumbar plexus block will provide good postoperative pain control for the hip.[38,39,49]

Thigh

The thigh is innervated by four nerves: the posterior femoral cutaneous nerve (a branch of the sciatic nerve) and three branches of the lumbar plexus: the lateral femoral cutaneous nerve, the obturator nerve, and the femoral nerve. The femoral nerve block may be ideal for surgery on the anterior thigh and upper femur, although for medial surgery including the medial femur only a psoas compartment block will reliably anesthetized the obturator nerve that innervates the medial femur and thigh.[39,49]

Knee

The femoral nerve innervates soft tissues and the lateral and middle part of the knee joint. The obturator nerve innervates the medial knee joint and is important for surgical anesthesia of the knee. The tibial branch of the sciatic nerve innervates the posterior knee joint. A posterior approach to the lumbar plexus must be used to reliably anes-

thetize the obturator nerve. The femoral nerve block is often sufficient for postoperative pain management.[39,49,60]

Lower Leg

The sciatic nerve innervates most of the leg. The saphenous nerve, branch of the femoral nerve and part of the lumbar plexus, innervates a small medial band on the leg. For a thigh tourniquet a high sciatic nerve block combined with a femoral injection is recommended. For a short procedure, a femoral nerve with a low sciatic nerve block (popliteal approach) is often sufficient for a thigh tourniquet in a cooperative patient or with light sedation.[39,49,60]

Ankle and Foot

The sciatic nerve and medially the saphenous nerve innervate the ankle. A popliteal fossa approach of the sciatic nerve combined to a saphenous nerve block is ideal for surgical anesthesia and postoperative analgesia of the ankle.[39] For a thigh tourniquet a femoral nerve block is often sufficient and will also cover the saphenous nerve.[49]

INTRAVENOUS REGIONAL ANESTHESIA

Intravenous regional anesthesia (IVRA), or Bier block, is often forgotten for lower-extremity surgeries. It is an easy, safe, and reliable technique for minor procedures of the upper extremity and has been proven to be likewise effective for lower-extremity procedures. It is important to remember, however, that this technique does not provide postoperative analgesia; thus, it is mostly indicated for less painful procedures and will benefit from wound infiltration techniques. The recommended maximum dose of lidocaine for lower-extremity IVRA is identical to that of the upper extremity. Reuben et al. have successfully added ketorolac 20 mg for IVRA with good results on postoperative pain and supplemental opioid requirement.[61]

WOUND INFILTRATION

Recent developments in wound infiltration are being implemented to improve postoperative pain control. Single injections with long-acting local anesthetics represent a safe and inexpensive supplement for pain control after procedures performed under GA, epidural anesthesia, spinal anesthesia, or IVRA. Continuous wound infiltration with a disposable infusion pump, with or without a patient-controlled bolus, may provide several days of analgesia.[26,62] Although these techniques may not be as potent as continuous PNBs, they are credited with being safe and very simple to use. They are optimal for mildly painful procedures (i.e., Achilles tendon repair) and can be easily combined with a single-injection PNB.[11,63]

EPIDURAL AND SPINAL ANESTHESIA

With recent advancements in PNB, the role of the central neuraxial blockade has diminished in ambulatory anesthesia for lower-extremity surgery. Though epidural and spinal anesthesia do not provide postoperative pain relief, they are optimal for procedures in which GA is preferably avoided and the surgery site cannot be efficiently anesthetized with a PNB.[64,65] For example, patients with severe lung dysfunction or unstable reactive airway disease often perform better under epidural or spinal anesthesia for hip surgery or bilateral procedures. Bilateral procedures of the lower extremity are rarely recommended for PNBs because the total dose of local anesthetic would most likely be unsafe and, furthermore, anesthetizing two plexuses in each extremity would be time-consuming and would seriously compromise early ambulation.

Though spinal anesthesia has the benefit of producing a fast and reliable block, the duration of the block is unpredictable unless lidocaine is employed.[64,66] Despite its short duration, however, the use of lidocaine should be restricted. The incidence of transient neurologic symptoms (TNS) with this drug, especially in the lithotomy position or after knee surgery, precludes its routine use for spinal anesthesia.[66–68] An alternative is to combine a low dose of bupivacaine with fentanyl or sufentanil to produce a shorter block.[64,69] Some preliminary data regarding chloroprocaine appear promising for short procedures under 45 min, but further studies are needed to confirm its safety profile.[70] The possibility of postdural puncture headache and urinary retention difficulties complicate the course of spinal anesthesia and rarely make it optimal for outpatient surgery.[69,71,72] Some recent studies show, however, that voiding may not be routinely required as a discharge criterion.[73]

Epidural anesthesia is often a good choice for ambulatory bilateral lower-extremity procedures or for surgeries where GA is inadvisable owing to patient conditions.[74] For this particular technique, drugs such as chloroprocaine and lidocaine are safe and their use does not need to be restricted. The placement of a catheter will permit the reinjection of local anesthetics and the "wash" of the epidural space with saline (10–30 mL) at the end of the operation, thereby accelerating the return of normal function and facilitating earlier discharge.[75]

SUMMARY

The application of a precise regimen with specific MPM and anesthesia techniques adapted to each patient, surgery, and institution will result in maximum benefits for lower-extremity surgical procedures. The traditional "no pain, no gain" theory of improvement should ultimately be usurped by its more productive antithesis: "no pain, max gain"— and not only for humanitarian reasons but because better perioperative pain control will reduce stress response, facilitate recovery, and bolster patient satisfaction. In this venue RA in general and particularly PNBs play crucial roles for painful surgery or for patients with chronic pain.

It must be remembered that prevention of central sensitization by preemptive analgesia is more efficient for limb surgery and, again, PNB is at the center for this venue. No pain will result in "max" gain. The vast majority of "novel" techniques in MPM are the result of an improvement, addition, or adaptation of previous, traditional methods. For example, PNBs have moved from a single-injection intraoperative anesthesia modality to a continuous postoperative PCRA at home. It is the duty of the anesthesiologist, as a perioperative physician, to use all available methods to provide both maximum patient safety and optimal care of the fifth vital sign—pain.[76]

REFERENCES

1. Pregler JL, Kapur PA. The development of ambulatory anesthesia and future challenges. Anesthesiol Clin North Am 2003;21:207–28.
2. Watcha MF, White PF. Economics of anesthetic practice. Anesthesiology 1997;86:1170–96.
3. Rhodes RS. Ambulatory surgery and the societal cost of surgery. Surgery 1994;116:938–40.
4. Felsher J, Chand B, Ponsky J. Minimally invasive surgery. Endoscopy 2003;35:171–77.
5. Wickham JE. Minimally invasive surgery: future developments. Br Med J 1994;308:193–96.
6. Deehan DJ, Pinczewski LA. Endoscopic anterior cruciate ligament reconstruction using a four strand hamstring tendon construct. J Roy Coll Surg Edinb 2002;47:428–36.
7. Fanelli G, Casati A, Garancini P, Torri G. Nerve stimulator and multiple injection technique for upper and lower limb blockade: failure rate, patient acceptance, and neurologic complications. Study Group on Regional Anesthesia. Anesth Analg 1999;88:847–52.
8. Bosenberg AT. Lower limb nerve blocks in children using unsheathed needles and a nerve stimulator. Anaesthesia 1995;50:206–10.
9. Casati A, Santorsola R, Aldegheri G, Ravasi F, Fanelli G, Berti M, Fraschini G, Torri G. Intraoperative epidural anesthesia and postoperative analgesia with levobupivacaine for major orthopedic surgery: a double-blind, randomized comparison of racemic bupivacaine and ropivacaine. J Clin Anesth 2003;15:126–31.
10. Klein SM, Nielsen KC, Greengrass RA, Warner DS, Martin A, Steele SM. Ambulatory discharge after long-acting peripheral nerve blockade: 2382 blocks with ropivacaine. Anesth Analg 2002;94:65–70.
11. Peng PW, Chan VW. Local and regional block in postoperative pain control. Surgi Clin North Am 1999;79:345–70.
12. Botte MJ, Gellman H, Meyer RS, Tafolla SE, Hoenecke HR Jr, Brage ME, Copp SN. Local and regional anesthesia for the management of pain in orthopaedic surgery. Instruct Course Lect 2000;49:523–40.
13. Gold BS, Kitz DS, Lecky JH, Neuhaus JM. Unanticipated admission to the hospital following ambulatory surgery. JAMA 1989;262:3008–10.
14. Bardiau FM, Taviaux NF, Albert A, Boogaerts JG, Stadler M. An intervention study to enhance postoperative pain management. Anesth Analg 2003;96:179–85.
15. Klein SM, Buckenmaier CC III. Ambulatory surgery with long acting regional anesthesia. Minerva Anestesiol 2002;68:833–41.
16. Greengrass RA. Regional anesthesia for ambulatory surgery. Anesthesiol Clin North Am 2000;18:341–53.
17. Rawal N. Postoperative pain management in day surgery. Anaesthesia 1998;53:(Suppl)2.
18. Apfelbaum JL, Chen C, Mehta SS, Gan TJ. Postoperative pain experience: results from a national survey suggest postoperative pain continues to be undermanaged. Anesth Analg 2003;97:5328–40.
19. Leon-Casasola OA. Cellular mechanisms of opioid tolerance and the clinical approach to the opioid tolerant patient in the post-

operative period. Best Pract Res Clin Anaesthesiol 2002;16: 521–25.

20. Wiebalck A, Zenz M. [Neurophysiological aspects of pain and its consequences for the anesthetist]. [German]. Anaesthesist 1997;46: (Suppl)53.

21. Rosaeg OP, Krepski B, Cicutti N, Dennehy KC, Lui AC, Johnson DH. Effect of preemptive multimodal analgesia for arthroscopic knee ligament repair. Reg Anesth Pain Med 2001;26:125–30.

22. Horlocker TT, Hebl JR, Kinney MA, Cabanela ME. Opioid-free analgesia following total knee arthroplasty—a multimodal approach using continuous lumbar plexus (psoas compartment) block, acetaminophen, and ketorolac. Reg Anesth Pain Med 2002;27:105–8.

23. Kehlet H, Wilmore DW. Multimodal strategies to improve surgical outcome. Am J Surg 2002;183:630–41.

24. Cousins MJ. Postoperative multimodal analgesia and intravenous nutrition. Reg Anesth Pain Med 2002;27:536.

25. Aida S, Baba H, Yamakura T, Taga K, Fukuda S, Shimoji K. The effectiveness of preemptive analgesia varies according to the type of surgery: a randomized, double-blind study. Anesth Analg 1999;89: 711–16.

26. Klein SM, Nielsen KC, Martin A, White W, Warner DS, Steele SM, Speer KP, Greengrass RA. Interscalene brachial plexus block with continuous intraarticular infusion of ropivacaine. Anesth Analg 2001;93:601–5.

27. Klein SM, Grant SA, Greengrass RA, Nielsen KC, Speer KP, White W, Warner DS, Steele SM. Interscalene brachial plexus block with a continuous catheter insertion system and a disposable infusion pump. Anesth Analg 2000;91:1473–78.

28. Klein SM, Greengrass RA, Gleason DH, Nunley JA, Steele SM. Major ambulatory surgery with continuous regional anesthesia and a disposable infusion pump. Anesthesiology 1999;91:563–65.

29. Ilfeld BM, Morey TE, Wang RD, Enneking FK. Continuous popliteal sciatic nerve block for postoperative pain control at home: a randomized, double-blinded, placebo-controlled study. Anesthesiology 2002;97:959–65.

30. Ilfeld BM, Enneking FK. A portable mechanical pump providing over four days of patient-controlled analgesia by perineural infusion at home. Reg Anesth Pain Med 2002;27:100–4.

31. Akatsuka M, Tanaka M, Otsuka M, Nakano H, Tanaka Y, Uda R, Rou N, Inamori K. The relief of postoperative pain by suppositories of buprenorphine or NSAID. [Japanese]. Masui Jpn J Anesthesiol 1996;45:298–303.

32. Kostarczyk M, Zabicka A, Machalica A, KuSnierczyk R. [Preoperative use of nonsteroidal anti-infective agents (NSAID) in treatment of postoperative pain]. [Polish]. Polski Merkuriusz Lekarski 2001;10: 12–15.

33. Weinbroum AA. A single small dose of postoperative ketamine provides rapid and sustained improvement in morphine analgesia in the presence of morphine-resistant pain. Anesth Analg 2003;96:789–95.

34. Sveticic G, Gentilini A, Eichenberger U, Luginbuhl M, Curatolo M. Combinations of morphine with ketamine for patient-controlled analgesia: a new optimization method. Anesthesiology 2003;98:1195–205.

35. Sinatra R. Role of COX-2 inhibitors in the evolution of acute pain management. J Pain Symptom Manag 2002;24:(Suppl)27.

36. Dutton R, Goldstein A. The Anesthesiologist's Guide to the OR: Prepped, 1st ed. Boston: Little, Brown, 1995.

37. Klein SM, Pietrobon R, Nielsen KC, Warner DS, Greengrass RA, Steele SM. Peripheral nerve blockade with long-acting local anesthetics: a survey of the Society for Ambulatory Anesthesia. Anesth Analg 2002;94:71–76.

38. Dilger JA. Lower extremity nerve blocks. Anesthesiol Clin North Am 2000;18:319–40.

39. Whitaker RH, Borley NR. Instant Anatomy, 2nd ed. Oxford, Boston: Blackwell Science, 2000.

40. McGrath B, Chung F. Postoperative recovery and discharge. Anesthesiol Clin North Am 2003;21: 367–86.

41. Horn JL, Gaebel BQ, Mollenholt PJ. Is regional anesthesia for upper extremity surgery time efficient? A 1278 patient retrospective study. Anesthesiology 2000;93:A884.

42. Enneking FK, Ilfeld BM. Major surgery in the ambulatory environment: continuous catheters and home infusions. Best Pract Res.Clin Anaesthesiol 2002;16:285–94.

43. Singelyn FJ, Deyaert M, Joris D, Pendeville E, Gouverneur JM. Effects of intravenous patient-controlled analgesia with morphine, continuous epidural analgesia, and continuous three-in-one block on postoperative pain and knee rehabilitation after unilateral total knee arthroplasty. Anesth Analg 1998;87:88–92.

44. Chelly JE, Greger J, Gebhard R, Coupe K, Clyburn TA, Buckle R, Criswell A. Continuous femoral blocks improve recovery and outcome of patients undergoing total knee arthroplasty. J Arthroplasty 2001;16:436–45.

45. Capdevila X, Barthelet Y, Biboulet P, Ryckwaert Y, Rubenovitch J, d'Athis F. Effects of perioperative analgesic technique on the surgical outcome and duration of rehabilitation after major knee surgery. Anesthesiology 1999;91:8–15.

46. Capdevila X, Macaire P, Dadure C, Choquet O, Biboulet P, Ryckwaert Y, d'Athis F. Continuous psoas compartment block for postoperative analgesia after total hip arthroplasty: new landmarks, technical guidelines, and clinical evaluation. Anesth Analg 2002; 94:1606–13.

47. Singelyn FJ, Aye F, Gouverneur JM. Continuous popliteal sciatic nerve block: an original technique to provide postoperative analgesia after foot surgery. Anesth Analg 1997;84:383–86.

48. Cousins MJ, Bridenbaugh PO. Neural Blockade in Clinical Anesthesia and Management of Pain, 3rd ed. Philadelphia: Lippincott Raven, 1998, pp. 179–180.

49. Chelly JE, Casati A, Fanelli G. Continuous Peripheral Nerve Block Techniques: An Illustrated Guide. London, New York: Mosby, 2001.

50. Paqueron X, Boccara G, Bendahou M, Coriat P, Riou B. Brachial plexus nerve block exhibits prolonged duration in the elderly. Anesthesiology 2002;97:1245–49.

51. Horlocker TT, Wedel DJ, Benzon H, Brown DL, Enneking FK, Heit JA, Mulroy MF, Rosenquist RW, Rowlingson J, Tryba M, Yuan CS. Regional anesthesia in the anticoagulated patient: defining the risks (the second ASRA Consensus Conference on Neuraxial Anesthesia and Anticoagulation). Reg Anesth Pain Med 2003;28:172–97.

52. Stevens RD, Van Gessel E, Flory N, Fournier R, Gamulin Z. Lumbar plexus block reduces pain and blood loss associated with total hip arthroplasty. Anesthesiology 2000;93:115–21.

53. Chelly JE, Greger J, Gebhard R. Ambulatory continuous perineural infusion: are we ready? Anesthesiology 2000;93:581–82.

54. Finucane BT. Complications of Regional Anesthesia. New York: Churchill Livingstone, 1999.

55. Eledjam JJ, Cuvillon P, Capdevila X, Macaire P, Serri S, Gaertner E, Jochum D, French Study Group. Postoperative analgesia by femoral nerve block with ropivacaine 0.2% after major knee surgery: continuous versus patient-controlled techniques. Reg Anesth Pain Med 2002;27:6028–11.

56. Barash PG, Cullen BF, Stoelting RK. Peripheral nerve blockade. In Handbook of Clinical Anesthesia, 4th ed. Philadelphia: Lippincott Williams & Wilkins, 2001, p. 715.

57. Mulroy MF, Larkin KL, Batra MS, Hodgson PS, Owens BD. Femoral nerve block with 0.25% or 0.5% bupivacaine improves postoperative analgesia following outpatient arthroscopic anterior cruciate ligament repair. Reg Anesth Pain Med 2001;26:228–29.

58. Lauwers MH, Vanlersberghe C, Camu F. Comparison of remifentanil and propofol infusions for sedation during regional anesthesia. Reg Anesth Pain Med 1998;23:628–70.

59. Mingus ML, Monk TG, Gold MI, Jenkins W, Roland C. Remifentanil versus propofol as adjuncts to regional anesthesia. Remifentanil 3010 Study Group. J Clin Anesth 1998;10:46–53.

60. Liu SS, Salinas FV. Continuous plexus and peripheral nerve blocks for postoperative analgesia. Anesth Analg 2003;96:263–72.

61. Reuben SS, Steinberg RB, Maciolek H, Manikantan P. An evaluation of the analgesic efficacy of intravenous regional anesthesia with lidocaine and ketorolac using a forearm versus upper arm tourniquet. Anesth Analg 2002;95:457–60.

62. Butterfield NN, Schwarz SK, Ries CR, Franciosi LG, Day B, MacLeod BA. Combined pre- and post-surgical bupivacaine wound infiltrations decrease opioid requirements after knee ligament reconstruction. Can J Anaesth 2001;48:245–50.

63. Shang AB, Gan TJ. Optimizing postoperative pain management in the ambulatory patient. Drugs 2003;63:855–67.

64. Liu SS. Drugs for spinal anesthesia: past, present, and future. Reg Anesth Pain Med 1998;23:3428–26.

65. Mulroy MF, Larkin KL, Hodgson PS, Helman JD, Pollock JE, Liu SS. A comparison of spinal, epidural, and general anesthesia for outpatient knee arthroscopy. Anesth Analg 2000;91:860–64.

66. Salinas FV, Liu SS. Spinal anaesthesia: local anaesthetics and adjuncts in the ambulatory setting. Best Pract Res Clin Anaesthesiol 2002;16:195–210.

67. Johnson ME. Potential neurotoxicity of spinal anesthesia with lidocaine. Mayo Clin Proc 2000;75:921–32.

68. Zaric D, Christiansen C, Pace NL, Punjasawadwong Y. Transient neurologic symptoms (TNS) following spinal anaesthesia with lidocaine versus other local anaesthetics. Cochrane Database Syst Rev 2003:CD003006.

69. Liu SS, McDonald SB. Current issues in spinal anesthesia. Anesthesiology 2001;94:888–906.

70. Neal JM, Deck JJ, Kopacz DJ, Lewis MA. Hospital discharge after ambulatory knee arthroscopy: a comparison of epidural 2-chloroprocaine versus lidocaine. Reg Anesth Pain Med 2001;26:35–40.

71. Mazze RI, Fujinaga M. Postdural puncture headache after continuous spinal anesthesia with 18-gauge and 20-gauge needles. Reg Anesth 1993;18:47–51.

72. Kamphius ET, Ionescu TI, Kuipers PW, de Gier J, van Venrooij GE, Boon TA. Recovery of storage and emptying functions of the urinary bladder after spinal anesthesia with lidocaine and with bupivacaine in men. Anesthesiology 1998;88:310–16.

73. Mulroy MF, Salinas FV, Larkin KL, Polissar NL. Ambulatory surgery patients may be discharged before voiding after short-acting spinal and epidural anesthesia. Anesthesiology 2002;97:315–19.

74. Pollock JE, Mulroy MF, Bent E, Polissar NL. A comparison of two regional anesthetic techniques for outpatient knee arthroscopy. Anesth Analg 2003;97:397–401.

75. Sitzman BT, DiFazio CA, Playfair PA, Stevens RA, Hanes CF, Herman TB, Yates HK, Leisure GS. Reversal of lidocaine with epinephrine epidural anesthesia using epidural saline washout. Reg Anesth Pain Med 2001;26:246–51.

76. Lanser P, Gesell S. Pain management: the fifth vital sign. Healthcare Benchmarks 2001;8:68–70.

Ambulatory Anesthesia for Laparoscopic Surgery

HOLLY A. MUIR · ADEYEMI J. OLUFOLABI

INTRODUCTION

For many years laparoscopic surgery had limited applications, even though its benefits in terms of recovery were well recognized. The expansion of laparoscopic surgery over the past two decades has led to an astronomic change in the scope of ambulatory surgery. Who could have dreamed even 25 years ago that cholecystectomy would become a routine outpatient procedure? This was a procedure that prior to the use of laparoscopy involved 5 or more days of hospitalization, largely for respiratory toiletry and pain management. We have seen similar trends with the broader application of these techniques in gynecologic surgery to include laparoscopic hysterectomy and oopherectomy. In recent years, we have been inundated with reports of the use of laparoscopic surgical techniques for ambulatory gastric fundoplication surgery.[1] A surgery once reserved for the most extreme cases of gastroesophageal reflux disease (GERD) is now done routinely in many ambulatory surgery centers with minimal complications. None of the advances in these ambulatory surgical techniques could have been possible without the concurrent advancement in the anesthetic management. The introduction of new antiemetic agents, short-acting opioids, new agents with reduced emetogenic potential, and non-opioid analgesic options has led to an improved ability to manage these patients as outpatients.

HISTORY OF LAPAROSCOPIC SURGERY

Pioneering laparoscopic surgery dates back to 1901 when Kelling, a surgeon with the aid of the Nitze cystoscope, utilized pressurized air to tamponade intestinal bleeding in dogs, the first use of pneumoperitoneum to facilitate laparoscopy.[2] Laparoscopy in humans is attributed to H.C. Jacobaeus, who in 1910 directly visualized both thorax and abdomen.[3] He also coined the term "Laparothorakoskopie." Otto Steiner, from Atlanta Georgia, utilized a trocar and cystoscope to view the abdominal cavity and introduced oxy-

gen insufflation.[4] Carbon dioxide (CO_2) insufflation was introduced in 1925.[5] Significant modifications and innovation were then introduced by the German Kalk, who invented dual trocars and the 135-degree lens system.[6] In 1937, the American John Ruddock, an internist, produced the first American landmark paper detailing 500 cases of laparoscopy and introduced the concept of laparoscopic biopsy.[7] A year later, the spring-loaded Veress needle was invented and is still currently used in its unchanged form.[8] About two decades later, the automated insufflator was produced by Kurt Semm in the 1960s.[9]

Advancement in modern laparoscopy is credited to primarily gynecologic procedures and the first series of laparoscopic sterilizations described by Power and Barnes in 1941.[10,11] However, it was not until the late 1970s that more advanced laparoscopic surgery was performed, especially for the treatment of endometriosis and infertility. The eventual acceptance of laparoscopy in general surgery was fueled partly by the development of the computer chip television camera, which introduced videolaparoscopy. The Frenchman Phillipe Mouret described the first laparoscopic cholecystectomy in 198s7 with the procedure being introduced to the United States in 1988, and since then, there has been an exponential proliferation of its indication in every aspect of surgery.[12]

Recent progress has seen developments in optics, laser, and electrosurgical technologies. Concern over gas embolism and effect on physiology has propelled research in alternative distending mediums, including inert gases and non-gas methods (gasless laparoscopy).[13,14] Revolutionary concepts such as robotic laparoscopy are gradually gaining ground but require further proof of patient and financial benefit.

Increased demand for laparoscopic training led to about 15,000 general surgeons trained from 1990 to 1992 in the United States, and more recently, guidelines for credentialing and training have been established.[15] A national registry that collated and disseminated clinical data and experience was set up in 1990.[16] Perception of improved safety has introduced new terms such as "minimally invasive surgery" or "minimal access surgery," coined to describe access, extensiveness, and safety features of the procedure. Current concerns have been stressed, however, over its proliferative use in surgeries without adequate evaluation.

DESCRIPTION OF THE SURGICAL PROCEDURE

Laparoscopy is the process of inspecting the abdominal cavity through an endoscope. Laparoscopic surgery is also known as minimally invasive surgery or endoscopic surgery. In the traditionally described technique, a pneumoperitoneum is first created using CO_2 insufflation into the abdomen. Most laparoscopists aim for an intra-abdominal pressure of 15 mmHg. The varied positions of Trendelenburg, reverse Trendelenburg, and lateral airplaning are used to facilitate surgical access and view. For the surgeon, laparoscopy requires special skills that may not be intuitive. Operating conditions require good hand-eye coordination, the use of visual cue to compensate for the loss of depth perception, and the relearning of basic surgical skills such as suturing. These requirements can make surgical times longer than with open procedures. Current ambulatory laparoscopy procedures are contrasted with those done as inpatient surgery in Table 29-1.[17]

Benefits

The benefits of using a laparoscopic approach to surgery have been well described. The primary gain is the reduction in tissue trauma. This results in decreased postoperative pain, an improvement in postoperative ventilatory mechanics, and a reduced time for both acute recovery and return to work. We have seen with time and experience the ability to move inpatient procedures to ambulatory facilities. Naturally, this can translate into significant cost saving to the health care system, even with the often increased

Table 29-1   Examples of Ambulatory versus Inpatient Laparoscopic Surgical Procedures

Ambulatory Procedures	Inpatient Procedures
Diagnostic laparoscopy	Splenectomy
Cholecystectomy	Nephrectomy
Nissen fundoplication	Adrenectomy
Fallopian tube surgery	Laparoscopic-assisted bowel resection
Inguinal hernia repair	Colostomy formation
Oopherectomy	Common bile duct exploration
Lysis of adhesions	Ventriculoperitoneal shunt
Oocyte retrieval	

Table 29-2   Complications of Trocar Insertion

Abdominal wall bleeding and hematoma

Abdominal wall hernia

Major vascular injury

Gastrointestinal tract perforation

Liver laceration

Bladder perforation

Extraperitoneal insufflation

cost of surgical equipment. With skilled surgeons, shorter operating room (OR) times can be attained, resulting in further reductions in cost. In addition, the shortened interval between surgery and resumption of work results in a global benefit to the work economy.

Risk

The morbidity and mortality rates associated with laparoscopic surgery are controversial. The available data largely come from case reports and retrospective surveys. Most injuries occur with the insertion of the trocar or Veress needle or as a complication of the pneumoperitoneum. Complications include subcutaneous emphysema, mediastinal emphysema, pneumothorax, bleeding, gastrointestinal perforation, solid visceral injury, avulsion of adhesions, cardiac arrhythmia, and incisional hernia at trocar insertion sites.

The incidence is variably reported to occur at a range from 0.05% to 0.38%.[18] Most of the available literature on complications comes from gynecologic experience. Complications related to needle and trocar insertion are listed in Table 29-2 and those of the pneumoperitoneum in Table 29-3. Some of these can be life-threatening.

Major vascular injury during the initiation of the pneumoperitoneum is well recognized, with a reported mortal-

Table 29-3   Complications of Pneumoperitoneum

Subcutaneous emphysema

Shoulder or back pain

Pneumothorax

Hypercarbia

Bradycardia

Oliguria

CO_2 gas embolism

Decreased cardiac output

Table 29-4 Cause of Death Associated with Trocar Injury

Cause	N	Percentage of Total Reported (32 deaths)
Bowel injury	6	19
Vascular injury:	26	81
Aorta or inferior vena cava	10	31
Iliac vessels	3	9
Other vessels	13	40

SOURCE: Bhoyrul S, Vierra MA, Nezhat CR, Krummel TM, Way LW. Trocar injuries in laparoscopic surgery. J Am Coll Surg 2001;192:677–83.

ity rate of 15%.[19] Its incidence has been variably reported, ranging from 0.02% in a French report[20] to 0.26% in both American and Canadian studies.[21,22]

In a recent study analyzing medical device–related incidents reported to the Food and Drug Administration, 629 trocar injuries occurred between 1993 and 1996, with 408 of these involving major blood vessels.[23] There were 32 deaths, with 81% of them as a result of a major blood vessel injury. The cause of death and the type of laparoscopic procedures are listed in Tables 29-4 and 29-5. Disturbingly, most of these procedures would be done routinely in an ambulatory setting where the resources to manage this situation may be limited. Minor vascular injuries occur slightly more frequently, with an incidence of 0.7–2.6%, but have significantly less morbidity associated with them.

Bowel injury is the third cause of death from laparoscopy after major vascular injury and anesthesia. Unlike major vascular injuries, which are usually recognized immediately, bowel perforation may go unrecognized, resulting in a delayed presentation in the postoperative period. The incidence of bowel injury is reported to range

Table 29-5 Laparoscopic Procedures Resulting in Fatal Injury

Procedure	N	Percentage of Total Deaths (32 deaths)
Cholecystecomy	16	50
Unspecified	8	25
Diagnostic laparoscopy	3	9
Tubal ligation	2	6
Appendectomy	2	6
Lymphadenectomy	1	3

SOURCE: Bhoyrul S, Vierra MA, Nezhat CR, Krummel TM, Way LW. Trocar injuries in laparoscopic surgery. J Am Coll Surg 2001;192:677–83.

from 0.05 to 0.3%.[18] An interesting, unusual complication reported with laparoscopy is the development of postoperative bowel obstruction secondary to herniation of bowel at the trocar insertion site. It is hypothesized that an outward pressure is produced as cannulas are removed, causing entrapment of bowel and producing a Richter hernia.

Bladder injury is a rare complication. This low incidence may be due to the routine of emptying the bladder prior to trocar placement. Distention of the urinary drainage bag by the insufflation gas may be the first sign.[18] Such injury risks are increased in patients with previous pelvic surgery.

It is difficult to estimate the incidence of intraoperative events such as pneumothorax, embolism, arrhythmia, or other cardiovascular/respiratory events. Most events are reported retrospectively as case reports, making it difficult to determine an overall incidence. A detailed discussion of the recognition and anesthesia management of intraoperative mishaps is given below. Conversion from laparoscopy to open surgery is 2.5–10% and is commonly due to uncontrolled bleeding, extensive tissue injury, or inadequate accessibility.[24]

PHYSIOLOGIC CHANGES ASSOCIATED WITH LAPAROSCOPY

The pneumoperitoneum and patient position needed for laparoscopic surgery can induce physiologic changes that can have widespread consequences. These result in ventilatory and respiratory alterations and changes in hemodynamics, including venous pooling, a decrease in cardiac output, and an increase in systemic vascular resistance; with potential alterations in renal, splanchnic, and cerebral blood flows. The respiratory and cardiovascular changes are the most significant and therefore will be the focus of our discussion.

The insufflation of CO_2 and the induction of a pneumoperitoneum are the events responsible for most of the physiologic changes and complications seen with laparoscopy. Although there are alternatives to both the use of CO_2 and the induction of a pneumoperitoneum, they have not gained widespread use. These include the use of an inert gas other than CO_2, such as helium or argon, and the use of abdominal lifting devices rather than pneumoperitoneum to allow for access and visualization (gasless laparoscopy).[25]

Arterial CO_2 partial pressure ($PaCO_2$) increases progressively to reach a plateau over the first 15–30 min of insufflation (any further increases once this plateau is reached should trigger concern that an untoward complication has occurred).[26] With the use of general anesthesia and controlled ventilation this is usually easily managed with hyperventilation. However, if the patient is anesthetized and breathing spontaneously, significant hypercarbia may ensue.[27] If the patient is having the procedure under local anesthesia, a normal physiologic response to hypercarbia is seen with an increase in the respiratory rate and thus a significant increase in minute ventilation.

Capnography should be used to monitor end-tidal carbon dioxide ($ETCO_2$). However, reports have suggested that the $PaCO_2$ to end-tidal carbon dioxide pressure ($PETCO_2$) difference may increase during CO_2 insufflation, thus reducing

Table 29-6   Cause of Increase in PaCO$_2$ During Laparoscopy

Absorption of CO$_2$

Ventilation/perfusion (V/Q) mismatch
  Abdominal rigidity
  Position of patient
  Intermittent positive pressure ventilation (IPPV)
  Reduced cardiac output

Increased production secondary to light anesthesia

Ventilatory depressants

Subcutaneous emphysema

Capnothorax

CO$_2$ embolism

the reliability of the ETCO$_2$ reading.[28] This is more pronounced in American Society of Anesthesiologists (ASA) physical status II and III patients.

Although the increase in PaCO$_2$ during laparoscopy is multifactorial (see Table 29-6), it is largely due to absorption of CO$_2$ during insufflation. It has been suggested that, as a result of the increase in arterial CO$_2$, release of a cascade of neurohumoral factors ensues, including catecholamines, renin-angiotension system factors, and vasopressin. All of these contribute to an increase in systemic vascular resistance. In addition, a fall in renal plasma flow has been documented in association with a 50% decrease in glomerular filtration rate.[29] The use of alpha-2 agonists such as clonidine and dexmedetomidine can attenuate some of these changes.[30,31]

The increase in PaCO$_2$ can also cause an increase in intracranial pressure due to CO$_2$-induced cerebral vascular dilatation.[32] Pneumoperitoneum, regardless of the agent used, causes decreased thoracopulmonary compliance by 30–50%.[33] Reductions in functional residual capacity due to diaphragmatic elevation and ventilation/perfusion (V/Q) mismatch secondary to increased airway pressure are also seen. In a healthy patient these changes are well tolerated; however, they may not be in patients with preexisting pulmonary disease.

In addition to the alterations in pulmonary function seen with pneumoperitoneum, significant changes in cardiac output occur. A decrease in cardiac output proportional to the increase in intra-abdominal pressure is seen.[34] This is largely a result of a decrease in venous return, although an increase in afterload may contribute. The increase in abdominal pressure leads to caval compression, pooling of blood in the lower extremities, and an increase in venous resistance, with a resulting decrease in left ventricular end diastolic volume. Ironically, this is associated with an increase in cardiac filling pressures, which may be explained by the increase in intrathoracic pressure induced by pneumoperitoneum.[34] This paradoxic response can affect the reliability of right atrial and pulmonary artery pressure monitoring.

Although a minor contributor to the physiologic disturbance seen with laparoscopy, positioning in lithotomy and steep head-down tilt can add to the dysfunction in respiratory mechanics. In addition, the head-down position can contribute to the development of atelectasis. The head-up position, used for laparoscopic cholecystectomy, can have more favorable respiratory dynamics, whereas the opposite is true of the effects of position on the negative effects of laparoscopy on cardiac function.[35]

SELECTION OF PATIENTS FOR THE AMBULATORY SETTING

In the past, young, healthy women having gynecologic surgery comprised the largest patient population undergoing laparoscopic surgery. These patients in general tolerate the physiologic changes seen in the cardiorespiratory systems. However, with the extension of laparoscopic techniques to gastrointestinal surgery, the patient population presenting for laparoscopic surgery has changed to include a much older, higher-risk, and generally debilitated cohort, thus making consideration of the risk of the laparoscopic procedure itself a significant consideration in deciding on both the appropriate route for the surgery (laparoscopic vs. open) and the location (ambulatory vs. inpatient). Owing to the significant physiologic changes associated with the laparoscopic technique, some patients may be unsuitable for care in an ambulatory setting. This may be further confounded by the availability of advanced monitoring techniques such as transesophageal echocardiography (TEE). Patients with severe congestive heart failure (left ventricular ejection fraction < 30%) or symptomatic valvular disease are at risk of developing cardiac complications. This may be reduced by use of invasive monitoring techniques such as an arterial line with blood gas sampling, pulmonary artery catheter, and TEE, none of which are part of routine care in an ambulatory setting. Patients with stable ischemic heart disease appear to be at less risk than those cited above. Patients with an FEV1 (forced expiratory volume in 1 second) less than 70% of predicted are at high risk of pulmonary complication with laparoscopy.[36] Interestingly, in patients with obstructive sleep apnea (generally regarded as high risk for ambulatory surgery), there is evidence that laparoscopy produces little sleep disturbance, especially when compared to laparotomy.[37]

Complications inherent to the surgical procedure itself can add to the patient selection issues. Major vascular injuries that more often occur on trocar insertion are more likely to occur in patients with prior abdominal surgery at risk for adhesions. Treatment of a major vascular injury can involve the need for massive blood and fluid resuscitation and often the help of a vascular surgeon, resources often not immediately available in an ambulatory surgery center.[38]

ANESTHETIC TECHNIQUES

General Anesthesia

The most common mode of anesthesia for this surgical approach is general anesthesia. Its major advantage is the flexibility it offers in terms of duration and the ability to handle surgical complications should they arise. Its major disadvantages are side effects and their influence on recovery time and the potential for anesthetic complications. For the most part, a standard approach to general anesthesia is recommended. Some controversy exists in the choice of "best" technique or agent, but to date no clear mode or agent has been shown to be superior.

An evolving controversy with general anesthesia that merits some discussion involves the use of a laryngeal mask airway (LMA) for laparoscopy. Although many in North America would fine it hard to imagine using an LMA for airway management in a laparoscopic procedure, in the United Kingdom it would be the preferred method for airway management of approximately 60% of anesthesiologists (in patients judged not to be at risk for aspiration).[39] In a recent survey of U.K. practice, use of the LMA for these procedures was highly endorsed although 89% of these anesthesiologists expressed concern about use in patients with obesity, GERD, or proven hiatal hernia. This opinion is supported by clinical investigations that have demonstrated the safety of the LMA.[40,41]

Choice of Anesthetic Agents

Muscle relaxants and reversal agents.   Good surgical conditions for this procedure require a still patient and some degree of muscle relaxation. A failure to achieve these conditions has been associated with surgical mishap.[23] In addition, many prefer endotracheal intubation for this procedure, which usually requires the use of muscle relaxants. The choice of muscle relaxant has been controversial. This has revolved largely around the use of succinylcholine. To date, this drug continues to offer significant advantages for ambulatory surgery in terms of rapidity of onset and duration of action; however, the side effect of myalgia can be somewhat troublesome for ambulatory patients, where the incidence seems to be highest.[42] Recent attempts to quantify the contribution of succinylcholine to this side effect in patients undergoing laparoscopy have produced mixed results. Substitution of a nondepolarizing agent for succinylcholine has not been shown to eliminate these myalgias, although it may reduce them slightly.[43,44] Alternatives to succinylcholine have been sought, with the limitations of onset time and duration of action making an ideal agent difficult to find. Rocuronium can be used as a good alternative, with the ability to achieve good intubating conditions in 90 sec. However, its duration of action after an intubating dose of 0.6 mg/kg can often exceed the length of the surgical procedure in the ambulatory setting and necessitate the use of reversal agents.[45] Mivacurium has been proposed as an alterative to rocuronium because of its shorter duration of action. Its onset time may be a limiting factor in its use as it requires > 200 sec to achieve good intubating conditions using a dose of 0.2–0.25 mg/kg.[46] Its duration of action, which facilitates spontaneous recovery of neuromuscular function, may offer the advantage of avoiding the use of muscle relaxants.

There is controversy regarding the effect of anticholinesterase drugs on the incidence of postoperative nausea and vomiting (PONV). Investigators have demonstrated both an increased[47] and decreased[48] PONV incidence with the use of these agents. A more recent study looking at the effects of reversal agents on PONV after laparoscopic surgery found an increased incidence of complaint of nausea in the patients who were administered neostigmine compare to those who were not; however, use of antiemetics, time to meet postanesthesia care unit (PACU) discharge criteria, and complaints of nausea or vomiting on 24-hr follow-up were not increased. Thus overall cost of care did not differ.[49] Similarly, in a study comparing the use of succinylcholine to rocuronium or mivacurium no difference in the incidence of PONV was found.[50] These investigators hypothesized that this was due to the use of edrophonium as the reversal agent. This concept has been supported in a small pediatric study.[51] Overall the effects of neostigmine on PONV are limited and therefore the decision to avoid the use of reversal agents or to use a short-acting agent (edrophonium) must be carefully balanced against the potential negative effects of residual neuromuscular block.

Nitrous oxide.   Nitrous oxide (N_2O) is a popular adjuvant to an anesthetic mixture because it is inexpensive, easy to administer, readily available in most OR settings, and reduces the use of other agents. Despite its popularity and frequency of use, controversy has continued to surround this agent. These controversies have involved some reports of adverse occupational effects on health care providers,[52,53] its contribution to PONV,[54,55] and its effects on expansion of air-filled spaces such as bowel, lung cyst, and air emboli.

The issue of potential toxicity of N_2O has been ongoing for a number of decades. Debate exists as to whether this is a real phenomenon or a function of the work environment in which it is used and is outside the scope of this discussion. There is, however, some evidence that N_2O may increase the incidence of PONV and thus delay discharge from the PACU. This may be a significant consideration when used as part of a laparoscopic procedure where the incidence of PONV is already a limiting factor in discharge readiness. Many of the earlier studies demonstrating this adverse effect were of such small sample size that they lack the statistical power to definitively determine an association between the adverse outcome of PONV and the administration of N_2O.

A recent publication that looked at a mixed population of female patients having both laparoscopic and nonlaparoscopic gynecologic procedures used an innovative approach to study this question. Using an anesthetic protocol based on the use of total intravenous anesthesia (TIVA), patients were randomized to receive either 65% N_2O/35% oxygen (O_2) or 100% O_2. Of the 1490 patients recruited, 490 had laparoscopic surgery (N_2O, n = 247; 100% O_2, n = 243). The known benefit of reduction in the use of anesthetic agents was demonstrated in this study with the mean dose of propofol being 25% less in the N_2O supplementation than in the 100% O_2 group (381.1 ± 137 mg vs. 456 ± 169 mg). In the primary outcome of this study, time to home readiness, no difference was noted in either subpopulation (laparoscopic and nonlaparoscopic surgery) regardless of their randomization. Similarly, there were no differences in maximum visual analog scale nausea scores between groups or in the incidence of vomiting in the laparoscopic group. The incidence of in-hospital use of antiemetics was similar in both groups (26.1% in N_2O and 28.9 in 100% O_2).[56] The study concluded that omission of N_2O in ambulatory surgery patients offered no benefit. Given the reduction in the dose of propofol in the N_2O group, however, one could infer a benefit to the use of this agent in terms of cost of anesthetic care.

Volatile agents. Isoflurane, sevoflurane, and desflurane are all suitable volatile agents available for ambulatory laparoscopy. Desflurane demonstrated quicker emergence and shorter time to extubation than isoflurane[57] or sevoflurane,[58] but cognitive recovery and discharge times were similar. In another study, sevoflurane demonstrated quicker eye opening and orientation compared to isoflurane but home discharge readiness times were similar.[59] In morbidly obese patients undergoing laparoscopic gastric banding, sevoflurane had shorter extubation, emergence, and response times compared to isoflurane, and patients were discharged earlier.[60] Using the Bispectral Index (BIS) monitor to titrate sevoflurane concentration, Nelskyla et al. demonstrated faster orientation and ability to drink and significantly less vomiting compared to control patients in whom sevoflurane was adjusted based on hemodynamic variables (30% had BIS reading < 40).[61] They also showed no difference in discharge times. Recart et al., using the auditory evoked potential monitor to assess depth of anesthesia, demonstrated a 25% reduced desflurane dose associated with a more rapid fast-track eligibility and shorter PACU stay during laparoscopy procedure.[62] Isoflurane and enflurane demonstrated similar incidence of emesis.[63] It would seem that significant differences in recovery profiles are seen in many of these studies without any consistent clinical benefit in discharge time. All the currently available volatile agents seem suitable for balanced anesthesia in ambulatory laparoscopy where provided dose is titrated to effect or depth of anesthesia and a suitable antiemetic is given.

Total intravenous anesthesia. TIVA has proven to be suitable alternative technique for ambulatory laparoscopy. Its advantages are, however, limited and mixed. Times to spontaneous neuromuscular recovery is delayed by 40–50% with sevoflurane and desflurane compared to propofol.[64] Desflurane and isoflurane produced shorter postoperative recovery (response, emergence) times compared to TIVA but psychomotor recovery times were mixed.[65–67] Discharge times were similar[65,68,69] or quicker with TIVA.[64]

In patients undergoing laparoscopic hysterectomy, TIVA and isoflurane anesthesia techniques were found suitable.[70] Early recovery profile (eye opening and orientation), however, was significantly faster in the isoflurane patients. Despite having more patients with sevoflurane (77%) and desflurane (94%) qualified to bypass PACU compared to propofol (44%), times to home readiness were similar.[71] Postural stability assessment postoperatively in patients who had TIVA showed residual balance deficits despite attaining postanesthesia discharge criteria.[72] Both the desflurane and propofol groups, however, demonstrated no difference in actual home discharge time. It was postulated that propofol-based anesthesia might be associated with vestibular disturbances. Criticism of this study and of many of the other comparable studies is the lack of assessment in the depth of anesthesia and whether similar dosing is given. Using hemodynamic parameters seems a crude method of determining anesthesia depth.

TIVA technique produces less PONV,[73–75] reducing delay in PACU discharge.[65,73,75] Preoperative ondansetron administration prior to desflurane anesthesia, however, produced similar low PONV incidence and early discharge criteria as in the TIVA group.[75] Similar observations were demonstrated when metoclopramide and ranitidine were given preoperatively.[76] Remifentanil/isoflurane-based anesthesia has also demonstrated similar low incidence of PONV compared to remifentanil/propofol anesthesia in laparoscopy and other ambulatory surgery.[77]

Spinal Anesthesia

The use of regional anesthesia for laparoscopic surgery is not widely practiced. Selective spinal anesthesia has been described in numerous publications.[78] This is defined as the practice of employing minimal doses of intrathecal agents so that only the nerve roots supplying a specific area and only the modalities that need to be anesthetized are affected. Many of these publications have involved the use of hypobaric solutions of 10–20 mg of lidocaine with the addition of either sufentanil 10 μg or fentanyl 25 μg. These solutions are reported to give good to excellent operating conditions with minimal motor block and a short recovery period. Side effects include pruritus in > 50% of patients (self-limiting, resolved without need for treatment), nausea with an incidence of 10–20%, and intraoperative shoulder tip pain in > 50% of cases. The authors use a combination of alfentanil and midazolam to treat the intraoperative shoulder tip pain. They report a zero incidence of conversion to general anesthesia for intraoperative pain.[79,80]

These techniques have also been called walk in–walk out spinal techniques, reflecting the very minor degree of motor block with these techniques. When formally studied, investigators were able to demonstrate the absence of motor block and an intact dorsal column function in 70% of patients on arrival in the PACU after spinal administration of a hypobaric solution of lidocaine 10 mg and sufentanil 10 μg, with an average surgical time of 22.5 ± 11.5 min.[81] In this same cohort of patients, 100% had normal motor and dorsal column function 60 min after arrival in the PACU. Discharge time from PACU was between 89 and 103 min in the majority of patients. The authors suggest that in the majority of patients, PACU could have been bypassed or "fast-tracked," thus resulting in cost savings to the health care system.

When a cost comparison between this technique and general anesthesia without fast-tracking was done, no difference in cost was demonstrated.[82] In a small Canadian study of 24 patients in the spinal group and 28 in the general anesthesia group, the costs of drugs and equipment were similar, anesthetic time was slightly longer in the spinal group (18 vs. 10 min), average PACU recovery time was 29 min longer in the spinal group, and the use of postoperative antiemetics was similar (8–14%). The only benefit demonstrated for the spinal technique in this study was a reduction in the use of postoperative analgesia (25 vs. 75%).[82] Noteworthy with this study was that the dose of lidocaine in the study group was slightly higher than that described in many of the walk in–walk out spinal studies (20–25 mg vs. 10 mg of lidocaine). Despite these findings, the authors suggested that if fast-tracking principles had been applied, the results may have been more favorable for the spinal technique.

Sufentanil has been described as having some local anesthetic properties and it had been speculated that laparoscopy could be performed using only spinal sufentanil. In a small randomized study, 20 μg of intrathecal sufentanil was compared with intrathecal lidocaine 10 mg and sufentanil 10 μg.[83] Forty percent of subjects in the sufentanil-only group required conversion to general anesthesia for inadequate block. In addition, the incidence of severe nausea in the sufentanil group was > 60%. These two observations led the investigators to actually terminate the study early and to conclude that sufentanil alone was ineffective for laparoscopic surgery.[83] Interestingly, in this study the investigators were able to demonstrate a sensory level to pinprick in the sufentanil-only group that was comparable to that in the lidocaine/sufentanil group (T5–T6). The limitation was the sensation of pain on trochar insertion. An interesting study might have been to use a smaller dose of sufentanil (10 μg) and enhance anesthesia at the trochar insertion site with local anesthetic infiltration.

Epidural Anesthesia

The use of epidural anesthesia has been described. However, induction time for epidural anesthesia for laparoscopic procedures is often longer than the surgical time itself. Epidural anesthesia did offer the advantage, however, of a lower incidence of postoperative nausea (4%) compared to general anesthesia (38%) in one study.[84] This incidence is lower than the 10–20% incidence seen with the intrathecal local anesthetic/opioid combinations and likely reflects the absence of opioids in the epidural solution. When surgical doses of local anesthetic are used, recovery times are also prolonged. An observation made at Virginia Mason Clinic, which at the time reported that 50% of their laparoscopic procedures were done using epidural block, was that not all patients having laparoscopic surgery are suitable for epidural block. Many patients have significant anxiety when the abdomen is insufflated and some respiratory compromise occurs.[85] In addition, many do not tolerate the head-down position or the shoulder tip pain that is common with gas insufflation. These issues will be fur-

ther confounded in our ever-expanding population of obese patients. In the studies discussed earlier using spinal anesthesia for laparoscopy, the largest patient included in the study cohorts was 87 kg.

Local Anesthesia

The use of local anesthesia for laparoscopic tubal ligation has been described since the early 1970s.[86] Many believe it is comparable in operating conditions to general anesthesia. The technique involves local infiltration of the skin with local anesthetic for trocar insertion with the simultaneous administration of intravenous sedation. Many advocate keeping insufflation volumes of gas low (< 0.5 L) and minimizing the time for and degree of Trendelenburg position. With the advent of smaller laparoscopy equipment, some surgeons have extended their use of laparoscopy for both tubal ligation and diagnostic purposes to the office setting.[87–89] A number of studies have demonstrated a reduced cost with the use of local anesthesia compared to general anesthesia. This is in terms of both cost of drug and equipment, and length of stay in hospital.[90–92] Many of these reports suggest the intraoperative use O_2 supplementation because of the high incidence of desaturation secondary to apnea from the deep sedation required. The need for conversion to general anesthesia was noted.[93] In one of the few published randomized studies, investigators cited many advantages for the use of local anesthesia; however, they recommend anesthetic surveillance as part of the protocol.[94] Other laparoscopic procedures with limited reports on use of local anesthesia include insertion of a peritoneal dialysis catheter and laparoscopic preperitoneal hernia repair.[95,96]

COMPLICATIONS

Intraoperative Complications

Despite being minimally invasive, leading to increased indication in high-risk patients, wider surgical specialties, and more extensive and longer-duration cases, complications dictate caution (Table 29-7).[97] Complications requiring surgical intervention occur in 1 in 660 cases, with a mortality of 1 in 2000 cases.[98,99] Other quoted series suggest a 0.38% morbidity, with a mortality rate of 0.05% and 0.28%,[100] with the majority being a consequence of pneumoperitoneum. Adequate training, reduced surgical duration, proven safer techniques, improved technology, a high index of suspicion, and prompt appropriate intervention will reduce these complications. In many serious life-threatening complications, deflation of the peritoneum may be indicated to ensure good outcome. Technically, lower intra-abdominal pressure, shorter surgical duration, and type of insufflating gas contribute to lower risks for complication.

Table 29-7   Complications of Laparoscopy

Respiratory	Cardiovascular	Other
Acidosis	Ventricular ectopic beats	Shoulder pain
Pneumothorax	Bradyarrhythmias	Retinal hemorrhage
Tension pneumothorax	Hypotension	Gastric hemorrhage
Atelectasis	Cardiovascular collapse	Ascites
Subcutaneous emphysema	Cardiac arrest	Oliguria
Tension hydropneumothorax	Cardiomyopathy	Transient ischemic attack
Pneumomediastinum	Deep vein thrombosis	Bowel ischemia
Pleural effusion	Pulmonary edema	Bowel edema
	Myocardial infarction	Hypothermia
	Myocardial ischemia	Necrotizing fasciitis
	Gas embolism	Tumor inoculation
	Pneumoperitoneum	Reflux esophagitis

SOURCE: Sharma KC, Kabinoff G, Ducheine Y, Tierney J, Brandstetter RD. Laparoscopic surgery and its potential for medical complications. Heart Lung 1997;26(1):52–67.

Cardiorespiratory Complications

A third of complications are due to the cardiorespiratory system.[97] Gas insufflation, abdominal distention and pressure, and positioning may contribute to ventilatory compromise and complication. Hypercarbia and acidosis can occur with extraperitoneal insufflation and absorption through transperitoneal/subcutaneous routes. Pneumothorax occurs in 0.03% of cases and usually requires no treatment.[101] Life-threatening pneumothorax will interfere with ventilation and oxygenation, requiring prompt intervention including deflating the peritoneum and possible tube thoracoscopy. Although surgical emphysema is routinely found in more than 50% of patients by computerized tomography (CT) scan, clinical subcutaneous emphysema occurs in 2–12 per 1000 cases and can extend to face, trunk, and neck.[102,103] It may be an indication of hypercarbia but usually resolves within 24 hr. Life-threatening surgical emphysema and hypercarbia can be a harbinger of pneumopericardium, although this complication has been reported without evidence of surgical emphysema.[104,105]

Other known complications include pneumomediastinum, atelectasis, pulmonary edema, and pleural effusions.

Arrhythmias are the most common cardiac intraoperative events, with a 47% incidence; with ventricular ectopy being the most common arrhythmia.[106] Beta blockers prevent this incidence but are not usually prescribed.[107] It is observed more with CO_2 insufflation and associated with acidosis and catecholamine release. Often, the presence of arrhythmia is evidence of a more serious underlying complication, such as pneumothorax, embolism, or hypoxemia.

Gas embolism occurs in 0.002–0.016% of cases and can be fatal.[108] It occurs usually within 10 min of initiating insufflation and is due to inadvertent vein cannulation or absorption via venous channels. CO_2 embolism has a safer profile than air or helium owing to its high solubility. Dysrrhythmia, pulmonary hypertension, raised central venous pressure, hypoxia, and cardiac arrest may occur. Pulmonary infarction is also reported.[109] Management requires prompt diagnosis, cessation of insufflation, attempt at emboli aspiration, and supportive therapy.

Surgical Complications

As described earlier, vascular and visceral injuries are the most common surgical complications. Conversion to open laparoscopy is required in 2.5–10% of cases and is commonly due to uncontrolled bleeding, extensive tissue injury, or inadequate accessibility.[110] The prevention and treatment of most surgical complications are, however, beyond the scope of this discussion.

Postoperative Complications

The two most common complaints after laparoscopic surgery are PONV and pain. The etiology and management of pain after laparoscopy will be discussed below. PONV after laparoscopic surgery has been the focus of countless clinical investigations, with numerous agents as the focus of study. Both patient and surgical risk factors for PONV have been identified, which seem to cumulatively increase risk of PONV. Patient factors include female gender, prior history of PONV or motion sickness, nonsmoker, and plan for postoperative opioid use. Laparoscopy figures prominently in the surgical risk factors, which also include laparotomy, plastic surgery procedures, major breast surgery, craniotomy, ear, nose, and throat surgery, and strabismus surgery. A patient is considered to be at mild to moderate risk if one or two of these factors are present, and it is recommended that they receive a single agent for prophylaxis against PONV. If three or four of these factors are present, the patient is considered high risk for PONV with the recommendation of two agents for prophylaxis. Patients considered very high risk for PONV would have more than 4 of these factors present. A multimodal approach is recommended with consideration of the use of TIVA with propofol.[111]

When a single agent is indicated, ondansetron has the most favorable results.[112–115] This is true for both in-hospital and postdischarge nausea and vomiting (PDNV). Low-dose droperidol compares favorably with ondansetron as an effective single agent for prevention of in-hospital PONV, but not for PDNV.[116] Combination therapy with more than one agent provides the most reduction in relative risk for PONV and PDNV.

POSTOPERATIVE PAIN MANAGEMENT

Pain that occurs after this procedure is much less and of shorter duration than after a similar procedure done with open laparotomy, thus allowing for earlier discharge from hospital. With the goal of early hospital discharge in mind, it is essential that the agents used to treat the pain post-operatively do not cause side effects that may delay discharge, such as PONV or somnolence.

Pain after laparoscopy may occur in the upper abdomen, lower abdomen, back, or shoulders regardless of the surgical site and may persist for many days postoperatively. The greatest incidence of pain is in the upper abdomen. The highest pain scores are reported in the first 24 hr after surgery, and usually then subside, but later may once again peak over the subsequent 24–72 hr.[117] Visceral pain related to the surgical site is most often reported in the first 24 hr; however, this usually subsides quickly, leaving complaints of shoulder and neck pain in subsequent days.

Rapid distention of the peritoneum may be associated with tearing of blood vessels, traumatic traction of nerves, and release of inflammatory mediators. The persistence of shoulder tip pain suggests excitation of the phrenic nerve. This has been shown to correlate with the presence of gas under the diaphragm.[118] Peritoneal inflammation or the presence of gas is probably also the origin of the upper-abdominal pain after lower-abdominal surgery or diagnostic laparoscopy.

Treatment modalities have included opioids, local anesthetics, and nonsteroidal anti-inflammatory drugs (NSAIDs). Potent opioids, such as fentanyl and morphine, can effectively treat the pain seen after laparoscopy. However, these agents are not suitable for continued use in the ambulatory setting owing to both their mode of administration and their undesirable side effects of nausea, vomiting, and somnolence.

Local anesthetics have been administered by a variety of methods with some success. A bilateral rectus sheath block performed above the umbilicus using 15 mL of 0.25% bupivacaine on each side has been demonstrated to reduce pain after diagnostic laparoscopy.[119] Shoulder tip pain and the other minor pain complaints after laparoscopy can be reduced by the application of local anesthetic below the diaphragm under direct vision, by peritoneal irrigation, or through the use of a subphrenic catheter. When peritoneal lavage is used, the addition of epinephrine can allow the use of a larger volume of local anesthetic with a reduced risk of toxicity. It seems that the head-down position to allow bathing of the phrenic nerve in local anesthetic increases the efficacy of intraperitoneal lavage techniques.[120–122] The pain following laparoscopic tubal ligation can be reduced by the direct application of

local anesthetic to the fallopian tube, regardless of the technique used for tube interruption.[123–124]

The efficacy of NSAIDs for the control of pain after laparoscopic surgery has been controversial. A recent review looked at 13 studies (total $n = 737$) that showed a benefit from the administration of NSAIDs by reducing the requirement for additional analgesic and compared these to 7 (total $n = 402$) that failed to show any reduction in analgesic requirement.[125] A variety of agents were administered by various routes, including oral, rectal, and IV. No clear advantage of one particular route of administration could be demonstrated; however, when oral or rectal routes were used, an effect was not demonstrable until, on average, 2 hr after administration. In some studies NSAIDs were shown to be efficacious in reducing global pain scores, but when each source of pain was examined individually, they were not more effective than placebo in controlling shoulder tip pain.[126,127]

The use of the newer cyclooxygenase-2 (COX-2) inhibitor agents has been studied for pain management in orthopedic surgery;[128,129] however, to date, there is little available literature documenting their use in laparoscopic surgery. COX-2 inhibitors are produced in both oral and IV forms but the IV preparations have not yet been released in the United States. These agents have reported advantages over other NSAIDs, with reduced gastric side effects, little effect on platelet functions, and possibly decreased effects on bone healing.[130–132] The use of rofecoxib 50 mg preoperatively in 10 patients having laparoscopic gastric banding surgery was compared retrospectively to 14 patients who did not receive rofecoxib. A decrease in the use of postoperative morphine in the rofecoxib group was observed. Four of the 10 patients, who received the COX-2 inhibitor drug, required no parenteral morphine postoperatively compared to an average dose of 36 mg in those who did. In the group of 14 patients not given rofecoxib, the average morphine dose was 66 mg. Although encouraging, the effects of these agents on postlaparoscopic shoulder tip pain are uncertain.[133]

No single mode of analgesia is ideal for the management of pain after laparoscopic surgery. A multimodal approach is therefore indicated, including the use of an NSAID or COX-2 inhibitor agent preoperatively, local infiltration of insertion sites with a long-acting local anesthetic, intraperitoneal lavage with a large volume of dilute local anesthetic solution containing epinephrine (a newer agent such as ropivacaine or levobupivacaine with reduced cardiotoxicity would be recommended), careful attention to elimination of insufflated gas by the surgeon, and the immediate postoperative use of potent short-acting opioids such as fentanyl.

FUTURE DIRECTIONS FOR LAPAROSCOPIC SURGERY

Laparoscopy has expanded to become a popular ambulatory procedure in surgical specialties owing to proven reduced postoperative pain, shorter hospital stay, reduced effect on patient home functionality, morbidity, and mortality. The burden of shifting postoperative care to patients and relatives and the financial benefit of early discharge to the hospital must be balanced with further patient education and continual patient support. Same-day discharge after more involved surgery may not always be welcomed by patients who desire longer hospital convalescence.[134,135]

The evolution and advancement of laparoscopy continue despite a dearth of proven advantage in many new indications. Comparative trials to conventional management are needed to confirm benefit. Furthermore, despite encouraging results, its use in high-risk patients requires further elucidation. It is anticipated that improving technology will facilitate improved safety, especially in areas of Veress needle/trocar insertion. More studies are needed to study insufflating gases and alternative forms of peritoneal visualization, such as the gasless laparoscopy technique. Management of postoperative pain, PONV, and home functionality are areas where anesthesiology can contribute to improve care.

SUMMARY

Over the past two decades we have seen an escalation in the use of laparoscopic techniques for ambulatory surgery. While it offers advantages in term of minimal tissue disruption, reduced postoperative pain, and acceleration in time to return to work, it comes with the risk of complications both minor and major. In addition, the patient population considered suitable for these techniques continues to change, with the presentation of higher-risk patients for these minimally invasive procedures. One must be familiar with the physiologic consequences of pneumoperitoneum and its effect on a variety of pathologic states. In the ambulatory setting a plan must be in place for management of complications of this procedure. The anesthesiologist must extend care to the postoperative period and preemptively address the issue of postprocedure pain and PONV, to facilitate a timely discharge from the PACU. As laparoscopic equipment becomes more refined, we expect to see more growth in the ambulatory patient population having laparoscopic surgery.

REFERENCES

1. Finley CR, McKernan JB. Laparoscopic antireflux surgery at an outpatient surgery center. Surg Endosc 2001;15:823–26.

2. Kelling G. Ueber Oesophagoskopie, Gastroskopie und Kölioskopie. Munch Med Wochenschr 1902;52:21–24.

3. Jacobaeus HC. Possibility of the use of cystoscope for investigation of serous cavities. Munch Med Wochenschr 1910;57:2090–92.

4. Steiner OP. Abdominoscopy. Surg Gynecol Obstet 1924;38:266–69.

5. Rubin JC. Uterine endoscopy, endometroscopy with the aid of uterine insufflation. Am J Obstet Gynecol 1926;10:313–27.

6. Kalk H. Erfahrungen mit der Laparoskopie. Z Klin Med 1929;111:303.

7. Ruddock JC. Peritoneoscopy. Surg Gynecol Obstet 1937;65:623.

8. Veress J. Neues Instrument zur Ausfuhrung von Brust- oder Bauchpunktionen und pneumothoraxbehandlung. Dtsch Med Wochenschr 1938;41:1480.

9. Semm K. *Operative Manual for Endoscopic Abdominal Surgery*. Chicago: Year Book Medical, 1987.

10. Power FH, Barnes AC. Sterilization by means of peritoneoscopic tubal fulguration. Am J Obstet Gynecol 1941;41:1038.

11. Chatman DL, Cohen MR. History of endoscopy. In: Martin DC (ed.), *Manual of Endoscopy*. Santa Fe Springs, CA: American Association of Gynecologic Laparoscopists, 1990, pp. 1–10.

12. Reddick EJ, Olsen DO. Laparoscopy laser cholecystectomy, a comparison with mini-lap cholecystectomy. Surg Lap Endosc 1990;1:2.

13. O'Boyle CJ. deBeaux AC. Watson DI. Ackroyd R. Lafullarde T. Leong JY. Williams JA. Jamieson GG. Helium vs carbon dioxide gas insufflation with or without saline lavage during laparoscopy. Surgical Endoscopy 2002;16(4):620–625.

14. Paolucci V, Schaeff B. *Gasless Laparoscopy in General Surgery and Gynecology*. Stuttgart: Thieme, 1996, pp. 115–36.

15. Society of American Gastrointestinal Endoscopic Surgeons: granting of privileges for laparoscopic general surgery. Am J Surg 1991;161:324.

16. White JV. Registry of laparoscopic cholecystectomy and new and evolving laparoscopic techniques. Am J Surg 1993;165:536.

17. Jones SB, Jones DB. Surgical aspects and future developments of laparoscopy. Anesthesiol Clin North Am 2001;19:107–24.

18. Philips P, Amaral JF. Abdominal access complications in laparoscopic surgery. J Am Coll Surg 2001;192:525–36.

19. Nordestgaard AG, Bodily KC, Osborne RW, Buttorff JD. Major vascular injuries during laparoscopic procedures. Am J Surg 1995;169:543–45.

20. Chapron C, Pierre F, Harchaoui Y, et al. Gastrointestinal injuries during gynaecological laparoscopy. Hum Reprod 1999;14:333–37.

21. Peterson HB, Hulka JF, Phillips JM. American Association of Gynecologic Laparoscopists 1988 membership survey on operative laparoscopy. J Reprod Med 1990;35:587–89.

22. Yuzpe A. Pneumoperitoneum needle insertion and trocar injuries in laparoscopy: a survey on possible contributing factors and prevention. J Reprod Med 1990;35:485–90.

23. Bhoyrul Sunil, Vierra Mark A, Nezhar Camran R, Krummed Thomas M, Way Lawrence W. Trocar injuries in laparoscopic surgery. J Am Coll Surg 2001;192:677–83.

24. Jones DB, Soper NJ. Complications of laparoscopic cholecystectomy. Annu Rev Med 1996;47:31–44.

25. Lindegren L, Koivusalo A-M, Kellokumpu I. Conventional pneumoperitoneum compared with abdominal wall lift for laparoscopic cholecystectomy. Br J Anaesth 1995;75:567.

26. Mullet CE, Viale JP, Sagnard PE et al. Pulmonary CO_2 elimination during surgical procedures using intra or extraperitoneal CO_2 insufflation. Anesth Analg 1993;76:622.

27. Hodgson C, McClelland RMA, Newton JR. Some effects of the peritoneal insufflation of carbon dioxide at laparoscopy. Anaesthesia 1970;25:382.

28. Fitzgerald SD, Andrus CH, Baudendistel LJ, et al. Hypercarbia during carbon dioxide pneumoperitoneum. Am J Surg 1992;163:186.

29. Hashikura Y, Kawasaki S, Munakata Y, et al. Effects of peritoneal insufflation on hepatic and renal blood flow. Surg Endosc 1994;8:759.

30. Joris JL, Chiche JD, Canivet JL, Jacquet NJ, Legros JJ, Lamy ML. Hemodynamic changes induced by laparoscopy and their endocrine correlates: effects of clonidine. J Am Coll Cardiol 1998;32(5):1389–96.

31. Aho M, Scheinin M, Lehtinen AM, et al. Intramuscularly administered dexmedetomidine attenuates hemodynamic and stress hormone responses to gynecologic laparoscopy. Anesth Analg 1992;75:932.

32. Kirkinen P, Hirovenen E, Kauko M, et al. Intracranial blood flow during laparoscopic hysterectomy. Acta Obstet Gynaecol Scand 1995;74:71.

33. Obeid F, Saba A, Fath J, et al. Increases in intra-abdominal pressure affect pulmonary compliance. Arch Surg 1995;130:544.

34. Ivankovich Ad, Miletich DJ, Albrecht RF, et al. Cardiovascular effects of intraperitoneal insufflation with carbon dioxide and nitrous oxide in the dog. Anesthesiology 1975;42:281.

35. Odeberg S. Ljungqvist O, Svenberg T, et al. Hemodynamic effects of pneumoperitoneum and the influence of posture during anesthesia for laparoscopic surgery. Acta Anaesthesiol Scand 1996;40:160.

36. Wittgen CM, Nauheim KS, Andrus CH, et al. Preoperative pulmonary function evaluation for laparoscopic cholecystectomy. Arch Surg 1993;128:880.

37. Rosenberg-Adamsen S, Skarbye M, Wildschiodtz G, et al. Sleep after laparoscopic cholecystectomy. Br J Anaesth 1996;77:572–75.

38. Querleu D, Chapron C. Complications of gynecologic laparoscopic surgery. Curr Opin Obstet Gynecol 1995;7:257–61.

39. Simpson RB, Russell D. Anaesthesia for daycase gynaecological laparoscopy: a survey of clinical practice in the United Kingdom. Anaesthesia 1999;54:51–85.

40. Swann DG, Spens H, Edwards SA, Chestnut RJ. Anaesthesia for gynaecological laparoscopy: a comparison between the laryngeal mask airway and tracheal intubation. Anaesthesia 1993;48:431–34.

41. Williams MT, Rice I, Ewen SP, Elliott SM. A comparison of the effect of two anaesthetic techniques on surgical conditions during gynaecological laparoscopy. Anaesthesia 2003;58:574–78.

42. Churchill-Davidson HC. Suxamethonium (succinylcholine) chloride and muscle pains. Br J Med 1954;1:74–75.

43. Zahl K, Apfelbaum JL. Muscle pain occurs after outpatient laparoscopy despite substitution of vecuronium for succinylcholine. Anesthesiology 1989;70:408–11.

44. Smith I, Ding Y, White P. Muscle pain after outpatient laparoscopy: influence of propofol versus thiopental and enflurane. Anesth Analg 1993;76:1181–84.

45. Hunter JM. New neuromuscular blocking drugs. N Engl J Med 1995;332:1691–99.

46. Frampton JE, McTavish D. Mivacurium: a review of its pharmacology and therapeutic potential in general anesthesia. Drugs 1993;45:1066–89.

47. King MJ, Milazkeiewicz R, Carli F, Deacock AR. Influence of neostigmine on postoperative vomiting. Br J Anaesth 1988;61:403–6.

48. Anhunen L, Tammisto T. Postoperative vomiting after different modes of general anaesthesia. Ann Chir Gynaecol 1972;61:152.

49. Ding Y, Fredman B, White P. Use of mivacurium during laparoscopic surgery: effect of reversal drugs on postoperative recovery. Anesth Analg 1994;78:450–54.

50. Tang J, Joshi GP, White P. Comparison of rocuronium and mivacurium to succinylcholine during outpatient laparoscopic surgery. Anesth Analg 1996;82:994–98.

51. Watcha MF, Safavi FZ, McCulloch DA, et al. Effect of antagonism of mivacurium-induced neuromuscular block on postoperative emesis in children. Anesth Analg 1995;80:713–17.

52. Dale O, Husum B. Nitrous oxide: a threat to personnel and global environment? Acta Anaesthesiol Scand 1994;38:777–79.

53. Baird PA. Occcupational exposure to nitrous oxide: not a laughing matter. N Engl J Med 1992;327:1026–27.

54. Fischer DM. Does nitrous oxide cause vomiting? Anesth Analg 1996;83:4–5.

55. Tramer M, Moore A, McQuay H. Omitting nitrous oxide in general anesthesia: meta-analysis of intraoperative awareness and post operative emesis in randomized controlled trials. Br J Anaesth 1996;76:186–93.

56. Arellano RJ, Pole ML, Rafuse SE, Fletcher M, Saad YG, Friedlander M, Norris A, Chung F. Omission of nitrous oxide from a propofol-based anesthetic does not affect the recovery of women undergoing outpatient gynecologic surgery. Anesthesiology 2000;93:332–39.

57. Jakobsson J. Rane K. Ryberg G. Anaesthesia during laparoscopic gynaecological surgery: a comparison between desflurane and isoflurane. Eur J Anaesthesiol 1997;14(2):148–52.

58. Nathanson MH, Fredman B, Smith I, White PF. Sevoflurane versus

desflurane for outpatient anesthesia: a comparison of maintenance and recovery profiles. Anesth Analg 1995;81(6):1186–90.

59. Eriksson H, Haasio J, Korttila K. Recovery from sevoflurane and isoflurane anaesthesia after outpatient gynaecological laparoscopy. Acta Anaesthesiol Scand 1995;39(3):377–80.

60. Torri G, Casati A, Albertin A, Comotti L, Bignami E, Scarioni M, Paganelli M. Randomized comparison of isoflurane and sevoflurane for laparoscopic gastric banding in morbidly obese patients. J Clin Anesth 2001;13(8):565–70.

61. Nelskyla KA, Yli-Hankala AM, Puro PH, Korttila KT. Sevoflurane titration using bispectral index decreases postoperative vomiting in phase II recovery after ambulatory surgery. Anesth Analg 2001;93(5):1165–69.

62. Recart A, White PF, Wang A, Gasanova I, Byerly S, Jones SB. Effect of auditory evoked potential index monitoring on anesthetic drug requirements and recovery profile after laparoscopic surgery: a clinical utility study. Anesthesiology 2003;99(4):813–18.

63. Horvoka J, Korttila K, Erkola O. Nitrous oxide does not increase nausea and vomiting following gynaecological laparoscopy. Can J Anaesth 1989;36(2):145–48.

64. Zhou TJ, Coloma M, White PF, Tang J, Webb T, Forestner JE, Greilich NB, Duffy LL. Spontaneous recovery profile of rapacuronium during desflurane, sevoflurane, or propofol anesthesia for outpatient laparoscopy. Anesth Analg 2000;91(3):596–600.

65. Green G, Jonsson L. Nausea: the most important factor determining length of stay after ambulatory anaesthesia: a comparative study of isoflurane and/or propofol techniques. Acta Anaesthesiol Scand 1993;37(8):742–46.

66. Graham SG, Aitkenhead AR. A comparison between propofol and desflurane anaesthesia for minor gynaecological laparoscopic surgery. Anaesthesia 1993;48(6):471–75.

67. Wilhelm W, Berg K, Langhammer A, Bauer C, Biedler A, Larsen R. [Remifentanil in gynecologic laparoscopy: a comparison of consciousness and circulatory effects of a combination with desflurane and propofol]. Anasthesiol Intensivmed Notfallmed Schmerzther 1998;33(9):552–56.

68. Van Hemelrijck J, Smith I, White PF. Use of desflurane for outpatient anesthesia: a comparison with propofol and nitrous oxide. Anesthesiology 1991;75(2):197–203.

69. Chung F, Mulier JP, Scholz J, Breivik H, Araujo M, Hjelle K, Upadhyaya B, Haigh C. A comparison of anaesthesia using remifentanil combined with either isoflurane, enflurane or propofol in patients undergoing gynaecological laparoscopy, varicose vein or arthroscopic surgery. Acta Anaesthesiol Scand 2000;44(7):790–98.

70. Nelskyla K, Eriksson H, Soikkeli A, Korttila K. Recovery and outcome after propofol and isoflurane anesthesia in patients undergoing laparoscopic hysterectomy. Acta Anaesthesiol Scand 1997;41(3):360–63.

71. Coloma M, Zhou T, White PF, Markowitz SD, Forestner JE. Fast-tracking after outpatient laparoscopy: reasons for failure after propofol, sevoflurane, and desflurane anesthesia. Anesth Analg 2001;93(1):112–15.

72. Song D, Chung F, Wong J, Yogendran S. The assessment of postural stability after ambulatory anesthesia: a comparison of desflurane with propofol. Anesth Analg 2002;94(1):60–64.

73. Van Hemelrijck J, Smith I, White PF. Use of desflurane for outpatient anesthesia: a comparison with propofol and nitrous oxide. Anesthesiology 1991;75(2):197–203.

74. Cheng KI, Chu KS, Fang YR, Su KC, Lai TW, Chen YS, Tang CS. Total intravenous anesthesia using propofol and ketamine for ambulatory gynecologic laparoscopy. Kaohsiung J Med Sci 1999;15(9):536–41.

75. Eriksson H, Korttila K. Recovery profile after desflurane with or without ondansetron compared with propofol in patients undergoing outpatient gynecological laparoscopy. Anesth Analg 1996;82(3):533–38.

76. Reigle MM, Leveque MA, Hagan AB, Gerbasi FR, Bhakta KP. Post-

operative nausea and vomiting: a comparison of propofol infusion versus isoflurane inhalational technique for laparoscopic patients. AANA J 1995;63(1):37–41.

77. Wilhelm W, Grundmann U, Van Aken H, Haus EM, Larsen R. A multicenter comparison of isoflurane and propofol as adjuncts to remifentanil-based anesthesia. J Clin Anesth 2000;12(2):129–35.

78. Vaghadia H, Viskari D, Mitchell GWE. Selective spinal anesthesia for outpatient laparoscopy. I. Characteristics of 3 hypobaric solutions. Can J Anaesth 2001;48:256–60.

79. Stewart AVG, Vaghadia H, Collins L, Mitchell GWE. Small-dose selective spinal anesthesia for short duration outpatient gynaecological laparoscopy: recovery characteristics compared with propofol anaesthesia. Br J Anaesth 2001;86:570–72.

80. Vaghadia H, Collins L, Sun H, Mitchell GWE. Selective spinal anesthesia for outpatient laparoscopy. IV. Population pharmacodynamic modeling. Can J Anaesth 2001;48:273–78.

81. Vaghadia H, Solylo MA, Henderson CL, Mitchell GWE. Selective spinal anesthesia for outpatient laparoscopy. II. Epinephrine and spinal cord function. Can J Anaesth 2001;48:261–66.

82. Chilvers CR, Goodwin A, Vaghadia H, Mitchell GWE. Selective spinal anesthesia for outpatient laparoscopy. V. Pharmaeconomic comparison vs general anesthesia. Can J Anaesth 2001;48:279–83.

83. Henderson CL, Schmid J, Vaghadia H, Fowler C, Mitchell GWE. Selective spinal anesthesia for outpatient laparoscopy. III. Sufentanil vs lisocaine-sufentanil. Can J Anaesth 2001;48:267–72.

84. Bridenbaugh LD, Soderstrom RM. Lumbar epidural block anesthesia for outpatient laparoscopy. J Reprod Med 1979;23:85.

85. Mulroy MF. Regional anesthesia: when, why, why not? In: Welcher BV (ed.), *Outpatient Anesthesia*. Problems in Anesthesia, vol 2. Philadelphia: Lippincott, 1988, p. 82.

86. Poindexter AN, Abduk-Malal M, Fast JE. Laparoscopic tubal sterilization under local anesthesia. Obstet Gynecol 1990;75:5–8.

87. Milki AA, Tazuke SI. Office laparoscopy under local anesthesia for gamete intrafallopian transfer: technique and tolerance. Fertil Steril 1997;68:128–32.

88. Haydon GH, Hayes PC. Diagnostic laparoscopy by physicians: we should do it. QJ Med 1997;90:297–304.

89. Zullo F, Pellicano M, Zupi E, Guida M, Mastrantonio P, Nappi C. Minilaparoscopic ovarian drilling under local anesthesia in patients with polycystic ovary syndrome. Fertil Steril 200;74:376–79.

90. DeQuattro N, Hibbert M, Buller J, Larsen F, Russell S, Poore S, Davis G. Microlaparoscopic tubal ligation under local anesthesia. J Am Assoc Gynecol Laparoscopy 1998;5:55–58.

91. Liscomb GH, Dell JR, Ling FW, Spellman JR. A comparison of the cost of local versus general anesthesia for laparoscopic sterilization in an operating room setting. J Am Assoc Gynecol Laparoscopy 1996;3:277–81.

92. Mazdisnain F, Plamieri A, Hakakha M, Cambridge C, Lauria B. Office microlaparoscopy for female sterilization under local anesthesia: a cost and clinical analysis. J Reprod Med 2002;47:97–100.

93. Duh QY, Senokozlieff-Englehart AL, Choe YS, Siperstein AE, Rowland K, Way LW. Laparoscopic gastrostomy and jejunostomy: safety and cost with local vs general anesthesia. Arch Surg 1999;134:151–56.

94. Bordhal PE, Raeder JC, Nordentoft J, Kirste U, Regsdal A. Laparoscopic sterilization: local or general anesthesia? A randomized study. Obstet Gynecol 1993;81:137–41.

95. Frezza EE, Ferzli G. Local and general anesthesia in the laparoscopic preperitoneal hernia repair. J Soc Laparosc Surg 2000;4:221–24.

96. Crabtree JH, Fishman A. A laparoscopic approach under local anesthesia for peritoneal dialysis access. Periton Dial Int 2000;20:757–65.

97. Sharma KC, Kabinoff G, Ducheine Y, Tierney J, Brandstetter RD. Laparoscopic surgery and its potential for medical complications. Heart Lung J Acute Crit Care 26(1):52–64.

98. Fishburne J. Anesthesia for laparoscopy: considerations, complications and techniques. J Reprod Med 1978;21:37–40.

99. Bongard F, Dubecz S, Klein S. Complications of therapeutic laparoscopy. Curr Probl Surg 1994;31:857–924.

100. Pearce DJ. Respiratory acidosis and subcutaneous emphysema during laparoscopic cholecystectomy. Can J Anaesth 1994;41:314–16.

101. Glauser FL, Bartlett RH. Pneumoperitoneum in association with pneumothorax. Chest 1974;66:536–40.

102. McAllister JD, D'Altorio RA, Snyder A. CT findings after uncomplicated percutaneous laparoscopic cholecystectomy. J Comput Assist Tomogr 1991;15:770–72.

103. Phillips JM. Complications in laparoscopy. Int J Gynecol Obstet 1977;95:157–62.

104. Know GB, Sung Y-F, Toledo A. Pneumopericardium associated with laparoscopy. J Clin Anesth 1991;3:56–59.

105. Barba MA, Saez L, Garcia-Molinero MJ, Aguilera M. Pneumopericardium without subcutaneous emphysema, pneumomediastinum, or pneumothorax after laparoscopy. Gastrointest Endosc 1993;39:740.

106. Myles PS. Bradyarrhythmias and laparoscopy: a prospective study of heart rate changes with laparoscopy. Aust NZ J Obstet Gynecol 1991;31:171–73.

107. Burns JM, Hart DM, Hughes RL, Kelman AW, Hillis WS. Effects of nadolol on arrhythmias during laparoscopy performed under general anaesthesia. Br J Anaesth 1988;61:345–46.

108. Bongard F, Dubecz S, Klein S. Complications of therapeutic laparoscopy. Curr Prob Surg 1994;31:857–932.

109. Seigismund K, Kreller E, Held HJ. Pulmonary gas embolism in laparoscopy: a rare complication [German]. Zentralbl Gynakol 1985;107:435–39.

110. Jones DB. Soper NJ. Complications of laparoscopic cholecystectomy. Annu Rev Med 1996;47:31–44.

111. Gan TJ. Post operative nausea and vomiting: can it be eliminated? JAMA 2002;287:1233–36.

112. Raphael JH, Norton AC. Antiemetic efficacy of prophylactic ondansetron in laparoscopic surgery: randomized, double-blind comparison with metoclopramide. Br J Anaesth 1993;71:845–48.

113. Bodner M, White PF. Antiemetic efficacy of ondansetron after outpatient laparoscopy. Anesth Analg 1991;73:250–54.

114. Sniadach MS, Alberts MS. A comparison of the prophylactic antiemetic effect of ondansetron and droperidol on patients undergoing gynecologic laparoscopy. Anesth Analg 1997;85:797–800.

115. Tang J, Wang B, White P, Watcha MF, Qi J, Wender R. The effect of timing of ondansetron administration on its efficacy, cost-effectiveness and cost-benefit as a prophylactic antiemetic in the ambulatory setting. Anesth Analg 1998;86:274–82.

116. Gupta A, Wu CL, Elkassabany N, Krug CE, Parker SD, Feisher LA. Does the routine prophylactic use of antiemetics affect the incidence of post discharge nausea and vomiting following ambulatory surgery: a systematic review of randomized controlled trials. Anesthesiology 2003;99:488–95.

117. Dobbs FF, Kumar V, Alexander JI, Hull MGR. Pain after laparoscopy related to posture and ring versus clip sterilization. Br J Obstet Gynaecol 1987;58:265–69.

118. Jackson SA, Laurence AS, Hill JC. Does post-laparoscopy pain relate to residual carbon dioxide? Anaesthesia 1996;51:485–87.

119. Smith BE, Suchak M, Siggins D, Challands J. Rectus sheath block for diagnostic laparoscopy. Anaesthesia 1988;43:947–48.

120. Goegler S, Blobner M, Busley R, Felber AR, Jelen-Esselbom S. Subphrenic catheter for postoperative analgesia after laparoscopic cholecystectomy. Anesthesiology 1993;79:A26.

121. Helvacioglu A, Weis R. Operative laparoscopy and post operative pain relief. Fertil Steril 1992;57:548–52.

122. Narchi P, Benhamou D, Fernandez H. Intraperitoneal local anesthetic for shoulder pain after day case laparoscopy. Lancet 1991;338:1569–70.

123. Kaplan P, Freund R, Squires J, Herz M. Control of immediate post-

operative pain with topical bupivacaine hydrochloride for laparoscopic ring tubal ligation. Obstet Gynecol 1990;76:798–802.

124. McKemzie R. Postoperative pain after laparoscopic sterilization. Anaesthesia 1989;44:450.

125. Alexander JI. Pain after laparoscopy. Br J Anaesth 1997;79:369–78.

126. Crocker S, Paech M. Preoperative rectal indomethacin for analgesia after laparoscopic sterilization. Anaesth Intens Care 1992;20: 337–40.

127. Van ER, Memrika DJ, Van der Lin CThM. Pain relief following day case diagnostic hysteroscopy-laparoscopy for infertility: a double blind randomized trial with pre-operative naproxen versus placebo. Obstet Gynecol 1993;82:951–54.

128. Gimbel JS, Brugger A, Zhao W, et al. Efficacy and tolerability of celecoxib versus hydrocodone/acetaminophen in the treatment of pain after ambulatory orthopedic surgery in adults. Clin Ther 2001;23(2):228–41.

129. Reuben SS, Phopatkar S, Maciolek H, et al. The preemptive analgesic effect of rofecoxib after ambulatory orthoscopic knee surgery. Anesth Analg 2002;94(1):55–59.

130. Noveck RJ, Laurent A, Kuss M, et al. Parecoxib sodium does not impair platelet function in healthy elderly and non elderly individuals. Clin Invest 2001;21:465–76.

131. Harder AT, An YH. The mechanisms of the inhibitory effects of nonsteroidal antiinflamatory drugs on bone healing: a concise review. J Clin Pharmacol 2003;43:807–15.

132. Whittle BJ. Gastrointestinal effects of nonsteroidal anti-inflammatory drugs. Fundam Clin Pharmacol 2003;17:301–13.

133. Meyer R. Rofecoxib reduces perioperative morphine consumption for abdominal hysterectomy and laparoscopic gastric banding. Anaesth Intens Care 2002;30:389–90.

134. Calland JF, Tanaka K, Foley E, Bovbjerg VE, Markey DW, Blome S, Minasi JS, Hanks JB, Moore MM, Young JS, Jones RS, Schirmer BD, Adams RB. Outpatient laparoscopic cholecystectomy: patient outcomes after implementation of a clinical pathway. Ann Surg 2001;233(5):704–15.

135. Lillemoe KD, Lin JW, Talamini MA, et al. Laparoscopic cholecystectomy as a "true" outpatient procedure: initial experience in 130 consecutive patients. J Gastrointest Surg 1993;3:44–49.

Ambulatory Anesthesia for Pediatrics

JOHN B. ECK   •   ALLISON K. ROSS

INTRODUCTION

Most pediatric surgeries and diagnostic procedures are well suited to the ambulatory environment. They are relatively minor in nature, do not involve major blood loss or fluid shifts, are of short duration, and do not require a prolonged recovery. They are usually performed on healthy patients. Children particularly benefit from convalescing at home in a comfortable setting. In addition, the ambulatory environment decreases costs, avoids exposure to hospital-acquired pathogens, and minimizes separation of children from their parents. Preoperative preparation, choice of anesthesia techniques, and postoperative care that focus on the unique needs of children are keys to success in this arena. This chapter will give an overview of particular strategies in anesthesia care that have been utilized to improve the experience for pediatric patients and their families.

PREOPERATIVE CONSIDERATIONS

Patient Selection

Common pediatric procedures performed on an outpatient basis are shown in Table 30-1. Most children presenting for ambulatory procedures should be generally healthy, American Society of Anesthesiologists (ASA) class I or II. Children with mild systemic disease must have their illnesses well controlled. Newer drugs and techniques of anesthesia and surgery have improved the recovery experience after ambulatory surgery and have encouraged consideration of ambulatory care for children who in the past would not have been considered outpatient candidates. Selected ASA III and IV patients may undergo ambulatory care after anesthesia but careful consideration should be given to the nature of the illness, the type of procedure, the kind of anesthesia, and the likely effects of these on their underlying medical conditions. The ability of their parents to care for them at home and recognize complica-

tions should be considered. In the face of complex surgeries being performed on sick patients on an ambulatory basis, anesthesiologists must be available for preoperative consultation with surgeons and to thoroughly evaluate patients prior to surgery in order to appropriately determine readiness for ambulatory surgery. The ability to admit a child to the hospital should always be an option when caring for pediatric patients, especially those with significant medical illnesses or for procedures where complications are common.

The minimum age for ambulatory pediatric anesthesia is controversial. Of particular concern is the risk of apnea after general anesthesia in infants. Although there have been case reports of apnea occurring in full-term infants,[1,2] this risk is generally exclusive to former premature infants, especially if they have ongoing apnea or are currently anemic.[3] Because most data in the scientific literature come from retrospective review and lack appropriate controls, specific age criteria for hospital admission for observation following anesthesia in infants differ between institutions. A conservative approach would be to plan hospital admission for all full-term infants less than 44 weeks postconceptual age (PCA) and all former preterm infants less than 60 weeks PCA. Premature infants between 50 and 60 weeks PCA may be discharged to home postoperatively after consideration of the health of the child, their response to anesthesia, and following consultation with the parents and the surgeon.

Perioperative complication rates are higher in infants than in older children and adults.[4,5] Because these complications in infants are more likely to be respiratory and cardiovascular in nature, the care of infants in the ambulatory environment should be very carefully considered. At Duke University Medical Center, only infants older than 6 months of age are cared for in our freestanding ambulatory surgery center (ASC). Younger infants, regardless of their ambulatory status, are cared for in the main pediatric hospital operating suite where backup is more readily available in the event of a problem and hospital admission is more easily accomplished.

Table 30-1   Common Pediatric Outpatient Procedures

General surgery
 Inguinal herniorrhaphy
 Umbilical herniorrhaphy
 Lymph node/breast/skin lesion biopsy

Urology
 Hydrocelectomy
 Orchiopexy
 Hypospadias repair

Otolaryngology
 Tonsillectomy
 Adenoidectomy
 Myringotomy with tube insertion
 Frenulectomy
 Sinus endoscopy

Orthopedic
 Club foot repair
 Osteotomy
 Fracture reduction
 Joint arthroscopy
 Supranumary digit removal
 Cast change

Ophthalmology
 Exam under anesthesia
 Strabismus repair
 Lacrimal duct probing
 Cryotherapy

Plastic/dermatology
 Laser therapy of skin lesions
 Congenital skin nevus excision

Gastrointestinal
 Upper/lower endoscopy

Pulmonary
 Bronchoscopy

Radiologic
 Computed tomography
 Magnetic resonance imaging

Table 30-2   American Academy of Pediatrics Guidelines for the Perioperative Anesthesia Environment

Medical staff policy issues
1. Written policies should delineate types and minimal annual volume of pediatric procedures and define clinical privileges of individuals.
2. Anesthesiology department should define which patients are at increased risk (includes patient age, physical status, and procedures).
3. Based on risk, determine whether anesthesiologists will require special clinical privileges to care for pediatric patients.

Facility issues
1. Separate pediatric preoperative section
2. Adequate laboratory and radiologic services
3. Wide selection of pediatric equipment
   a. Airway
   b. Ventilation
   c. Monitoring
   d. Vascular access
   e. Resuscitation
   f. Temperature maintenance
   g. Ventilation
4. Policy regarding effective pediatric pain management
5. Policy for nursing personnel training and experience
6. Policy for postanesthesia care of children
7. Quality of pediatric care should be periodically evaluated.

SOURCE: Hackel A, Badgwell JM, Binding RR, Dahm LS, Dunbar BS, Fisher CG, et al. Guidelines for the pediatric perioperative anesthesia environment. Pediatrics 1999;103:512–15.

lines are intended to supplement the Standards and Guidelines of the ASA. Included in the AAP guidelines are outlines for policies relating to medical staff privileges, categorization of pediatric patients and procedures, and minimum volume of cases to maintain clinical competency of anesthesia providers. It also specifies essential support staff, equipment, and drug availability (Table 30-2). The AAP guidelines are an excellent method for ensuring a safe environment for children.

Ambulatory Environment

Whether performed in the main surgical suite of a hospital or in a separate ASC, most pediatric patients can be safely cared for in a perioperative environment that is primarily designed for adults. However, special consideration should be given to additional elements that ensure a safe experience for children. The American Academy of Pediatrics (AAP), section on Anesthesiology has developed guidelines for the pediatric perianesthesia environment that delineate specific features of the facilities, equipment, and personnel that aim to minimize the risks to children in this setting.[6] These guide-

Preoperative Preparation

Preoperative preparation for pediatric patients undergoing ambulatory surgery includes history and physical examination, appropriate laboratory tests, and psychologic preparation. Systems need to be in place for this to occur prior to the day of surgery, if necessary. Screening laboratory exams for preoperative preparation are generally inefficient.[7] The decision to obtain tests should be guided by a thorough evaluation of the child's medical condition and planned surgical procedure and are not routinely obtained unless there are specific indications. For example, measurement of hemoglobin should be reserved for patients undergoing procedures associated with significant potential blood loss or for children whose age, gender, or medical condition suggests the possibility of anemia (e.g., infants at 2–3 months of age with physiologic anemia or menstruating females). Other laboratory studies, such as electrolyte examinations or assessment of coagulation, should be performed only if there is a clinical suspicion of abnormality, especially if the results may alter the procedure or the anesthetic technique.

Routine pregnancy testing is controversial. Because of the high costs and low yield associated with testing every postmenarchal female adolescent, some centers have abandoned this practice. However, adolescent girls interviewed in the presence of their parent or guardian may not be forthcoming about their sexual activities. They are also more likely to miss or deny the physical manifestations of pregnancy. Although a thorough preoperative history has been shown to be predictive of current pregnancy,[8] routine testing has demonstrated about a 1% rate of missed pregnancy using history alone.[9,10] Therefore, when possible, adolescent females should be interviewed separate from their parent or guardian. The date of their last menstrual period should be determined and information on sexual activity and use of contraceptives should be sought. Urine or serum beta-HCG testing should be obtained if the dates are unknown, equivocal, or if there is any suspicion of pregnancy based on the history. If conservatively employed, this type of directed approach using the judgment of the clinician can be very successful and cost-effective, but may still not be 100% reliable. Alternatively, routine testing can be employed. The cost versus benefit of this practice may make it prohibitive and it is best employed in settings with high-risk adolescents.

Psychologic preparation may play an important role in improving the ambulatory experience for children and their parents. This preparation may involve reading materials or video presentations about anesthesia, personal or phone conversations with anesthesia providers, or more formal presentations by specialists in child life. These interactions have been shown to improve knowledge, decrease parental anxiety, and minimize behavioral changes postoperatively.[11,12] The benefits of these programs in relation to the costs have not been adequately studied.

Preoperative Fasting

The ASA has published guidelines for preoperative fasting (Table 30-3).[13] These guidelines liberalize oral intake compared to older schemes and particularly benefit children and their families. They are also ideal for the ambulatory setting because they are specifically intended for healthy patients undergoing elective procedures. The guidelines do not distinguish between infants and older children. This simplicity may promote compliance. The recommendations are based on studies of gastric volume in adults and children after fasting. Clear liquids consistently empty from the stomach within 2 hr after ingestion, whereas breast milk and infant formula take more than 2 hr to pass. Solid foods prolong gastric emptying time further. Nonhuman milk is similar to solids in its gastric emptying time.

Table 30-3 American Society of Anesthesiologists Guidelines for Preoperative Fasting

Ingested Material	Minimum Fasting Period (hr)
Clear liquids	2
Breast milk	4
Infant formula, nonhuman milk, light meal	6

SOURCE: Practice guidelines for preoperative fasting and the use of pharmacologic agents to reduce the risk of pulmonary aspiration: application to healthy patients undergoing elective procedures. Anesthesiology 1999; 90:896–905.

A light meal (toast and clear liquid) is accepted up to 6 hr prior to anesthesia, but large meals, especially those fried or with high fat content, may require 8 hr to pass from the stomach. Following these guidelines does not guarantee complete gastric emptying. Despite their usefulness in a healthy ambulatory population, the amount and type of food and the child's medical condition should ultimately determine the appropriate fasting time.

Premedication

Administration of medications prior to induction of anesthesia is very common in children and serves to alleviate anxiety, provide perioperative amnesia, and improve cooperation[14] (Table 30-4). The most effective and most frequently used premedication is the benzodiazepine midazolam. Midazolam has a short elimination half-life of 1.2 hr[15] and may reduce the incidence of postoperative nausea and vomiting (PONV),[16] making it particularly suitable for ambulatory surgery. It provides good anxiolysis in most cases and may also help to reduce behavioral changes in children after hospital discharge.[17]

Although midazolam can be given via the intravenous, intranasal, or rectal routes, the oral method is the most common. Oral midazolam is often combined with oral analgesics to mask the flavor of the medication and to provide pain control after short procedures. Although effec-

Table 30-4 Pediatric Premedication Agents

Drug	Route	Dose (mg/kg)
Midazolam	Oral	0.5
	Nasal	0.2–0.3
	Rectal	0.5–1
Fentanyl Oralet	Oral	0.005–0.01
Ketamine	Oral	6
	Intramuscular	2

tive, midazolam can delay recovery after short (less than 30 min) anesthetics, but it should not affect the quality of recovery in these patients.[18]

COMMON PEDIATRIC CONDITIONS

Reactive Airway Disease

Children with a history of reactive airway disease (RAD) or asthma often present for ambulatory surgery and anesthesia which may exacerbate their condition. However, they can be cared for safely if the following guidelines are followed. Children should be maintained on their medical therapies throughout the perioperative period. They should have a prophylactic treatment with a beta-2 agonist (e.g., albuterol) on the morning of their surgery and should have no active wheezing on the day of surgery. They should be free of respiratory infections, which may exacerbate RAD. Instrumentation of the airway should be avoided whenever it is safe to do so and drugs associated with histamine release should similarly be avoided. Bronchodilators should be available in the recovery room and discharge should not take place until the child has no evidence of active wheezing or compromised breathing. Around-the-clock bronchodilator therapy for 24 hr after surgery should be considered.

Respiratory Infection

Children with an active upper respiratory infection (URI) are up to seven times more likely to have a respiratory-related adverse event in the perioperative period compared to children who do not have a URI.[19] Children who require intubation are at particular risk. Signs and symptoms of URI that should alert the practitioner include fever, active wheezing, thick nasal discharge, and/or a persistent nonproductive cough. A productive cough may represent a lower respiratory tract infection and is particularly concerning. Generally speaking, greater than 2 weeks should pass following a URI before elective surgery is undertaken. Four to six weeks of recovery may be necessary if the lower respiratory tract is involved. If this delay is not possible owing to frequency of infections or other considerations, the patient should be treated as if he/she has RAD and special attention should be paid to the respiratory system perioperatively.

Prematurity

Depending on the degree of prematurity, the child may have multiorgan system manifestations of prematurity that must be considered. Chronic lung disease is the most worrisome of these problems and may result in ventilation/perfusion mismatching in the lung presenting as baseline hypercarbia and hypoxemia. If the degree of pulmonary compromise is significant, the infant should be admitted postoperatively for observation. Evidence of other important conditions associated with prematurity should be sought, including hydrocephalus and gastroesophageal reflux.

POSTOPERATIVE CONSIDERATIONS

Postoperative Nausea and Vomiting

PONV is a particularly troublesome problem in the setting of ambulatory surgery where associated delays in discharge and possible hospital admission can drive up costs. In addition, the distress to the child can be significant and may reduce patient and parental satisfaction.[20] Because the incidence of vomiting is twice as frequent among children compared to adults, appropriate and reasonable efforts to reduce the incidence of PONV in the pediatric population are crucial to success in the ambulatory environment. A thorough understanding of the pathophysiology and treatment options available to children is imperative. Because nausea is difficult to diagnose in younger children, only active vomiting is typically studied (and treated) in this population. General anesthesia can increase the risk of PONV by 11-fold compared to regional anesthetic techniques. Since children are often not candidates for a straight regional anesthetic, other measures must be employed.

The routine use of antiemetic therapies is not necessary for all pediatric patients in the ambulatory environment. The decision to prophylactically treat children with antiemetic therapy should be individualized and targeted at high-risk patients. Risk factors include age, gender, type of procedure, use of opioids, history of motion sickness,[21] or history of previous PONV. In particular, risk of PONV increases with age and then decreases after puberty. Children less than 2 years of age have a low overall incidence of PONV (5%).[22] Preschool children are at somewhat higher risk (20%) and school children have a peak incidence of up to 50% overall.[4] Gender differences do not become apparent until after puberty. Boys over 13 years are less likely to vomit after anesthesia compared to girls over 13 years, who vomit frequently after surgery.[23] Risk also increases significantly with specific operations. Patients undergoing surgery of the head and neck are at particular risk. For example, whereas procedures that exclude the head and neck may have an incidence of PONV of around 10% overall,[24] common procedures such as tonsillectomy and strabismus repair can approach rates of 70–80%.[25] Other procedures associated with a higher incidence of PONV include orchiopexy, herniorrhaphy, and laparotomy.[26] Prolonged duration of anesthesia may also increase the risk.[27]

Halothane is associated with a higher incidence of vomiting compared to newer halogenated anesthetic agents like sevoflurane.[21,28] Omission of nitrous oxide has been shown to reduce the incidence of vomiting but not nausea in adult patients.[26] A similar small reduction in postoperative vomiting (POV) in children undergoing dental restorations has been reported, but only for a limited period postoperatively.[29] An overall reduction in vomiting has yet to be established in pediatric patients with omission of nitrous oxide. Propofol has been associated with a lower incidence of PONV (especially early in the postoperative period),[26] but this has not been fully established in children.

Table 30-5   Pediatric Antiemetic Doses

Drug	Intravenous Dose (mg/kg)	Maximum Dose (mg)
Ondansetron	0.05–0.1	4
Dexamethasone	0.15	8
Dolasetron	0.35	12.5
Dimenhydrinate	0.5	50
Promethazine	0.25–0.5	25
Droperidol	0.05–0.075	1.25

Pain can affect gastric emptying time and may contribute to PONV. The severity of pain is positively correlated with the incidence of vomiting in children after ambulatory surgery.[30] In addition, opioids used to treat pain can significantly increase the incidence of PONV.

Recommended antiemetics for children are listed in Table 30-5. Antiemetic drugs can be very effective in pediatric patients but important differences exist between adults and children in the usefulness of individual agents. For example, a meta-analysis of the literature has revealed that the 5-hydroxytryptamine type 3 (5-HT$_3$) receptor antagonist drug ondansetron is more effective than droperidol in treating POV in children, despite equal effectiveness in adults.[31] Also, children may be more prone to side effects associated with antiemetic agents.[25] Despite their higher cost, newer agents with better side-effect profiles may therefore be preferred in children. In particular, numerous studies in the literature have confirmed the effectiveness of the 5-HT$_3$ receptor antagonists in controlling POV in children. Because these drugs have greater efficacy in preventing vomiting than nausea, they should be used as first-line therapy in children. Although ondansetron has been studied most commonly in children, there is no evidence of any difference in safety or efficacy when comparing the different agents in the 5-HT$_3$ receptor antagonist class. These drugs are best administered prophylactically near the end of the procedure.[32]

Dexamethasone is an older, less expensive drug that has few side effects and has been shown to be quite effective in the prevention and treatment of pediatric POV. It has also been associated with an earlier return to a regular diet after tonsillectomy in children.[33] Dexamethasone may have extended prophylactic effects as well. Pappas et al.[34] showed that children administered large doses of dexamethasone (1 mg/kg, maximum 25 mg) after tonsillectomy showed no difference in PONV in the recovery area compared to children who received placebo. However, during the 24 hr after discharge, more children in the placebo group experienced PONV compared to the steroid group (64% vs. 24%). There were also fewer returns to the hospital for management when dexamethasone was given. Other studies have shown good results with lower doses of dexamethasone (0.15 mg/kg), which may be preferable.[35]

Combination therapy with antiemetic agents of different classes may be particularly effective in children. For example, 5-HT$_3$ receptor antagonists and dexamethasone should complement each other by providing both short- and long-term prophylaxis for PONV with few side effects. Splinter and Rhine[36] compared ondansetron alone (0.15 mg/kg) to a combination of ondansetron (0.05 mg/kg) plus dexamethasone (0.15 mg/kg) for children undergoing strabismus repair. Children in the combination group had a 1% incidence of vomiting in the hospital and only 9% after discharge versus 7% in hospital and 28% after discharge in the ondansetron-only group. Similar results have been shown with combination of tropisetron and dexamethasone.[37]

Droperidol is an effective antiemetic in children. Unfortunately, droperidol has been associated with rare cases of QT-interval prolongation and torsades de pointes in adults and is therefore being used less frequently. Given the increased risk for extrapyramidal symptoms and its propensity to cause sedation, droperidol is best reserved for children who have failed all other therapies and who will require hospital admission.[32] Metoclopromide has little effect on the incidence of PONV in children and should similarly be avoided in favor of more effective agents.[38]

Anesthetic techniques and medications can have a significant effect on the incidence of PONV. For example, techniques that minimize pain and allow the avoidance of opioids can decrease the incidence of PONV.[26] Avoiding gastric distension may also help. Since patients who vomit immediately after surgery usually do so after drinking for the first time, the traditional practice of requiring oral fluids in the recovery room prior to discharge may actually promote POV.[39] Adequate perioperative hydration should help to reduce the need for oral intake after surgery and therefore may decrease vomiting during recovery.

The association between the cholinesterase inhibitor neostigmine and nausea and vomiting is controversial and has not been fully evaluated in children. This association has recently been questioned in the setting of ambulatory surgery in adults.[40] One of the difficulties in evaluating this association is the common use of anticholinergic medications in conjunction with the cholinesterase inhibitor, the differential effects of which have been shown to influence the incidence of PONV in adults.[41] The incidence of vomiting is significantly lower in children when atropine is used in combination with neostigmine compared to glycopyrrolate.[42] This is likely due to the central antiemetic effect of atropine afforded by its ability to cross the blood-brain barrier. The quaternary structure of glycopyrrolate does not allow this.

Postoperative Pain

Providing appropriate analgesia is one of the most important considerations for pediatric patients undergoing ambulatory surgery. Children who have poorly controlled pain after surgery are more likely to be more difficult to care for at home and are more likely to experience PONV.[43]

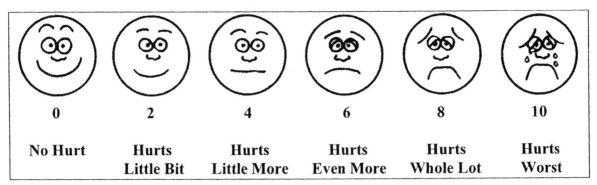

0	2	4	6	8	10
No Hurt	**Hurts Little Bit**	**Hurts Little More**	**Hurts Even More**	**Hurts Whole Lot**	**Hurts Worst**

Figure 30-1   Wong-Baker FACES pain rating scale for pediatric pain assessment. (From Wong DL, Hockenberry-Eaton M, Wilson D, Winkelstein ML, Schwartz P. *Wong's Essentials of Pediatric Nursing,* 6th ed. St. Louis: Mosby 2001, p. 1301. Copyrighted by Mosby, Inc. Reprinted by permission.)

The increasing number of ambulatory surgeries in children has significantly increased the need to optimize strategies for pain control that can be utilized at home.

Appropriate assessment of pain is the first step in treatment. Although self-assessment is superior to assessment by observers, it is not reliable in young children. The FACES pain scale (Fig. 30-1) is now widely used as an assessment tool by observers, as well as for self-assessment by older children. It is preferred by children and is superior to behavioral or physiologic means of assessing pain.[44]

Many ambulatory pediatric surgeries will result in pain that will require opioid analgesics and these should be prescribed liberally for home use when appropriate. With proper dosing, oral opioids are unlikely to cause significant respiratory depression and children should not be undermedicated for fear of this side effect. However, because opioids are associated with PONV, many practitioners have attempted to either reduce or eliminate the need for opioids by using nonopioid analgesics. These drugs should be given around the clock for 24–48 hr postoperatively and supplemented with opioids only as needed. Acetaminophen is the most commonly used of these agents. Rectal dosing recommendations have recently increased. The suggested minimum effective single dose of rectal acetaminophen is 30–40 mg/kg.[45] Doses in this range are associated with a significant opioid-sparing effect and a reduction in the incidence of PONV after surgery in children.[46] Subsequent rectal doses of 20 mg/kg every 6 hr for the first 24 hr after surgery have been recommended for children 2–12 years of age.[47] A higher-than-usual single dose of oral acetaminophen (40 mg/kg) may also be more effective and safe in children perioperatively, but more studies need to be undertaken to confirm this before it can be recommended.[48]

Nonsteroidal analgesics may also be particularly effective for pain control for ambulatory surgery in children. For example, oral ibuprofen (10 mg/kg every 6–8 hr) is very effective and can be dosed less frequently than acetaminophen. Ketorolac can be used orally, intramuscularly, or intravenously and is very effective at doses of 0.25–0.5 mg/kg (up to 30 mg) every 6 hr. However, ketorolac can nonselectively inhibit prostaglandin synthesis at the cyclooxygenase (COX)-1 and COX-2 sites and may be associated with decreased platelet function and bleeding. Newer agents that selectively inhibit the COX-2 site are available and should not alter platelet function. Although preliminary studies show promise, they have not been fully evaluated for use in children.[49]

Regional anesthetic techniques can be very effective for children undergoing ambulatory surgery. Among the possible benefits are improved postoperative analgesia, exposure to fewer emetogenic agents, and shortened recovery stay. Although the caudal block remains the most common regional anesthetic technique in children, peripheral nerve blocks are being used more frequently, especially for extremity surgery. Most of the blocks that are performed in adults (see Chapter 36) can also be utilized in children. Although continuous regional anesthesia techniques utilizing catheters for home use can be very effective in select adult ambulatory patients (see Chapter 46), these techniques have not been fully evaluated in children. When regional anesthesia is utilized, a specific plan for postblock analgesia should be made and discussed with the patient and the family, as block resolution is likely to occur at home. In the absence of a regional anesthetic technique, simple wound infiltration at the end of surgery should be used whenever possible.

Discharge Criteria

Children should be discharged to home when they are awake, their vital signs are stable, their protective reflexes have returned, their pain is controlled, and there is no evidence of nausea, vomiting, or excessive bleeding. There should be no absolute requirement for oral intake or voiding prior to discharge, except in particular cases. Parents should have written instructions on the expected postoperative course at home, specific complications to look out for, and a plan for treating pain. They should also be instructed where to call if problems arise at home.

SUMMARY

Children benefit significantly by recovering at home whenever it is possible to do so safely. With proper preoperative evaluation, appropriately sized equipment, suitably trained staff, and anesthesia techniques that minimize side effects and emotional distress for children and their families, ambulatory anesthesia for pediatric patients can be tremendously successful. Consideration of the unique perspective and needs of children is one of the most important facets of this endeavor.

REFERENCES

1. Cote CJ, Kelly DH. Postoperative apnea in a full-term infant with a demonstrable respiratory pattern abnormality. Anesthesiology 1990;72:559–61.

2. Tetzlaff JE, Annand DW, Pudimat MA. Postoperative apnea in a full-term infant. Anesthesiology 1988;69:426–28.

3. Welborn LG. Postoperative apnea in the former preterm infant: a review. Paediatr Anaesth 1992;2:37–43.

4. Cohen MN, Cameron CB, Duncan PG. Pediatric anesthesia morbidity and mortality in the perioperative period. Anesth Analg 1990; 70:160–67.

5. Tiret L, Nivoche Y, Hatton F. Complications related to anaesthesia in infants and children: a prospective study of 40,240 anaesthetics. Br J Anaesth 1988;61:263–69.

6. Hackel A, Badgwell JM, Binding RR, Dahm LS, Dunbar BS, Fischer CG, et al. Guidelines for the pediatric perioperative anesthesia environment. Pediatrics 1999;103:512–15.

7. O'Connor ME, Drasner K. Preoperative laboratory testing of children undergoing elective surgery. Anesth Analg 1990;70:176–80.

8. Malviya S, D'Errico C, Reynolds P, Huntington J, Voepel-Lewis TD, Pandit UA. Should pregnancy testing be routine in adolescent patients prior to surgery? Anesth Analg 1996;83:854–58.

9. Wheeler M, Cote CJ, Kelly DH. Preoperative pregnancy testing in a tertiary care children's hospital: a medico-legal conundrum. J Clin Anesth 1999;11(1):56–63.

10. Azzam FJ, Padda GS, DeBoard JW, Krock JL, Kolterman S. Preoperative pregnancy testing in adolescents. Anesth Analg 1996;82(1):4–7.

11. Margolis JO, Ginsberg B, Dear G, Ross AK, Goral JE, Bailey AG. Paediatric preoperative teaching: effects at induction and postoperatively. Paediatr Anaesth 1998;8(1):17–23.

12. Cassady JF Jr, Wysocki TT, Miller KM, Cancel DD, Izenberg N. Use of a preanesthetic video for facilitation of parental education and anxiolysis before pediatric ambulatory surgery. Anesth Analg 1999; 88(2):246–50.

13. Practice guidelines for preoperative fasting and the use of pharmacologic agents to reduce the risk of pulmonary aspiration: application to healthy patients undergoing elective procedures. Anesthesiology 1999;90:896–905.

14. Kain Z, Mayes LC, Bell C, Weisman S, Hofstadter MB, Rimar S. Premedication in the United States: a status report. Anesth Analg 1997; 84:427–32.

15. Payne K, Mattheyse FJ, Liebenberg D, Dawes T. The pharmacokinetics of midazolam in paediatric patients. Pharmacology 1989;37: 267–72.

16. Splinter WM, Macneill HB, Menard EA, Rhine EJ, Roberts DJ, Gould MH. Midazolam reduces vomiting after tonsillectomy in children. Can J Anaesth 1995;42:201–3.

17. Kain Z, Mayes LC, Wang S, Hofstadter MB. Postoperative behavioral changes in children: effects of sedative premedication. Anesthesiology 1999;90(3):758–65.

18. Viitanen H, Annila P, Viitanen M, Tarkkila P. Premedication with midazolam delays recovery after ambulatory sevoflurane anesthesia in children. Anesth Analg 1999;89:75–79.

19. Cohen MM, Cameron CB. Should you cancel the operation when a child has an upper respiratory tract infection? Anesth Analg 1991; 72:282–88.

20. Derrico C, Voepel-Lewis TD, Siewert M, Malviya S. Prolonged recovery stay and unplanned admission of the pediatric surgical outpatient: an observational study. J Clin Anesth 1998;10:482–87.

21. Busoni P, Sarti A, Crescioli M, Agostino MR, Sestini G, Banti S. Motion sickness and postoperative vomiting in children. Paediatr Anaesth 2002;12:65–68.

22. Karlsson E, Larsson LE, Nilsson K. Postanaesthetic nausea in children. Acta Anaesthesiol Scand 1990;34:515–18.

23. Heyland K, Dangel P, Gerber AC. Postoperative nausea and vomiting (PONV) in children. Eur J Paediatr Surg 1997;7:230–33.

24. Villeret I, Laffon M, Duchalais MH, Blond MH, Lecuyer AI, Mercier C. Incidence of postoperative nausea and vomiting in paediatric surgery. Paediatr Anaesth 2002;12:712–17.

25. Baines D. Postoperative nausea and vomiting in children. Paediatr Anaesth 1996;6:7–14.

26. Rose JB, Watcha MF. Postoperative nausea and vomiting in paediatric patients. Br J Anaesth 1999;83(1):104–17.

27. Rowley MP, Brown TCK. Postoperative vomiting in children. Anaesth Intens Care 1982;10:309–13.

28. Busoni P, Crescioli M, Agostino MR, Sestini G. Vomiting and common paediatric surgery. Paediatr Anaesth 2000;10:639–43.

29. Splinter WM, Komocar L. Nitrous oxide does not increase vomiting after dental restorations in children. Can J Anaesth 1997;84: 506–8.

30. Kotiniemi LH, Ryhanen PT, Valanne J, Jokela R, Mustonen A, Poukkula E. Postoperative symptoms at home following day-case surgery in children: a multicentre survey of 551 children. Anaesthesia 1997;52:963–69.

31. Domino KB, Anderson EA, Polissar NL, Posner KL. Comparative efficacy and safety of ondansetron, droperidol and metoclopromide for preventing postoperative nausea and vomiting: a meta-analysis. Anesth Analg 1999;88(6):1370–79.

32. Gan TJ, Meyer T, Apfel CC, Chung F, Davis PJ, Eubanks S, et al. Consensus guidelines for managing postoperative nausea and vomiting. Anesth Analg 2003;97:62–71.

33. Caitlin FI, Grimes WJ. The effect of steroid therapy on recovery from tonsillectomy in children. Arch Otolaryngol 1991;117:649–52.

34. Pappas AL, Sukhani R, Hotaling AJ, Mikat-Stevens M, Javorski JJ, Donzelli J, et al. The effect of preoperative dexamethasone on the immediate and delayed morbidity in children undergoing adenotonsillectomy. Anesth Analg 1998;87:57–61.

35. Splinter WM, Roberts DJ. Dexamethasone decreases vomiting by children after tonsillectomy. Anesth Analg 1996;83:913–16.

36. Splinter WM, Rhine EJ. Low-dose ondansetron with dexamethasone more effectively decreases vomiting after strabismus surgery in children than does high dose ondansetron. Anesthesiology 1998; 88:72–75.

37. Holt R, Rask P, Coulthard K, Sinclair M, Van Der Walt J, MacKenzie V, et al. Tropisetron plus dexamethasone is more effective than tropisetron alone for the prevention of postoperative nausea and vomiting in children undergoing tonsillectomy. Paediatr Anaesth 2000;10:181–88.

38. Lawhorn CD, Kymer PJ, Stewert FC. Ondansetron dose response curve in high-risk pediatric patients. J Clin Anesth 1997;9:637–42.

39. Kearney R, Mack C, Entwistle L. Withholding oral fluids from children undergoing day surgery reduces vomiting. Paediatr Anaesth 1998;8:331–36.

40. Joshi GP, Garg SA, Hailey A, Yu SY. The effects of antagonizing residual neuromuscular blockade by neostigmine and glycopyrrolate on nausea and vomiting after ambulatory surgery. Anesth Analg 1999; 89:628–31.

41. Salmenpera M, Kuoppamaki R, Salmenpera A. Do anticholinergic agents affect the occurrence of postanaesthetic nausea? Acta Anaesthesiol Scand 1992;36:445–48.

42. Chhibber AK, Listik SJ, Thakur R, Francisco DR, Fickling KB. Effects of anticholinergics on postoperative vomiting, recovery, and hospital stay in children undergoing tonsillectomy with or without adenoidectomy. Anesthesiology 1999;90:697–700.

43. Munro HM, Malviya S, Lauder GR, Veopel-Lewis T, Tait AR. Pain relief in children following outpatient surgery. J Clin Anesth 1999; 11:187–91.

44. Goddard JM, Pickup SE. Postoperative pain in children. Anaesthesia 1996;51:588–91.

45. Birmingham PK, Tobin MJ, Henthorn TK, Fisher DM, Berkelhamer MC, Smith FA, et al. Twenty-four hour pharmacokinetics of rectal acetaminophen in children: an old drug with a new recommendation. Anesthesiology 1997;87:244–52.

46. Korpela R, Korvenoja P, Meretoja OA. Morphine-sparing effect of acetaminophen in pediatric day-case surgery. Anesthesiology 1999; 91(2):442–47.

47. Birmingham PK, Tobin MJ, Fisher DM, Henthorn TK, Hall SC, Cote CJ. Initial and subsequent dosing of rectal acetaminophen in children: a 24-hour pharmacokinetic study of new dose recommendations. Anesthesiology 2001;94:385–89.

48. Bolton P, Bridge HS, Montgomery CJ, Merrick PM. The analgesic efficacy of preoperative high dose (40mg/kg) oral acetaminophen after bilateral myringotomy and tube insertion. Paediatr Anaesth 2002;12:29–35.

49. Joshi W, Connely NR, Reuben S, Wolckenhaar M, Thakkar N. An evaluation of the safety and efficacy of administering rofecoxib for postoperative pain management. Anesth Analg 2003;97:35–38.

Ambulatory Anesthesia for Cosmetic Surgery

DIANNE L. SCOTT

INTRODUCTION

The popularity of cosmetic surgery has increased significantly over the past 5 years. The five most common plastic surgical procedures in 2002 included liposuction, breast augmentation, face lift, nose reshaping, and eyelid surgery. This statistic also correlates with the top five cosmetic surgical procedures performed on women.[1] In the past this secret surgery was limited mostly to those of significant celebrity or financial means. Owing to the popularity of reality television and emphasis on physical perfection in society, the average citizen is now considering cosmetic surgery. These patients actively and openly seek enhancement of their physical appearance. A total of 6.6 million people had cosmetic plastic surgery in the year 2002. Women continue to represent the largest population having these procedures (85%). Not surprisingly, 35–50-year-olds made up 45% of all cosmetic surgical patients (Fig. 31-1). Males are gaining in their representation in the cosmetic surgery arena. Nose reshaping is most popular in this group (Fig. 31-2). There was a 7% increase in popularity of this procedure in males from 2001 to 2002. Thirty-seven percent of all cosmetic plastic surgery patients were repeat patients. The number of minorities having cosmetic procedures remains constant since 2001, with African-Americans representing 6%, Hispanics 7%, and Asian-Americans 3%.[1] Oddly enough, since 1999, there has been a slight decreasing trend in abdominoplasties, while nose-reshaping surgery has increased. There are increasing financial pressures to perform these cosmetic procedures outside of conventional hospital settings. It is therefore crucial that the standard of patient care not relax when the hospital environment is not being used.

The concept of office-based anesthesia continues to be evaluated for its efficacy and safety for these procedures. Fifty percent of cosmetic surgical procedures are performed in the office-based setting. Seventeen percent of cosmetic surgical procedures are performed in freestanding ambulatory surgical facilities and 32% are done in the hospital. Although there is a tendency of patients, the me-

dia, and cosmetic surgeons to minimize the risk of these procedures, cosmetic surgery is considered major surgery from an anesthetic perspective. Anesthesiologists should always adhere to guidelines provided by accreditation agencies such as the Joint Commission on Accreditation of Healthcare Organizations (JCAHO) when providing services in any of these surgical environments.[2]

Anesthesia for cosmetic surgery has been provided traditionally with use of local anesthesia with or without sedation.[3] Regional anesthesia has been used under certain conditions.[4] However, owing to the increasing complexity of these procedures and thus increased duration of surgery, general anesthesia is becoming more popular. Almost one-third of all patients (32%) had multiple cosmetic procedures during a single session. Old fears regarding dangers of general anesthesia have been dispelled owing to the advent of anesthetic agents with a safe and fast recovery profile.[5]

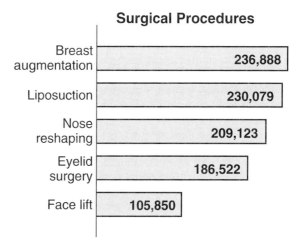

Figure 31-1 Top five female cosmetic procedures, 2002 (N = 5,623,056). (Adapted from American Society of Plastic Surgeons statistics. www.plasticsurgery.org, 2002.)

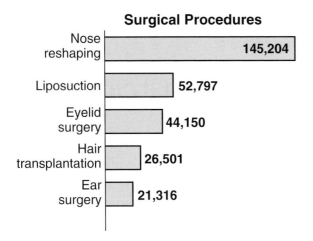

Figure 31-2 Top five male cosmetic procedures, 2002 (N = 966,821). (Adapted from American Society of Plastic Surgeons statistics. www.plasticsurgery.org, 2002.)

PATIENT SAFETY

Regardless of the environment in which cosmetic plastic surgery is performed, patient safety should be the most important factor when defining patient suitability. The American Society of Plastic Surgery Task Force on Patient Safety in Office-Based Surgery Facilities convened in 2002 to address this matter. The task force included representatives from the American Society of Anesthesiologists (ASA) and various related plastic surgery organizations: the American Society of Plastic Surgeons (ASPS) and American Society of Aesthetic Plastic Surgeons (ASAPS).[6] Recommendations were based on scientific literature published as a result of research performed in the hospital-based setting. Although the hospital does not represent the setting in which most cosmetic surgery is performed, it is the arena that best represents the office setting. By all accounts, the preoperative history and physical examination is extremely important. Not only does it provide baseline medical information but it also identifies comorbidities that will influence the environment in which the procedure is performed (inpatient vs. outpatient vs. office). There should also be an evaluation for a history and/or presence of venous thrombosis as this entity is one of the most common surgical complications seen in this patient population undergoing general anesthesia. This is due to the high percentage of women between the ages of 35 and 50 undergoing cosmetic surgery. This increased incidence of venous thrombosis also corresponds with this entity occurring mostly in women over 40 who are taking oral contraceptives or hormone replacement therapy for menopause (Table 31-1).[6]

Although there has been some question as to whether the anesthesiologist has a role in evaluating these cosmetic patients,[7] the preanesthetic evaluation should be performed not only to obtain medical information that would impact anesthetic management but also to minimize the likelihood of surgical cancellations due to unresolved medical concerns. In addition, lessening anxiety about anesthesia in the preoperative interaction will result in an overall positive surgical experience for patients. This preoperative anesthetic interaction should occur prior to the day of surgery. The

Table 31-1   Risk Rating and Prophylaxis for Thromboembolic Events

Risk rating for thrombosis and embolism
Low risk   Patients with no risk factors. Under age 40.

Moderate risk
   Patients 40 years or older with no additional risk factors.
   Procedure duration greater than 30 min.
   Patients who use oral contraceptives or hormone replacement for menopause.

High risk
   Patients over the age of 40 with at least one risk factor.
   Procedure duration greater than 30 min under general anesthesia.
   Other risk factors.

Prophylaxis for thrombosis or embolism
Low risk   Comfortable positioning with knees slightly flexed.
Moderate risk   In addition to low-risk recommendations, these patients should receive intermittent pneumatic compression devices on the calf and ankle. The devices should be placed prior to induction of general anesthesia and remain in place until emergence and patient resumes spontaneous movement.

High risk
   In addition to the above recommendations, a hematology consultation should be obtained. Consider preoperative and postoperative anticoagulation therapy.
   Review family history for past thromboembolic events, edema in legs, and history of venous insufficiency.

Source: Adapted from Iverson RE, Lynch DJ. ASPS Task Force on Patient Safety in Office-Based Surgery Facilities. Patient safety in office-based surgery facilities: II. Patient selection. Plast Reconstr Surg 2002;110(7): 1785–90.

preoperative screening can be performed in various ways including (1) facility visit prior to the day of surgery; (2) office visit prior to the day of surgery; (3) review of health questionnaire provided to patients on the day that they schedule their procedure; and (4) computer-assisted information-gathering system.[8-10] Adequate patient education is imperative to assure a high level of satisfaction.

Who Should Not Have Surgery?

Any patient who has financial means will consider herself/himself a candidate for outpatient cosmetic surgery. It is the anesthesiologist's role to determine patients who are not suitable for outpatient cosmetic surgery. There should never be a relaxation of preanesthetic criteria simply because cosmetic surgery is contemplated. Patients will minimize their medical history, and sometimes resort to deception, to pursue their quest for perfection. This surgery is the ultimate elective surgery. None of it is necessary and medical rules and common sense should not be ignored to accommodate a patient. Patients may think that the risk is worth it. Anesthesiologists do not. Intuitively, one would think that only patients with physical status ASA I and II would be candidates for these procedures on an outpatient basis. It is, however, appropriate for patients with ASA III and IV classifications to undergo these procedures as well. Natof concluded in a prospective study of 13,000 patients that ASA III patients with well-controlled medical conditions were at no higher risk to undergo outpatient surgery than those of ASA I and II.[11] This of course must be considered along with the type of procedure that the patient is to undergo. Over time, a group of patients has been identified who are clearly not candidates for outpatient anesthesia of any kind. These guidelines hold true for patients undergoing cosmetic surgery as well, including:

Unstable ASA III and IV Patients

All patients undergoing outpatient cosmetic surgery should have written medical clearance by their primary care physician or subspecialist. This clearance should specifically include suitability for general anesthesia even when local anesthesia is proposed. This extent of clearance will assure that complete medical assessment of all comorbidities has been done. Although a surgeon may consider the patient medically sound, he/she may not be from an anesthetic perspective and will present significant risk.

Obesity

De Jong states that body mass index (BMI) represents a predictor for sensitivity to respiratory depressants. Body mass index ≥ 30 represents heightened respiratory sensitivity to sedation and general anesthesia. In patients who are morbidly obese, with BMI ≥ 35, the risk of obstructive sleep apnea may confound the morbidity.[12] The BMI should therefore be one of the factors that is strongly considered when deciding whether overnight admission is appropriate, assuming all other conditions are equal.

Psychological Distress

There is the general impression among physicians not involved with surgical patients that individuals undergoing cosmetic surgery are psychologically different from the average patient undergoing outpatient surgery. This perception is not entirely unfounded. Meninguad[13] published the results of a prospective multicenter study indicating that there was a 20% higher incidence of depression in patients undergoing cosmetic surgery than controls. Social anxiety was higher in patients undergoing cosmetic surgery. This

Table 31-2   Disorders That Accompany Body Dysmorphic Diagnosis

Major depression
Avoidant personality
Social phobia
Obsessive compulsive disorder
Delusional disorder
Anorexia nervosa
Gender identity disorder

SOURCE: Adapted from Rohrich RJ. The who, what, when, and why of cosmetic surgery: do our patients need a preoperative psychiatric evaluation? Plast Reconstr Surg 2000;106(7):1605–7.

study also indicated that 50% of cosmetic patients had already taken psychiatric treatment, for which 27% were on antidepressants. This begs the question as to whether patients undergoing cosmetic surgery should have a preoperative psychiatric evaluation. Certainly not. There is a small population of patients, however, who do represent a surgical and anesthetic risk. Sarwer wrote in 1998 that cosmetic surgery patients were no more likely to demonstrate dissatisfaction than controls. Seven percent of cosmetic patients did represent those who have diagnostic criteria for body dysmorphic disorder. These are patients who are not only capable of suing their physicians but who are also capable of physical harm to their physicians.[14] These patients should not undergo elective surgery of any kind. It is important that the anesthesiologist elicit careful history that can reveal this personality. Usually the psychiatric and/or medication history is an indicator. Even when all other aspects of the preoperative assessment are "clean," this kind of psychiatric information is a cause for pause (Table 31-2).[15]

Herbal Medications Intake

It must be assumed that all patients who value their appearance will also represent those who are in pursuit of perfect health as well. These patients assume that all "natural" products are safe. These products can in fact prove fatal when combined with general anesthesia or surgery. Complications such as bleeding, arrhythmias, stroke, and delayed awakening from anesthesia can occur. These herbal medications should be discontinued 2–3 weeks prior to surgery (Table 31-3).[16]

Aspirin Products and Nonsteroidal Anti-inflammatory Drugs Intake

The use of aspirin and nonsteroidal anti-inflammatory drugs (NSAIDs) is a relative contraindication to surgery in most circumstances, depending on the surgeon's discretion. The use of aspirin or products that contain aspirin and NSAIDs can prove disastrous in cosmetic surgery. It is

Table 31-3   Common Herbs and Foods to Be Avoided Two Weeks Prior to Surgery

Alfalfa: anticoagulant effect from coumarin

Angelica (root of the Holy Ghost): anticoagulant and antiplatelet effects

Anise: anticoagulant effect

Arnica (leopard's bane, wolf's bane, mountain tobacco): anticoagulant effect

Asafetida (gum, giant fennel, devil's drug): anticoagulant effect

Aspen (*Populi cortex, populi folium*): antiplatelet effect from salicylate constituent

Black cohosh (bugwort, black snakeroot, baneberry): antiplatelet effect

Bogbean (water shamrock, buckbean, marsh trefoil): anticoagulant effect

Boldo (*Peumus boldus*, boldine): anticoagulant effect from coumarin constituents

Bromelain: anticoagulant effect from enzyme

Capsicum (*Capsicum frutescen*, African pepper, cayenne, chili pepper): antiplatelet effect

Celery: antiplatelet effect

Clove: antiplatelet effect

Dong quai: anticoagulant and antiplatelet effects

Feverfew (bachelor's button, featherfew, midsummer daisy): antiplatelet effect

Fish oils (omega-3 fatty acids): antiplatelet effect, vasodilatation, prolonged bleeding time

Fucus (kelp, black tang, bladderwrack, cutweed): anticoagulant effect

Garlic (nectar of the gods, stinking rose): inhibition of platelet aggregation

Ginger: anticoagulant effect

Gingko (*Gingko biloba*, maidenhair): inhibits platelet aggregation and decreases blood viscosity

Gingeng (*Panax ginseng*, Asian ginseng, Korean red, jintsam): anticoagulant and antiplatelet effects

Goldenseal (eye balm, yellow puccoon): coagulant effect

Horse chestnut (Venostat, *Aesculus hippocastanum*, escine): anticoagulant effect

Horseradish (pepperroot, mountain radish, *Armoracia rusticana*): anticoagulant effect

Licorice (sweet root, *Glycyrrhiza*): antiplatelet effect

Onion (*Allium cepa*): antiplatelet effect

Papain (*Carica papaya*): bleeding risk

Plantain (plantago major, common plantain): coagulant effect from vitamin K constituent

Red clover (*Trifolium praetense*, trefoil, cow clover, beebread): anticoagulant effect

Safflower (saffron, zaffer, *Carthamus tinctorium*): anticoagulant effect from safflower

Tumeric (Indian saffron, *Curcumaa longa*): antiplatelet effect

Vitamin E (alpha-tocopherol): inhibits platelet aggregation and interferes with clotting

Wild lettuce (green endive, lettuce opium, *Latuca virosa*): anticoagulant effect from coumarin constituent

Willow bark (*Salix alba*, white willow, silbereide): antiplatelet effect from salicylate constituent

Yarrow (*Achillea millefolium*, wound wort, thousand-leaf): coagulant effect

SOURCE: Adapted from Shiffman MA. Warning about herbals in plastic and cosmetic surgery. Plast Reconstr Surg 2001;108(7):2180–81.

considered an absolute contraindication to cosmetic surgery owing to the risk of bleeding. Intraoperative and postoperative bleeding can result in ischemia, necrosis, and loss of skin flaps on the face, breast, and abdomen. It can result in blindness in the setting of blepharoplasties. Surgeons should be alerted to any history of use of these products elicited on the day of surgery. Preanesthetic instructions should always include elimination of these products 2 weeks prior to surgery.

Malignant Hyperthermia

Any patient with a history or family history of malignant hyperthermia should not undergo anesthesia in an office. Their anesthesia should be performed in a facility that is equipped to manage all of the medical issues associated with this syndrome. If surgery is contemplated in an ambulatory facility, the facility should be equipped to fully stabilize the patient followed by immediate transfer to an inpatient hospital.

Monoamine Oxidase Inhibitors

Owing to the hemodynamic instability that is seen with the use of these drugs, the author recommends discontinuation of these medications for 2 weeks prior to surgery. If for some psychiatric reason these medications cannot be discontinued, the surgery and anesthesia should be performed in an inpatient setting or well-equipped ambulatory setting. Under no circumstances should this patient undergo cosmetic surgery in an office. Intensive hemodynamic monitoring is crucial for these patients. An office setting cannot provide this.

PREOPERATIVE LABORATORY TESTING

Since cosmetic surgery is minimally invasive in nature, and is performed on healthy or medically stable patients, there are no preset requirements for preanesthetic laboratory exams. The requirement for screening laboratory information should be based on the patient's preexisting medical history. This means that healthy patients with a negative medical history can undergo cosmetic surgery without any laboratory work done. The temptation for knee-jerk laboratory requirements should be avoided. At the same time, patients with significant baseline medical problems should have the same preoperative laboratory assessment as that required for surgery in an inpatient facility.[17] This is especially important when surgery in a freestanding ambulatory facility or a physician's office is being considered. In these environments, there is the temptation to minimize laboratory scrutiny to avoid the appearance and feeling of a hospital. The lack of vigilance in this matter can prove deadly.

INFORMED CONSENT

Written informed consent for anesthesia for cosmetic surgery should be the same as that used for inpatient surgery.

There is no place for a watered-down version simply because surgery is being performed in a physician's office or a freestanding ambulatory facility. This full consent provides valuable information to the patient regarding risks of anesthesia. Acceptance of these risks also solidifies in the patient and surgeon's mind that they are accepting the risk for anesthesia for major surgery. This consent should be obtained by the person who is trained to answer questions regarding the anesthesia—the anesthesiologist or his/her designee. This recommendation is in keeping with the recommendations made by the ASPS Task Force.[6]

ANESTHESIA TECHNIQUES FOR COSMETIC SURGERY

Cosmetic surgery can be performed using local anesthesia with sedation, regional anesthesia, or general anesthesia. Surgeon and anesthesiologist's skills as well as historical practice will dictate the choice. However, owing to the complexity of current cosmetic surgical procedures, general anesthesia is gaining in popularity. The technique presented is used at the author's institution[18] and it has proven suitable in all cosmetic surgical procedures and satisfies the requirement of quick onset, quick offset, and high level of patient comfort, safety, and satisfaction. It is a primary opioid technique using intravenous (IV) fentanyl at a dose up to 5 μg/kg with a maximum of 10 μg/kg for abdominoplasties. Propofol is used at 2 mg/kg for general anesthesia induction, followed by a background infusion of propofol at 65–70 μg/kg/min. Intravenous midazolam is also used as a single dose of 0.015 mg/kg at induction. Ventilation is controlled. Nausea is treated preemptively using IV promethazine 0.625 mg following induction and IV ondansetron 4 mg 30 minutes prior to emergence. Care should be taken that the patient maintains normal temperature during these procedures. Hypothermia is often overlooked owing to the erroneous opinion that cosmetic procedures are not serious surgical procedures. Hypothermia can lead to poor anesthetic metabolism, prolonged muscle relaxation effect, and increased postoperative sedation. All of these factors can contribute to slow return to baseline in the recovery period. Anesthetic morbidity and death can be directly correlated with lack of nursing vigilance and lack of attention to temperature homeostasis.

CONSIDERATIONS FOR SPECIFIC COSMETIC PROCEDURES

Breast Augmentation/Lift (Mastopexy)/Reductions

These procedures are usually performed on healthy or medically stable patients. The exception in the setting is reconstructive surgery after breast cancer. These procedures can be performed with an opioid-based general anesthetic technique[18] with regional anesthesia[3] or with local anesthesia in combination with IV sedation.[4] The latter two techniques depend on special skills of both the anesthesiologist and surgeon. Regardless of technique, the monitoring should include standard ASA monitors. Additional monitoring is dictated by the patient's physical status. In all situations, field avoidance is necessary. Patient position will change intermittently from supine to sitting to assess the effect of gravity on the final surgical product. The anesthetic technique chosen should assure the maintenance of airway integrity. Blood loss is minimal in these procedures. The exception is breast reduction, where blood loss varies according to the size of the breast being reduced. Blood loss can be significant, particularly in a situation where reduction reaches 800–1000 g/side of breast tissue.[19] Autologous blood transfusion is extremely rare in the cosmetic population. Pain control is very important in these patients, particularly when a submuscular/subpectoral breast implant is placed. No anesthetic technique has an advantage for postoperative analgesia and patient satisfaction. It is important that patients receive appropriate analgesia for their body weight, not for the facility in which they are receiving surgery. There should never be preset amounts of analgesia that a patient receives.

Rhytidectomy (Face and Neck Lift)

This procedure is designed to rejuvenate the face and neck. It is achieved by tightening the muscles and skin in the face and neck. This procedure can be performed using local anesthetic infiltration and oral or IV sedation. Surgical time can range from 3 to 6 hr. Because of increasing demand for more complex and time-consuming procedures, general anesthesia has fallen back into favor among cosmetic surgeons. In the past, there was unfounded fear of general anesthesia owing to perceived increased risk of pain, nausea, bleeding, and excessive postoperative sedation. Due to the advent of safe anesthetics (short-acting, fast emergence),[20] and technologic advances in monitoring of anesthetic depth with the development and implementation of bispectral index (BIS) monitoring, there is no need to fear the use of adequate general anesthesia in cosmetic patients.[21] This recent technologic advance, however, should not be an excuse for decreased vigilance and administration of inadequate levels of anesthesia. To further dispel this fear in the surgical community, Hoefflin reported a retrospective evaluation of 23,000 patients undergoing cosmetic plastic surgery under general anesthesia over an 18-year period. There were no postoperative deaths or significant complications.[5] Since this surgery is performed around the head and neck, care should be used to avoid injury to the eyes. When corneal protectors are used, note of insertion and removal should be made. Since this is not a high-volume-blood-loss procedure, IV fluids should be restricted to avoid edema in the face. Intravenous fluids should be titrated to achieve a urine output of 0.5 mL/kg/hr. Blood pressure control is crucial to avoid excessive bleeding and loss of facial skin flaps.

Coughing and bucking should be prevented as well. This can be achieved by maintenance of a deep plane of anesthesia and/or use of a small amount of muscle relaxant, titrated to a train-of-four ratio of 2/4. This amount of titration will allow the surgeon to stimulate the facial nerve

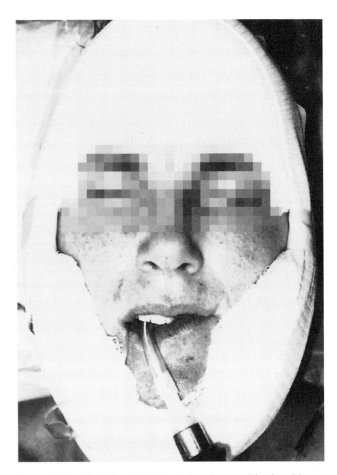

Figure 31-3   Traditional bulk head dressing used for face lift procedures.

during dissection if desired. The use of muscle relaxant should be discussed with the surgeon in advance. Emergence from anesthesia and endotracheal extubation should be cautiously and skillfully done. While coughing and bucking should be avoided, premature extubation can prove disastrous. The traditional bulky head dressing used for face lift procedures makes external maintenance of airway patency with jaw lift or oral airway insertion almost impossible. The patient must therefore demonstrate full return of protective airway reflexes and response to commands prior to endotracheal extubation (Fig. 31-3).

Eyelid Surgery (Blepharoplasty)

This procedure is designed to improve drooping eyelids and removal of bags below the eyes. This is achieved by removal of fat, muscle, and skin in the eyelids. The procedure can be as brief as 30 min or as long as 180 min. Most procedures are performed on an outpatient basis unless there is some other confounding medical condition. Excessive bleeding may require an overnight admission. The anesthetic technique is local infiltration with oral or IV sedation. General anesthesia is used in situations of excessive patient anxiety or in those combined with more extensive surgery. Blood pressure control is crucial to avoid excessive bleeding and potential blindness. If patients are unable to remain still or avoid coughing, sneezing, or Valsalva maneuvers, then general anesthesia should be used. A fine line must be walked if an attempt is made to avoid these intraoperative problems with the use of sedation alone. Common sense should always prevail. Excessive sedation can prove more dangerous than a well-controlled general anesthetic. Nausea should be treated preemptively to avoid postoperative nausea and vomiting (PONV), and subsequent rising of blood pressure and bleeding.

Nose Reshaping Surgery (Rhinoplasty)

This procedure is performed on patients of all ages; however, young to middle-aged patients comprise the majority of patients. It was the most popular cosmetic surgical procedure for men in 2002, representing a 7% increase from 2001.[1] It is designed to reshape the nose. This is achieved by changing the size or shaping the tip and bridge of the nose. This is usually an outpatient procedure and can be performed under local anesthesia with sedation. Awake patients should be advised of the potential for swallowing blood during the procedure. In situations of excessive patient anxiety or surgeon's preference, general anesthesia is advised. If general anesthesia is used, endotracheal intubation is advised to avoid aspiration of blood. Throat packs can be placed by the surgeon in awake patients or those under general anesthesia. These packs must be removed and documentation of this removal should be made at the end of the procedure. Failure to remove throat packs can result in aspiration of the pack into the airway. Gauze soaked in vasoconstrictive agents (oxymetazoline, cocaine, or phenylephrine) is commonly used intranasally to achieve hemostasis. This can result in elevation of blood pressure. Blood pressure control is crucial to avoid excessive bleeding. Coughing and bucking are to be avoided during emergence. Since the patient has essentially a full stomach owing to swallowing of blood, full return of airway reflexes should be evident prior to extubation. If this procedure is performed with local anesthesia and sedation, sedation should be titrated to avoid loss of protective airway reflexes.

Forehead Lift (Browlift)

Browlifts are done to minimize forehead wrinkles, drooping eyebrows, and eyelid hooding. This is achieved by tightening forehead skin and adjusting forehead muscles. The procedure can be performed endoscopically or with an open, coronal incision. This procedure is performed on middle-aged to elderly patients. The surgical time can range from 1 to 3 hr. Anesthesia can be achieved with local infiltration and selective nerve blocks with IV sedation or general anesthesia for endoscopic browlift, and general anesthesia for open browlift. There can be injury to the facial nerve and alopecia as a result of this surgery.[22] Patients should be advised of these possibilities as they may attribute their hair loss to the anesthetic technique rather than the surgical procedure. Use of the coronal incision is in-

herently associated with blood loss owing to the rich blood supply of the scalp. Care should be made to control blood pressure to avoid this problem. Adequate hydration should be the goal in these patients to avoid postoperative hypotension and orthostasis.

Abdominoplasty ("Tummy Tuck")

This procedure is designed to flatten the abdomen by removing excessive fat and skin and tightening abdominal muscles. This procedure is performed on overweight patients of all ages. The number of men undergoing abdominoplasty tripled between 2001 and 2002 with numbers increasing from 1940 to 5145, respectively.[1] Female patients of normal weight will have this procedure to correct abdominal laxity associated with childbirth. Surgical time can last from 2 to 5 hr. This is the procedure that the morbidly obese patient or one who has achieved recent extensive weight loss is likely to have. Care should be taken that these patients have returned to nutritional and metabolic homeostasis. Their weight should be stable for 6 months. Preoperative electrolytes, automated blood count, liver function tests, and electrocardiogram (ECG) should be obtained. If there are coexisting issues such as type 2 diabetes, requiring insulin, or history of obstructive sleep apnea or the planned surgery is extensive with anticipated blood loss; the surgery should be performed in a facility that allows overnight monitoring. An obese patient such as this should never have surgery in a physician's office. All things being equal, postoperative pain is the most important factor to be addressed. These procedures can be performed with use of local anesthesia and IV sedation[23] or an opioid-based general anesthetic. Use of regional anesthesia such as epidural anesthesia is counterproductive as far as postoperative analgesia is concerned. It will result in a delay in discharge owing to pain control, as there is no way to titrate analgesia while the epidural block is in effect.

Laser Facial Resurfacing

Laser resurfacing is designed to smooth fine facial lines due to sun damage. This procedure uses carbon dioxide (CO_2) laser. It can be performed in limited areas such as under the eyes and perioral or involve the entire face. Anesthesia performed by an anesthesia provider is not necessary when these limited areas are involved. Local anesthesia is usually adequate. When full-face laser is anticipated, anesthesia with local anesthetic infiltration and IV sedation or general anesthesia is used. If sedation is to be used, it should be considerable. The burn and intraoperative pain produced by this laser is equivalent to that of a second-degree burn. If general anesthesia is used, adequate intraoperative analgesia should be provided. That being said, the amount of postoperative pain associated with this procedure is small. This is the one procedure where the ultrashort-acting opioid analgesics such as alfentanil and remifentanil are appropriate. Regardless of the anesthetic technique, institutional precautions that are generally mandated with laser use should be followed. The surgical field should be draped with moist towels and endotracheal tubes designed for laser use should be used when laser work is done on the facial area. The lowest inspiratory oxygen fraction (FiO_2) tolerated by the patient should be used. Avoidance of contact of the laser beam with oxygen is crucial to avoid ignition.

Liposuction (Suction Lipectomy)

Liposuction remains in the top five cosmetic surgical procedures in the past 5 years among men and women. It was designed to remove exercise-resistant fat deposits. These resistant fat deposits can be removed from cheeks, chin, buttocks, neck, upper arms, breasts, abdomen, buttocks, thighs, hips, knees, calves, and ankles. Unfortunately, not all surgeons adhere to this strict indication. There are a number of surgeons who perform single-session, large-volume (greater than 5000 mL aspirate) liposuction with the goal of weight reduction and total body resculpting. This is the scenario that breeds trouble. For liposuction in fibrous body areas such as male breast tissue, ultrasound-assisted lipoplasty (UAL) is used. This procedure involves using an ultrasound probe beneath the skin to heat and thus liquefy the fat prior to suctioning. A complication of this technique is thermal injury from the ultrasonic probe. This procedure can be performed using local anesthetics, regional anesthesia such as epidural anesthesia, and general anesthesia.

Traditional liposuction uses the tumescent technique which was first described by Klein.[24] Simply put, this technique involves infusion of a saline solution containing very dilute local anesthetic (0.05–0.1% lidocaine) and epinephrine 1:1,000,000 subcutaneously for pain control, prior to suctioning using cannulas of varying sizes. The solution contains adrenaline for hemostasis. In Klein's strictest of definition, this tumescent technique precludes the use of any further anesthetic or sedation or IV fluids and is therefore declared "safer."

No matter how simple liposuction may appear, it is by no means without risks. Since its initial description, the safety of this technique has been challenged. De Jong[25] asserts that the majority of complications related to liposuction are preventable. They are related to inadequate patient observation during the intraoperative and postoperative periods. There is also underestimation of the impact of sedation, large-dose lidocaine, and fluid absorption and hypothermia on patient morbidity. All of these problems are indeed preventable if care is used in the perioperative management of patients. Emphasis should be on patient safety and not on quick-discharge criteria. To that end, the ASPS recommends that anesthesia services should be used in situations where significant liposuction (greater than 5000 mL) is planned and/or conscious sedation is being used.

Review of the literature indicates that the most common causes of death in this patient population are pulmonary thromboemboli, fat emboli, fluid overload, and lidocaine and epinephrine toxicity.[26–27] Liposuction morbidity has been the topic of many debates. It is so controversial that this topic was specifically addressed by the ASPS Task Force for patient safety in office-based procedures in 2002. Their recommendation is that high-volume liposuction (greater than 5000 mL aspirate) should not be combined with other surgical procedures as this combination is associated with significant morbidity. The ASPS also recommends that liposuction can be performed safely in the office setting when the total aspirate is limited to 5000 mL or less.[21] Some states have legislated more rigorous control of liposuction owing to morbidity. Florida determined in 2001 that liposuction can be performed in combination with other surgical procedures if (1) combined with abdominoplasty, with the aspirate volume not exceeding 1000 mL; (2) aspirate may not exceed 1000 mL when directly related to other surgical procedures; and (3) major liposuction (greater than 1000 mL) may not be performed in a remote location from any other surgical procedure.[28] Although there is no controlled study to support this rigid stance, the information used to formulate this recommendation is real, although anecdotal.[29]

It is very important that the anesthesiologist understands the type of technique proposed by the surgeon. Semantics can certainly prove catastrophic if everyone is not clear regarding the technique. The tumescent technique described above takes advantage of the known tissue-binding capacity of lidocaine (1 mg/g, implying that 1 g of tissue can bind 1 mg of lidocaine). With such a dilute concentration of local anesthetic (0.05–0.1%), there is a slow but steady trickle of local anesthetic out of the tissues with serum lidocaine concentrations peaking as late as 10–14 hr after infiltration and then gradually declining over the next 6–14 hr. With this technique, the recommended dose of lidocaine has been 45–55 mg/kg. This recommendation has been declared safe based on scattered serum samples indicating that the plasma lidocaine is well below the cardiotoxic 5 μg/mL.[30] It should be made clear that this high-dose lidocaine recommendation applies only to this particular circumstance where dilute lidocaine (0.05–0.1% with epinephrine 1 mg/L) is being used. As previously mentioned, its safety depends on the ability of l g of tissue to bind 1 mg of lidocaine. Safety also depends on normal liver function. Using any higher concentration of lidocaine will outstrip this tissue-buffering capacity, thus leaving free lidocaine to enter the serum and thus rise according to classic kinetics of rapid rise and slow decline. Any other use of lidocaine such as out-of-the-bottle use for regional or infiltration anesthesia should adhere to the Food and Drug Administration recommendation for maximum dosing of 7 mg/kg.

The original tumescent anesthetic description dictates that no IV fluids should be provided. In situations, however, where large-volume liposuctions (> 4000 mL) are contemplated, it is recommended that IV fluids should not only be provided but effective monitoring of urine output by continuous urinary catheter is required.[31–32] Fluid resuscitation is a balancing act and there are no exact recipes for this. When the dry technique is used, no wetting solution is used and the intraoperative fluid requirement can be significant (Table 31-4).[33] When the superwet technique is used, an equal amount of wetting solution is infused to that expected to be aspirated. The fluid requirement may be reduced in this circumstance. The recommended fluid resuscitation is as follows: (1) small

Table 31-4 Fluid Requirements for Dry Liposuction

Amount of Aspirate (mL)	Amount of Fluid
1. < 500	2 L crystalloid
2. 500–1000	3 L crystalloid
3. 1000–1500	3 L crystalloid + Hetastarch (1)
4. 1500–2000	3 L crystalloid + 1 U blood
5. 2000–2500	3 L crystalloid + 2 U blood
6. 2500–3000	4 L crystalloid + 3 U blood
Consider overnight admission in 5 and 6.	

SOURCE: Adapted from Hetter, G. Aspirative lipoplasty. In: Georgiade NG et al. (eds.), *Elements of Plastic, Maxillofacial, and Reconstructive Surgery*, 3rd ed. Philadelphia: Williams & Wilkins, 1997.

Table 31-5 Causes of Death From Liposuction

Cause of Death	Death (N)	Percentage (%)
Thromboembolism	30	22.1
Abdomen/viscus perforation	19	14.6
Anesthesia/sedation/medication	13	10
Fat embolism	11	8.5
Cardiorespiratory arrest	7	5.4
Massive infection	7	5.4
Bleeding	6	4.6
Unknown	37	28.5
Total	130	100

SOURCE: Adapted from Grazer FM, De Jong RH. Fatal outcomes from liposuction: census survey of cosmetic surgeons. Plast Reconstr Surg 2000;105(1):436–46.

volume liposuction (< 4 L aspirate) is maintenance fluid + tumescent wetting solution; (2) large volume liposuction (≤ 4 L aspirate) is maintenance fluid + tumescent wetting solution + 0.25 mL IV crystalloid per mL of aspirate removed after 4 L.[31] Regardless of the proposed technique, fluid resuscitation remains empiric. Although it may appear that solution is infused and immediately suctioned, in fact 60% of the solution infused remains in the tissues and is ultimately absorbed into the intravascular compartment. In addition to obvious suction aspirate volumes, consideration must also be given to the amount of tissue trauma from suctioning and subsequent third spacing of fluid into the remaining surgical cavity that occurs with this procedure. Under- or overestimation of this fluid mobilization can result in pulmonary edema or hypovolemic shock. It is generally accepted that aspirate of less than 4000 mL of wetted tissue is relatively benign.[31]

Pulmonary fat embolism is a common complication of this procedure owing to mobilization of fat with the suction cannula. Fat is even more likely to enter the circulation after it has been emulsified as with UAL.[34] To compound this risk is the age and gender groups that are most likely to have this procedure. It is known that women (88% of patients) aged between 25 and 55 are most likely to undergo extensive liposuction. This demographic information correlates with those patients who will use birth control pills or hormone replacement therapy for menopause. In addition to fat emboli, this population is at significant risk for venous thromboembolic events. The thromboembolic complication is a delayed event that is managed by surgeons. This issue has been addressed somewhat with the prophylactic use of intermittent pneumatic leg compressive devices during general anesthesia. The "boots" should be applied and activated prior to the induction of general anesthesia.[35] Any intraoperative catastrophe should include pulmonary fat embolism in the differential diagnosis. Other complications include viscus perforation, pulmonary edema, vascular perforation, local anesthetic

toxicity, and hypothermia (Table 31-5). Liposuction, although seemingly simple in execution, is a serious surgery. The mortality rate is 1 in 5224 (or 19/100,000) compared to 3/100,000 for hernia operations.[27] These deaths may have been prevented if dedicated nursing and anesthesia personnel had been involved.

POSTANESTHESIA CARE

Postanesthesia care for cosmetic patients follows the guidelines described by the ASA for Phase 2 level of care. Using the anesthetic technique described above, patients are able to qualify for bypass PACU Phase 1. While in the operating room, patients must be able to meet all discharge criteria necessary for transfer from PACU Phase 1 to Phase 2 (Table 31-6).[20] Certainly, if for some reason this is not the case, patients should receive Phase 1 level of care un-

Table 31-6 Criteria for Immediate Transfer to Phase 2 PACU

Minimal/no pain
Patient alert
Minimal/no nausea
Patient able to hold head lift for 5 sec
Patient able to stand
Oxygen saturation greater than 94% on room air

SOURCE: Adapted from Apfelbaum JL. Eliminating intensive postoperative care in same day surgery patients using short acting anesthetics. Anesthesiology 2002;97(1):66–74.

til stable. It is likely that if a cosmetic patient does not immediately qualify for PACU Phase 2, there has been some breech in the screening process for outpatient or office surgery. It is crucial that patients are screened appropriately for outpatient or office-based cosmetic surgery to avoid untoward postanesthetic events.

All personnel involved in caring for patients in the PACU should have advanced cardiac life support (ACLS) certification. Nursing and physician staffs should be present and immediately available to the patient. The staff should not have any duties other than the care of the recovering patient. Monitoring should be performed using standard ASA monitors. Detailed records of vital signs and fluid intake and output should be kept. Family members should be given detailed instructions on postoperative care. During this period, oral intake should be established with clear liquids. Initial oral postoperative pain medications should be started if needed. Assessment and treatment of PONV should be completed. Orthostatic blood pressure will assure adequate volume status. This is especially important after liposuction. Patients should satisfy all standard, institutional criteria appropriate for discharge from any inpatient or ambulatory facility. The Ramsey score is used in the author's facility. There should not be any shortcutting of the above discharge criteria. Predetermined discharge times are not appropriate. Patient safety and adequate home readiness are the adherence to the above recommendations that will assure a safe outpatient cosmetic surgical experience.

REFERENCES

1. Plastic Surgery Information Service Web page. American Society of Plastic Surgeons. www.plasticsurgery.org, 2002.
2. Iverson RE. ASPS Task Force on Patient Safety in Office-Based Surgery Facilities. Patient safety in office-based surgery facilities: I. Procedures in the office-based surgery setting. Plast Reconstr Surg 2002;110(5):1337–42.
3. Ahlstrom KK, Frodel JL. Local anesthetics for facial plastic procedures. Otolaryngol Clin North Am 2002;35(1):29–53.
4. Klein SM, Bergh A, Steele SM, Georgiade GS, Greengrass RA. Thoracic paravertebral block for breast surgery. Anesth Analg 2000; 90(6):1402–5.
5. Hoefflin SM, Bornstein JB, Gordon M. General anesthesia in an office-based plastic surgical facility: a report on more than 23,000 consecutive office-based procedures under general anesthesia with no significant anesthetic complications. Plast Reconstr Surg 2001; 107(1):243–51.
6. Iverson RE, Lynch DJ. ASPS Task Force on Patient Safety in Office-Based Surgery Facilities. Patient safety in office-based surgery facilities: II. Patient selection. Plast Reconstr Surg 2002;110(7):1785–90.
7. Friedberg BL. A role for the anesthesiologist in elective cosmetic surgery? Plast Reconstr Surg 2003;111(2):953–55.
8. Apfelbaum, JL. Current Controversies in Adult Outpatient Anesthesia. ASA Refresher Course Lectures 2003;152:1–7.
9. Apfelbaum JL, Roizen MF. Initial clinical trials of a computerized HEALTHQUIZ to suggest preoperative laboratory test. Anesthesiology 1988;69:A717.
10. Borkowski RG, Maurer WG, Tetzlaff JE, Androjna C, Che MS, Parker BM. Cost analysis of using a computerized patient assessment program in a preoperative anesthesia clinic. Anesthesiology 2000;93:A39.
11. Natof HE. Pre-existing medical problems: ambulatory surgery. IMJ Ill Med J 1984;166(2):101–4.
12. De Jong RH. Body mass index: risk predictor for cosmetic day surgery. Plast Reconstr Surg 2001;108(2):556–61.
13. Meningaud JP, Benadiba L, Servant JM, Herve C, Bertrand JC, Pelicier Y. Depression, anxiety and quality of life among scheduled cosmetic surgery patients: multicentre prospective study. J Maxillofac Surg 2001;29(3):177–80.
14. Sarwer DB, Wadden TA, Pertschuk MJ, Whitaker LA. Body image dissatisfaction and body dysmorphic disorder in 100 cosmetic surgery patients. Plast Reconstr Surg 1998;101(6):1644–49.
15. Rohrich RJ. The who, what, when, and why of cosmetic surgery: do our patients need a preoperative psychiatric evaluation? Plast Reconstr Surg 2000;106(7):1605–7.
16. Shiffman MA. Warning about herbals in plastic and cosmetic surgery. Plast Reconstr Surg 2001;108(7):2180–81.
17. Roizen, MF. Preoperative evaluation. In Miller RD (ed.), *Anesthesia*, 4th ed. New York: Churchill Livingstone, 1994, pp. 24, 827–83.
18. Scott, DL. Personal Communication. Director of Anesthesia at the Duke Aesthetic Center, Durham, NC 27710, 2003.
19. Georgiade NG, Georgiade GS, Riefkohl R. *Aesthetic Surgery of the Breast*. Philadelphia: W.B. Saunders, 1990.
20. Apfelbaum, JL. Eliminating intensive postoperative care in same day surgery patients using short acting anesthetics. Anesthesiology 2002;97(1):66–74.
21. O'Connor MF, Daves SM, Tung A, Cook RI, Thisted R, Apfelbaum J. BIS monitoring to prevent awareness during general anesthesia. Anesthesiology 2001;94(3):520–22.
22. Dominguez E, Eslinger MR, McCord SV. Postoperative (pressure) alopecia: report of a case after elective cosmetic surgery. Anesth Analg 1999;89(4):1062–63.
23. Rosenberg MH, Palaia DA, Bonanno PC. Abdominoplasty with procedural sedation and analgesia. Ann Plast Surg 2001;46(5):485–87.
24. Klein J. The tumescent technique for liposuction surgery. Am J Cosmetic Surg 1987;4:263.
25. De Jong RH, Grazer FM. Perioperative management of cosmetic liposuction. Plast Reconstr Surg 2001;107(4):1039–44.
26. Platt MS, Kohler LJ, Ruiz R, Cohle SD, Ravichandran P. Deaths associated with liposuction: case reports and review of the literature. J Forensic Sci 2002;47(1):205–7.
27. Grazer FM, De Jong RH. Fatal outcomes from liposuction: census survey of cosmetic surgeons. Plast Reconstr Surg 2000;105(1):436–46.
28. Florida Board of Medicine. 64B8-9.009 Rule. Standard of Care for Office Surgery, February 27, 2001.
29. Hughes CE III. Reduction of lipoplasty risks and mortality: an ASAPS survey. Aesthetic Surg Journal 2001;21(2):120–24.
30. Ostad A, Kageyama N, Moy RL. Tumescent anesthesia with a lidocaine dose of 55 mg/kg is safe for liposuction. Dermatol Surg 1996; 22(11):921–27.
31. Trott SA, Beran SJ, Rohrich RJ, Kenkel JM, Adams WP Jr., Klein KW. Safety considerations and fluid resuscitation in liposuction: an analysis of 53 consecutive patients. Plast Reconstr Surg 1998; 102(6):2220–29.
32. Teimourian B, Adham MN. A national survey of complications associated with suction lipectomy: what we did then and what we do now. Plast Reconstr Surg 2000;105(5):1881–84.
33. Hetter, G. Aspirative lipoplasty. In: Georgiade NG et al. (eds.), *Elements of Plastic, Maxillofacial, and Reconstructive Surgery*, 3rd ed. Philadelphia: Williams & Wilkins, 1997.
34. Rohrich RJ, Morales DE, Krueger JE, Ansari M, Ochoa O, Robinson J Jr., et al. Comparative lipoplasty analysis of in vivo-treated adipose tissue. Plast Reconstr Surg 2000;105(6):2152–58.
35. McDevitt NB. Deep vein thrombosis prophylaxis. American Society of Plastic and Reconstructive Surgeons. Plast Reconstr Surg 1999; 104(6):1923–28.

Paravertebral Blocks for Chest, Truncal, and Abdominal Procedures

SUGANTHA GANAPATHY

INTRODUCTION

Pain following thoracic, abdominal, and chest wall surgeries can be significant, necessitating opioid administration via the parenteral route and admission to the hospital for adequate pain control. Regional anesthesia techniques that reduce opioid requirements for such procedures include epidural analgesia, intrathecal opiates, and paravertebral and intercostal blocks. More patients are undergoing a variety of surgical procedures on the chest and abdomen as ambulatory surgical patients, dictated by economic impact of such procedures on health care utilization. With the video-assisted pulmonary resection and thoracic sympathectomy, more patients undergoing thoracic procedures will be ambulatory surgical candidates. Central neuraxial techniques including neuraxial opiates do not lend themselves to be applied in the ambulatory setting. Hugo Sellheim introduced thoracic paravertebral block (PVB) almost a century ago and Kappis refined this technique for use in abdominal surgery in early 1919.[1] Eason and Wyatt revived this technique in 1979.[2] While investigators used it extensively in Europe in patients admitted to the hospital, Wood et al.[3] reported on its use in ambulatory patients for the first time in 1981. It is only since the report of Weltz et al.[4] in 1995 on the management of breast cancer surgery as an ambulatory surgical procedure that the use of this technique is widely adopted for many ambulatory surgical procedures. Although much scientific information had been published about PVBs, mainly derived from the work performed on patients admitted to the hospital, application of these principles in the ambulatory setting requires careful attention to detail. This chapter will review some of the basic principles on the use of PVBs for chest, truncal, and abdominal surgery with particular reference to ambulatory surgical procedures. There are excellent reviews on this topic,[1,5–8] and the reader is encouraged to study them to develop a comprehensive knowledge of this subject.

ANATOMIC BACKGROUND

The paravertebral space is a wedge-shaped space on either side of vertebrae bound anterolaterally by the parietal pleura, posteriorly by the superior costotransverse ligaments, and its base is formed by the vertebrae, intervertebral discs, intervertebral foramina, and its contents. The apex of the space continues laterally as the intercostal space. The superior costotransverse ligaments run from the top of the ribs to the lower border of the transverse process above. The endothoracic fascia, a fibroelastic structure that anchors the pleura to the vertebral body, lines the chest between the superior costotransverse ligament and the parietal pleura (Fig. 32-1 and 32-2). It is closely applied to the ribs and fuses with the periosteum at the midpoint of the vertebral body. Loose connective tissue called subserous fascia fills the space between the endothoracic fascia and the parietal pleura (Fig. 32-3 and 32-4). Radiopaque contrast injected via the catheters positioned under direct vision following thoracotomies in this location by Sabanathan et al.[9] has been shown to allow vertical spread of contrast along the paravertebral gutter. Karmakar et al.,[10] in a radiologic study, have shown that contrast delivered ventral to the endothoracic fascia can track to the contralateral paravertebral gutter via the prevertebral space. Magnetic resonance imaging (MRI) (Fig. 32-5 and 32-6; unpublished personal data) reveals a similar path for contralateral spread and no spread via the epidural route after an injection of 20 mL of saline via thoracic paravertebral catheters. Thus for a multisegment block the injections have to be ventral to the endothoracic fascia. Anatomically it signifies that the paravertebral space is divided into two fascial compartments by the endothoracic fascia, namely the anterior "extrapleural" space and a posterior subendothoracic compartment.[10]

Drugs delivered in the posterior subendothoracic compartment do move vertically to the adjacent two to four segments (restricted by heads and necks of ribs), but for

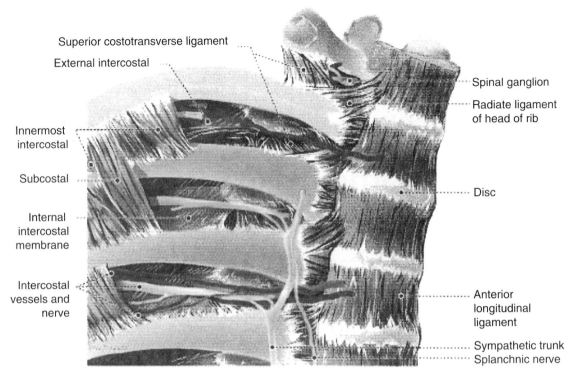

Figure 32-1   Anatomy of paravertebral space viewed from inside the chest. Note how the head and necks of ribs can inhibit vertical spread of drugs unless delivered more anteriorly closer to the vertebral body.

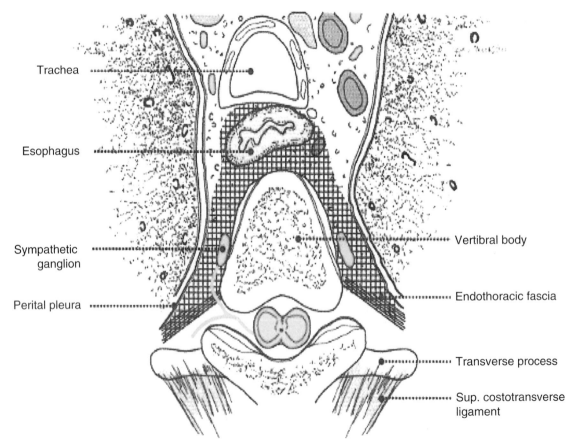

Figure 32-2   Schematic diagram of the cross section of chest depicting the endothoracic fascia, the subserous compartment, and the communication prevertebrally of the extrapleural paravertebral space to the contralateral side.

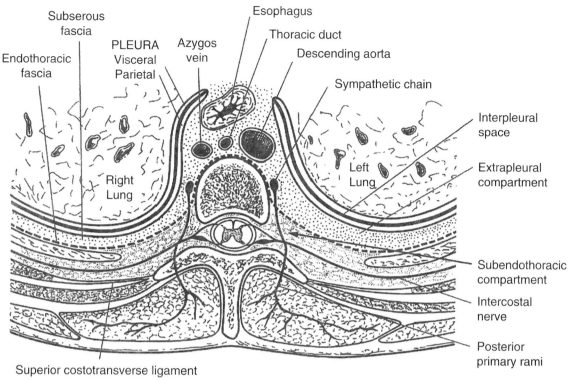

Figure 32-3   Endothoracic fascia divides the paravertebral space into subserous and extrapleural spaces. Note the attachment of endothoracic fascia to the vertebral body. (Reprinted with permission from Karmakar MK. Thoracic paravertebral block. Anesthesiology 2001;95:771–80. Copyright 2000–2003 Ovid Technologies, Inc.)

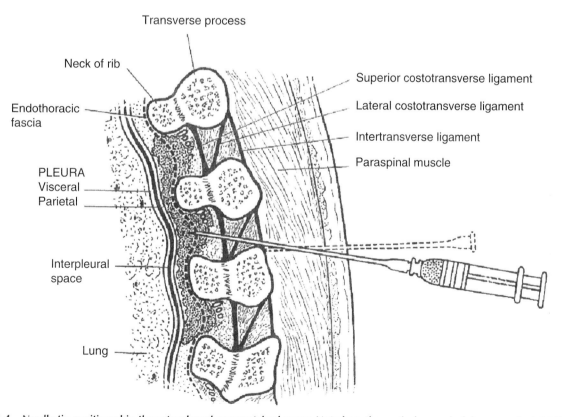

Figure 32-4   Needle tip positioned in the extrapleural paravertebral space. Note how the vertical spread of drugs can be inhibited by the necks of ribs dorsal to the endothoracic fascia. (Reprinted with permission from Karmakar MK. Thoracic paravertebral block. Anesthesiology 2001;95:771–80. Copyright 2000–2003 Ovid Technologies, Inc.)

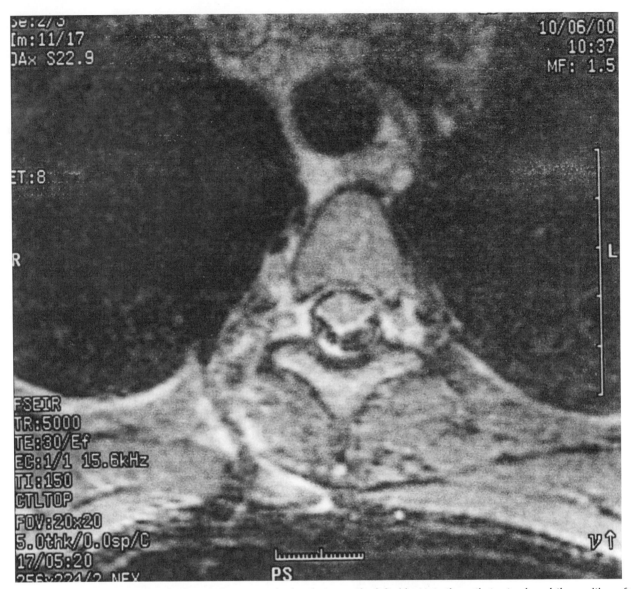

Figure 32-5   Magnetic resonance imaging of T3 paravertebral catheter on the left side. Note the catheter track and the position of the catheter tip closer to the side of the spine. This image is taken prior to injection of saline via the catheter. Note the proximity of pleura to the catheter.

extensive unilateral and contralateral blocks the drugs have to be delivered in the anterior extrapleural compartment. Although epidural spread was documented to account for contralateral spread by Purcell-Jones et al.,[11] a number of authors have documented prevertebral spread as the cause of contralateral analgesia.[10,12] It is likely that injections under pressure in the posterior subendothoracic compartment may follow the path of least resistance into the epidural space along the nerve roots to produce the epidural spread seen clinically with weakness in legs lasting several hours. Whether lower-limb weakness will occur as a consequence of prevertebral spread is currently unknown.

The second important fact is the communication between the thoracic and lumbar paravertebral spaces. Using cadavers, Saito et al.[13] have shown that injection into the lower thoracic paravertebral spaces "under" the endotho-

racic fascia tracks to the retroperitoneal area via the medial and lateral arcuate ligaments behind the transversalis fascia where the spinal nerves lie. Although there is a lot of ambiguity with regard to terminology, clinical experience suggests that injections ventral to the endothoracic fascia result in extensive multisegment blocks with communications between the thoracic and lumbar areas[14] as well as limited contralateral spread. However, injections dorsal to the endothoracic fascia result in a much more restricted vertical spread of more or less three segments. Intuitively, advancement of the needle between pleura and the endothoracic fascia can risk pleural puncture and resultant pneumothorax. In the ambulatory setting avoiding pleural puncture is of paramount importance.

The third important anatomic detail is the level of the transverse process in relation to the palpable superior aspect of the spinous process. In the lumbar area the trans-

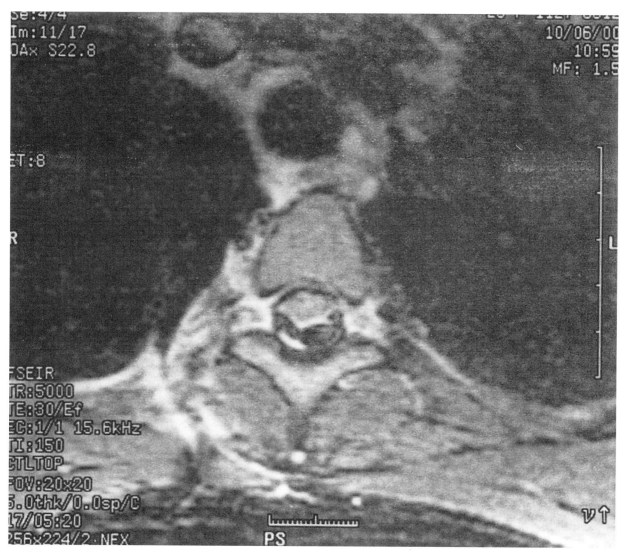

Figure 32-6   Magnetic resonance imaging of T3 paravertebral catheter after 20 mL of saline has been injected via the catheter. Note increased signal prevertebrally and on the contralateral side extrapleurally.

verse processes may be at the same horizontal level as the spinous process. However, in the thoracic area, the transverse process belongs to the vertebra one level below the level of the palpated spinous process owing to the oblique angle of the thoracic spinous process. For example, the superior aspect of T7 spinous process may be at the level of the transverse process of T8 vertebra. Similarly, the superior aspect of C7 vertebra corresponds to the transverse process of T1 vertebra and the T1 nerve root travels under the transverse process of T1 vertebra (Fig. 32-7). This is important to know when T1 block is planned to cover axillary node dissection during breast surgery.

Thus with drugs delivered in the paravertebral space, vertical, contralateral, and epidural spread can occur depending on the location of the needle tip in relation to endothoracic fascia and volume and force of injections. Further studies are needed to verify these observations.

A number of muscles covering the chest, such as the pectoral muscles, serratus anterior, and latissimus dorsi, are supplied by branches of brachial plexus and therefore are not anesthetized by PVBs. This is why patients feel discomfort with a functioning PVB when the pectoral muscles are dissected during mastectomy. Supraclavicular nerves that are branches of the cervical plexus are involved in cutaneous innervation down to the second intercostal space anteriorly as well as the anterior shoulder. This results in sparing of the upper chest with PVBs necessitating a superficial cervical plexus block for complete anesthesia of the anterior chest wall.

TECHNIQUE

A number of techniques have been used to initiate and maintain PVBs. In the original technique described by Eason and Wyatt,[2] the point of needle entry was 2–3 cm lateral to the superior aspect of the spinous process, perpendicular to the skin until the transverse process was contacted. The needle was walked superior to the transverse process to enter the paravertebral space. The supe-

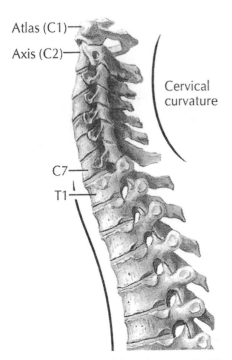

Atlas (C1)

Axis (C2)

Cervical
curvature

C7

T1

Figure 32-7   Lateral view of the spine. Note that the C7 spinous process top corresponds to the T1 vertebral transverse process. The angulations of mid to low thoracic spines make the spinous process correspond to the transverse processes of at least one vertebra lower. (From Netter FH [ed.], *Atlas of Human Anatomy*. King of Prussia, PA: Rittenhouse Book Distributors, 1997.)

rior angulation was suggested, as it was more likely to contact the intercostal nerves to elicit paresthesia. Later modifications included "walking" caudad to the transverse process for a fixed depth of 1–1.5 cm. A graduated 22 gauge Tuohy needle is used for this purpose. This modification probably is the reason behind reduced incidence of pneumothorax with the series from Greengrass et al.[8,15] and therefore is particularly useful in ambulatory surgical patients. It is likely that the posterior paravertebral space is broader inferiorly than closer to the lower border of the transverse process. The true incidence of pneumothorax is probably unknown, as none of the series reported so far have done prospective radiologic evaluations of patients to identify pneumothoraces not apparent on clinical examination. Loss-of-resistance to saline or local anesthetic is used additionally to confirm correct localization of the space.

Ultrasonography has been used to identify the depth of transverse process from the skin and estimate the safe depth that the needle can be inserted.[16] Richardson et al.[17] have described the use of pressure transducer to identify entry into the paravertebral space. The paraspinal muscles and the superior costotransverse ligament produce a positive-pressure wave during expiration and inspiration. Entry into the paravertebral space results in reduction in expiratory pressure. Entry into the pleural cavity produces negative pressures during inspiration and expiration. Tenicela and Pollan[18] have reported a more medial approach of walking laterally on the lamina until the needle

slips into the paravertebral space. Intuitively, the chances of puncture of dural sleeve, epidural spread, and pleural puncture should be higher with this technique, however there are no studies that have evaluated this technique comparatively to other techniques. In their series of 384 blocks in 130 patients they document one dural puncture and two intrathecal spreads. They also noted a 1.3% incidence of bilateral blocks and evidence of epidural spread in the form of motor sensory blocks of legs with thoracic paravertebral injections. This incidence is similar to the lateral approach described by Eason et al. modified by Naja and Lönnqvist[19] (1% intrathecal or epidural spread, 0.5% pneumothorax, and 0.8% pleural puncture).

Catheterization of the posterior paravertebral space is challenging and usually only 2–3 cm of the catheter can be advanced with difficulty. Buckenmaier et al.[20] have recently reported on the use of such a technique using a continuous catheter delivery system called Contiplex (B. Braun Medical Incorporated, Bethlehem, PA) to provide extended analgesia after breast surgery. The advantage of using this continuous catheter delivery system, according to these authors, is the potential to avoid entraining air should a pleural puncture occur.

Catheterization of the extrapleural paravertebral space is often done using loss of resistance to saline with the same landmarks. After the superior costotransverse ligament is punctured, the needle is advanced toward the vertebral body until loss of resistance to saline injection is felt. Often there is a subtle "pop" of entering the endothoracic fascia. In this location, inspiratory efforts by the patient do not suck in the fluid from the loss of resistance syringe, but there is loss of resistance to injection of saline. Often 5–6 cm of the catheter can be inserted in this location after initial distension of the area with local anesthetic. The use of peripheral nerve stimulators to identify needle location was initially reported by Bonica and Buckley[21] and has been used clinically by a few investigators.[22,23] Fine-tuning needle tip position with the nerve stimulator might also result in increased chances of pleural puncture compared to advancing the needle a fixed length after the transverse process is contacted. This is evident in the paper published by Naja and Lonnqvist.[19]

Sabanathan et al. created an extrapleural pocket paravertebrally and positioned a percutaneously inserted catheter in this pocket to provide continuous PVB after thoracotomies and esophagogastrectomies (Fig. 32-8). A similar technique is used in infants and children after thoracotomies. This technique will obviously not be applicable in the ambulatory setting.

In ambulatory surgical patients the technique that one should adopt must be easy and quick to perform with predictable success and lowest incidence of complications. The operative site should have uniform surgical anesthesia unless the technique is used for analgesic purposes. The multiple-injection technique popularized by Greengrass et al.[8,15] fulfills these criteria well. The patient is usually seated with the assistant providing the support to flex the thoracic and cervical spine. This assistant also helps with the injections and therefore it is important to train the supporting nursing staff with regard to the resistance of injection into the paravertebral space. Routine monitors are applied and the patient is sedated with intravenous (IV) fentanyl